Learning Medical Terminology

Learning Medical Terminology

A Worktext

Miriam G. Austrin, B.A., R.N.
Consultant in Allied Health Careers and Medical Office Management;
former Coordinator-Director, Medical Assistant Program,
St. Louis Community College,
St. Louis, Missouri

Harvey R. Austrin, Ph.D.
Diplomate in Clinical Psychology,
American Board of Professional Psychology;
Emeritus Professor of Psychology, St. Louis University,
St. Louis, Missouri

EIGHTH EDITION
with 106 *illustrations*

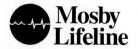

St. Louis Baltimore Berlin Boston Carlsbad Chicago London Madrid
Naples New York Philadelphia Sydney Tokyo Toronto

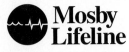

Dedicated to Publishing Excellence

Publisher: David T. Culverwell
Editor: Richard A. Weimer
Development Editor: Julie Scardiglia
Editorial Assistant: Kay Beard
Project Manager: Carol Sullivan Weis
Senior Production Editor: Shannon Canty
Senior Designer: Betty Schulz
Manufacturing Supervisor: Karen Lewis

8th Edition

Printed in the United States of America
Composition by: The Clarinda Company
Printing/binding by: Von Hoffmann Press

Mosby-Year Book, Inc.
11830 Westline Industrial Drive
St. Louis, Missouri 63146

Library of Congress Cataloging in Publication Data

Austrin, Miriam G., 1925–
    Learning medical terminology : a worktext. -- 8th ed. / Miriam G.
Austrin, Harvey R Austrin.
        p. cm.
    Includes bibliographical references and index.
    ISBN 0-8016-8050-6
    1. Medicine--Terminology.   I. Austrin, Harvey R.   II. Title.
    [DNLM: 1. Nomenclature.   W 15 A938L 1994]
R123.Y6 1994
610′.14-dc20
DNLM/DLC
for Library of Congress   94-30060
                                                                                              CIP

To
Sarah and Benjamin Austrin-Willis
and
Brian and Bradley Austrin

Preface

In this eighth edition of LEARNING MEDICAL TERMI-NOLOGY we have maintained the basic structure of previous editions. Dividing the book into sections has been well received and generally found conducive to effective learning. Section I (the first four chapters) is devoted to introducing the student to the basics of medical language. These chapters list word parts in easily read chart form. Some schools utilize these four chapters alone as the basis for a short course in medical terminology, using the additional chapters as an enrichment resource. Users have found particularly helpful the extensive lists of prefixes, suffixes, roots and combining forms. The roots and their combining forms are arranged into categories (external and internal anatomy), and groupings (verbs and adjectives, body fluids, substances, chemicals, and colors). Since medical language is inexorably linked to the body, we have continued to use the system approach, which ties basic explanations of the anatomy of each system to the language. Revisions include an interesting relevant fact at the beginning of most chapters. New questions have been added to the reviews and exercises throughout the book. Content has been rearranged within selected chapters, and an additional chapter has been added. Substantial revisions of some chapters have been necessary to reflect current knowledge.

In accord with current views, the Lymphatic System has been removed from the Cardiovascular System chapter and integrated into the Immune System chapter, because of its importance in this area. Many medical authorities believe that the immune system and its diseases will be of utmost significance and concern in the future, and this revision reflects that belief.

The final chapter consists of a glossary of Multiple-System diseases, with extensive descriptions, arranged under headings consistent with the other glossaries in the book.

Each chapter concludes with a glossary based on the material within that chapter, with phonetic pronunciation guides, and has been revised, deleting obsolete material. These glossaries contain large numbers of additional medical terms, which can pique student interest, helping them enjoy the learning process and further reinforcing their understanding of the text. There are listings and descriptions of anatomic parts, diseases and disorders, surgical procedures, and laboratory tests, reflecting current knowledge. Chapter material and the glossary together optimize interest, understanding, and satisfaction.

Over 1500 review and exercise questions (with answers) are included in the text to assist the student in learning the chapter contents. Additionally, we have included a crossword puzzle and a hidden word puzzle for chapters 1 through 16, for reinforcing enjoyment in the learning process. There are 16 full-color anatomic plates at the front of the book for reference.

Overall, this text is designed so that a motivated student can use it as a self-teaching instrument, with minimal or no supervision.

An instructor's manual and an audio tape pronunciation guide are available from the publisher. The manual contains tips on teaching, including setting up courses of different lengths ranging from a short 3 month course to a 2 semester one. Medical historical background and folklore are included in the manual, as well as a chapter-by-chapter test file of about 1000 questions.

We are indebted to cartoonist Mike Peters for allowing us to use a strip from "Mother Goose and Grimm" relating (in its own unique way) to medical terminology. Special thanks are due to Dr. Harold Burton of the Anatomy and Neurobiology Departments at Washington University in St. Louis for his assistance in clarifying some fine points, and to John Ashby, Susan Sonderman, and Angela Pitts of St. Louis University's media departments for their help in researching medical language sources. Additionally, our appreciation and very special thanks to Richard Weimer, Executive Editor of Mosby-Year Book, Inc., for his many suggestions and continuous help, to Julie Scardiglia, Developmental Editor, for her sense of humor and patience, to Kay Beard for always being available to pick up the pieces, to Shannon Canty for smiling through the production process, and to the entire team at Mosby Lifeline. Last, but by no means least, we would like to express our gratitude to those instructors and students who generously provided us with constructive criticism and suggestions.

Miriam G. Austrin
Harvey R. Austrin

Contents

Section One: The Basic Foundation of Medical Terminology

1 An Introduction to Medical Terminology

Objective, 3
Specific Suggestions for Learning Medical Terminology, 4
Pronunciation of Medical Terms, 4
Plurals, 4
Spelling, 4
Exercises, 5

2 Building a Medical Vocabulary

Step 1: Prefixes and Suffixes, 10
Prefixes, 10
Suffixes, 14
Exercises, 18

3 Adding to the Foundation

Step 2: Roots and Combining Forms, 23
External Anatomy, 23
Internal Anatomy, 26
Exercises, 29

4 Completing the Foundation

Step 3: Additional Roots and Combining Forms, 33
Verbal Roots and Combining Forms, 33
Adjectival Roots and Combining Forms, 36
Body Fluids, 39
Body Substances and Chemicals, 40
Colors, 40
Exercises, 42

Section Two: The Body Shell and Its Supports

5 Understanding the Body and Its Structure

Study of the Body, 49
Basic Structure, 49
Characteristics of Living Matter, 49
Cells, 50
Tissues, 51
Organs, 54
Systems, 54
Directions, Anatomic Planes, and Positions, 55
Body Regions, 56
Exercises, 59
Glossary, 64

6 The Skeletal System: *The Framework of the Body*

The Skeleton, 65
Classification of Bones, 66
Structural Descriptive Terms of Bones, 69
Axial Skeleton, 69
Vertebral Column, 71
Ribs, 71
Sternum, 71
Appendicular Skeleton, 72
Joints, 73
Bursae, 74
Types of Movement, 75
Exercises, 77
Glossary, 92

7 The Muscular System: *The Moving Force*

Muscles, 99
Allied Muscular Structures, 99
Composition of Muscle, 100

Classification of Muscles, 100
Attachment of Muscles, 101
Movement of Muscles, 101
How Muscles Are Named, 101
Adjectives For Muscles, 102
Muscle Groups, 103
Exercises, 109
Glossary, 119

8 **The Integumentary System:**
   The Skin and its Accessory Structures

Skin, 123
   Composition of the Skin, 124
   Structure of the Skin, 124
   Hair, 125
   Sweat Glands, 125
   Sebaceous Glands, 125
   Ceruminous Glands, 125
   Nails, 126
Exercises, 127
Glossary, 134

Section Three: The Internal Mechanisms of the Body

9 **The Cardiovascular System:**
   The Transports of the Body

The Cardiovascular System, 141
The Heart, 141
Types of Blood Vessels, 143
Blood, 144
Blood Pressure, 147
The Pulse, 147
Circulation of the Blood, 148
The Major Blood Vessels of Circulation, 149
Exercises, 152
Glossary, 165

10 **The Respiratory System:**
    The Breath of Life

Structures and Functions, 175
Organs of the Upper Respiratory Tract, 175
Organs of the Lower Respiratory Tract, 177
The Process of Respiration, 178
Exercises, 180
Glossary, 190

11 **The Gastrointestinal System:**
    The Food Processor

Structures and Functions, 195
The Mouth, 195
The Pharynx, 199
The Esophagus, 199

The Process of Swallowing, 199
The Stomach, 199
The Digestive Process, 200
The Abdominal Cavity, 200
The Pancreas, 201
The Liver, 201
Exercises, 203
Glossary, 214

12 **The Genitourinary System:**
    Liquid Waste Processing and Human Reproduction

The Urinary System, 224
   The Kidneys, 224
   The Ureters, 225
   The Urinary Bladder, 226
   The Urethra, 226
The Male Reproductive Organs, 228
The Female Reproductive Organs, 230
The Menstrual Cycle, 233
Pregnancy, 233
Exercises, 235
Glossary, 247

Section Four: The Adaptive and Defense Mechanisms of the Body

13 **The Endocrine System:**
    The Chemical Stimulators

The Endocrines, 261
   The Pituitary Gland, 261
   The Hypothalamus, 263
   The Thyroid, 263
   The Parathyroid Glands, 264
   The Adrenal Glands, 265
   The Pineal Gland, 265
   The Pancreas, 265
   The Gonads, 265
Thymus, 267
Exercises, 268
Glossary, 277

14 **The Nervous System:**
    The Central Processing Unit

Characteristics of the Nervous System, 281
Central Nervous System, 283
   The Meninges, 283
   The Brain, 284
   The Functional Areas of the Cerebral Cortex, 286
   Hemispheric Differences in Function, 286
   Cerebrospinal Fluid, 287
Spinal Cord, 287
The Peripheral Nervous System, 290

Cranial Nerves, 290
Spinal Nerves, 291
The Autonomic Nervous System, 292
Exercises, 294
Glossary, 302

15   The Special Senses:
The Sources of Information

The Sense of Vision, 320
The Sense of Hearing, 324
The Sense of Smell, 326
The Sense of Taste, 326
Touch and Other Cutaneous Senses, 327
Exercises, 329
Glossary, 339

16   The Lymphatic and Immune Systems:
The Defenders of the Body

The Lymphatic System, 347
The Immune System, 349
   Nonspecific Immune Mechanisms, 349
   Specific Immune Mechanisms, 350
   Acquired Immunity, 352
   Immune System Problems, 352
Exercises, 354
Glossary, 363

17   Multiple-System Diseases:
A Glossary of Conditions Affecting
Multiple Systems

Section Five: Adding to the Structure

Appendix

A.   **Abbreviations and Symbols, 377**

B.   **Latin and Greek Combining Forms for**
     English Numbers, 384

C.   **The Metric System and Equivalents, 385**

D.   **Medical Specialties, 386**

E.   **Hospital Records and Reports, 388**

F.   **Medical Insurance, 397**

Bibliography, 404

Index, 405

Color Plates

Skeletal System

Anterior View of Skeleton, A-1
Posterior View of Skeleton, A-2
Thorax and Ribs, A-3
Male Pelvis, A-3
Female Pelvis, A-3
Lateral View of Vertebral Column, A-4
Individual Vertebra, A-4
Microscopic Structure of Bone, A-5

Muscular System

Anterior View, A-6
Posterior View, A-7

Lymphatic System

Spleen, A-8
Location and Gross Anatomy of Thymus, A-8

Respiratory System

Organs of Respiratory System and Associated
    Structures, A-9
Structure of Nose, A-10
Structures of Nasal Passages and Throat, A-10

Digestive System

Organs of Digestive System and Some Associated
    Structures, A-11
Location of Salivary Glands, A-12
Sources of Intestinal Secretions, A-13

Reproductive System

Female Reproductive Organs and Associated
    Structures, A-13
Female Perineum, A-13

Urinary System

Urinary System and Some Associated Structures, A-14

Special Senses

Hearing

Gross Anatomy of the Ear in Frontal Section, A-15
Impedence-Matching Components of Inner Ear,
A-15

Sight

Cross-Sectional View of Right Eye, A-16
Normal Structure of Eye, A-16

ANTERIOR VIEW OF SKELETON

Axial skeleton is shown in blue. Appendicular system is bone colored.

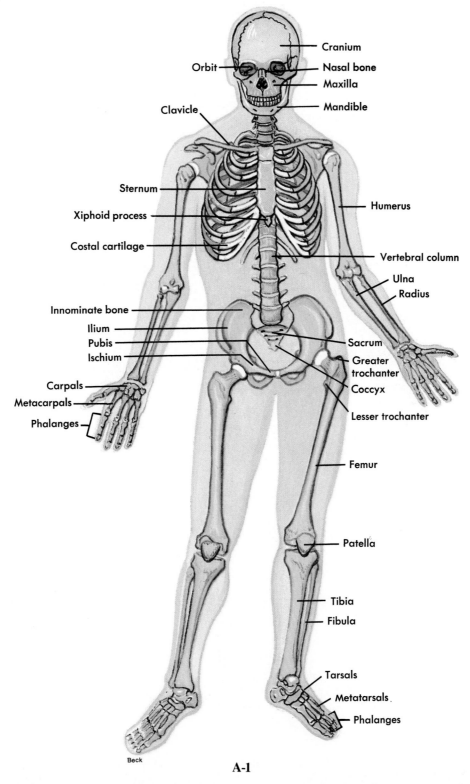

Cranium

Orbit

Nasal bone

Maxilla

Mandible

Clavicle

Sternum

Humerus

Xiphoid process

Costal cartilage

Vertebral column

Ulna

Radius

Innominate bone

Ilium

Pubis

Sacrum

Ischium

Greater trochanter

Coccyx

Carpals

Metacarpals

Lesser trochanter

Phalanges

Femur

Patella

Tibia

Fibula

Tarsals

Metatarsals

Phalanges

Beck

A-1

POSTERIOR VIEW OF SKELETON
Axial skeleton is shown in blue. Appendicular system is
bone colored.

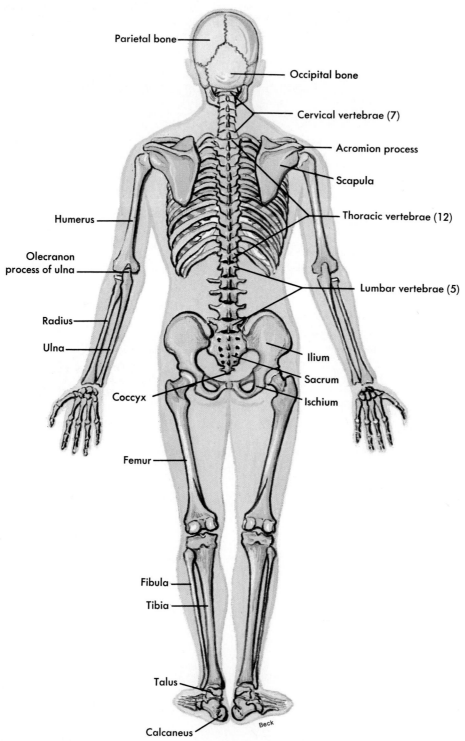

Parietal bone

Occipital bone

Cervical vertebrae (7)

Acromion process

Scapula

Humerus

Thoracic vertebrae (12)

Olecranon
process of ulna

Lumbar vertebrae (5)

Radius

Ulna

Ilium

Sacrum

Coccyx

Ischium

Femur

Fibula

Tibia

Talus

Calcaneus

Beck

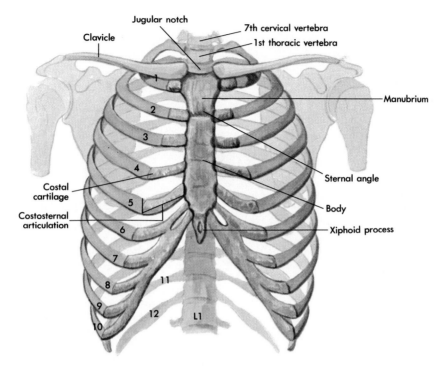

THORAX AND RIBS

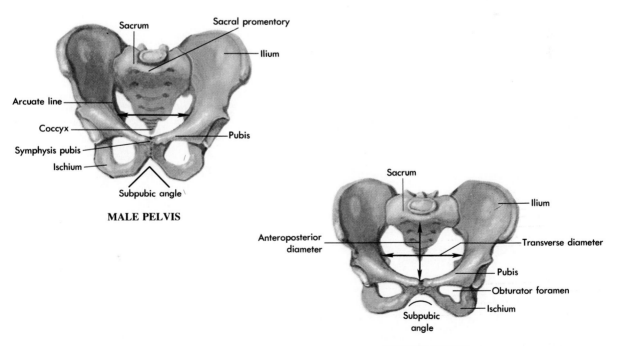

MALE PELVIS

FEMALE PELVIS

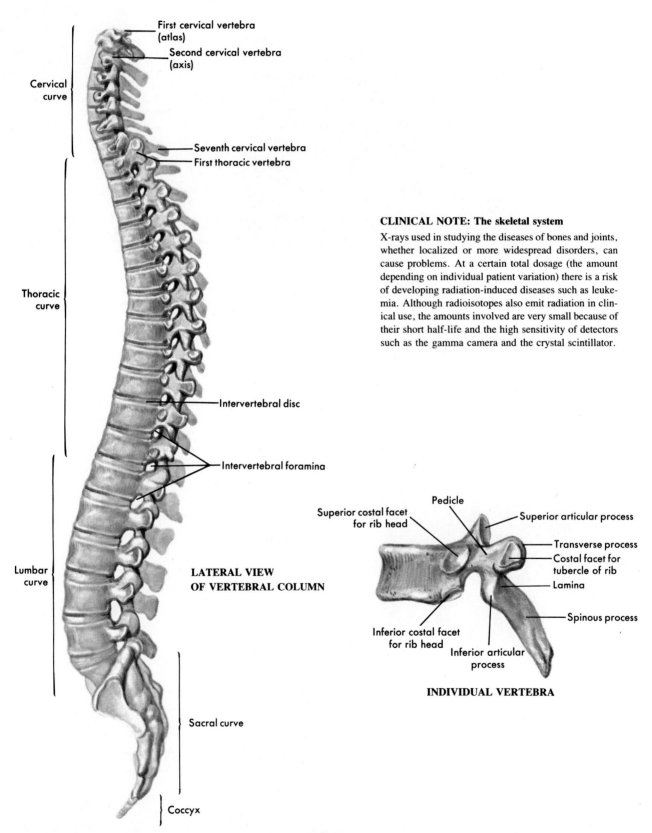

First cervical vertebra
(atlas)

Second cervical vertebra
(axis)

Cervical curve

Seventh cervical vertebra

First thoracic vertebra

Thoracic curve

Intervertebral disc

Intervertebral foramina

Lumbar curve

LATERAL VIEW OF VERTEBRAL COLUMN

Sacral curve

Coccyx

Superior costal facet for rib head

Pedicle

Superior articular process

Transverse process

Costal facet for tubercle of rib

Lamina

Spinous process

Inferior costal facet for rib head

Inferior articular process

INDIVIDUAL VERTEBRA

CLINICAL NOTE: The skeletal system

X-rays used in studying the diseases of bones and joints, whether localized or more widespread disorders, can cause problems. At a certain total dosage (the amount depending on individual patient variation) there is a risk of developing radiation-induced diseases such as leukemia. Although radioisotopes also emit radiation in clinical use, the amounts involved are very small because of their short half-life and the high sensitivity of detectors such as the gamma camera and the crystal scintillator.

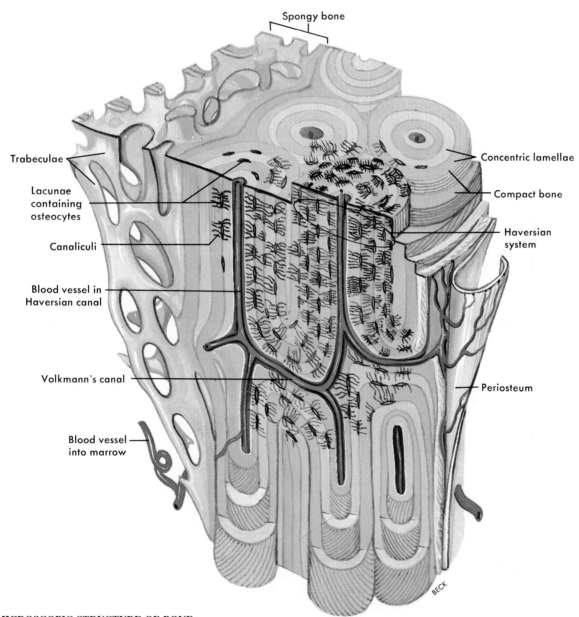

Spongy bone

Trabeculae

Lacunae
containing
osteocytes

Canaliculi

Blood vessel in
Haversian canal

Volkmann's canal

Blood vessel
into marrow

Concentric lamellae

Compact bone

Haversian
system

Periosteum

BECK

MICROSCOPIC STRUCTURE OF BONE
Haversian systems, several of which are shown here,
compose compact bone. Note the structures that make
up one haversian system: concentric lamellae, lacunae,
canaliculi, and a haversian canal. Shown bordering the
compact bone on the left is spongy bone, a name
descriptive of the many open spaces that characterize
it.

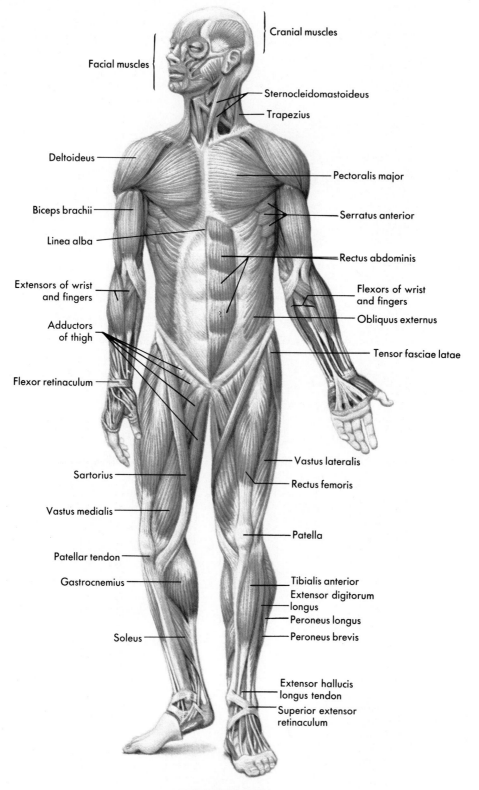

Cranial muscles

Facial muscles {

Sternocleidomastoideus

Trapezius

Deltoideus

Pectoralis major

Biceps brachii

Serratus anterior

Linea alba

Rectus abdominis

Extensors of wrist
and fingers

Flexors of wrist
and fingers

Adductors
of thigh

Obliquus externus

Flexor retinaculum

Tensor fasciae latae

Vastus lateralis

Sartorius

Rectus femoris

Vastus medialis

Patella

Patellar tendon

Tibialis anterior

Gastrocnemius

Extensor digitorum
longus

Peroneus longus

Soleus

Peroneus brevis

Extensor hallucis
longus tendon

Superior extensor
retinaculum

ANTERIOR VIEW

A-6

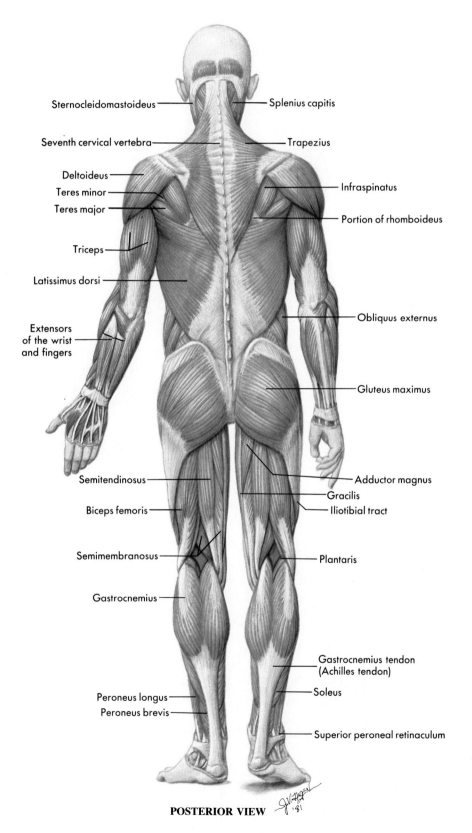

Sternocleidomastoideus

Splenius capitis

Seventh cervical vertebra

Trapezius

Deltoideus

Teres minor

Teres major

Infraspinatus

Portion of rhomboideus

Triceps

Latissimus dorsi

Obliquus externus

Extensors
of the wrist
and fingers

Gluteus maximus

Semitendinosus

Adductor magnus

Gracilis

Biceps femoris

Iliotibial tract

Semimembranosus

Plantaris

Gastrocnemius

Gastrocnemius tendon
(Achilles tendon)

Soleus

Peroneus longus

Peroneus brevis

Superior peroneal retinaculum

POSTERIOR VIEW

A-7

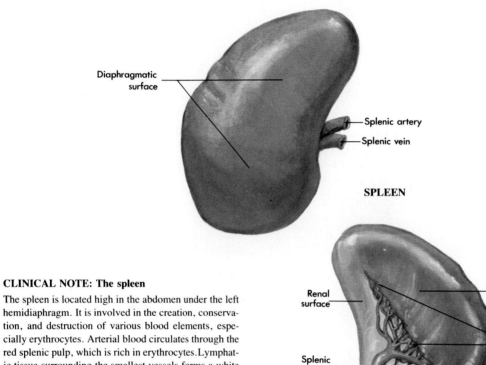

Diaphragmatic surface

Splenic artery

Splenic vein

SPLEEN

Renal surface

Gastric surface

Hilus

Splenic artery

Splenic vein

CLINICAL NOTE: The spleen

The spleen is located high in the abdomen under the left hemidiaphragm. It is involved in the creation, conservation, and destruction of various blood elements, especially erythrocytes. Arterial blood circulates through the red splenic pulp, which is rich in erythrocytes. Lymphatic tissue surrounding the smallest vessels forms a white pulp material.

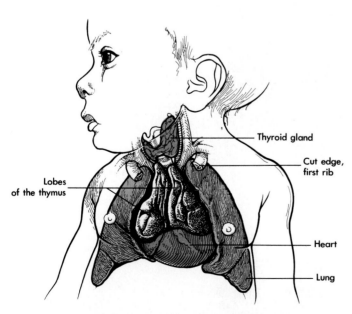

Thyroid gland

Cut edge, first rib

Lobes of the thymus

Heart

Lung

LOCATION AND GROSS ANATOMY OF THYMUS

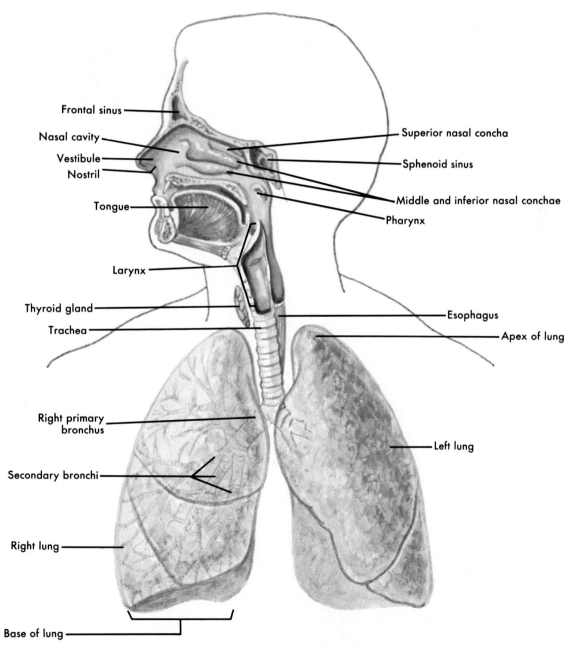

Frontal sinus

Nasal cavity

Vestibule

Nostril

Tongue

Larynx

Thyroid gland

Trachea

Right primary bronchus

Secondary bronchi

Right lung

Base of lung

Superior nasal concha

Sphenoid sinus

Middle and inferior nasal conchae

Pharynx

Esophagus

Apex of lung

Left lung

**ORGANS OF RESPIRATORY SYSTEM
AND ASSOCIATED STRUCTURES**

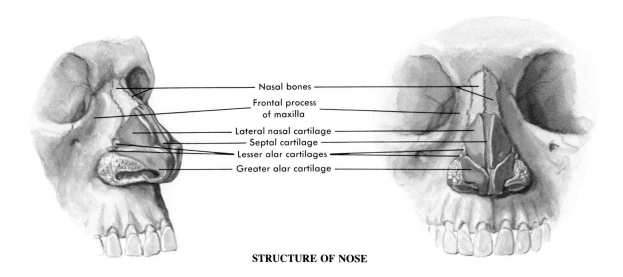

Nasal bones

Frontal process
of maxilla

Lateral nasal cartilage

Septal cartilage

Lesser alar cartilages

Greater alar cartilage

STRUCTURE OF NOSE

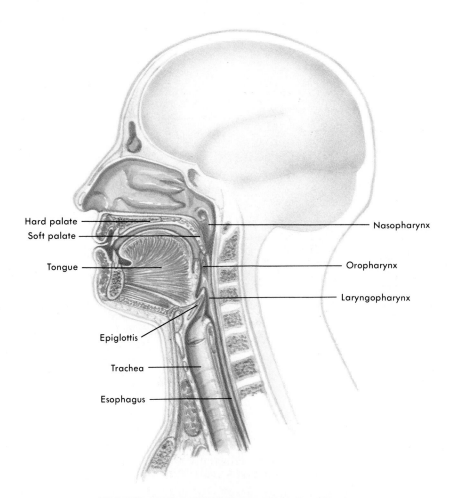

Hard palate

Soft palate

Tongue

Epiglottis

Trachea

Esophagus

Nasopharynx

Oropharynx

Laryngopharynx

STRUCTURES OF NASAL PASSAGES AND THROAT

A-10

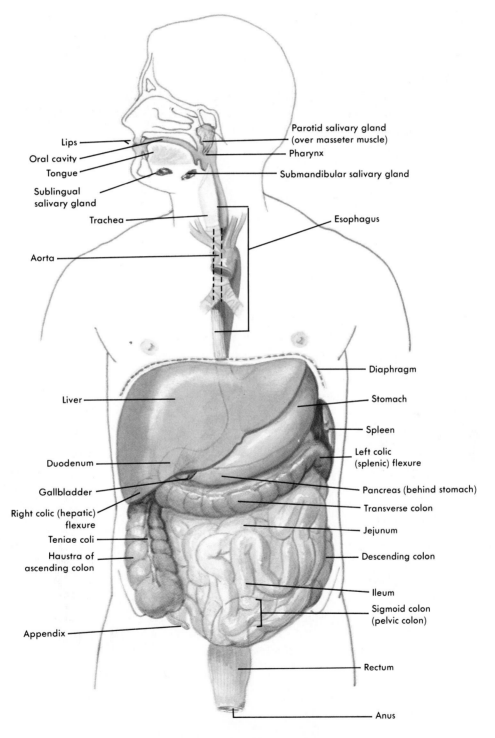

Lips

Oral cavity

Tongue

Sublingual
salivary gland

Trachea

Aorta

Parotid salivary gland
(over masseter muscle)

Pharynx

Submandibular salivary gland

Esophagus

Diaphragm

Liver

Stomach

Spleen

Left colic
(splenic) flexure

Duodenum

Gallbladder

Right colic (hepatic)
flexure

Teniae coli

Haustra of
ascending colon

Pancreas (behind stomach)

Transverse colon

Jejunum

Descending colon

Ileum

Sigmoid colon
(pelvic colon)

Appendix

Rectum

Anus

**ORGANS OF DIGESTIVE SYSTEM AND
SOME ASSOCIATED STRUCTURES**

A-11

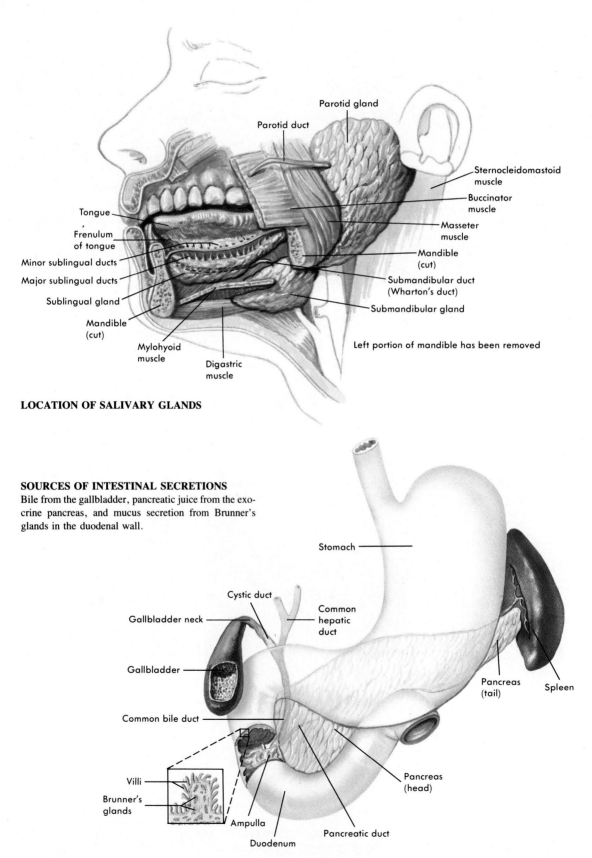

Parotid gland

Parotid duct

Sternocleidomastoid muscle

Buccinator muscle

Masseter muscle

Mandible (cut)

Submandibular duct (Wharton's duct)

Submandibular gland

Tongue

Frenulum of tongue

Minor sublingual ducts

Major sublingual ducts

Sublingual gland

Mandible (cut)

Mylohyoid muscle

Digastric muscle

Left portion of mandible has been removed

LOCATION OF SALIVARY GLANDS

SOURCES OF INTESTINAL SECRETIONS

Bile from the gallbladder, pancreatic juice from the exocrine pancreas, and mucus secretion from Brunner's glands in the duodenal wall.

Stomach

Cystic duct

Gallbladder neck

Common hepatic duct

Gallbladder

Pancreas (tail)

Spleen

Common bile duct

Villi

Brunner's glands

Ampulla

Duodenum

Pancreatic duct

Pancreas (head)

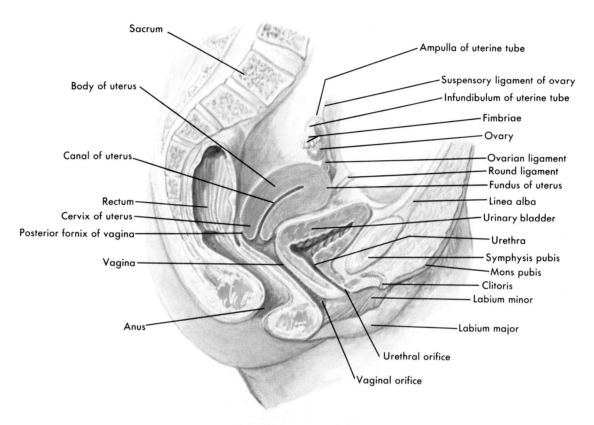

Sacrum

Body of uterus

Canal of uterus

Rectum

Cervix of uterus

Posterior fornix of vagina

Vagina

Anus

Ampulla of uterine tube

Suspensory ligament of ovary

Infundibulum of uterine tube

Fimbriae

Ovary

Ovarian ligament

Round ligament

Fundus of uterus

Linea alba

Urinary bladder

Urethra

Symphysis pubis

Mons pubis

Clitoris

Labium minor

Labium major

Urethral orifice

Vaginal orifice

**FEMALE REPRODUCTIVE ORGANS AND
ASSOCIATED STRUCTURES**

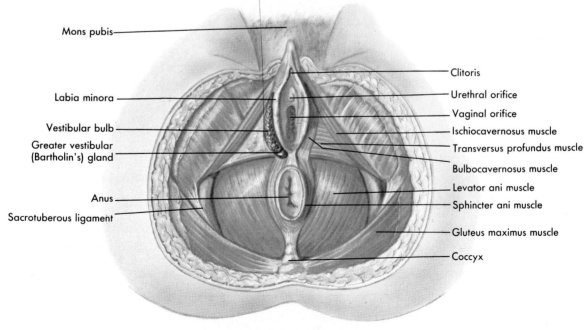

Mons pubis

Labia minora

Vestibular bulb

Greater vestibular
(Bartholin's) gland

Anus

Sacrotuberous ligament

Clitoris

Urethral orifice

Vaginal orifice

Ischiocavernosus muscle

Transversus profundus muscle

Bulbocavernosus muscle

Levator ani muscle

Sphincter ani muscle

Gluteus maximus muscle

Coccyx

FEMALE PERINEUM

A-13

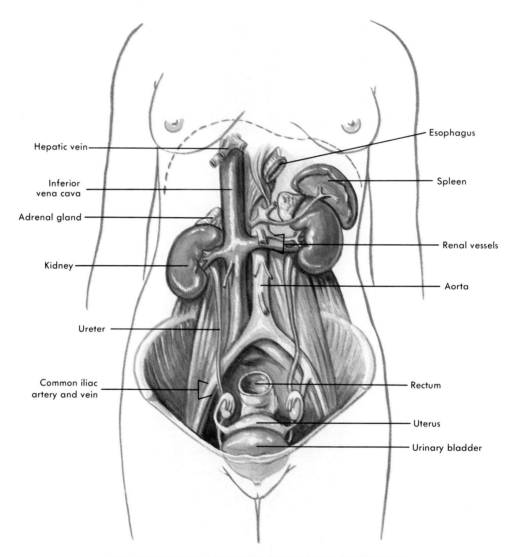

Hepatic vein

Inferior
vena cava

Adrenal gland

Kidney

Ureter

Common iliac
artery and vein

Esophagus

Spleen

Renal vessels

Aorta

Rectum

Uterus

Urinary bladder

URINARY SYSTEM AND SOME ASSOCIATED STRUCTURES

Hearing

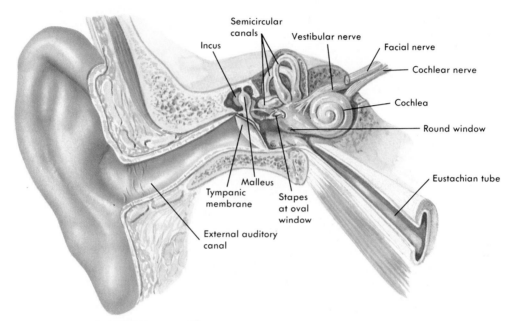

GROSS ANATOMY OF THE EAR IN FRONTAL SECTION

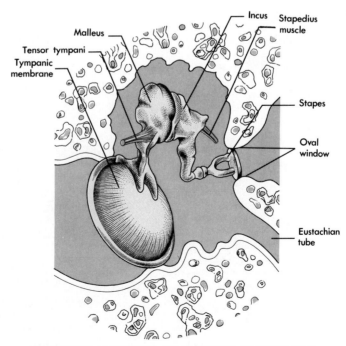

IMPEDENCE-MATCHING COMPONENTS OF INNER EAR

Sight

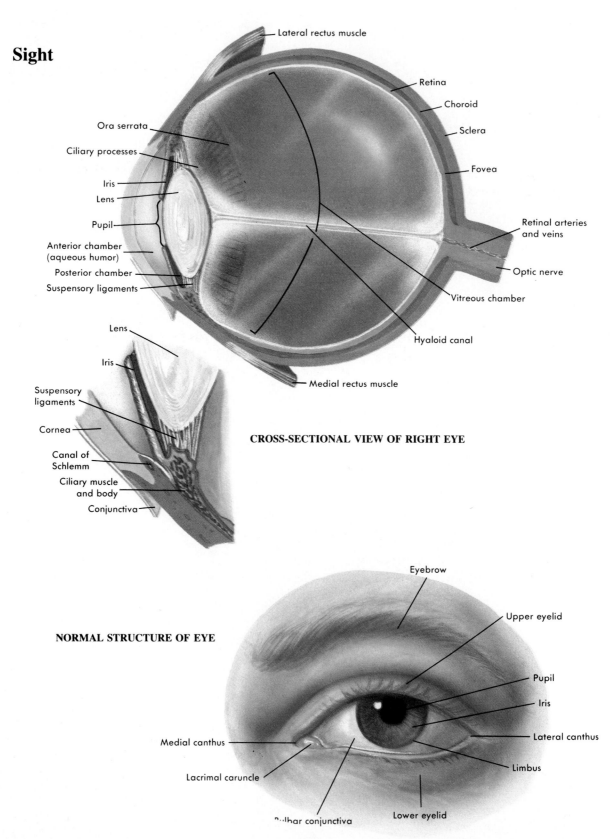

Lateral rectus muscle

Retina

Choroid

Sclera

Fovea

Ora serrata

Ciliary processes

Iris

Lens

Pupil

Retinal arteries and veins

Anterior chamber (aqueous humor)

Posterior chamber

Suspensory ligaments

Optic nerve

Vitreous chamber

Hyaloid canal

Medial rectus muscle

Lens

Iris

Suspensory ligaments

Cornea

Canal of Schlemm

Ciliary muscle and body

Conjunctiva

CROSS-SECTIONAL VIEW OF RIGHT EYE

NORMAL STRUCTURE OF EYE

Eyebrow

Upper eyelid

Pupil

Iris

Lateral canthus

Medial canthus

Limbus

Lacrimal caruncle

Bulbar conjunctiva

Lower eyelid

A-16

The Basic Foundation of Medical Terminology

This is the first of the five sections of **LEARNING MEDICAL TERMINOLOGY.** This section contains four chapters to introduce the student to the basic foundation of medical language.

Chapter 1 is a brief introduction to the separate parts of words, with examples to help the student understand the construction of medical terms.

Chapter 2 presents the initial step in building and learning the vocabulary. The most essential components of the language, prefixes and suffixes, are conveniently arranged in chart form with meanings and examples.

Chapter 3 is the second step in building the vocabulary by the addition of the roots and combining forms that relate to the structures of the body. The chapter is divided into two sections, external and internal anatomy, arranged in chart form, with pronunciations and identification of the specific body parts.

Chapter 4 is the third step in the development of the foundation. It contains descriptive words, roots and combining forms, divided into separate sections. These sections cover actions, conditions, characteristics, body fluids and substances, chemicals, and colors. Each section is presented in chart form with meanings clearly shown.

MOTHER GOOSE & GRIMM / By Mike Peters

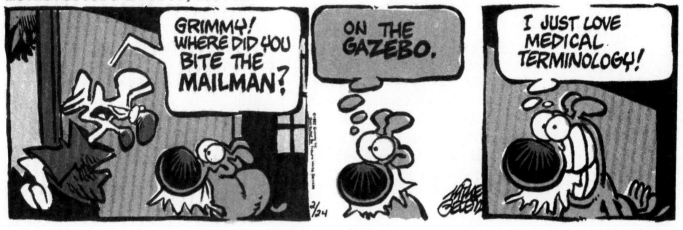

Chapter 1

An Introduction to Medical Terminology

CHAPTER OVERVIEW

This chapter introduces word elements (prefixes, suffixes, and roots and combining forms), their meanings, and ways of combining them to build medical terms. Basic pronunciation rules are presented, with pertinent examples.

OBJECTIVE

The primary objective of this book is to enable you, the student, to learn medical terminology. When first confronted with medical terms one is bewildered by their strange spelling and pronunciation. This is understandable when one considers that approximately 75% of these terms are based on either Greek or Latin. New terms are constantly being coined, but most are derivatives of Greek or Latin words. The Greeks were the founders of modern medicine, although Latin has become the universal source of medical language.

When you complete this worktext, you will have a basic, workable vocabulary, applicable to any branch of medicine. You do not need prior knowledge of Greek, Latin, anatomy, or physiology to build a medical vocabulary. The knowledge you do need is presented step by step in this worktext and will help you to learn, and be comfortable with, medical language.

This is accomplished by:

1. breaking a word apart and identifying its parts (prefix, suffix, and root and combining form).
2. describing the structure and functions of each of the body systems.
3. relating applicable words and their parts to each of the body systems.
4. using illustrations, diagrams, and charts to assist in the learning process.
5. reviewing text material using questions (and answers) throughout and at the end of each chapter.

Most medical terms are a combination of two or more word parts. The definition of a word involves a search for the meaning of each of its parts. When they are translated separately and combined, the parts give the essential meaning of the entire word.

The fundamental method of building a medical vocabulary, as it is outlined in this book, consists of breaking down a word and identifying its parts: prefix, suffix, root or roots, and combining form. A prefix is the beginning part of a word, and a suffix is the end part. A root is the foundation, or basic meaning, of a word, and may appear with a prefix, with a suffix, or between a prefix and suffix. Prefixes and suffixes can never stand alone; they must always be attached to a root. A combining form is a root with an added vowel (known as a combining vowel) that connects the root with a suffix or with another root. For example:

In the word *antisepsis*:
the *prefix* anti- means against
the *root* sepsis means infection
antisepsis means against infection

In the word *rhinitis*:
the *root* rhin- means nose
the *suffix* -itis means inflammation
rhinitis means inflammation of the nose

In the word *glycohemia*:
the *root* glyc- means sugar or sweet
when we add the *combining vowel "o"* to glyc-
it becomes the *combining form* glyco-
the *root* hem- means blood
the *suffix* -ia means state or condition
glycohemia means sugar in the blood

Some words contain more than one root, each of which retains its basic meaning. Such words, called compounds, are very common in medicine. *Glycohemia*, shown above as an example of a combining form, is also an example of a compound word. Another example of a compound word is *osteoarthritis*. The combining form *osteo-* comes from the root *oste-*, which means bone; the root arthr- means joint or joints; and the suffix *-itis* means inflammation. Therefore, the compound word *osteoarthritis* means inflammation of the bone joints.

Specific Suggestions for Learning Medical Terminology

The identification of prefixes, suffixes, and roots of words pertaining to anatomy is the first step in building a medical vocabulary. The next step is to learn to recognize the most common roots referring to conditions, actions, characteristics, body fluids, body substances and chemicals, and colors. This will help you to understand anatomic structures, diseases, procedures, and other descriptive terms by simply breaking each word into its components, defining the components separately, and then combining them to discover the meaning of the word as a whole. If you practice analyzing medical words that you see or hear, you will find, in time, that you are able to define words at a glance, much the same as you would learn a foreign language.

It is possible to memorize some medical words without regard to a breakdown of their components, but you cannot memorize the entire medical dictionary. Although most medical terms can be learned easily from their components, there is no way to use components to analyze those terms that are derived from proper names. Use your medical dictionary when you do not recognize a term that bears a proper name, when you cannot arrive at a definition by analysis, or when the meaning is not clear. This book does not pretend to break down all medical terms into components, but it does give you the key to analysis by listing over 500 specific roots and combining forms of the type you will find in the majority of medical words. Treat each medical word as if it were a puzzle you are attempting to solve, and you will see how enjoyable and rewarding it will be to define the word without reference to a medical dictionary.

Pronunciation of Medical Terms

Medical terms are hard to pronounce, especially if you have never heard them spoken. Here are some shortcuts you will find helpful:

ch is sometimes pronounced like *k*
Examples—chromatin, chronic

ps is pronounced like *s*
Examples—psychiatry, psychology

pn is pronounced with only the *n* sound
Examples—pneumonia, pneusis

c and *g* are given the soft sounds of *s* and *j*, respectively, before *e*, *i*, and *y*
Examples—generic, giant, cycle, cytoplasm

c and *g* have a hard sound before other letters
Examples—cast, cardiac, gastric, gonad

ae and *oe* are pronounced *ee*
Examples—fasciae, coelom

i at the end of a word is pronounced *eye* (to form a plural)
Examples—alveoli, glomeruli, fasciculi

es, at the end of a word, is often pronounced as a separate syllable
Examples—stases (stay′ seez), nares (nah′ reez)

To help in pronunciation, the phonetic spelling of words is used, where necessary, in the glossaries.

Plurals

The plural of most English words is formed by adding *s* or *es*, but in medical terms the plural may be formed by changing the ending. Some examples are:

ae, as in fasciae (singular, *fascia*)
ia, as in crania (singular, *cranium*)
i, as in glomeruli (singular, *glomerulus*). If the singular form ends in *us*, the plural is made by dropping the *us* and adding *i*
ata, as in adenomata (singular, *adenoma*)

Spelling

Rules for pronunciation and the formation of plurals are essential for spelling, but it is very important that you consult a medical dictionary if you are not sure. Phonetic spelling has no place in medicine. Some terms sound alike but are spelled differently. For example, the *ileum* is a part of the intestinal tract, but the *ilium* is a pelvic bone. A misspelled word may lead to the wrong meaning, creating confusion and possibly an incorrect diagnosis.

CHAPTER 1 EXERCISES

AN INTRODUCTION TO MEDICAL TERMINOLOGY

Exercise 1: List the four principal parts of a medical word.

1. _____   3. _____

2. _____   4. _____

Exercise 2: Identify the place and/or purpose of the four parts above.

1. _____

2. _____

3. _____

4. _____

Exercise 3: Matching:

____ **1.** -ia   **A.** inflammation

____ **2.** anti-   **B.** nose

____ **3.** -itis   **C.** blood

____ **4.** -sepsis   **D.** joint

____ **5.** rhin-   **E.** bone

____ **6.** glyc-   **F.** against

____ **7.** oste-   **G.** infection

____ **8.** hem-   **H.** state or condition

____ **9.** arthr-   **I.** sugar

Exercise 4: For the following statements indicate T for true or F for false in the space provided.

____ **1.** Ps and pn are pronounced with a silent p.

____ **2.** Phonetic spelling is acceptable in medical language.

____ **3.** The medical dictionary is an unimportant tool.

____ **4.** The letters c and g always have a hard sound.

____ **5.** Like English, the plurals of medical terms end in s or es.

CHAPTER 1 CROSSWORD PUZZLE

Across

1. Many roots relate to the _____ of the body.

2. The plural suffix of fascia.

7. Beginning word part.

8. Founders of modern medicine.

9. A word part.

13. Science related to the study of the parts of the body.

14. A suffix meaning state or condition.

15. Words that come from proper names or other words.

18. A type of visual aid to assist in learning.

21. Type of dictionary.

22. A root meaning nose.

23. A prefix meaning against.

25. Means bone.

Down

1. Infection.

3. First.

4. Opposite of teach.

5. Words with more than one root.

6. Phonetic sounding out of a word.

10. Means sugar or sweet.

11. Learning medical terminology is the _____ of this text.

12. Additional visual aids to assist in learning.

16. Ending word part.

17. Source of medical language.

19. Means blood.

20. Part of intestinal tract that sounds like a pelvic bone.

22. A foundation word part.

23. A root meaning joint.

24. Inflammation.

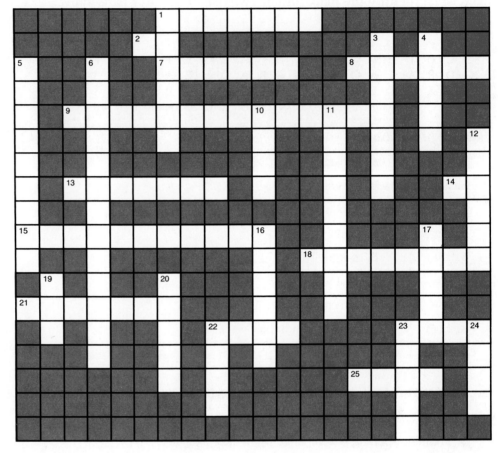

Chapter 1 Hidden Word Puzzle

```
W  P  V  F  C  R  P  B  M  J  E  Q  A  X  T  E  J  B  T  H  B  F  W
D  W  O  K  J  O  E  E  K  X  W  U  C  I  X  Y  N  O  I  O  Q  P  E
Q  F  A  W  S  I  L  B  E  C  X  G  T  N  B  Y  O  S  N  M  G  Z  W
M  H  R  S  Y  M  T  O  P  J  N  V  I  D  N  Q  R  B  M  T  R  F  Q
E  O  N  E  P  P  L  W  R  H  L  L  O  E  A  S  P  U  X  V  W  G  Z
D  I  A  G  R  A  M  S  Q  S  O  A  N  S  L  N  A  V  P  V  U  I  R
I  F  G  C  O  N  D  I  T  I  O  N  S  E  B  R  P  A  D  T  I  Y  X
C  T  K  V  N  D  Q  P  V  N  U  G  E  P  F  M  U  I  H  G  Q  P  K
A  E  E  I  U  Q  Y  V  O  G  N  U  P  T  E  F  W  P  J  A  I  X  B
L  L  S  S  N  O  K  Q  T  U  O  A  L  W  I  L  L  O  L  X  M  H  C
D  T  W  C  C  O  H  D  D  L  Q  G  R  Z  N  C  L  O  Q  G  S  L  U
S  O  C  U  I  H  C  K  A  A  U  E  P  A  E  S  F  I  Q  J  X  F  C
V  G  D  R  A  F  A  O  F  R  Q  G  K  A  D  L  E  A  N  O  F  E  J
M  N  X  X  T  E  R  M  I  N  O  L  O  G  Y  N  P  R  G  J  S  U
N  L  Q  O  I  B  Y  F  A  P  U  V  I  D  E  O  W  N  F  D  F  P  X
E  V  Y  N  O  Q  A  T  J  C  O  X  B  G  I  X  N  T  I  N  Y  R  A
L  V  U  T  N  W  N  X  C  B  T  N  V  Q  Z  K  S  L  V  M  V  A  I
U  E  W  S  X  X  D  L  H  O  R  E  E  V  D  K  L  I  C  H  E  O  P
H  R  I  L  V  H  A  C  X  F  X  N  R  N  F  I  W  T  M  A  K  M  X
D  Y  J  V  E  Z  I  F  Q  D  C  O  H  I  T  H  A  N  A  L  Y  Z  E
N  H  G  J  W  W  S  J  W  E  F  S  Z  A  S  S  P  G  D  F  O  T  M
V  B  N  X  N  C  G  M  B  F  O  U  N  D  A  T  I  O  N  X  P  B  R
M  D  E  M  W  S  E  I  E  I  Q  B  P  H  Y  S  I  O  L  O  G  Y  L
T  F  M  C  J  Y  U  S  E  N  W  S  M  M  L  P  X  C  M  T  S  Z  Y
G  H  F  G  R  E  H  D  B  E  K  T  T  G  I  W  Q  W  S  U  N  I  Q
G  W  Y  O  E  F  C  D  V  O  C  A  B  U  L  A  R  Y  X  X  H  T  S
L  G  Q  X  S  L  I  M  J  Q  N  N  O  N  M  J  G  C  K  G  Y  X  Q
G  B  U  G  A  B  X  M  S  D  K  C  G  H  A  I  C  Z  K  S  E  E  Y
G  P  G  W  I  C  Y  K  Q  Q  B  E  E  R  U  T  U  U  V  B  B  A  K
T  W  U  I  F  Y  M  T  W  J  E  S  I  N  M  X  Y  I  I  D  N  L  V
```

Can you find the 20 words hidden in this puzzle? All hidden word puzzles will have words running from top to bottom, left to right, and diagonally downward.

CHARACTERISTICS	PRONUNCIATION	TERMINOLOGY	COMPONENTS
CONDITIONS	FOUNDATION	PHYSIOLOGY	SUBSTANCES
VOCABULARY	DIAGNOSIS	DIAGRAMS	LANGUAGE
PHONETIC	SINGULAR	SPELLING	ACTIONS
ANALYZE	MEDICAL	COLORS	DEFINE

Chapter 1 Answers

Exercise 1
In any order:
1. prefix
2. suffix
3. root
4. combining form

Exercise 2
In any order:
1. prefix: beginning or first part of a word
2. suffix: ending or last part of a word
3. root: foundation of a word
4. combining form: root with combining vowel to attach to another root or a suffix

Exercise 3
1. H
2. F
3. A
4. G
5. B
6. I
7. E
8. C
9. D

Exercise 4
1. T
2. F
3. F
4. F
5. F

Answers: Chapter 1 Crossword Puzzle

Answers: Chapter 1 Hidden Word Puzzle

```
. . . . C . . . . . . A . . . . . . . . .
. . . . . O . . . . . C . . . . . . . . .
. . . . . L . . . T . . . . . . . . .
M . . . . . O P . . . I . . . . . . .
E . . P . . . R H . L O . . . . . . .
D I A G R A M S . S O A N . . . . . . .
I . . C O N D I T I O N S . . . . . . .
C . . N . . . N . G E P . . . . . . .
A . . U . . . G . U . T E . . . . . .
L . N . . . . U . A . . I L . . . . .
. . . . C . . . L . G . . . C L . . . .
. . . I H C . . A . E . . . . I . . .
. . . A . A O . R . . . . . . . . N . .
. . . . T T E R M I N O L O G Y . . . G . . .
. . . . I . . . A P . . . . . . .
. . . . O . . . C O . . . . . .
. . . . N . . . . T N . . . . .
. . . . . . . . . E E . D . . .
. . . . . . . . . R N . I . . .
. . . . . . . . D . . . I T . A N A L Y Z E
. . . . . . . . E . S . . S S . G . . .
. . . . . . . . F O U N D A T I O N . . .
. . . . . . . . I . B P H Y S I O L O G Y .
. . . . . . . . N . S . . . . . C . . S . . .
. . . . . . . . E . T . . . . . . S . I .
. . . . . . . . V O C A B U L A R Y . . . . S
. . . . . . . . N . . . . . .
. . . . . . . . C . . . . . .
. . . . . . . . E . . . . . .
. . . . . . . . S . . . . . .
```

Words:

\ CHARACTERISTICS	\/ PRONUNCIATION	> TERMINOLOGY	\ COMPONENTS
> CONDITIONS	> FOUNDATION	> PHYSIOLOGY	\/ SUBSTANCES
> VOCABULARY	\ DIAGNOSIS	> DIAGRAMS	\/ LANGUAGE
\ PHONETIC	\/ SINGULAR	\ SPELLING	\/ ACTIONS
> ANALYZE	\/ MEDICAL	\ COLORS	\/ DEFINE

Chapter 2

Building a Medical Vocabulary

CHAPTER OVERVIEW

In this chapter the student becomes familiar with prefixes (the beginnings of words) and suffixes (the endings of words) by means of definitions and word examples. These word parts are listed alphabetically in chart form to enhance learning.

STEP 1: PREFIXES AND SUFFIXES

The next three chapters present the basic building blocks of a medical vocabulary. Your ability to break down medical terms into their separate parts, or to recognize a complete word, depends on your learning of the roots and combining forms that appear in medical terms and the prefixes and suffixes that alter or modify the meaning and usage of a term.

By learning the meanings of the word parts given in these chapters, you will find that you can define most of the medical words in subsequent chapters. The meanings of the word parts presented in these chapters will generally *not* be repeated; however, these chapters can be used for reference whenever you do not recognize the meaning of a word part.

Prefixes

A prefix consists of one or more syllables placed at the beginning of a word. A prefix never stands alone. It is placed in front of a verb, adjective, or noun to modify its meaning. Most prefixes are parts of words in ordinary language and do not specifically refer to medical terminology. However, many prefixes do occur frequently in medical language, and studying them is an important first step in learning medical terms. The principal prefixes used in medical terminology are given in Table 2-1.

Table 2-1   PREFIXES

Prefix	Meaning	Examples
a-, an-	without, lack of, not	Aphasia (without speech) Anemia (lack of blood)
ab-	away from	Abductor (leading away from) Aboral (away from mouth)
ad-	toward, to, near	Adductor (leading toward) Adrenal (near the kidney)
ambi-, ampho-	both	Ambidextrous (ability to use both hands equally) Amphogenic (producing young of both sexes)
amphi-	on both sides, double	Amphibious (living both on land and in water) Amphithymia (dual mental state of depression and elation)
ana-	up, toward, apart	Anatomy (to cut apart) Anacatharsis (vomiting up)
ante-	before, in front of, forward	Antecubital (before the elbow) Anteflex (to bend forward)
anti-	against, opposing	Antisepsis (against infection) Anticarious (against cavities)
ap-, apo-	separated from, derived from	Apobiosis (death of a part) Apocleisis (aversion to food)
aut-, auto-	self	Autoanalysis (self-analysis) Autoerotism (sexual self-love)
bi-	two, double, twice	Bifocal (two foci) Biarticulate (double joint)
cata-	down, under, lower, against	Catabolism (breaking down) Catalepsy (reduced movement)
circum-	around	Circumflex (winding around) Circumarticular (around a joint)
co-,* com-,** con-	with, together	Commissure (coming together) Conductor (leading together)
contra-	opposed, against	Contralateral (opposite side) Contraception (prevention of conception)
de-	down, from	Dehydrate (remove water from) Decay (breakdown)
di-	two, twice	Dicephalous (two-headed) Dichromic (having two colors)
dia-	between, through, apart, across, completely	Diapedesis (ooze through) Diaphragm (wall across) Diagnosis (complete knowledge)
dis-	apart from, free from	Disinfection (free from infection) Dissect (cut apart) Disarticulation (separation at a joint)
dys-	difficult, bad, painful	Dyskinesis (difficult motion) Dyspepsia (bad digestion) Dyspareunia (painful coitus)

*co- before a vowel
**com- before b, m, and p

Continued.

Table 2-1 PREFIXES — cont'd.

Prefix	Meaning	Examples
e-, ec-, ex-	out of, from, away from	Enucleate (remove whole from) Ectopic (out of place) Exostosis (outgrowth of bone)
ect-, ecto-, exo-	outer, outside, situated on	Ectal (on the surface) Ectoderm (outer skin) Ectocytic (outside of the cell) Exogenic (originating outside)
em-,* en-	in	Empyema (pus in a body cavity) Encranial (in the cranium)
end-, endo-, ent-, ento-	within, inner	Endaural (within the ear) Endocranial (within the cranium) Entiris (inner eye color) Entocele (internal hernia)
ep-, epi-	upon, on, over	Epicostal (upon a rib) Epidermis (outer skin layer) Eponychia (infection over the nail bed)
eu-	normal, good, well, healthy	Eucrasia (normal health) Euplastic (healing well)
extra-, extro-	outside of, beyond, outward	Extraoral (outside of the mouth) Extroversion (turning inside out)
hemi-	half	Hemiepilepsy (epilepsy on one side of the body) Hemilingual (half of the tongue)
hyper-	excessive, above, beyond	Hyperactive (overactive) Hypertension (above-normal blood pressure)
hyp-, hypo-	under, deficient, beneath	Hypalgia (reduced pain sense) Hypothyroidism (deficiency of thyroid activity)
im-,** in-	in, into, within	Implant (insert into) Injection (forcing fluid into)
im-,** in-	not	Immature (not mature) Involuntary (not voluntary)
infra-	below, beneath	Infraorbital (beneath the eyes) Infracostal (below a rib)
inter-	between	Intercostal (between ribs) Internodal (between nodes)
intra-	within	Intracardiac (within the heart) Intraocular (within the eye)
intro-	into, within	Introversion (turning inward) Introrsus (turned in)
mes-, meso-	middle	Mesencephalon (midbrain) Mesonasal (middle of the nose)
meta-	change, beyond	Metachrosis (color change) Metabasis (disease changes)
micr-, micro-	small	Micracoustic (faint sounds) Microbe (minute organism)
mult-, multi-	many	Multiarticular (many joints) Multiform (many shapes)
neo-	new, recent	Neoblastic (new tissue growth) Neonatal (newborn)
pan-	all, entire	Panacea (cure-all) Pantalgia (entire-body pain)

*em- before b, m, and p
**im- before b, m, and p

Table 2-1   PREFIXES — cont'd.

Prefix	Meaning	Examples
para-	beside, beyond, after	Paracardiac (beside the heart) Paracyesis (pregnancy outside the uterus)
per-	through, excessive	Permeable (may pass through) Peracute (excessively sharp)
peri-	around	Periosteum (membrane around bone) Peribulbar (around the eye bulb)
poly-	many, much, excessive	Polycystic (with many cysts) Polydipsia (excessive thirst)
post-	after, behind	Postoperative (after surgery) Postocular (behind the eye)
pre-, pro-	before, in front of	Prenatal (before birth) Project (throw forward)
pseud-, pseudo-	false	Pseudarthrosis (false joint) Pseudocyesis (false pregnancy)
re-	again, backward	Reflex (bend back) Regurgitation (vomiting)
retro-	backward, behind	Retrograde (going backward) Retrolingual (behind the tongue)
semi-	half	Semiconscious (partly aware) Seminormal (half normal)
sub-	under, beneath	Subcutaneous (under the skin) Subungual (beneath the nail)
super-, supra-	above, superior, excess	Superactivity (overactivity) Suprarenal (above the kidneys)
sym-,* syn-	together, with	Symmelia (fusion of limbs) Synclinal (bent together)
trans-	across, through	Transection (cut across) Transaortic (through the aorta)
ultra-	beyond, excess	Ultravirus (very small virus) Ultrasonic (beyond the upper limit of human hearing)

*sym- before b, m, p, and ph

Review Questions: Prefixes

Complete the following:

1. A prefix _____ stands alone.

2. The prefix ante- means _____.

3. A prefix meaning two or twice is _____.

4. A prefix meaning around is _____ or _____.

5. A prefix for half is _____ or _____.

6. Super- has a similar meaning to the prefix _____.

7. The prefix sym- is used before _____.

8. The prefix for false is _____.

9. The prefix pan- means _____.

10. The prefixes mes- and meso- mean _____.

Matching

____	**1.** a-, an-	**A.** self
____	**2.** ambi-, ampho-	**B.** difficult, bad
____	**3.** contra-	**C.** apart, free from
____	**4.** dys-	**D.** without, lack of, not
____	**5.** ep-, epi-	**E.** below, beneath
____	**6.** aut-, auto-	**F.** upon, on, over
____	**7.** multi-	**G.** opposed, against
____	**8.** dis-	**H.** both
____	**9.** infra-	**I.** normal
____	**10.** eu-	**J.** many

Answers to Review Questions: Prefixes

Completion
1. never
2. before, in front of
3. bi-, di-
4. circum-, peri-
5. hemi-, semi-
6. supra-
7. b, m, p, and ph

8. pseud-, pseudo-
9. all, entire
10. middle

Matching
1. D
2. H
3. G

4. B
5. F
6. A
7. J
8. C
9. E
10. I

Suffixes

A suffix consists of one or more syllables placed at the end of a word. Like a prefix, a suffix never stands alone. Suffixes are added to the roots of words to modify their meanings. To make pronunciation easier, the last letter or letters of the root may be changed before adding the suffix. For this purpose, two general rules may be followed:

1. The last vowel of the root may be changed to another vowel. Usually, but not always, an "o" or another vowel may be inserted between the root and a suffix that begins with a consonant. This vowel is known as a *combining vowel.* For example:

   Cardiology means study of the heart.
   To the *root* cardi-, meaning heart,
   the *combining vowel* "o" is added,
      producing
   the *combining form* cardio-, to which is
      added
   the *suffix* -logy, which means study of.

2. When a suffix begins with a vowel, the last vowel of the root may be dropped before adding the suffix. For example:

   Carditis means inflammation of the heart.
      The ending vowel "i" of
      the *root* cardi- is dropped before adding
      the *suffix* -itis, which means inflammation.

Most suffixes are in common use, but some are specific to medical language. The most common suffixes encountered are listed in Table 2-2, with those used in ordinary language in italics.

Table 2-2   SUFFIXES

Suffix	Meaning	Examples
-ac, -al, -ic, *-ous, -tic*	pertaining to, relating to	Cardiac (pertaining to the heart) Neural (pertaining to nerves) Hemorrhagic (relating to bleeding) Delirious (relating to mental disturbance) Acoustic (pertaining to sound)
-algia, -dynia	pain	Neuralgia (pain in nerves) Mastodynia (pain in the breast)
-ate, -ize	use, subject to	Impregnate (to make pregnant) Visualize (to use the imagination)
-cele	protrusion (hernia)	Cystocele (bladder hernia) Rectocele (protrusion of the rectum into the vagina)
-centesis	surgical puncture to remove fluid	Paracentesis (removal of fluid from a body cavity) Thoracentesis (removal of fluid from the chest cavity)
-cle, -cule, *-ole, -ola,* *-ule,* -ulum, -ulus	small	Follicle (small sac) Molecule (small unit of matter) Arteriole, arteriola (small artery) Nodule (small node) Ovulum (small egglike structure) Homunculus (small human)
-cyte	cell	Leukocyte (white blood cell) Erythrocyte (red blood cell)
-ectomy	cutting out	Lobectomy (cutting out of a lobe) Appendectomy (cutting out of the appendix)
-emesis	vomit	Hematemesis (vomiting of blood) Hyperemesis (excessive vomiting)
-emia	blood condition	Leukemia (malignant disease of the blood) Anemia (lack of red blood cells)
-ent, -er, *-ist, -or*	person or agent	Recipient (one who receives) Examiner (one who examines) Oculist (eye physician) Donor (one who donates)
-esis, -ia, -iasis, *-ism,* *-ity,* -osis, -sis, *-tion,* -y	state or condition	Paresis (partial paralysis) Anesthesia (loss of sensation) Psoriasis (skin condition) Priapism (persistent erection) Acidity (excess acid) Narcosis (drugged state) Inhalation (state of inhaling) Therapy (treatment condition)
-form, -oid	resembling, shaped like	Fusiform (spindle-shaped) Ovoid (egg-shaped)
-genesis	beginning process, origin	Pathogenesis (origin of disease) Homogenesis (young same as parent)
-gram, -graphy	recording, written record	Mammogram (X-ray of the breast) Cardiography (heart action record)

Continued.

Table 2-2   SUFFIXES — cont'd.

Suffix	Meaning	Examples
-graph	instrument that records	Cardiograph (instrument for measuring heart action) Encephalograph (instrument for measuring brain function)
-ible, -ile	capable, able	Flexible (capable of bending) Contractile (able to contract)
-ites, -itis	inflammation	Tympanites (drumlike swelling of the abdomen) Adenitis (inflammation of a gland)
-logy	science, study of	Biology (science of life) Histology (study of tissues)
-oma	tumor	Carcinoma (malignant growth) Sarcoma (cancerous tumor)
-penia	deficiency of, lack of	Glycopenia (sugar in tissues) Leukopenia (white blood cells)
-pexy, -pexis	fixation, storing	Nephropexy (of floating kidney) Glycopexis (glycogen in liver)
-phagia, -phagy	eating, devouring	Geophagia (eating dirt or clay) Aerophagy (swallowing air)
-phobia	abnormal fear or intolerance	Acrophobia (fear of heights) Photophobia (of light)
-plasty	surgical shaping or formation	Rhinoplasty (nose formation) Otoplasty (external ear)
-pnea	breathing	Apnea (absence of breathing) Dyspnea (difficult breathing)
-ptosis	prolapse, downward displacement	Proctoptosis (prolapse of anus) Nephroptosis (prolapse of kidney)
-rrhage, -rrhagia	excessive flow	Hemorrhage (excessive blood flow) Metrorrhagia (abnormal menses)
-rrhaphy	suturing in place	Herniorrhaphy (repair of hernia) Osteorrhaphy (wiring of bone)
-rrhea	flow or discharge	Rhinorrhea (nasal discharge) Galactorrhea (breast milk)
-rrhexis	rupture	Enterorrhexis (intestinal rupture) Metrorrhexis (rupture of uterus)
-stomy	surgical opening	Colostomy (colon to body surface) Gastrostomy (into stomach)
-scope	instrument for examining	Microscope (minute objects) Cystoscope (urinary bladder)
-scopy	act of examining	Microscopy (minute objects) Cystoscopy (urinary bladder)
-tome	instrument for	Cystotome (cutting into bladder) Neurotome (dissecting nerves)
-tomy	cutting, incision	Cystotomy (of urinary bladder) Phlebotomy (incision of vein)

Review Questions: Suffixes

Complete the following:

1. A suffix _____ stands alone.

2. A suffix is added to a root to _____ its meaning.

3. A suffix meaning pain is _____.

4. A suffix for protrusion is _____.

5. State or condition may be indicated by one of several suffixes, two of which are

   _____ and _____.

6. A suffix meaning instrument that records is

   _____.

7. The suffixes -ites and -itis mean

   _____.

8. The suffix _____ means tumor.

9. The suffix for prolapse or downward displacement

   is _____.

10. The suffix -phobia means _____.

Matching:

____ **1.** -al, -ic

____ **2.** -ectomy

____ **3.** -penia

____ **4.** -scopy

____ **5.** -emesis

____ **6.** -centesis

____ **7.** -stomy

____ **8.** -logy

____ **9.** -rrhage, -rrhagia

____ **10.** -form, -oid

A. surgical puncture

B. vomit

C. resembling, shaped like

D. excessive flow

E. act of examining

F. deficiency of, lack of

G. pertaining to

H. surgical opening

I. science of, study of

J. cutting out

Answers to Review Questions: Suffixes

Completion:
1. never
2. modify
3. -algia, -dynia
4. -cele
5. -esis, -ia, -iasis, -ity, -osis, -sis, -tion, -y
6. -graph

7. inflammation
8. -oma
9. -ptosis
10. abnormal fear or intolerance

Matching:
1. G
2. J
3. F
4. E
5. B
6. A
7. H
8. I
9. D
10. C

CHAPTER 2 EXERCISES

BUILDING A MEDICAL VOCABULARY

Step 1: Prefixes and Suffixes

The following exercises constitute an additional opportunity to review and use the preceding prefixes and suffixes. As in the review questions, the answers are provided at the end of the questions. To make the best use of these exercises, if you find that you cannot answer a given question, we strongly suggest that you look it up in the preceding text material. You should use the answers provided only to check your accuracy, and not as a short route to completion of the exercises.

Exercise 1: In the blank following each pair of prefixes and suffixes, indicate whether their meaning is the *same* or *opposite*.

1. dys-
   eu- _____

2. ecto-
   endo- _____

3. semi-
   hemi- _____

4. hyper-
   hypo- _____

5. -algia
   -dynia _____

6. a-
   an- _____

7. circum-
   peri- _____

8. -iasis
   -osis _____

9. bi-
   di- _____

10. -ectomy
    -rrhaphy_____

11. -ac
    -al _____

12. anti-
    contra-_____

13. -ible
    -ile _____

14. -gram
    -graphy_____

15. ante-
    anti- _____

Exercise 2: Define the following prefixes.

1. post- _____

2. dys- _____

3. a- _____

4. infra- _____

5. retro- _____

6. endo- _____

7. inter- _____

8. para- _____

9. ambi- _____

10. cata- _____

Exercise 3: Define the following suffixes.

1. -ate _____

2. -genesis _____

3. -itis _____

4. -oma _____

5. -phobia _____

6. -cele _____

7. -logy _____

8. -tome _____

9. -rrhea _____

10. -phagia _____

Exercise 4: Matching:

____1. -cyte

____2. -ic

____3. hemi-

____4. -ptosis

____5. con-

____6. -emia

____7. ab-

____8. -emesis

____9. auto-

____10. -rrhexis

____11. dia-

____12. -scope

____13. -oid

____14. epi-

____15. -pnea

A. blood condition

B. away from

C. instrument

D. rupture

E. between, through

F. breathing

G. upon, on, over

H. resembling, shaped like

I. prolapse

J. with, together

K. cell

L. pertaining to

M. half

N. self

O. vomit

Chapter 2 Crossword Puzzle

Across

1. before birth
5. ability to use both hands equally
9. suffix meaning small
13. prefix meaning not
15. beneath the eye
16. prefix meaning without
17. prefix meaning out of
18. suffix meaning blood condition
20. prefix meaning up or apart
21. prefix meaning under or beneath
22. prefix meaning difficult
23. prefix meaning new
24. prefix meaning separation from

Down

1. suffix meaning fixation
2. prefix meaning away from
3. prefix meaning in
4. prefix meaning two or twice
5. against infection
6. prefix meaning down or from
7. suffix meaning state or condition
8. under the skin
10. cut across
11. pain in nerves
12. not voluntary
14. excessive thirst
19. suffix for resembling

Chapter 2 Hidden Word Puzzle

```
V I U S F I A U H X L X L I C S D A F J M I J W A P C J D B
W W Y I S L H P H Y U I O O Y V X V Q C D S U K U X X E O V
W I B V Q Z J Z C I P T W L S K N V V M J G H R Q E M N G J
I C L G L I D N C J G E N C T N O J G D O Y Y Y Q K X O P P
J E H H I G R P D W W R R V O V A M F X N E U L C I E B T E
D B F T E P I D E R M I S T C V I Q X G R J Y X S K O G O P
Z Y A Y I M R W W Z Q F R S E G L I B U H I Q L H P D I X I
I C S N V D O M Y I R D P E L N F R N O P Y S M O D J E Y U
Y V S P E N T R I N T R O V E R S I O N R R G E I T L P B L
X T V N E S S S R F Y D Q M F D E I N M P C J B B P J G Y S
S M O D F P T R F H F A J M F V M X O E Q M E Y T S Y G G T
S M Y F U P S H E M A T E M E S I S B N C Y W X J K U W Q O
P R U S L O J I E L K G O U I D C N L R E H R W A R U V O N
B B H Y V W J N A S B D E N T J O L J V D E C A Y C R A P O
K B C H D W N O E E I E W R W G N N L E D M A N E M I A Z D
Q F M N R J L P Q M O A X C V T S E O V C L R P J M J T E U
M L H P M D W L D B L I S N G D C P U R I T D R G G X T P L
O Y U I C Q I A L O O E F I M C I P W R S U I M M A T U R E
L Q V J F M H S I Q G I J P Q B O N M Y A M A O E U P C F O
E H G P O O B T S S Y D N U V M U F I Q K L C Y N V D F C K
W T C O F V C Y B E O L J Y N O S L C Q Z X G K T U E X P N
V V I Y R V V G W P C T U F T F B V U J Y G O I P B D S Q N
D R F V F N S J Q N I T H D N B W F Z O V Y W S A F T D P D
```

Can you find the 20 words hidden in this puzzle? All hidden word puzzles will
have words running from top to bottom, left to right, and diagonally downward.

SEMICONSCIOUS	HYPERTENSION	INTROVERSION	HEMATEMESIS
RHINOPLASTY	ANESTHESIA	HEMORRHAGE	CYSTOCELE
DYSPEPSIA	EPIDERMIS	INJECTION	NEURALGIA
IMMATURE	BIOLOGY	CARDIAC	DISSECT
ANEMIA	NODULE	DECAY	DONOR

CHAPTER 2 ANSWERS

Exercise 1

1. opposite
2. opposite
3. same
4. opposite
5. same
6. same
7. same
8. same
9. same
10. opposite
11. same
12. same
13. same
14. same
15. opposite

Exercise 2

1. behind
2. bad, difficult
3. without
4. below
5. behind
6. within
7. between
8. around
9. both
10. down, under

Exercise 3

1. use, subject to
2. beginning process, origin
3. inflammation
4. tumor
5. abnormal fear, intolerance
6. protrusion
7. science of, study of
8. instrument
9. flow or discharge
10. eating, devouring

Exercise 4

1. K
2. L
3. M
4. I
5. J
6. A
7. B
8. O
9. N
10. D
11. E
12. C
13. H
14. G
15. F

Answers: Chapter 2 Crossword Puzzle

Answers: Chapter 2 Hidden Word Puzzle

```
.   .   .   .   .   .   H   .   .   .   .   C   .   .   .   .   .   .   .   .   .   .   .   .   .   .
.   .   .   .   .   .   .   Y   .   .   .   Y   .   .   .   .   .   .   .   .   .   .   .   .   .   .
.   .   .   .   .   .   .   .   P   .   .   S   .   .   .   .   .   .   .   .   .   .   .   .   .   .
.   .   .   .   .   .   .   .   .   E   .   T   .   .   .   .   .   .   .   .   .   .   .   .   .   .
.   .   .   H   .   .   .   .   .   .   R   .   O   .   .   .   .   .   .   .   .   .   .   .   .   .
D   .   .   E   P   I   D   E   R   M   I   S   T   C   .   .   .   .   .   .   .   .   .   .   .   .
.   Y   A   .   .   M   .   .   .   .   .   .   .   E   .   .   .   .   .   .   .   .   .   .   .   .
.   .   S   N   .   .   O   .   .   .   .   .   .   L   N   .   .   .   .   .   .   .   .   .   .   .
.   .   .   P   E   .   .   R   I   N   T   R   O   V   E   R   S   I   O   N   .   .   .   .   .   .
.   .   .   .   E   S   .   .   R   .   .   .   .   .   .   E   I   .   .   .   .   .   .   .   .   .
.   .   .   .   .   P   T   R   .   H   .   .   .   .   .   M   .   O   .   .   .   .   .   .   .   .
.   .   .   .   .   .   S   H   E   M   A   T   E   M   E   S   I   S   .   N   .   .   .   .   .   .
.   .   .   .   .   .   .   I   E   .   .   G   .   .   D   C   N   .   .   .   .   .   .   .   .   N
.   .   .   .   .   .   .   N   A   S   B   .   E   .   .   .   O   .   J   .   D   E   C   A   Y   .   .   .   O
.   .   .   .   .   .   .   O   .   .   I   .   .   .   .   N   N   .   E   .   .   A   N   E   M   I   A   .   D
.   .   .   .   .   .   .   P   .   .   O   A   .   .   .   S   E   O   .   C   .   R   .   .   .   .   U
.   .   .   .   D   .   L   .   L   .   .   .   .   C   .   U   R   .   T   D   .   .   .   .   L
.   .   .   I   A   .   O   .   .   .   .   I   .   R   .   I   M   M   A   T   U   R   E
.   .   .   .   S   .   G   .   .   .   .   O   .   .   A   .   A   O   .   .   .   .   .   .
.   .   .   .   T   S   .   Y   .   .   .   .   U   .   .   .   L   C   .   N   .   .   .   .
.   .   .   .   Y   .   E   .   .   .   .   .   S   .   .   .   .   .   G   .   .   .   .   .
.   .   .   .   .   .   C   .   .   .   .   .   .   .   .   .   .   I   .   .   .   .   .
.   .   .   .   .   .   T   .   .   .   .   .   .   .   .   .   A   .   .   .   .   .
```

Words:

∨ SEMICONSCIOUS	\ HYPERTENSION	> INTROVERSION	> HEMATEMESIS
∨ RHINOPLASTY	\ ANESTHESIA	\ HEMORRHAGE	∨ CYSTOCELE
\ DYSPEPSIA	> EPIDERMIS	\ INJECTION	\ NEURALGIA
> IMMATURE	∨ BIOLOGY	∨ CARDIAC	\ DISSECT
> ANEMIA	∨ NODULE	> DECAY	\ DONOR

Chapter 3

Adding to the Foundation

CHAPTER OVERVIEW

In this chapter the student is presented with lists of roots and their combining forms, grouped according to relationship to external or internal anatomy. External anatomy refers to any visible part of the body, and internal anatomy refers to organs, bones, and other tissues within the body.

STEP 2: ROOTS AND COMBINING FORMS

This chapter consists of extensive lists of roots and combining forms pertaining to the structure of the body (anatomy). You will remember that a root is the foundation or basic meaning of a word. A combining form is a root with an added combining vowel, attaching the root to a suffix or another root. The first list, Table 3-1, relates to external body structure (that which can be seen with the naked eye). Each root is listed alphabetically with its pronunciation and associated body part. Each combining form is divided by a slash mark (/) separating the root and the combining vowel, which is usually, but not always, an "o."

Table 3-1 EXTERNAL ANATOMY

Root/Combining Form	Pronunciation	Body Part
blephar/o-	blef'ahr-o	Eyelid or eyelash
brachi/o-	bra'ke-o	Arm
bucc/o-	buk'o	Cheek
canth/o-	kan'tho	Corner of the eye
capit/o-	kap'it-o	Head
carp/o-	karp'o	Wrist
cephal/o-	sef'al-o	Head
cervic/o-	ser'vik-o	Neck (also refers to necklike projection of the cervix uteri, which is internal anatomy)
cheil/o-, chil/o-	kile'o	Lip
cheir/o-, chir/o-	ki'ro	Hand
cili/o-	sil'ee-o	Eyelid, eyelash, or small hairlike processes
cor/e-, cor/o-	kor'ee, kor'o	Pupil of eye
dactyl/o-	dak'til-o	Finger, sometimes toe
dent/i-, dent/o-	dent'ee, dent'o	Tooth or teeth
derm/a-, derm/o-, dermat/o-	derm'a, derm'o, derm'at-o	Skin
dors/i-, dors/o-	dor'see, dor'so	Posterior or back
faci/o-	fa'shee-o	Face

Continued.

Table 3-1   EXTERNAL ANATOMY – cont'd.

Root/Combining Form	Pronunciation	Body Part
gingiv/o-	jin′jiv-o	Gums
gloss/o-	glos′o	Tongue
gnath/o-	nath′o	Jaw
irid/o-	ir′id-o	Iris of eye
labi/o-	lay′bee-o	Lip, especially lips of mouth
lapar/o-	lap′ahr-o	Loin or flank, sometimes abdomen
later/o-	lat′er-o	Side
lingu/o-	ling′wo	Tongue
mamm/a-, mamm/o-	mam′ah, mam′o	Breast
mast/o-	mast′o	Breast
mel/o-	mel′o	Limb
nas/o-	naze′o	Nose
occipit/o-	ok-si′pit-o	Back of head
ocul/o-	ok′ule-o	Eye
odont/o-	o-dont′o	Tooth or teeth
om/o-	o′mo	Shoulder
omphal/o-	om′fah-lo	Navel or umbilicus
onych/o-	on′ik-o	Nail or nails
ophthalm/o-	of-thal′mo	Eye or eyes
or/o-	or′o	Mouth
ot/o-	oh′toe	Ear
papill/o-	pah-pill′o	Nipple or nipple-shaped projection
phall/o-	fal′o	Penis
pil/o-	pile′o	Hair
pod/o-	pod′o	Foot or foot-shaped part
rhin/o-	rine′o	Nose
somat/o-, somatic/o-	so-mat′o, so-mat′ik-o	Body
steth/o-	steth′o	Chest
stom-, stomat/o-	sto′mah-toe	Mouth
tal/o-	tal′o	Ankle or ankle bone
tars/o-	tahr′so	Instep of foot or eyelid edge
thel/o-	theel′o	Nipple
thorac/o-	tho′rah-ko	Chest or thorax
trachel/o-	trake′el-o	Neck or necklike structure
trich/o-	trik′o	Hair or hairlike structure
ventr/i-, ventr/o-	ven′tree, ven′tro	Front of body or belly

Review Questions: External Anatomy Roots and Combining Forms

Complete the following:

1. Blepharo- and cilio- mean _____.

2. The combining forms for head are

   _____ and _____.

3. A combining form for hair is _____.

4. A combining form for lip is _____.

5. Rhino- and naso- both refer to _____.

6. Two combining forms for breast are

   _____ and _____.

7. Cervico- and trachelo- mean _____.

8. A combining form for mouth is

   _____.

9. Ophthalmo- and _____ are combining forms for eye.

10. Stetho- and _____ are combining forms for chest.

Matching:

____ 1. carpo-

____ 2. derma-, dermo-, dermato-

____ 3. brachio-

____ 4. glosso-

____ 5. ventri-, ventro-

____ 6. oto-

____ 7. core-, coro-

____ 8. occipito-

____ 9. podo-

____ 10. bucco-

A. tongue

B. pupil of eye

C. ear

D. back of head

E. foot

F. cheek

G. wrist

H. arm

I. skin

J. front of body or belly

Answers to Review Questions: External Anatomy Roots and Combining Forms

Completion:
1. eyelid or eyelash
2. capito-, cephalo-
3. tricho-, pilo-
4. cheilo-, chilo-, labio-
5. nose
6. mamma-, mammo-, masto-
7. neck (or necklike structure)
8. oro-, stomato-
9. oculo-
10. thoraco-

Matching:
1. G
2. I
3. H
4. A
5. J
6. C
7. B
8. D
9. E
10. F

Table 3-2 relates to internal body structure (that which is inside the body). Each root is listed alphabetically with its pronunciation and associated body part. The combin-ing form is divided with a slash mark (/) separating the root and the combining vowel, which is usually, but not always, an "o."

Table 3-2 INTERNAL ANATOMY

Root/combining form	Pronunciation	Body part
aden/o-	ad'e-no	Gland
adren/o-	ad-ree'no	Adrenal gland
angi/o-	an'jee-o	Vessel, usually a blood vessel
arteri/o-	ar-te're-o	Artery
arteriol/o-	ar-te're-o"lo	Arteriole
arthr/o-	ar'thro	Joint
atri/o-	a'tree-o	Atrium or upper heart chamber
balan/o-	bal'ah-no	Glans penis or glans clitoridis
bronch/i-, bronch/o-	brong'kee, brong'ko	Bronchus
bronchiol/o-	brong'kee-olo	Bronchiolus
cardi/o-	kar'dee-o	Heart
cerebell/o-	ser"e-bel'o	Cerebellum of brain
cerebr/i-, cerebr/o-	ser'e-bree, ser'e-bro	Cerebrum of brain
choledoch/o-	ko-lee'dok-o	Common bile duct
chondr/i-, chondr/io-, chondr/o-	kon'dree, kon'dree-o, kon'dro	Cartilage
chord/o-	kor'do	Vocal cord or spermatic cord
cleid/o-	kli'do	Clavicle (collar bone)
colp/o-	kol'po	Vagina
cost/o-	kos'to	Rib
cyst/i-, cyst/o-	sis'tee, sis'to	Bladder, cyst, or sac
cyt/o-	si'to	Cell
duoden/o-	du"o-de'no	Duodenum of intestine
encephal/o-	en-sef'ah-lo	Brain
enter/o-	en'ter-o	Intestine
episi/o-	e-peez'e-o	Vulva
fibr/o-	fie'bro	Fiber
gastr/o-	gas'tro	Stomach
gli/o-	glee'o	Neuroglia, or gluey substance
hepat/ico-, hepat/o-	he-pat'i-ko, he-pat'o	Liver
hist/o-	his'to	Tissue
hyster/o-	his'ter-o	Uterus
ile/o-	il'ee-o	Ileum of intestine
ili/o-	il'ee-o	Ilium (upper part of hip bone)
jejun/o-	je-joo'no	Jejunum of intestine
kerat/o-	ker'ah-to	Horny tissue or cornea of eye

Table 3-2 INTERNAL ANATOMY – cont'd.

Root/combining form	Pronunciation	Body part
laryng/o-	lah-ring′go	Larynx (voice box)
lien/o-	li′en-o	Spleen
lymph/o-	lim′fo	Lymphatic vessels or lymphocytes
mening/o-	me-ning′go	Membranes covering brain and spinal cord
metr/a-, metr/o-	me′trah, me′tro	Uterus
myel/o-	my′el-o	Bone marrow or spinal cord
my/o-	my′o	Muscle
myring/o-	my-ring′o	Eardrum
nephr/o-	nef′ro	Kidney
neur/o-	nu′ro	Nerve, nerves, or nervous system
oophor/o-	o-of′or-o	Ovary
orchi/o-, orchi/do-	or′kee-o, or′ki-do	Testis or testes
osche/o-	os′kee-o	Scrotum
oss/eo-, oss/i-, ost/e-, ost/eo-	os′see-o, os′see, os′tee, os′tee-o	Bone or bones
palat/o-	pal′ah-to	Palate (roof of mouth)
pharyng/o	fah-ring′go	Pharynx (throat)
phleb/o-	fleb′o	Vein or veins
phren/i-, phren/ico-, phren/o-	fren′ee, fren′i-ko, fren′o	Diaphragm or mind
pleur/o-	ploor′o	Pleura or rib
pneum/a-, pneum/o-, pneum/ato-, pneum/ono-	nu′mah, nu′mo, nu-mat′o, nu-mon′o	Lungs or respiration (air, breath)
proct/o-	prok′to	Rectum or anus
pulm/o-	pul′mo	Lungs
pyel/o-	py′el-o	Pelvis of kidney
rachi/o-	ra′kee-o	Spine
rect/o-	rek′to	Rectum
ren/i-, ren/o-	ren′ee, ren′o	Kidney
sacr/o-	sa′kro	Sacrum
salping/o-	sal-ping′go, sal-pin′jo	Fallopian tube or Eustachian tube
sarc/o-	sar′ko	Flesh or muscular substance
splanchn/ee-, splanchn/o-	splank′nee, splank′no	Viscera or splanchnic nerve
splen/o-	splen′o	Spleen
spondyl/o-	spon′di-lo	Vertebra or spinal column
stern/o-	stern′no	Sternum (breastbone)
tend/o-, ten/o-, tenont/o-	ten′doe, ten′o, ten′on-toe	Tendon
thym/o-	thy′mo	Thymus gland
thyr/o-	thy′ro	Thyroid gland
trache/o-	tra′kee-o	Trachea
ureter/o-	u-ree′ter-o	Ureter (tube from kidney to bladder)

Continued.

Table 3-2   **INTERNAL ANATOMY** – cont'd.

Root/combining form	Pronunciation	Body part
urethr/o-	u-ree'thro	Urethra (tube from bladder to outside)
vas/o-	vaz'o	Vessel or duct
ven/e-, ven/i-, ven/o-	vene'eh, vene'ee, vene'o	Vein or veins
vesic/o-	ves'i-ko	Bladder or blister
viscer/o-	vis'er-o	Viscera

Review Questions: Internal Anatomy Roots and Combining Forms

Complete the following:

1. The combining form for gland is

   _____.

2. A combining form for uterus is

   _____.

3. Ileo- is the combining form meaning

   _____.

4. Gastro- is the combining form meaning

   _____.

5. The combining form for common bile duct is

   _____.

6. Pneuma- or pulmo- refers to _____.

7. The combining form for spleen is

   _____.

8. Osteo- refers to _____.

9. A combining form for vein is _____.

10. Cleido- is a combining form meaning

   _____.

Matching:

____ 1. urethro-

____ 2. procto-

____ 3. tracheo-

____ 4. splanchni-

____ 5. sarco-

____ 6. myelo-

____ 7. rachi-

____ 8. kerato-

____ 9. myo-

____ 10. reni-

A. viscera

B. spine

C. kidney

D. bone marrow or spinal cord

E. muscle

F. urethra

G. trachea

H. flesh

I. rectum or anus

J. horny tissue

Answers to Review Questions: Internal Anatomy Roots and Combining Forms

Completion:
1. adeno-
2. hystero-, metra-, or metro-
3. ileum
4. stomach
5. choledocho-
6. lungs
7. lieno- or spleno-

8. bone
9. phlebo-, vene-, veni-, or veno-
10. clavicle

Matching:
1. F
2. I
3. G

4. A
5. H
6. D
7. B
8. J
9. E
10. C

CHAPTER 3 EXERCISES

ADDING TO THE FOUNDATION

Step 2: Roots and Combining Forms
The following exercises provide further opportunities for learning the roots and combining forms presented in this chapter. Once again, we urge you to consult the answers only after you have completed the exercises.

Exercise 1: In the blank following each pair of roots or combining forms, indicate whether their meaning is *similar* or *different*.

1. blepharo- facio- _____	**8.** rhino- naso- _____	**15.** coro- iridio- _____
2. angio- vas- _____	**9.** splanchno- viscero- _____	**16.** phlebo- veno- _____
3. capito- cephalo- _____	**10.** pilo- tricho- _____	**17.** rachio- spondilo- _____
4. lieno- ileo- _____	**11.** myo- myelo- _____	**18.** colpo- hystero- _____
5. oculo- ophthalmo- _____	**12.** linguo- glosso- _____	**19.** omphalo- papillo- _____
6. oro- oto- _____	**13.** odonto- dento- _____	**20.** stetho- thoraco- _____
7. talo- tarso- _____	**14.** reno- nephro- _____	

Exercise 2: Fill in the combining form for each of the following body parts.

1. cartilage _____	**11.** nose _____
2. bladder or blister _____	**12.** muscle _____
3. membranes covering brain and spinal cord _____	**13.** horny tissue _____
4. fibers _____	**14.** kidney pelvis _____
5. common bile duct _____	**15.** larynx _____
6. tendon _____	**16.** thyroid gland _____
7. lip _____	**17.** breast _____
8. eye _____	**18.** ankle _____
9. wrist _____	**19.** body _____
10. finger _____	**20.** ear _____

Exercise 3: Define the following roots and combining forms.

1. bucco- _____	**6.** gnatho- _____
2. cheilo- _____	**7.** somato- _____
3. dactylo- _____	**8.** omo- _____
4. latero- _____	**9.** stomato- _____
5. onycho- _____	**10.** podo- _____

Exercise 4: Matching:

____ **1.** brachio-   **A.** back of head

____ **2.** cantho-   **B.** gum

____ **3.** carpo-   **C.** head

____ **4.** gingivo-   **D.** arm

____ **5.** derma-   **E.** nipple

____ **6.** melo-   **F.** neck

____ **7.** occipito-   **G.** skin

____ **8.** talo-   **H.** limb

____ **9.** trachelo-   **I.** front of body or belly

____**10.** ventro-   **J.** wrist

____**11.** thelo-   **K.** either corner of the eye

____**12.** cephalo-   **L.** ankle

Chapter 3 Crossword Puzzle

Across

1. heart
3. finger or toe
5. nose
7. bronchus
9. mouth
10. ear
11. skin
14. heart
15. common bile duct
16. hair
19. nail(s)
21. jaw
23. artery
25. eardrum

Down

1. angle at ends of eyelid
   slits
2. tooth or teeth
4. cartilage
6. vertebra or spinal column
7. arm
8. neck
12. pharynx
13. eyelid or eyelash
17. duodenum
18. larynx
20. vein
21. gums
22. liver
24. shoulder

Chapter 3 Hidden Word Puzzle

```
I   D   Y   N   H   W   B   L   P   H   C   A   F   S   I   U
I   H   I   D   E   R   M   Y   U   I   V   N   R   Z   J   W
J   A   J   G   P   X   J   Y   V   I   W   H   A   O   J   R
P   O   N   N   A   D   E   N   J   U   D   O   W   Y   R   E
P   N   D   A   T   S   M   S   D   V   J   I   V   J   W   R
C   O   S   T   S   D   T   B   P   E   C   L   D   H   T   O
T   S   S   H   X   C   E   R   V   I   C   W   I   Q   O   D
U   W   S   C   L   D   A   C   T   Y   L   T   W   U   Y
P   U   R   R   U   E   N   C   E   P   H   A   L   I   Y   M
S   F   Z   U   X   I   I   H   H   N   N   X   B   A   F   G
Y   Q   R   B   X   D   C   I   S   O   M   A   T   S   B   F
V   B   T   O   M   F   K   S   L   I   N   G   U   B   R   I
S   T   I   X   Y   E   A   R   Q   U   H   D   D   N   Q   R
Q   G   Z   C   H   B   S   C   C   M   C   A   R   P   E   P
C   X   R   S   A   U   G   P   Y   L   Y   G   B   J   X   T
Y   M   H   W   F   O   D   I   N   Z   S   B   J   D   Y   V
B   E   Z   P   K   L   I   E   F   R   T   S   V   X   S   L
```

Can you find the 20 words hidden in this puzzle? All hidden word puzzles will
have words running from top to bottom, left to right, and diagonally downward.

ENCEPHAL	BRACHI	CERVIC	CHONDR
DACTYL	CLEID	GASTR	GNATH
HEPAT	LINGU	SOMAT	ADEN
CARP	COST	CYST	DERM
LABI	NAS	OSS	MY

CHAPTER 3 ANSWERS

Exercise 1
1. different
2. similar
3. similar
4. different
5. similar
6. different
7. different
8. similar
9. similar
10. similar
11. different
12. similar
13. similar
14. similar
15. different
16. similar
17. similar
18. different
19. different
20. similar

Exercise 2
1. chondri-, chondrio-, chondro-
2. vesico-
3. meningo-
4. fibro-
5. choledocho-
6. tendo-, teno-, tenonto-
7. cheilo-, chilo-, labio-
8. oculo-
9. carpo-
10. dactylo-
11. rhino-, naso-
12. myo-
13. kerato-
14. pyelo-
15. laryngo-
16. thyro-
17. mammo-, mamma-, masto-
18. talo-
19. somato-, somatico-
20. oto-

Exercise 3
1. cheek
2. lip
3. finger
4. side
5. nail (s)
6. jaw
7. body
8. shoulder
9. mouth
10. foot

Exercise 4
1. D
2. K
3. J
4. B
5. G
6. H
7. A
8. L
9. F
10. I
11. E
12. C

Answers: Chapter 3 Crossword Puzzle

	¹C	A	R	²D	I			³D	⁴A	C	T	Y	L
	A			E						H			
	N		⁵N	A	⁶S		⁷B	R	O	N	⁸C	H
	T		T		P	⁹O	R		N		E	
	H				¹⁰O	T	A		¹¹D	E	R	M
		¹²P		¹³B	N		¹⁴C	O	R		V	
	¹⁵C	H	O	L	E	D	O	C	H		¹⁶P	I	L
¹⁷D		A		E	Y			I				C
U		R		P					¹⁸L		
¹⁹O	N	Y	C	H		²⁰V	²¹G	N	A	T	²²H
D		N		²³A	R	T	E	R	I		R	E
E		G		R			N		N		Y	P
N						²⁴O		G		N		A
						²⁵M	Y	R	I	N	G	T
								V				

Answers: Chapter 3 Hidden Word Puzzle

```
. . . . . H . . . . . . . . .
. . . D E R M . . . . . . . .
. . . G P . . Y . . . . . . .
. . N N A D E N . . . . . . .
. . . A T S . . . . . . . . .
C O S T S . T B . . . . . . .
. . S H . C E R V I C . . . .
. . . S . L D A C T Y L . . .
. . . . . E N C E P H A L . .
. . . . . I . H H . . . . A . .
. . . . . D . I S O M A T . B .
. . . . . . . L I N G U . . I
. . . . . . . . D . . . .
. . . . . . . . C A R P . .
. . . . . . . . Y . . . .
. . . . . . . . S . . . .
. . . . . . . . T . . . .
```

Words:

> ENCEPHAL	∨ BRACHI	> CERVIC	\ CHONDR
> DACTYL	∨ CLEID	\ GASTR	∨ GNATH
∨ HEPAT	> LINGU	> SOMAT	> ADEN
> CARP	> COST	∨ CYST	> DERM
\ LABI	\ NAS	\ OSS	\ MY

Chapter 4

Completing the Foundation

CHAPTER OVERVIEW

This chapter presents five additional lists of roots and their combining forms, grouped as verbs; adjectives; body fluids; body substances and chemicals; and colors.

STEP 3: ADDITIONAL ROOTS AND COMBINING FORMS

The following lists of roots and combining forms relate to action or description. Table 4-1 lists verbal (verb-based) roots and combining forms that show an activity, a condition, or an action. Each combining form is divided by a slash mark (/) between the root and its combining vowel.

Table 4-1 **VERBAL ROOTS AND COMBINING FORMS**

Root/Combining Form	Meaning	Examples
audi/o-	hearing	Audiometer (hearing test device) Audiology (study of hearing)
bio-	life	Biology (study of living things) Biogenesis (origin of life)
caus-, caut-	burn	Causalgia (burning pain) Cautery (device to scar or burn)
clas-	break	Osteoclasis (surgical fracture) Clastothrix (splitting of hair)
-duct-	lead	Abduct (lead away from) Duct (tube leading to or from)
-ectas-	dilate	Phlebectasia (dilation of veins) Venectasia (dilation of veins)
-edem-	swelling	Cephaledema (swelling of head) Edematous (swollen)
-esthes-	sensation	Anesthesia (without sensation) Esthesiogenic (producing sensation)
fiss-	split, cleft	Fissure (cleft or groove) Fissile (capable of being split)
-flect-, flex-	bend	Anteflect (bend forward) Flexion (bending)
gen/o-	producing	Genesis (origin or beginning) Genophobia (fear of sexuality)
-iatr/o-	treatment	Geriatrics (treatment of aging) Pediatrics (treatment of children)

Continued.

Table 4-1   VERBAL ROOTS AND COMBINING FORMS —cont'd.

Root/Combining Form	Meaning	Examples
kin/e-, kin/o-	movement, motion	Kinetogenic (producing movement) Kinomometer (device to measure motion)
ly/o-, lys/o-	dissolve	Lyotropic (readily soluble) Lysogen (producing dissolution)
morph/o-	form, structure, shape	Amorphous (having no definite form) Polymorphic (having many forms)
-op/ia	vision	Myopia (nearsightedness) Hyperopia (farsightedness)
opt/ico-, opt/o-	seeing	Opticokinetic (pertaining to eye movement) Optometer (device for refraction)
phag/o-	eating	Phagomania (food craving) Phagophobia (fear of eating)
phan/ero-	visible, manifest	Phanerosis (process of becoming visible) Phantasm (unreal mental image)
-phas-	speech	Aphasia (loss of speech functions) Dysphasia (difficulty in speaking)
phil-	affinity, love for	Philanthropy (love of humankind) Philoneism (love of change)
-plegia	paralysis	Hemiplegia (one-sided paralysis) Paraplegia (paralysis of lower trunk and legs)
-poiesis	formation, production	Hemopoiesis (blood cell formation) Leukopoiesis (white blood cell production)
schist/o-, schiz/o-	split, cleft, division	Schistocystis (bladder fissure) Schizonychia (splitting of nails)
spasm/o-	spasm	Spasmogenic (causing spasms) Spasmolysis (relieving a spasm)
-stasis	standing still, stoppage	Epistasis (film on standing liquid) Hemostasis (stoppage of blood flow)
top/o-	place, location	Topalgia (localized pain) Toponarcosis (localized anesthesia)
troph/o-	nourishment, food	Trophism (nutrition) Dystrophy (defective nutrition)

Review Questions: Verbal Roots and Combining Forms

Complete the following:

1. Verb-based roots show an activity, an action, or a

_____ .

2. The combining form audi- means

_____ .

3. The combining form _____ means
dilate.

4. The combining form caus- means

_____.

5. The combining form for speech is

_____.

6. The combining form _____means
eating.

7. _____means affinity or love for.

8. The combining form for standing still is

_____.

9. _____ means place or location.

10. The combining form meaning treatment is

_____.

Matching:

____ **1.** duct-	**A.** break
____ **2.** phanero-	**B.** sensation
____ **3.** optico-	**C.** movement
____ **4.** edem-	**D.** lead
____ **5.** fiss-	**E.** dissolve
____ **6.** esthes-	**F.** formation
____ **7.** lyso-	**G.** visible
____ **8.** clas-	**H.** swelling
____ **9.** -poiesis	**I.** split, cleft
____ **10.** kine-	**J.** seeing

Answers to Review Questions: Verbal Roots and Combining Forms

Completion:
1. condition
2. hearing
3. ectas-
4. burn
5. phas-
6. phago-
7. phil-
8. -stasis
9. topo-
10. iatro-

Matching:

1. D	**6.** B
2. G	**7.** E
3. J	**8.** A
4. H	**9.** F
5. I	**10.** C

Table 4-2 lists adjectival (adjective-based) roots and combining forms that describe a quality or characteristic.

Each combining form is divided by a slash mark (/) between the root and its combining vowel.

Table 4-2   ADJECTIVAL ROOTS AND COMBINING FORMS

Root/Combining Form	Meaning	Examples
ankyl/o-	bent, crooked, stiff, fixed	Ankyloglossia (tongue-tie) Ankylosis (stiff or fixed joint)
brachy-	short	Brachydactylia (short fingers) Brachygnathous (receding underjaw)
brady-	slow	Bradycardia (slow heartbeat) Bradypepsia (slow digestion)
brev/i-	short	Brevicollis (short neck) Breviflexor (short flexor muscle)
cel-, coel-	hollow, cavity	Celiac (pertaining to the abdominal cavity) Coelom (body cavity of embryo)
cry/o-	cold	Cryotherapy (treatment using cold) Cryoanesthesia (freezing of a body part)
crypt/o-	hidden	Cryptorchidism (undescended testis) Cryptomnesia (subconscious memory)
dextr/o-	right, right side	Dextrocardia (heart on right side) Dextromanual (right handed)
dipl/o-	double, twice	Diplocoria (double pupil in eye) Diplopia (double vision)
dolich/o-	long	Dolichocephalic (long head) Dolichoderus (long neck)
eso-	within, inward	Esophoria (crossed eye) Esodeviation (a turning inward)
eury-	wide, broad	Eurysomatic (thickset body) Eurycephalic (unusually broad head)
glyc/o-	sugar, sweet	Glycemia (glucose in the blood) Glycogeusia (sweet taste)
hapl/o-	simple, single	Haploid (single or half set of chromosomes) Haplopathy (uncomplicated disease)
heter/o-	other, different	Heterocellular (pertaining to different cells) Heterohypnosis (induced by another)
hom/eo-, hom/o-	same, alike	Homeomorphous (similar in shape) Homozygous (having identical genes)
hydr/o-	wet, water	Hydremia (excess water in blood) Hydroadipsia (absence of thirst)
is/o-	equal, alike	Isocellular (having similar cells) Isocoria (equal-sized pupils)
lei/o-	smooth	Leiodermia (smooth, glossy skin) Leiotrichous (smooth hair)
lept/o-	slender, small, thin	Leptodactylous (slender fingered) Leptodermic (thin-skinned)
lev/o-	left, to the left	Levoduction (eyes turn left) Levorotation (turning to the left)
macr/o-	large	Macrencephaly (large brain) Macrobiosis (long life)

Table 4-2 ADJECTIVAL ROOTS AND COMBINING FORMS —cont'd.

Root/Combining Form	Meaning	Examples
mal-	ill, bad	Malady (illness) Malaise (general discomfort)
malac/o-	soft, softening	Malacia (softening) Malacotomy (incision of soft parts)

meg/a-,
  meg/alo-,
  meg/aly-
	large, oversized	Megalgia (severe pain)
		Megalomania (grandiose delusions)
		Hepatomegaly (enlarged liver)

mi/o-	less, decrease	Miopragia (decreased activity) Miosis (contraction of pupil)
necr/o-	death	Necrophobia (fear of death) Necropsy (autopsy)
olig/o-	few, little	Oligomenorrhea (scanty menses) Oligosymptomatic (having few symptoms)
opisth/o-	backward, behind, dorsal	Opisthocheilia (recession of lips) Opisthoporeia (walking backward)
orth/o-	straight, normal, correct	Orthodontics (straightening of teeth) Orthograde (walking erect)
oxy-	sharp, quick	Oxyesthesia (overly acute senses) Oxyrhine (sharp-pointed nose)
pachy-	thick	Pachyderma (abnormally thick skin) Pachyonychia (overly thick nails)
pale/o-	old, primitive	Paleogenetic (originating in past) Paleologic (primitive reasoning)
platy-	flat, wide	Platyglossal (wide, flat tongue) Platycephaly (flattened skull)
ple/o-	more	Pleonexia (excessive greediness) Pleonosteosis (excessive bone growth)
poikil/o-	irregular, varied	Poikiloderma (mottled skin) Poikilothermic (cold-blooded)
-scler/o-	hardness	Sclerosis (hardening) Arteriosclerosis (hardening of artery)
scoli/o-	twisted, crooked	Scoliokyphosis (curvature of spine) Scoliosis (crooked spine)
sinistr/o-	left, to the left	Sinistrocular (left-eyed) Sinistromanual (left-handed)
sten/o-	narrow	Stenosed (narrowed, contracted) Stenostomia (narrow oral cavity)
stere/o-	solid, three-dimensional	Stereoscopic (solid appearance) Stereopsis (three-dimensional vision)
tachy-	rapid, fast	Tachyphagia (bolting one's food) Tachylogia (rapid speech)
tel/e-, tel/o-	distant, end	Telalgia (pain from another area) Telencephalon (end brain)
therm/o-	heat	Thermogenic (producing heat) Thermolabile (alteration or destruction by heat)
xer/o-	dry	Xerochilia (dry lips) Xerostomia (dry mouth)

Review Questions: Adjectival Roots and Combining Forms

Complete the following:

1. Adjectival roots and combining forms describe

   _____.

2. The combining form _____ means short.

3. The combining form meaning double is

   _____.

4. The combining form dolicho- means

   _____.

5. The combining form eury- means

   _____.

6. Hetero- means _____.

7. Homeo- means _____.

8. A combining form meaning large is

   _____.

9. The combining form necro- means

   _____.

10. The combining form _____ means rapid or fast.

Matching:

____	**1.** thermo-	**A.** thick
____	**2.** steno-	**B.** left
____	**3.** mal-	**C.** simple, single
____	**4.** sclero-	**D.** cold
____	**5.** pachy-	**E.** slow
____	**6.** malaco-	**F.** heat
____	**7.** haplo-	**G.** soft
____	**8.** levo-	**H.** hardness
____	**9.** brady-	**I.** ill, bad
____	**10.** cryo-	**J.** narrow

Answers to Review Questions: Adjectival Roots and Combining Forms

Completion:
1. quality or characteristic
2. brachy-, brevi-
3. diplo-
4. long
5. wide, broad
6. different
7. same, alike
8. macro-, mega-, megalo-, -megaly
9. death
10. tachy-

Matching:

1. F	**6.** G
2. J	**7.** C
3. I	**8.** B
4. H	**9.** E
5. A	**10.** D

Tables 4-3 to 4-5 list a number of additional terms used in medical language. Collectively, these terms complete the basic foundation for learning medical terminology. They are presented as words, roots, and combining forms, in separate tables relating to body fluids, body substances and chemicals, and colors. Each combining form is divided by a slash mark (/) between the root and its combining vowel.

Table 4-3   BODY FLUIDS

Word, root/combining form	Meaning
aqua, hydr/o-	water
chol/e-, chol/o-	bile
chyle	milky fluid (product of digestion)
dacry/o-, lacrima	tears
galact/o-, lac	milk
hem/a-, hemat/o-, hem/o-	blood
hidr/o-, sudor	sweat
lymph/o-	lymph
mucus	secretion of mucous membranes
myx/o-	mucus
plasma	fluid portion of blood
ptyal/o-	saliva
pus	liquid product of inflammation
py/o-	pus
sangui-, sanguin/o-	blood, bloody
serum	clear portion of blood fluid
sial/o-	saliva, salivary glands
ur/e-, ur/ea-, ur/eo-, ur/in-, ur/ino-, ur/o-	urine, urea

Table 4-4   BODY SUBSTANCES AND CHEMICALS

Word, root/combining form	Meaning
adip/o-	fat
amyl/o-	starch
cerumen	earwax
collagen	fibrous protein of connective tissue, cartilage, bone, and skin
ele/o-, ole/o-	oil
ferrum	iron
glyc/o-, sacchar/o-, sacchar/i-	sugar
hal/o-	a salt
heme	iron-based, pigmented part of hemoglobin
hormone	body-produced chemical substance
hyal/o-, hyalin	glassy, translucent substance
lapis	stone
lip/o-, lipid	fat, fatty acids
lith/o-	stone or calculus
mel/i-	honey or sugar
natrium	sodium
petrous	stony hardness
sal	salt
sebum	sebaceous gland secretion

Table 4-5   COLORS

Word, root/combining form	Meaning
albus	white
chlor/o-, chloros	green
chrom/o-	color (as compared with no color)
cirrhos	orange-yellow
cyan/o-	blue
erythr/o-	red
leuc/o-, leuk/o-	white
lutein	saffron yellow
melan/o-	black
poli/o-	gray (pertaining to gray matter of the nervous system)
rhod/o-	red
ruber, rubor	red, redness
xanth/o-	yellow, yellowish

Review Questions: Body Fluids, Body Substances and Chemicals, and Colors

Complete the following:

1. A word meaning water is _____ .

2. A combining form for mucus is

   _____ .

3. The combining form for pus is

   _____ .

4. The clear portion of blood fluid is

   _____ .

5. The combining form hidro- means

   _____ .

6. A combining form for milk is _____ .

7. The word _____ means earwax.

8. A combining form for fat is _____ .

9. The combining form for blue is

   _____ .

10. The combining form for black is

    _____ .

Matching:

____	**1.** rubor	**A.**	stony hardness
____	**2.** leuko-	**B.**	saliva
____	**3.** polio-	**C.**	sugar
____	**4.** meli-	**D.**	salt
____	**5.** chole-	**E.**	white
____	**6.** petrous	**F.**	iron
____	**7.** glyco-	**G.**	red
____	**8.** ptyalo-	**H.**	bile
____	**9.** sal	**I.**	honey or sugar
____	**10.** ferrum	**J.**	gray

Answers to Review Questions: Body Fluids, Body Substances and Chemicals, and Colors

Completion:
1. aqua
2. myxo-
3. pyo-
4. serum
5. sweat
6. galacto-
7. cerumen
8. lipo-, adipo-
9. cyano-
10. melano-

Matching:

1. G	**6.** A
2. E	**7.** C
3. J	**8.** B
4. I	**9.** D
5. H	**10.** F

CHAPTERS 2, 3, AND 4 EXERCISES

THE COMPLETE FOUNDATION

The following exercises provide a review of the foundation material. The word parts are not necessarily clustered according to use, as was done in the preceding exercises. Approach the exercises as a challenge. You may find it necessary to look back through Chapters 2 and 3, as well as this one, to locate answers. Once more, try to avoid using the answer page except as a final check.

Exercise 1: In the blank following each pair of words, roots, or combining forms, indicate whether their meaning is the *same* or *opposite*.

1. myxo-
mucus _____

2. macro-
-megaly _____

3. lepto-
pachy- _____

4. levo-
dextro- _____

5. erythro-
rhodo- _____

6. homeo-
iso- _____

7. sinistro-
levo- _____

8. hydro-
xero- _____

9. leuko-
albus _____

10. hema-
sangui-_____

Exercise 2: This exercise will help you to learn to break medical words into their component parts in order to define them. Define each component and then define the word. Do not define those suffixes following a slash mark (/).

1. Postocular:

post _____

ocul/ar _____

_____

2. Aphasia:

a _____

phas/ia _____

_____

3. Proctoptosis:

procto _____

ptosis _____

_____

4. Microscope:

micro _____

scope _____

_____

5. Oophorectomy:

oophor _____

ectomy _____

_____

6. Hematopoiesis:

hemato _____

poiesis _____

_____

7. Endocardium:

endo _____

cardi/um _____

_____

8. Intercostal:

inter _____

cost/al _____

_____

9. Paraurethral:

para _____

urethr/al _____

_____

10. Osteomalacia:

osteo _____

malac/ia _____

_____

11. Xerostomia:

xero _____

stom/ia _____

_____

12. Schizonychia:

schiz _____

onych/ia _____

_____

13. Diplopia:

dipl _____

opia _____

_____

14. Pleomorphism:

pleo _____

morph/ism _____

_____

15. Hydronephrosis:

hydro _____

nephr _____

osis _____

_____

16 Retrocervical:

retro _____

cervic/al _____

_____

17. Leukorrhea:

leuko _____

rrhea _____

_____

18 Leiomyoma:

leio _____

my _____

oma _____

_____

Exercise 3: Fill in the appropriate word, root, or combining form.

1. bile _____

2. sweat _____

3. saliva _____

4. iron _____

5. fluid portion of blood _____

6. salt _____

7. sugar _____

8. oil _____

9. starch _____

10. sebaceous gland secretions _____

Chapter 4 Crossword Puzzle

Across

1. meaning of therm
4. root for black
7. root for formation
8. root for salt
11. meaning of the root ptyal
13. chemical substance produced by the body
15. meaning of the root mal
16. word meaning lead away from
20. root meaning paralysis
21. root meaning break
22. root meaning form, shape, structure
23. root meaning smooth

Down

2. root meaning hearing
3. root meaning stone
5. root meaning dilate
6. a cleft or groove
8. root meaning hardness
9. root meaning milk
10. root meaning twisted or crooked
12. word for earwax
13. root for wet or water
14. root for standing still
17. meaning of the root chrom
18. meaning of the root pachy
19. root meaning fast
20. root for eating
22. root meaning less or decrease

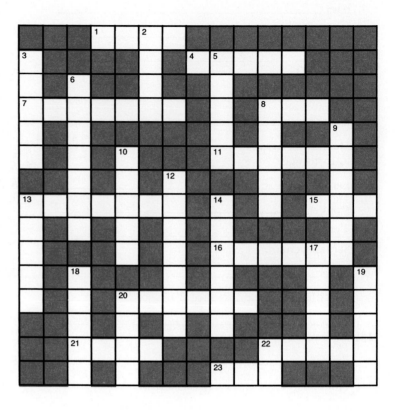

Chapter 4 Hidden Word Puzzle

Can you find the 20 words hidden in this puzzle? All hidden word puzzles will have words running from top to bottom, left to right, and diagonally downward.

PLEGIA	BRADY	MELAN	AMYL
BREV	CHOL	CLAS	CYAN
FISS	FLEX	LITH	PHAS
SIAL	STEN	BIO	CRY
HEM	KIN	LIP	OP

```
Y  E  C  R  Y  S  F  K  K  L  X  I  U  M
S  I  A  L  K  Z  P  T  L  I  P  V  T  Z
V  Q  M  S  A  M  Y  L  C  T  N  K  B  D
E  Y  V  F  I  S  S  O  E  H  E  M  T  W
G  C  H  I  D  D  G  K  K  G  O  E  D  G
S  P  K  Y  Z  U  U  X  C  W  I  L  X  C
Y  D  Q  E  P  A  S  F  W  B  R  A  D  Y
X  D  J  J  P  H  A  S  L  R  I  N  N  A
F  N  U  U  S  H  X  S  T  E  N  O  P  N
L  C  O  C  G  O  Z  N  Z  V  X  D  X  E
```

CHAPTERS 2, 3, AND 4 ANSWERS

Exercise 1

1. same	**4.** opposite	**7.** same
2. same	**5.** same	**8.** opposite
3. opposite	**6.** same	**9.** same
		10. same

Exercise 3
1. chole-, cholo-
2. hidro-, sudor
3. sialo-, ptyalo-
4. ferrum
5. plasma
6. sal
7. glyco-, saccharo-, sacchari-
8. eleo-, oleo-
9. amylo-
10. sebum

Exercise 2
1. behind; referring to eye—behind the eye
2. without; speech—without speech
3. rectum or anus; falling—prolapse of rectum or anus
4. small; examining instrument—instrument to examine small objects
5. ovary; excision of—surgical excision of ovary or ovaries
6. blood; formation—formation of blood
7. within or inner; heart—inner heart lining
8. between; referring to ribs—between the ribs
9. beside or near; referring to urethra—near the urethra
10. bone; softening—softening of bone
11. dry; mouth—dry mouth
12. split; nail(s)—split nail(s)
13. double; referring to vision—double vision
14. more; form—more than one form
15. water; kidney; condition—collection of fluid in kidney(s)
16. behind; referring to cervix—behind the cervix (uterine)
17. white; discharge or flow—white discharge (from the vagina)
18. smooth; muscle; tumor—smooth muscle tumor

Answers: Chapter 4 Crossword Puzzle

Answers: Chapter 4 Hidden Word Puzzle

```
. . C R Y . . . K L . . . . .
S I A L . . P . L I P . . . .
. . . . A M Y L C T N . . . .
. . . F I S S . E H E M . . .
. . . . . . . . . G O E . . .
. . . . . . . . . I L . C
. . . . . . . F . B R A D Y
. . . . . P H A S L R I N . A
. . . . . . . S T E N O P N
. . . . . . . . V X . . . .
```

Words:

\ PLEGIA	> BRADY	\/ MELAN	> AMYL
\/ BREV	\ CHOL	\ CLAS	\/ CYAN
> FISS	\ FLEX	\/ LITH	> PHAS
> SIAL	> STEN	\ BIO	> CRY
> HEM	\ KIN	> LIP	> OP

Section Two

The Body Shell and Its Supports

This is the second of the five sections of **LEARNING MEDICAL TERMINOL-OGY.** This section contains four chapters introducing the student to the language of the body structure, and the systems that support, move, and protect it.

Chapter 5 acquaints the student with the six branches of science that deal with the study of the body, the basic structure of the body, and the terms used to describe directions, planes, positions, and regions of the body. Beginning with this chapter, a glossary of medical terminology relating to the material in the text will be found at the very end of each chapter.

Chapter 6 describes the Skeletal System and its function as a supporting framework for the body.

Chapter 7 describes the Muscular System, and how it produces movement of the body in conjunction with the Skeletal System.

Chapter 8 describes the Integumentary System and its many functions.

Drawings within the chapters illustrate the principal anatomic parts for that chapter. In addition, there are colored plates at the front of the text which provide more vivid detail.

Chapter 5

Understanding the Body and Its Structure

It's a Fact:
There are more than 50 trillion cells in the average adult body.

CHAPTER OVERVIEW

A jokester once said that the human body is a remarkably intricate and complex apparatus manufactured by the unskilled labor of two workers.

In this chapter we describe the basic structures of the human body, their characteristics and composition, and descriptive anatomic terms are introduced in chart form.

STUDY OF THE BODY

Six branches of science deal with the study of the body. They are anatomy, physiology, pathology, embryology, histology, and biology:

Anatomy, which literally means cutting apart, is the study of the structure of the body and the relationship of its parts. It derives its name from the fact that the structure of the human body is learned mainly from dissection.
Physiology is the study of the normal functions and activities of the body.
Pathology is the study of the changes caused by disease in the structure or functions of the body.
Embryology is the study of the origin and development of an organism. After conception, the period from the second through the eighth week is called the embryonic stage. After this, the developing organism is referred to as the fetus.
Histology is the microscopic study of the minute structure, composition, and function of normal cells and tissues.
Biology is the study of all forms of life.

BASIC STRUCTURE

The human body may be compared to a machine, its many parts working together to promote good health, growth, and life itself. It is a combination of organs and systems supported by a framework of muscles and bones, with an external covering of skin for protection

The *cell* is the smallest unit of life from which tissues, organs, and systems are constructed (*cyt-* is the root for cell). Cells similar in structure and function form a mass called a *tissue*. Groups of different tissues combine to form an *organ* of the body (for example, the liver, heart, or lungs), each of which performs a special function. The organs are grouped into *systems* for the purpose of performing specific and more complicated functions.

CELL
V
A GROUP OF CELLS
V
FORM A TISSUE
V
A GROUP OF TISSUES
V
FORM AN ORGAN
V
A GROUP OF ORGANS
V
FORM A SYSTEM

CHARACTERISTICS OF LIVING MATTER

The body is maintained by a process called *metabolism* (*meta-* means change; *bolus* refers to mass; *-ism*

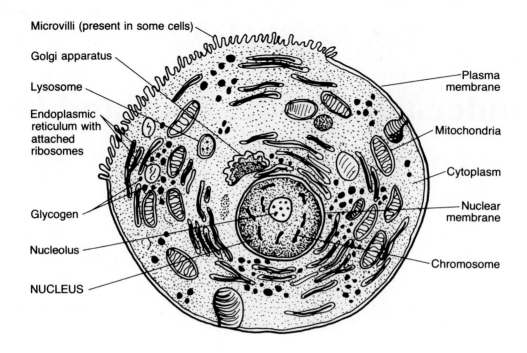

Microvilli (present in some cells)
Golgi apparatus
Lysosome
Endoplasmic reticulum with attached ribosomes
Glycogen
Nucleolus
NUCLEUS
Plasma membrane
Mitochondria
Cytoplasm
Nuclear membrane
Chromosome

Figure 5-1.   Diagram of a cell showing cellular structures, as seen with the electron microscope

means condition). Metabolism is the sum total of the process of **anabolism** (**ana-** means building up) and **catabolism** (**cata-** means breaking down). When metabolism ceases, the organism dies.

All living matter is irritable and excitable— it reacts to stimulation. With appropriate stimulation, nerve cells conduct impulses; muscle cells contract; and gland cells secrete substances.

CELLS

Understanding the structure and function of the body begins with the smallest unit of life, the cell. Specialized cells carry out the functions of growth, secretion, excretion, irritability, nutrition, and reproduction. They are activated by mechanical, chemical, or nervous stimulation.

Composition of Cells

Each cell of the body is enclosed by a membrane called the **plasma membrane**. This membrane protects the internal structure of the cell and regulates the passage of materials in and out of the cell. Inside the membrane is a jellylike substance, **cytoplasm**, surrounding a centrally located body, the **nucleus** (Fig. 5-1).

The cytoplasm contains **fibers** that provide a lattice-type framework for the cell and also contains huge numbers of **organelles** (little organs) outside the nucleus, including the following:

The **endoplasmic reticulum** is a network of canals consisting of smooth and rough portions. The smooth portion manufactures carbohydrates and some fats. Attached to the rough portion are thousands of granules called **ribosomes**, made up of ribonucleic acid (**RNA**). The ribosomes make proteins before passing them on to the Golgi apparatus.

The **Golgi apparatus** consists of vesicles, or small sacs, believed to manufacture carbohydrates and combine them with protein in a closed globule that is secreted by the cell.

The **mitochondria** are microscopic sacs with enzyme molecules attached to their membranous walls. These enzymes are considered to be the "power plants" of the cell, supplying its energy.

The **lysosomes** are membranous closed sacs containing enzymes capable of digesting large molecules and particles for use by the cell. They also protect the cell by digesting invading bacteria by **phagocytosis** (**phago-** means eating).

The **nucleus**, enclosed in a membrane called the **nuclear membrane**, is a spheroid (round), centrally located body that is highly specialized, regulating growth and reproduction. It contains deoxyribonucleic acid (**DNA**) molecules, which determine heredity. During cell division, the DNA molecules become short and rod-like and are then called **chromosomes**.

There are 46 chromosomes (23 pairs) in all human cells, with the exception of mature sex cells, which only have half this number (23). At conception, the mature male and female reproductive (sex) cells unite, each contributing a chance combination of 23 chromosomes out of innumerable possible combinations. This explains why no two individuals are alike, except in the case of identical twins.

The **nucleolus** is a round body within the nucleus, consisting mainly of RNA. Its function is to combine RNA with protein to form the ribosomes.

Review A

Complete the following:

1. The six branches of science that deal with the study of the body are _____, _____, _____, _____, _____, and _____.

2. The smallest unit of life is _____.

3. The body is maintained by a process called _____.

4. Specialized cells are activated by _____, _____, or _____ stimulation.

5. The _____ determine heredity.

6. There are _____ chromosomes in a mature sex cell.

7. The nucleus regulates _____ and _____.

8. Cells similar in structure and function form a _____.

9. All living matter is _____ and _____.

10. The membrane enclosing each cell of the body is the _____ membrane.

TISSUES

Tissues are groups of specialized cells that are similar in structure and function but have different characteristics in accordance with their function. The basic types of tissue are **epithelial**, **connective**, **muscle**, and **nervous**.

Epithelial Tissue

Epithelial tissue (**epi-** means upon, on, or over) is found throughout the human body. It makes up the outer covering of external and internal body surfaces such as the skin; mucous membranes; serous membranes; and the lining of the digestive, respiratory, and urinary tracts.

The main functions of epithelial tissue are to protect, absorb, and secrete. For example, the skin protects underlying structures; other types allow substances to pass through them and serve as absorbing tissue (lungs and intestines) or secreting tissue (mucous membranes and glands).

A special type of epithelial tissue called **endothelium** (**endo-** means within or inner) lines the heart, blood and lymph vessels, and other serous body cavities. **Mesothelium** (**meso-** means middle), another type of epithelial tissue, covers the surface of serous membranes (pleura, pericardium, and peritoneum).

There are various types of epithelial tissue, classified according to the number of layers of cells:

Simple epithelial tissue has one layer of cells.
Stratified epithelial tissue has three or more layers of cells.
Pseudostratified epithelial tissue has one layer of cells but appears to have more.

Epithelial tissue is also classified according to the shape of the surface layer of the cells:

Squamous cells have a flat appearance.
Cuboidal cells have a cubelike appearance.
Columnar cells resemble columns.
Transitional cells vary from squamous to cuboidal because they are found only in the urinary tract and change appearance according to the amount of pressure to which they are subjected.

Three types of epithelial tissue are illustrated in Fig. 5-2. All types are composed largely or entirely of cells that undergo **mitosis** (cell division) for the replacement of old or damaged cells.

Connective Tissue

Connective tissue, the most widespread tissue, props and shapes the body, holds organs in place, and connects

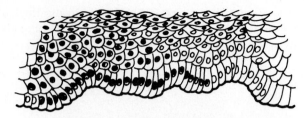

Stratified squamous epithelium

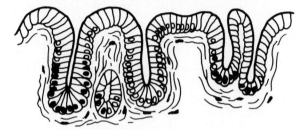

Simple columnar epithelium

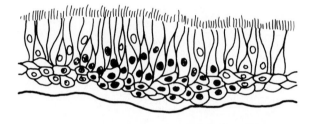

Pseudostratified ciliated columnar epithelium

Figure 5-2.   Types of epithelial tissue.

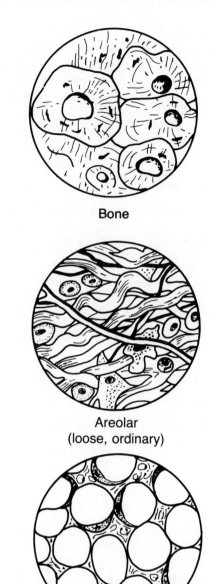

Bone

Areolar
(loose, ordinary)

Adipose (fat)

Figure 5-3.   Three types of connective tissue.

body parts to each other (Fig. 5-3). The main types of connective tissue are:

Bone: hard and unbendable—supports and protects the body.
Cartilage: firm, but bendable—found throughout the body.
Dense fibrous: strong, bendable—mostly tendons and ligaments.
Areolar (loose, ordinary): elastic, stretchable, weblike network of fibers and cells providing support for internal organs.
Adipose: fatty tissue—pads and protects organs, stores excess fat, and insulates against body heat loss.
Hematopoietic: specialized connective tissue that forms both red and white blood cells.
Blood: although liquid, classified as connective tissue.

Muscle Tissue

There are three types of muscle tissue—***skeletal***, which is striated (striped) and voluntary (movable at will); ***visceral***, which is nonstriated (smooth) and involuntary; and ***cardiac***, which is striated but involuntary.

Skeletal muscles move bones. Visceral muscles are located in the walls of hollow internal structures (blood vessels, intestines, and the uterus). Cardiac muscle makes up the heart (Fig. 5-4).

The main function of muscle tissue is to contract. Muscle cells are long and slender and are called fibers. The fibers decrease in length and increase in thickness during contraction of a muscle.

Hematopoietic Tissue

Hematopoietic (blood-forming) tissue is found in bone marrow (Chapter 6) and the lymphatic system (Chapter 16).

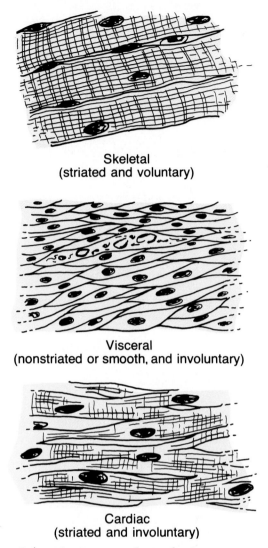

Skeletal
(striated and voluntary)

Visceral
(nonstriated or smooth, and involuntary)

Cardiac
(striated and involuntary)

Figure 5-4.   Three types of muscle tissue.

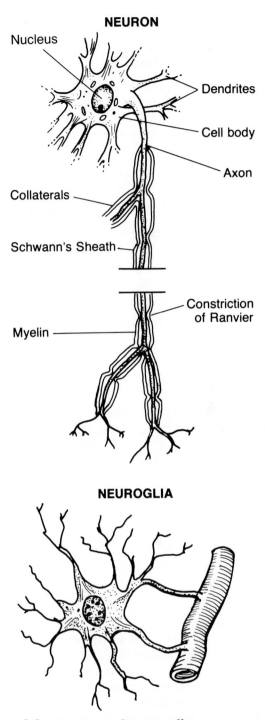

Figure 5-5.   Structure of nerve cells.

Blood Tissue

Blood tissue is found in the blood vessels (Chapter 9).

Nervous Tissue

Nervous tissue is composed of nerve cells called ***neurons***, nerve fibers, and supporting tissue between the cells and fibers to keep them in position. The supporting structure of nervous tissue is ***neuroglia*** (***neuro-*** means nerve; ***-glia*** means glue). Nervous tissue is the most highly specialized tissue in the body, requiring more oxygen and more nutrition than any other body tissue (Fig. 5-5).

Review B

Complete the following:

1. The basic types of tissue are _____, _____, _____, and

   _____.

2. The most widespread tissue in the body is _____ tissue.

3. Three types of epithelial tissue classified by numbers of layers of cells are _____,

   _____, and _____.

4. The three types of muscle tissue are _____, _____, and _____.

5. _____ is the supporting structure of nervous tissue.

6. _____ tissue is found in bone marrow.

7. Striated means _____.

8. The main functions of epithelial tissue are to _____, _____, and _____.

9. A type of cell varying from squamous to cuboidal is a _____ cell.

10. Nervous tissue is composed of nerve cells called _____.

ORGANS

In the body, groups of cells form tissues, and similar tissues form organs (for example, the heart, lungs, liver, and kidneys). Organs, although they act as individual units, do not function independently; several combine to form a system, with each system having a special function.

SYSTEMS

A system is a combination of organs that performs a particular function. The systems of the body and their functions are:

Skeletal: framework of the body, supporting organs and furnishing a place of attachment for muscles.
Muscular: permits motion and movement of the body.
Integumentary: includes skin, hair, nails, and sweat and sebaceous glands; covers and protects the body, aids in temperature regulation, and has functions in sensation and excretion.
Cardiovascular: transports the blood.
Lymphatic: retrieves plasma and tissue fluids and has a role in the immune system.
Respiratory: absorbs oxygen and discharges carbon dioxide.
Gastrointestinal: digests and absorbs food and excretes waste.
Genitourinary: reproduction and urine excretion.
Endocrine: manufactures hormones.
Nervous with the *special senses*: processes stimuli and enables the body to act and respond.
Immune: protects the body from invading organisms and disease.

DIRECTIONS

anterior—ventral (or front) surface of the body

posterior—dorsal (or back) surface of the body

medial—nearer to or toward the midline

lateral—farther from the midline or to the side of the body

internal—inside

external—outside

proximal—nearer to the point of origin or closer to the body

distal—away from the point of origin or away from the body

superior—above

inferior—below

cranial—toward the head

caudal—toward the lower end of the body (*cauda* means tail)

DIRECTIONS, ANATOMIC PLANES, AND POSITIONS

A number of anatomic terms are used in describing the body and determining direction. The terms listed in the accompanying boxes refer to the anatomic position, with the body standing erect and the arms hanging to the side, palms facing forward (Fig. 5-6).

ANATOMIC PLANES

frontal (coronal) plane—a section through the side of the body, passing at right angles to the median plane and dividing the body into anterior and posterior portions.

median (midsagittal, midline) plane—an imaginary plane that passes from the front to the back through the center of the body and divides the body into right and left equal portions.

sagittal plane—a section parallel to the long axis of the body or parallel to the median plane, dividing the body into right and left unequal parts.

transverse plane—a horizontal plane passing at right angles to both the frontal and median planes and dividing the body into cranial and caudal parts.

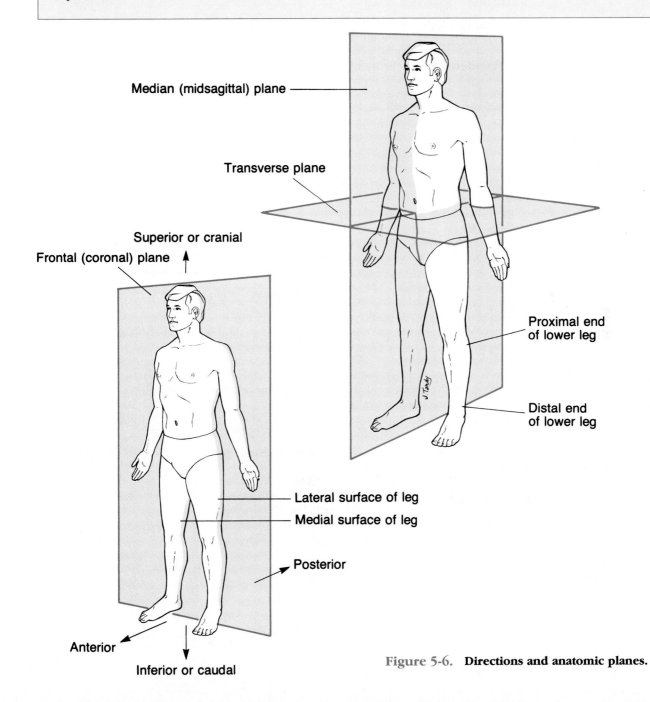

Figure 5-6. **Directions and anatomic planes.**

ANATOMIC POSITIONS

There are numerous terms to describe anatomic positions. Some of the more frequently used ones are listed below.

erect—standing position

Fowler's—head of bed raised, knees elevated

knee-chest (genupectoral)—kneeling, with chest resting on same surface

lateral recumbent (Sim's)—lying on left side with right thigh and knee drawn up

prone—lying face down

semi-Fowler's—head of bed raised, upper half of body inclined

Trendelenburg—inclined, with head lower than body and legs

supine (dorsal)—lying flat on back

BODY REGIONS (Fig. 5-7, A and B)

HEAD

auricular—around the ears

buccal—the cheeks

infraorbital—immediately below the eyes

mental—the chin

occipital—covering the occipital bone

orbital—around the eyes

submaxillary—on either side of the submental region, below the ramus of the mandible

submental—below the chin

supraorbital—above the eyebrows

THORAX AND ABDOMEN

axillary—axilla (armpit) and its borders

clavicular—on either side of the sternum (breastbone), extending the length of the clavicle (collarbone)

epigastric—within the costal (rib) arch, located in the median part of the abdomen

hypochondriac—right and left areas on either side of the epigastric region

hypogastric—in the lower abdomen between the inguinal regions, between and below the iliac spines

infraclavicular—below the clavicle

inguinal (iliac)—triangular area on either side of the hypogastric region

lateral abdominal (lumbar)—on either side of the umbilical region

mammary—breasts, on either side of the chest between the third and sixth ribs, extending below the lower margins of the pectoralis major muscles on either side

pubic—the central portion of the hypogastric region, above the pubis

BODY REGIONS (Fig. 5-7, A and B)

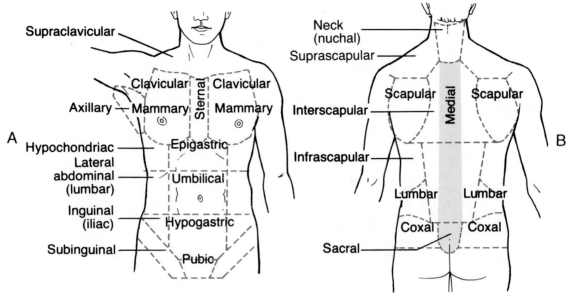

Figure 5-7.   Body Regions.   *A*, Anterior view;   *B*, Posterior view.

BODY REGIONS (Fig. 5-7, A and B)

sternal—over the front of the sternum

subinguinal—just below the inguinal region

supraclavicular—above the clavicle

umbilical—medial abdominal region, above the hypogastric region

POSTERIOR TRUNK

coxal—just below the lumbar regions in the back, and lateral abdominal regions on either side; bordered by gluteal regions (area over the buttocks)

infrascapular—below the scapulae (shoulder blades), extending down to the last ribs

interscapular—part of the medial region of the back, between the scapulae, on either side of the vertebral column

lumbar—immediately below the infrascapular region, extending down to the crest of the ilium

medial region of back—central zone of the back, extending from the neck as far down as the base of the sacrum

nuchal—back of the neck, beginning just below the occipital (back of head) region, extending down to the spine of the seventh cervical vertebra

sacral—area over the sacrum at the base of the median region

scapular—areas on either side, covering the scapula

suprascapular—areas on either side above the scapular region, extending to the curve of the neck

REVIEW C

Complete the following:

1. The systems of the body are the _____

   _____

   _____ .

2. Cranial means _____ .

3. Distal is the opposite of _____ .

4. The four anatomic planes of the body are _____ , _____ , _____ , and

   _____ planes.

5. Prone means _____ .

6. The _____ region is between the scapulae on either side of the vertebral column.

7. _____ refers to the region around the ears.

8. Several _____ combine to form a system.

9. The genupectoral is also called the _____ position.

10. The framework of the body is formed by the _____ system.

Answers to Review Questions: Understanding the Body and Its Structure

Review A
1. anatomy, physiology, pathology, embryology, histology, biology
2. the cell
3. metabolism
4. mechanical, chemical, nervous
5. DNA molecules or chromosomes
6. 23
7. growth, reproduction
8. tissue
9. irritable, excitable
10. plasma

Review B

1. epithelial, connective, muscle, nervous
2. connective
3. simple, stratified, pseudostratified
4. skeletal, voluntary, or striated; visceral, involuntary, nonstriated, or smooth; cardiac, involuntary, or striated
5. neuroglia
6. hematopoietic
7. striped
8. protect, absorb, secrete
9. transitional
10. neurons

Review C

1. skeletal, muscle, integumentary, cardiovascular, lymphatic, respiratory, gastrointestinal, genitourinary, endocrine, nervous, immune
2. toward the head
3. proximal
4. frontal or coronal; median, midsagittal, or midline; sagittal; transverse
5. lying face down
6. interscapular
7. auricular
8. organs
9. knee-chest
10. skeletal

CHAPTER 5 EXERCISES

UNDERSTANDING THE BODY AND ITS STRUCTURE

Exercise 1: Complete the following:

1. Specialized cells that are similar in structure and functions are assembled into a(n) _____.

2. Groups of different tissue are combined to form a(n) _____.

3. For the purpose of performing specific functions, the organs are grouped into a(n) _____.

4. The smallest unit of life and the building block for tissues, organs, and systems is called a(n)

   _____.

5. The body is maintained by a process called _____.

6. A special type of epithelial tissue, called _____, lines the heart, blood and lymph vessels, and other serous body cavities.

7. The most highly specialized tissue in the body is _____ tissue.

8. Cells arranged in three or more layers are called _____.

9. The connective tissue of the body making up tendons and ligaments is called _____.

10. The number of chromosomes in a human cell is _____.

Exercise 2: Matching:

____ **1.** ventral	**A.** face down
____ **2.** distal	**B.** head
____ **3.** cranial	**C.** standing up
____ **4.** caudal	**D.** ends of fingers
____ **5.** prone	**E.** front
____ **6.** supine	**F.** right and left epigastric area
____ **7.** erect	**G.** either side of umbilical region
____ **8.** hypochondriac	**H.** breast area of chest
____ **9.** lateral abdominal	**I.** face up
____**10.** mammary	**J.** lower end of body

Chapter 5 Crossword Puzzle

Across

1. breast
3. smooth involuntary muscle tissue
5. one of four basic types of tissue
7. above
8. jelly-like substance of cells
9. inside
11. below the clavicles
15. another of four basic types of tissue
18. face down
20. standing position
22. study of all forms of life
23. centrally located body in cell
24. region around the eyes
27. region between scapula and ilium
28. nerve cells
29. what a group of cells form

Down

2. ribonucleic acid
4. voluntary striped muscle tissue
6. study of the body's normal functions and activities
10. ventral or front surface of body
12. 23 pairs in each cell
13. what a group of organs form
14. the process by which the body is maintained
16. below
17. fatty tissue
19. area over breastbone
21. region of the cheeks
25. type of hard connective tissue
26. these molecules become chromosomes during cell division

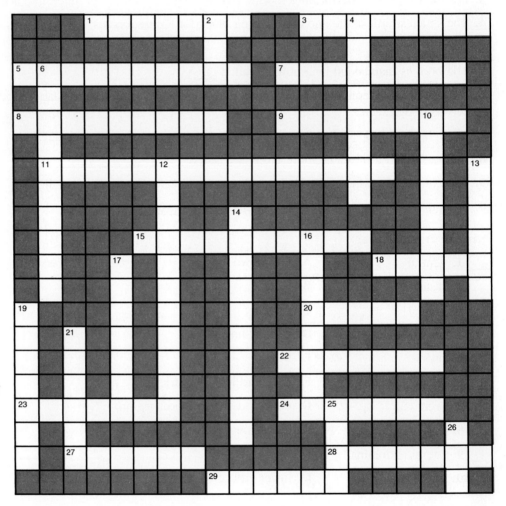

Chapter 5 Hidden Words Puzzle

```
J  O  Q  D  U  Y  N  R  T  U  F  J  O  A  B  Q  V  L  K  Y  T  H  H  A  Q
O  R  J  F  L  X  R  R  I  C  A  B  F  P  X  T  M  T  V  I  G  E  Q  X  R
P  E  Y  W  F  D  D  M  S  H  N  N  G  N  U  C  L  E  U  S  Q  P  F  L  J
R  T  X  T  J  N  N  U  S  X  A  V  T  E  L  Y  W  G  Q  B  F  Y  T  C  Y
F  N  K  H  O  T  W  R  U  F  T  Q  F  R  B  H  H  F  R  R  T  X  X  N  N
X  B  H  W  O  V  X  E  E  K  O  M  Q  V  Y  I  A  P  U  M  T  O  I  Y  S
W  L  C  H  R  O  M  O  S  O  M  E  S  O  D  S  P  C  L  U  O  A  H  P  L
C  O  N  N  E  C  T  I  V  E  Y  R  N  U  J  T  T  K  S  A  R  I  Y  F  I
E  O  D  B  M  M  G  V  V  Y  P  H  Y  S  I  O  L  O  G  Y  D  G  N  M  C
L  D  B  K  B  K  A  C  J  V  F  I  S  J  F  L  G  N  S  I  R  D  M  U  D
L  A  D  A  R  I  M  T  Y  V  M  E  T  A  B  O  L  I  S  M  X  R  R  E  W
Z  B  H  Y  Y  T  G  S  O  E  C  W  E  H  W  G  R  A  W  U  D  Z  D  V  V
J  O  H  P  O  T  I  N  T  P  G  F  K  E  E  Y  M  E  O  H  T  B  C  H  F
N  K  Q  O  L  K  D  L  K  L  O  M  U  S  C  L  E  L  G  J  M  B  N  U  K
W  O  F  R  O  A  X  Y  O  A  R  I  O  K  B  U  I  P  K  I  S  V  R  M  J
M  S  E  N  G  R  N  D  F  U  S  Q  E  T  Z  I  P  A  T  H  O  L  O  G  Y
X  A  Z  P  Y  P  V  E  I  J  I  W  V  T  C  N  O  L  L  X  R  N  E  D  E
Q  W  S  J  I  D  L  E  S  C  Q  N  K  H  I  K  S  L  O  J  K  N  S  W  M
X  N  M  D  X  W  O  Z  J  R  E  E  D  W  H  C  I  B  O  X  H  X  Y  X  F
O  S  V  J  Y  L  H  O  Z  S  K  G  X  F  Q  X  T  U  W  G  V  Y  H  H  N
L  K  M  O  Q  X  M  X  N  T  Y  U  H  P  B  V  I  Q  B  K  Y  Y  Y  O  V
V  S  D  V  I  M  U  H  M  P  W  X  J  V  V  M  O  T  O  X  L  I  T  X  X
U  W  Y  S  T  F  V  W  G  H  K  E  Y  U  G  Z  N  P  L  R  R  L  I  C  S
C  K  A  L  P  I  H  W  U  I  Q  A  Y  O  E  B  S  K  Q  N  D  W  L  W  E
```

Can you find the 20 words hidden in this puzzle? All hidden word puzzles will have words running from top to bottom, left to right, and diagonally downward.

HEMATOPOIETIC	CHROMOSOMES	CONNECTIVE	EMBRYOLOGY
EPITHELIAL	METABOLISM	PHYSIOLOGY	HISTOLOGY
PATHOLOGY	POSITIONS	ANATOMY	BIOLOGY
NERVOUS	NUCLEUS	REGIONS	TISSUES
MUSCLE	PLANES	BLOOD	CELL

CHAPTER 5 ANSWERS

Exercise 1
1. tissue
2. organ
3. system
4. cell
5. metabolism
6. endothelium
7. nervous
8. stratified epithelial tissue
9. dense fibrous
10. 46

Exercise 2
1. E   6. I
2. D   7. C
3. B   8. F
4. J   9. G
5. A   10. H

Answers: Chapter 5 Crossword Puzzle

A crossword puzzle answer grid with the following filled-in words:

Across:
- 1. MAMMARY
- 3. VISCERAL
- 5. EPITHELIAL
- 7. SUPERIOR
- 8. CYTOPLASM
- 9. INTERNAL
- 11. INFRACLAVICULAR
- 15. CONNECTIVE
- 18. PRONE
- 20. ERECT
- 22. BIOLOGY
- 23. NUCLEUS
- 24. ORBITAL
- 27. LUMBAR
- 28. NEURONS
- 29. TISSUE

Down:
- 2. ANNOY (A-N...)
- 4. SKELETAL
- 6. PHYSIOLOGY
- 10. ANTERIOR
- 12. CHROMATIN
- 13. SYSTEM
- 14. METABOLISM
- 16. CONNECTIVE (vertical)
- 17. ADIPOSE
- 19. STEREN...
- 21. BUCCA
- 25. ROBON
- 26. DA

Answers: Chapter 5 Hidden Words Puzzle

```
.  .  .  .  .  .  .  .  T  .  .  .  .  .  .  .  .  .  .  .  .
.  .  .  .  .  .  .  .  I  .  A  .  .  .  .  .  .  .  .  .  .
.  .  .  .  .  .  .  .  S  .  N  .  .  N  U  C  L  E  U  S  .  .  .  .  .
.  .  .  .  .  .  .  .  S  .  A  .  .  E  .  .  .  .  .  .  .  .
.  .  .  .  .  .  .  .  U  .  T  .  .  R  .  H  .  .  .  .  .  .  .
.  B  .  .  .  .  .  .  E  .  O  .  .  V  .  I  .  .  .  .  .  .  .
.  L  C  H  R  O  M  O  S  O  M  E  S  O  .  S  .  .  .  .  .  .  .
C  O  N  N  E  C  T  I  V  E  Y  .  .  U  .  T  .  .  .  .  .  .
E  O  .  .  M  M  .  .  .  P  H  Y  S  I  O  L  O  G  Y  .  .  .  .  .
L  D  .  .  B  .  A  .  .  .  .  I  .  .  .  L  .  .  .  .  .  .
L  .  .  .  R  .  T  .  .  M  E  T  A  B  O  L  I  S  M  .  .  .  .  .
.  .  .  .  Y  .  .  O  .  .  .  .  H  .  G  R  .  .  .  .  .  .
.  .  .  P  O  .  .  .  P  .  .  .  E  Y  .  E  .  .  .  .  .  .
.  .  .  .  L  .  .  .  .  O  M  U  S  C  L  E  .  G  .  .  .  .  .
.  .  .  .  O  A  .  .  .  .  I  .  B  .  I  .  I  .  .  .  .  .
.  .  .  .  G  .  N  .  .  .  .  E  .  .  I  P  A  T  H  O  L  O  G  Y
.  .  .  .  Y  .  E  .  .  .  .  T  .  .  O  .  L  .  N  .  .  .  .
.  .  .  .  .  .  .  .  S  .  .  .  .  I  .  S  L  .  .  .  S  .  .
.  .  .  .  .  .  .  .  .  .  .  .  .  C  I  .  O  .  .  .  .  .
.  .  .  .  .  .  .  .  .  .  .  .  .  T  .  G  .  .  .  .
.  .  .  .  .  .  .  .  .  .  .  .  .  I  .  .  Y  .  .  .
.  .  .  .  .  .  .  .  .  .  .  .  .  O  .  .  .  .  .
.  .  .  .  .  .  .  .  .  .  .  .  .  N  .  .  .  .  .
.  .  .  .  .  .  .  .  .  .  .  .  .  S  .  .  .  .  .
```

Words:

\ HEMATOPOIETIC	> CHROMOSOMES	> CONNECTIVE	V EMBRYOLOGY
\ EPITHELIAL	> METABOLISM	> PHYSIOLOGY	V HISTOLOGY
> PATHOLOGY	V POSITIONS	V ANATOMY	\ BIOLOGY
V NERVOUS	> NUCLEUS	\ REGIONS	V TISSUES
> MUSCLE	\ PLANES	V BLOOD	V CELL

Beginning with this chapter, a glossary (word list with definitions), with phonetic pronunciation guides, will be found at the end of each chapter to help the student understand the terms that relate to the preceding mate-rial. Each glossary is organized according to its text, with some review material and some additions, including anatomic terms, diseases, conditions, procedures, and other descriptive terms.

CHAPTER 5 GLOSSARY

adipose tissue (ad′i-pos): fatty connective tissue such as that found in the buttocks and abdominal walls.

areolar tissue (ah-re′o-lar): type of connective tissue consisting of stretchable, weblike networks of fibers and cells providing support for internal organs.

axon (ak′son): essential conducting part of a nerve fiber.

bony tissue: dense connective tissue that forms the skeletal framework of the body.

cardiac muscle tissue: heart muscle.

cartilage (kar′ti-lij): firm, elastic, somewhat dense connective tissue that forms many parts of the skeleton.

centrosome (sen′tro-som): area of cell cytoplasm near the nucleus, containing centrioles (minute cells), which play an important part in mitosis (cell division).

chromosomes (kro′mo-somz): rodlike bodies in the nucleus, composed mainly of DNA and containing the genes, which transmit the hereditary codes.

collaterals: small side branches of an axon.

columnar epithelium (ko-lum′nar ep″i-the′le-um): cells arranged in one layer, resembling columns.

connective tissue: forms the framework of the body, holds organs in place, and connects body parts to each other.

cuboidal epithelium: surface layer of cells, having a cubelike appearance.

cytoplasm (si′to-plazm″): jellylike substance of a cell, within the plasma membrane, surrounding the nucleus.

dense fibrous tissue: strong, pliant connective tissue of the body, found where organs are subjected to stress or strain.

deoxyribonucleic acid (DNA) (de-ok′se-ri″bo-nu-kle′ic): large molecule that is the main constituent of chromosomes.

endothelium (en″do-the′le-um): layer of simple squamous cells lining the inner surfaces of the circulatory organs and serous body cavities.

enzyme (en′zim): protein able to catalyze (speed up or change) chemical reactions in living cells.

epithelium (ep″i-the′le-um): epithelial tissue covering the external and internal body surfaces.

Golgi apparatus (gol′je): cellular component of the cytoplasm, believed to condense substances before they leave the cell as secretions.

inorganic matter: mineral.

invertebrate (in-ver′te-brate″): division of the animal kingdom, including all organisms with no backbone.

involuntary muscle tissue: muscle tissue that cannot be controlled at will; types are visceral (nonstriated—smooth), and cardiac (striated—striped).

lysosomes (li′so-somz): microscopic membranous sacs in the cytoplasm that contain enzymes capable of phagocytosis (digestion for nutrition and protection of the cell).

mesothelium (mes″o-the′le-um): epithelial tissue covering the serous membranes that line the abdominal and chest cavities.

metabolism (me-tab′o-liz″m): sum of all physical and chemical processes by which living organisms are maintained.

mitochondria (mi″to-kon′dre-ah): component of the cytoplasm, containing enzymes that are considered to be the source of supply of energy for the cell (also called *chondriosomes*).

mitosis (mi-to′sis): process of cell division.

molecule (mol′e-kul): chemical combination of two or more atoms that form a specific chemical substance (DNA and RNA are molecules).

nervous tissue: tissue composing nerves and nerve centers.

nucleolus (nu-kle′o-lus): spherical body within the nucleus, composed mainly of RNA and some protein (plural, *nucleoli*).

nucleus (nu′kle-us): spheroid body in the cell, containing the chromosomes and nucleoli (plural, *nuclei*).

organic matter: animal and vegetable (living) matter.

phagocytosis (fag″o-si-to′sis): ingestion and digestion of particulate matter by cells.

ribonucleic acid (RNA) (ri″bo-nu-kle′ik): a nucleic acid, similar to DNA, that relates to the function of the ribosomes.

ribosomes (ri′bo-somz): organelles (tiny organs) in the cytoplasm, attached to the endoplasmic reticulum, that build and transmit proteins.

squamous epithelium (skwa′mus): flat epithelial cells arranged in one or more layers.

stratified epithelium: cells arranged in three or more layers; may be columnar or squamous.

striated (stri′at-ed): striped.

transitional epithelium: a tissue made up of cells varying from squamous to cuboidal according to the amount of pressure to which they are subjected.

vertebrate (ver′te-brate): division of the animal kingdom comprising all animals that have a vertebral column or backbone, including mammals, reptiles, fish, and birds.

voluntary muscle tissue: striated muscle tissue that can be controlled at will (also called skeletal muscle).

Chapter 6

The Skeletal System

The Framework of the Body

CHAPTER OVERVIEW

In this chapter we describe the bones of the body, which make up the skeleton, and the ways in which they connect and are moved, relative to structure, classification, and location.

THE SKELETON

The skeleton is the jointed framework, made up of 206 bones, that supports and gives shape to the body. This framework helps to protect vital and delicate organs from external injury and furnishes attachment points for muscles, ligaments, and tendons, making movement possible. Bones store mineral salts, and some bones contain the hematopoietic (blood cell-forming) red bone marrow.

The study of bone is called *osteology* (*oss-* and *ost-* are roots meaning bone).

Composition of Bone

Bone (osseous tissue), a specialized form of connective tissue, is about 50% water and 50% solid matter. Part of the solid matter consists of inorganic (mineral) salts, which give bone its hardness. When the embryonic skeleton is first formed, it is made of cartilage and fibrous membrane in the shape of bones, which harden and become bone before birth. Because this ossifying process takes up to 25 years to complete, the bones of children

are more flexible and less subject to fracture than mature adult bones. The inorganic matter that gives bone its hardness contains higher proportions of lime as the body ages, causing the bones to become brittle and more easily fractured in old age.

Structure of Bone

The bone structure consists of a hard outer shell called *compact bone tissue* and an inner, spongy, latticelike structure called *cancellated* or *cancellous bone*. The dense compact bone is thick in the midshaft to prevent bending under stress and tapers to paper thinness at the ends. When a long bone in an adult is sectioned longitudinally, the *medullary cavity* (innermost part) of the *diaphysis* (shaft) is seen to be filled with yellow marrow, which stores fat. The yellow marrow has replaced red marrow, which is hematopoietic (red blood cell-forming) tissue containing red blood cells in various stages of growth (Fig. 6-1). In the adult, red marrow has mostly disappeared, except for that found in spaces in cancellated bone such as the flat bones of the skull, pelvis, vertebrae, ribs, and sternum, and the upper ends of the shafts of the humerus and femur.

The surfaces of bone, with the exception of the cartilage-covered articular surfaces, are covered by a tough, fibrous, vascular membrane called the *periosteum*, which is very thick except where muscles are attached to the bone. The outer layer is vascular, and the inner layer in the growing bone is lined with *osteoblasts* (immature bone cells). The deposition of bone from this layer of osteoblasts on the surface of the shaft provides for growth of bone and for repair when a bone is fractured. The periosteum also provides a confining membrane for the bone. It contains numerous blood vessels that enter the canals of the bone to supply it with nutrients. If the periosteum is removed, the bone is deprived of its nutrition and dies. Periosteum is regenerative, except in the

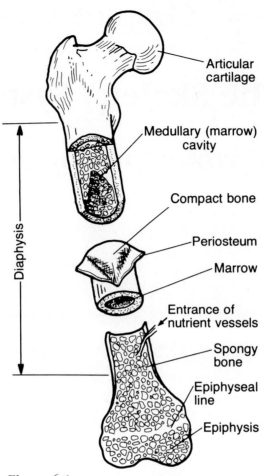

Figure 6-1.   **Structure of bone.**

skull, where if a section is removed, a plate must be used to fill the gap. Numerous nerves in the periosteum account for the pain experienced after an injury to a bone.

Arteries that nourish bone tunnel into the medullary (bone marrow) cavity, and make **anastomoses** (connections) with the numerous blood vessels of the periosteum. The bones have a poor capillary network but have many minute arterioles. Venous blood of the marrow and bone is returned to the circulation by numerous large veins that leave the bone by **foramina** (openings) at the extremities.

Growth of Bone

The long bones grow in length at the junctions of the **epiphyses** (ends of the developing bones) and the **diaphyses** (shafts) and grow in thickness, through the activity of the osteoblasts, in the deep layers of the periosteum. Growth of the long bones is produced by the growth of cartilage followed by deposits of bone to the diaphyses along the epiphyseal line. Growth of bone is controlled by a hormone secreted by the anterior lobe of the pituitary gland.

Growth of bone is precisely balanced through the teamwork of the osteoblasts and **osteoclasts** (large phagocytic cells). The osteoblasts produce bony tissue, and the osteoclasts eat away bony tissue in the medullary cavity, preventing the bone from becoming too thick. Healthy bone is constantly being broken down, reabsorbed, and repaired, but the process slows down with increasing age.

CLASSIFICATION OF BONES

Bones are classified according to their shape—long, flat, short, and irregular. The **femur** (bone between the hip joint and the knee) and the **humerus** (bone between the shoulder and the elbow) are examples of long bones. Short bones are those of the **carpals** (wrist), and **tarsals** (ankle bones). Flat bones are those of the **sternum** (breastbone), **scapula** (shoulder blade), and **pelvis**. The **vertebrae** are examples of irregular bones.

The skeleton of the human body (Figs. 6-2 and 6-3) is divided into two main parts, **axial** and **appendicular**. The axial skeleton has 80 bones and forms the vertical

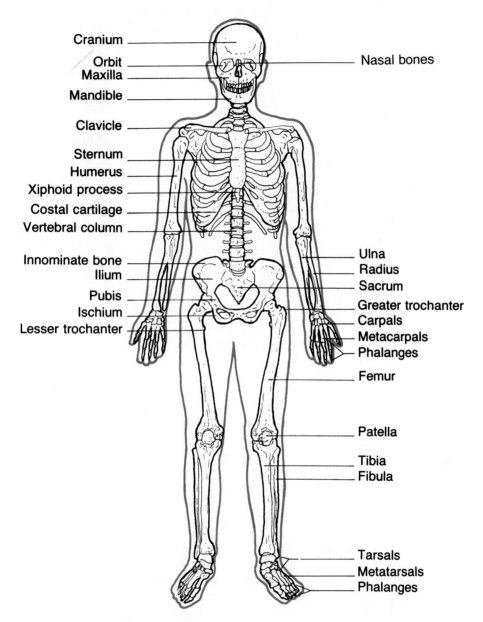

Figure 6-2.   Skeleton, anterior view (anatomic position).

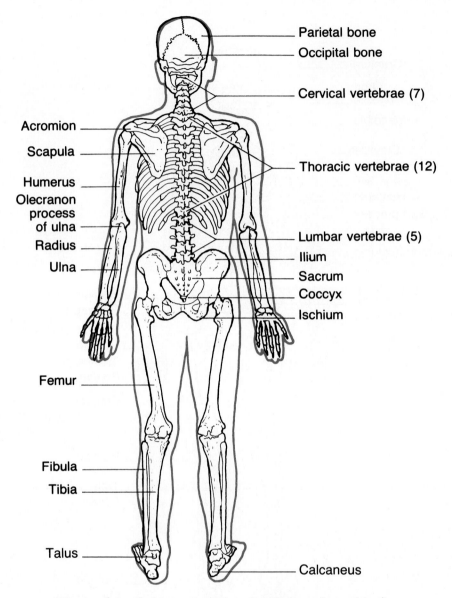

Figure 6-3.   Skeleton, posterior view (anatomic position).

axis of the body. These bones include the 28 bones of the *skull*, the *hyoid* bone (U-shaped bone located in the neck), the *vertebral column*, *ribs*, and *sternum*. The appendicular skeleton is made up of the 126 bones that support the extremities: *clavicle*, *scapula*, *humerus*, *radius*, *ulna*, *carpals*, *metacarpals*, *phalanges* (fingers), *pelvic girdle*, *femur*, *patella*, *tibia*, *fibula*, *tarsals*, *metatarsals*, and *phalanges* (toes).

Review A

Complete the following:

1. The skeleton is made up of _____ bones.

2. The shaft of long bones is called the _____.

3. Bone marrow is contained in the _____ cavity of long bones.

4. The outer membrane covering bones is called _____.

5. Immature bone cells are called _____.

6. Bones are classified according to shapes, which are _____

   _____.

7. The humerus is an example of a _____ bone.

8. The carpals and tarsals are classified as _____ bones.

9. The two main parts of the skeleton are the _____ and the _____.

10. The U-shaped bone in the neck is called the _____ bone.

AXIAL SKELETON

Skull

The skull includes two major segments, the *cranium* (brain case), and the facial framework. There are 8 bones in the cranium, 14 in the face, and 6 *ossicles* (small bones) in the ears (Fig. 6-4). The skull protects the brain and the organs of special sense—hearing, sight, taste, and smell. All the bones of the skull are immobile except the *mandible* (lower jawbone).

The bones of the skull are united by *sutures* (seams). In the newborn there are membranes covering two areas where bony tissue has not yet formed, leaving soft spots called *fontanels* (little fountains). The *coronal suture* separates the *frontal bone* from the two *parietal bones* and leaves a membrane-covered, diamond-shaped area, called the *anterior fontanel*, which can be seen rising and falling with the heartbeat of the infant. At the age of 10 to 18 months this fontanel closes. The *occipital fontanel*, located at the back of the head, closes by 2 months of age. The sutures, which initially are joined by cartilage to permit the growth of the brain, ossify by about 26 years of age.

Within the bones of the skull and the face are hollows called *sinuses*, which lessen the bone weight, provide resonating chambers for the voice, and moisten and warm incoming air.

STRUCTURAL DESCRIPTIVE TERMS OF BONES

canal—tunnel

condyle—rounded projection

crest, crista—high ridge

facet—small, smooth area

foramen—(plural: foramina) opening or hole

fossa, fovea—basinlike depression

head—rounded eminence or projection

line—low ridge

meatus—passage or opening

process—any projection

sinus—cavity or channel

spine—sharp projection

sulcus—open, ditchlike groove

suture—seam

trochanter—broad, flat process

tubercle—small, rounded eminence

tuberosity—protuberance (swelling or knob)

Cranial Bones

The **_frontal_** bone forms the forehead and helps form the **orbits** (eye sockets) and the front part of the cranial floor. The two cavities within this bone are called the **_frontal sinuses_**. The **coronal suture** separates the frontal from. . .

Two **_parietal_** bones, forming the roof of the skull and upper part of each side, that are separated from each other by the **_sagittal suture_**. These bones are separated from. . .

The **_occipital_** bone by the **_lambdoid suture_**. The occipital bone forms the back of the skull as well as the base. In the base is a large opening, the **_foramen magnum_** (meaning large hole or opening), for the passage of the spinal cord from the skull into the spine.

Two **_temporal_** bones form part of the cranial floor and the lower part of the sides. These bones contain the middle and inner ear structures, and the **_mastoid sinuses_**.

The **_sphenoid_**, a butterfly-shaped bone at the base of the skull, extends laterally to support parts of the orbits, and forms the lateral walls of the skull. It contains the **_sphenoid sinuses_**.

The **_ethmoid_** bone lies in front of the sphenoid but behind the nasal bones of the face, forming the front of the base of the skull, the medial walls of the orbits, and part of the roof and lateral walls of the nose. It contains the **_ethmoid sinuses_**.

Facial Bones

Two **_maxillary_** bones form the upper jaw, nose, orbits, and roof of the mouth. Located within these bones are the **_maxillary sinuses_**, which connect with the nose.

Two **_zygomatic_** or **_malar_** bones (cheekbones) have chewing muscles attached to them.

Two **_lacrimal_** bones located at the inner corners of the eyes form bony channels through which tear ducts drain into the nasal cavity.

Two **_nasal_** bones form the upper part of the bridge of the nose.

The **_vomer_** is the thin, flat bone that forms the lower part of the nasal septum. (The tip of the nose and the nostrils are composed of cartilage.)

Two **_inferior nasal conchae_** (**_turbinates_**) are ledges that form the side and lower wall of each nasal cavity.

Two **_palatine_** bones form the posterior portion of the hard palate, and the sides of the nasal cavity.

The **_mandible_**, which forms the lower jaw, is the only movable bone in the skull and is the largest and strongest bone of the face.

Hyoid Bone

The **_hyoid_** bone is a U-shaped bone in the neck. It does not form a joint with any other bone. It is located above the larynx and below the mandible and is suspended from the temporal bones by ligaments. It serves for the insertion of muscles of the tongue (hyoglossus) and floor of the mouth (mylohyoid and geniohyoid).

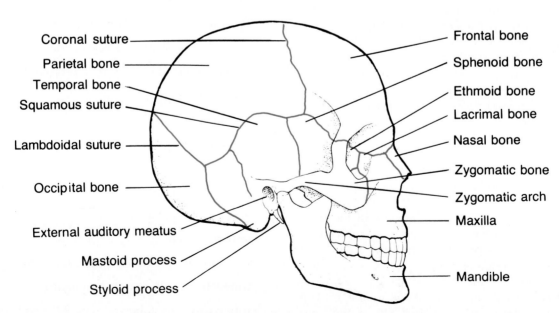

Figure 6-4.   Principal bones and sutures of the skull.

VERTEBRAL COLUMN

The vertebral or spinal column (backbone) is made up of 24 *vertebrae* (plural of *vertebra*), the *sacrum*, and the *coccyx*.

The vertebral column shelters the spinal cord, supports the skull and thorax, lends stiffening to the trunk, anchors the pelvic girdle, and provides attachment points for many of the main muscles. It is made up of:

The 7 *cervical* (neck) vertebrae, the first of which is the *atlas*, which supports the skull and rotates on the second cervical vertebra, the *axis*;

The 12 *thoracic* (chest) vertebrae, to which the ribs are attached;

The 5 *lumbar* (lower back) vertebrae, which support the lower trunk;

The *sacrum*, which is a triangular bone formed by the fusion of five vertebrae, to which the pelvic girdle is attached;

The *coccyx* (tailbone), located at the extreme tip of the vertebral column, is the result of fusion of several rudimentary vertebrae.

Each vertebra has a *body* (anterior portion) and an *arch* (posterior portion). The body bears the weight, and the arch helps to form the canal that houses the spinal cord. Between the vertebrae are *intervertebral disks*, which are made up of cartilage and serve as shock absorbers, or cushions (Figs. 6-2 and 6-3).

RIBS

There are twelve pairs of ribs, which are flat, curved bones attached posteriorly to the thoracic portion of the vertebral column. The first seven pairs are known as the *true ribs* because of their connection to the sternum by *costal* (referring to ribs) cartilages. The remaining five pairs are called *false ribs*, with the eighth, ninth, and tenth pairs joined to the cartilage of the seventh rib, and the eleventh and twelfth pairs, the so-called *floating ribs*, are unattached anteriorly. The ribs form the chest wall and protect the heart and lungs.

STERNUM

The *sternum* (breastbone) is a flat, swordshaped bone, located in the midline of the chest, to which are attached the two *clavicles* (collar bones), one on each side, and the anterior ends of the first seven pairs of ribs. The thoracic vertebrae, the ribs and costal cartilages, and the sternum make up the thoracic cage, the bony structure that protects vital organs of the chest and allows it to expand and contract during *respiration* (breathing).

Review B

Complete the following:

1. An opening or passage in bone is called a _____.

2. A sharp projection is called a _____.

3. All skull bones are immobile except for the _____.

4. _____ unite the bones of the skull.

5. The butterfly-shaped bone at the base of the skull is the _____ bone.

6. The zygomatic (malar) bones are also called _____.

7. The spinal column is made up of vertebrae, _____, and _____.

8. The three groups of vertebrae in the spinal column are the _____, _____, and _____.

9. There are _____ pairs of ribs.

10. The cushions of cartilage between the vertebrae are known as _____.

APPENDICULAR SKELETON

Upper Extremities

The bones of the upper extremities are:

The two **clavicles** (collarbones), flat bones attached, one on each side, to the scapulae laterally, and to the sternum anteriorly, forming the **sternocla-vicular joint**;

The two **scapulae** (shoulder blades), large triangular bones at the back of the thorax, one on each side, which form the shoulder girdle together with the clavicles;

The two **humerus** bones, long bones, one in each arm, extending from the shoulder to the elbow, articulating (joining) with the scapula at the shoulder, and the ulna and radius at the elbow;

The two **ulna** bones, medial long bones of the forearms, that form the elbow joints by articulation with the humerus bones at the **olecranon processes** (Fig. 6-5);

The two **radius** bones, lateral long bones of the forearms, articulate with the ulna at both ends, the humerus at the elbow, and some wrist bones to form the wrist joint.

The **wrists** (Fig. 6-5), composed of eight small, irregularly shaped **carpal** bones in two rows. The proximal row has four carpals, articulating with the radius and ulna.

Beginning on the radial side, these are:

> **scaphoid** or **navicular** (boat-shaped)
> **lunate** or **semi-lunar** (crescent-shaped)
> **triquetrum** or **pyramidale** (wedge-shaped)
> **pisiform** or **lentiform** (pea-shaped)

The distal row of four carpals, on the radial side are:

> **trapezium** or **greater multangular**
> **trapezoid** or **lesser multangular**
> **capitate** (rounded head)
> **hamate** (hooklike)

The **hands** (Fig. 6-5), are made up of:

> **metacarpals**, five long bones that articulate with the carpals, forming the palm of the hand, and articulating with the
> **phalanges** (finger bones), long bones forming the knuckle joints. Each finger has three phalanges, except for the thumb, which has two.

Lower Extremities

The bones of the lower extremities include those of the hip, thigh, leg, ankle and foot (Figs. 6-2, 6-3, and 6-6).

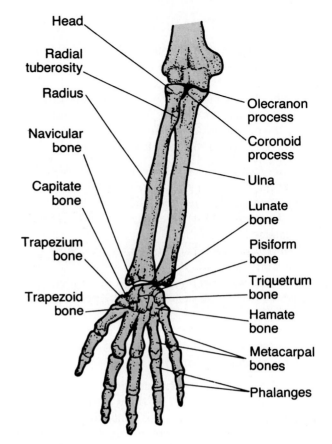

Figure 6-5.   Bones of the forearm and hand.

The **pelvic girdle** (2 **innominate bones**—hip bones) consists of three pairs of bones that fuse early in life into one solid, irregular bone. This girdle connects to the sacrum and coccyx and forms a basinlike structure that supports the trunk, affords an attachment for the lower limbs, and protects the lower abdominal organs. These three pairs of bones that fuse are:

> the **ilium**, uppermost and largest pair, flaring to the side;
> the **ischium**, lowest, strongest, and posterior pair;
> the **pubis**, most anterior pair, meets at the **symphysis pubis**, a cartilaginous joint.

The **femur** (thigh bone), the longest bone in the body, articulates with the **acetabulum** (hip socket) at the proximal end, and with the **tibia** (a lower leg bone) at the distal end. The **greater** and **lesser trochanters** are two processes on the femur, for attachment of muscles. The **lateral** and **medial condyles**, two bony prominences at the lower end of the femur, articulate with the tibia and **patella**.

The **patella** (kneecap) is a small, flat bone (resembling a thick saucer), overlapping the distal

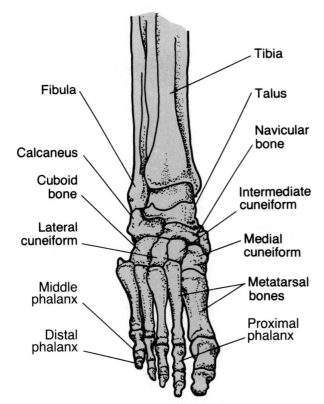

Figure 6-6. Bones of the ankle and foot.

Fibula
Calcaneus
Cuboid bone
Lateral cuneiform
Middle phalanx
Distal phalanx

Tibia
Talus
Navicular bone
Intermediate cuneiform
Medial cuneiform
Metatarsal bones
Proximal phalanx

(2) *intermediate cuneiform*—smallest of the three;

(3) *lateral cuneiform*.

The *cuboid* has a cube shape.

The *foot* bones resemble those of the hands, having:

5 *metatarsals*, forming the foot, and articulating with the *tarsals* and the *phalanges*, with the first metatarsal (on the big toe side) being the heaviest and the most weight-bearing.

14 *phalanges*, with structure and arrangement similar to those of the fingers, the great toe having two and the others three each.

JOINTS

The term applied to the study of the joints is *arthrology* (*arthr-* means joint). A joint is an articulation between bones, or bones and cartilage, held in place by ligaments of connective tissue, and may or may not permit motion between them.

Joints are classified according to the degree of movement they permit and their tissue structure, and there is a direct relationship between these two classifications.

(1) Degree of movement:

synarthroses—allow no movement.

amphiarthroses—allow slight movement.

diarthroses—freely permit movement.

(2) Tissue structure:

fibrous (synarthroses) joints contain fibrous tissue that unites bones and permits no movement. An example of this type is found in the sutures of the skull.

cartilaginous (amphiarthroses) joints contain cartilage that connects the bones and permits slight movement. Examples of this type are found in the vertebrae and the symphysis pubis.

synovial (diarthroses) joints are freely movable, the most numerous, and the most complex in the body. They have six characteristic structures:

a) *joint capsule*—forms a covering around the articulating ends of the bones, holding them to each other.

b) *synovial membrane*—lines the joint capsule, and secretes synovial fluid lubricating opposing surfaces of the bones.

c) *joint cavity*—space between the opposing surfaces of bones of the joint.

d) *articular cartilage*—thin covering of cartilage that cushions the articulating bone surfaces.

e) *ligaments*—cords of white, dense fibrous tissue that help to bind the bones together.

f) *articular disks*—pads of cartilage between articulating surfaces in some synovial joints.

end of the femur and proximal end of the tibia, and protecting the knee joint.

The *tibia* (shin bone) is the larger, more weight-bearing and medially placed bone of the two lower leg bones, articulating at its proximal end with the femur, and at its distal end with the *fibula* and the *talus*, the ankle joint bone, forming the bony prominence on the inside of the ankle, the *medial malleolus*.

The *fibula* (splint bone) is a long, slender, lateral bone, articulating on the proximal end with the tibia, and at the distal end with the tibia and talus, forming the bony prominence on the outside of the ankle, the *lateral malleolus*.

The *tarsals* (ankle bones) are seven short bones, resembling those of the wrist in structure and function, which articulate with the tibia and fibula.

The *talus* (*astragalus*) forms the ankle joint with the tibia and fibula.

The *calcaneus*, the largest tarsal, forms the heel.

The *navicular* or *scaphoid* has a boat-shape.

The *cuneiforms*, three wedge-shaped bones forming the arch of the foot and numbered from the medial side:

(1) *medial cuneiform*—largest of the three;

The movable joints are further divided into subtypes (Fig. 6-7):

hinge joints—those that permit movement in only one direction, as in the elbow and the knee.

ball-and-socket joints—the round head of one bone fits into a cuplike cavity of another, permitting movement in different directions, as in the joint of the femur and the hipbone.

gliding joints—the least movable of this group, in which the adjacent bone surfaces glide upon each other to permit movement, such as that of the wrists and ankles.

pivot (rotary) joints—one bone pivots around a stationary bone, such as the axis and atlas (cervical vertebrae).

condyloid (knuckle) joints—the oval head of one bone fits into a shallow depression in another, such as the union between the radius and the carpal bones.

Not all joints can perform all the movements listed in the accompanying box. The immovable joints are incapable of performing any of them. Of the freely movable joints, only the ball-and-socket can perform all the movements listed. The hinge joints are able to perform only flexion and extension. The slightly movable joints can perform rotation.

BURSAE

The ***bursae*** are sacs of connective tissue lined with synovial membrane and filled with synovial fluid. Synovial fluid relieves pressure between moving parts. Bursae become inflamed (bursitis) in areas such as the patella (housemaid's knee) and the olecranon process (tennis elbow).

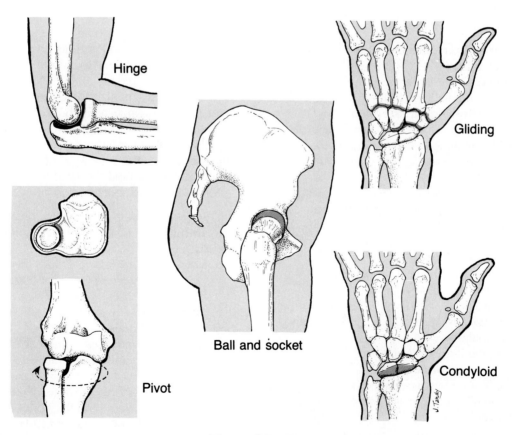

Figure 6-7.   Joints.

TYPES OF MOVEMENT

The following are descriptive terms for defining the different types of motion.

flexion—bending at a joint, as the forearm or elbow.

extension—straightening, or unbending, of a joint; this movement is the opposite of flexion.

abduction—movement that draws a body part away from the midline of the body, such as the extension of the arms straight out from the shoulders.

adduction—movement that draws the body part toward the midline of the body, such as returning the extended arms.

rotation—movement that turns a body part on its own axis; for example, the turning of the head.

pronation—turning down or downward; for example, turning the palm of the hand downward.

supination—turning upward; for example, turning the palm upward.

eversion—turning outward.

inversion—turning inward.

circumduction—a movement describing a circle, such as with an outstretched arm.

Review C

Complete the following:

1. The collar bones are called _____.

2. The shoulder blades are called _____.

3. The long bones of the arm are the _____, _____, and _____.

4. The eight carpal bones are located in the _____.

5. The pelvic girdle is formed by the _____, _____, and _____.

6. The patella is the _____.

7. The seven ankle bones are called _____.

8. Fibrous joints allow _____ movement, cartilaginous joints allow _____ movement, and synovial joints allow _____ movement.

9. The most movable type of joint in the body is the _____ joint.

10. The bending of a joint is called _____.

Answers to Review Questions: The Skeletal System

Review A
1. 206
2. diaphysis
3. medullary
4. periosteum
5. osteoblasts
6. long, flat, short, irregular
7. long
8. short
9. axial, appendicular
10. hyoid

Review B
1. meatus
2. spine
3. mandible (lower jaw bone)
4. sutures
5. sphenoid
6. cheekbones
7. sacrum, coccyx
8. cervical, thoracic, lumbar
9. 12
10. Intervertebral disks

Review C
1. clavicles
2. scapulae
3. humerus, ulna, radius
4. wrist
5. ilium, ischium, pubis
6. kneecap
7. tarsals
8. no, slight, free
9. ball-and-socket
10. flexion

CHAPTER 6 EXERCISES

SKELETAL SYSTEM: THE FRAMEWORK OF THE BODY

Exercise 1: Complete the following:

1. The hard outer shell of bone is called _____.

2. The inner lattice-like, spongy structure of bone is called _____ bone.

3. The shaft of long bone is called _____.

4. The developing ends of long bones are called _____.

5. The names of the anatomic classifications of the skeleton are _____ and _____.

Exercise 2: Classify the following bones according to shape.

1. humerus _____

2. wrist _____

3. ankle bone _____

4. sternum _____

5. scapula _____

Exercise 3: Multiple choice:
1. Which of the following bones is the only movable one in the skull?
   a. frontal
   b. mandible
   c. ear ossicles
   d. maxillary
2. In which of the following bones are the mastoid sinuses located?
   a. frontal
   b. parietal
   c. temporal
   d. sphenoid
3. Which is the butterfly-shaped bone of the skull?
   a. ethmoid
   b. sphenoid
   c. occipital
   d. frontal
4. Which bones form the posterior portion of the hard palate?
   a. turbinates
   b. palatines
   c. lacrimals
   d. zygomatics
5. What does the sagittal suture separate?
   a. the eye sockets
   b. the parietals
   c. frontal sinuses
   d. the temporals

Exercise 4: Matching:

____ 1. periosteum   A. seam

____ 2. red bone marrow   B. tough fibrous membrane covering

____ 3. osteoblast   C. phagocytic cell

____ 4. osteoclast   D. immature bone cell

____ 5. fossa   E. small, smooth area

____ 6. sulcus   F. basin-like depression

____ 7. facet   G. high ridge

____ 8. crista   H. hematopoietic tissue

____ 9. suture   I. opening or hole

____10. foramen   J. open, ditch-like groove

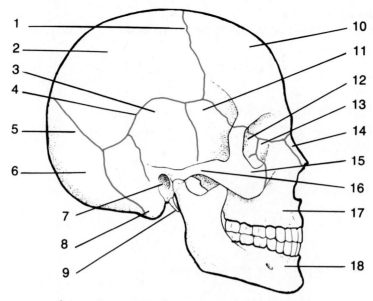

Figure 6-8.   Principal bones and sutures of the skull.

Exercise 5: Using the list of terms below, identify each part in Fig. 6-8 by writing its name in the corresponding blank.

Coronal suture	1. _____
Maxilla	2. _____
Zygomatic bone	3. _____
Parietal bone	4. _____
Squamous suture	5. _____
External auditory meatus	6. _____
Lacrimal bone	7. _____
Sphenoid bone	8. _____
Nasal bone	9. _____
Occipital bone	10. _____
Mastoid process	11. _____
Zygomatic arch	12. _____
Temporal bone	13. _____
Lambdoidal suture	14. _____
Frontal bone	15. _____
Styloid process	16. _____
Ethmoid bone	17. _____
Mandible	18. _____

Exercise 6: Using the list of terms below, identify each bone in Figs. 6-9 and 6-10 by writing its name in the corresponding blank. (Some of these terms may be shown more than once.)

Acromion
Carpals
Cervical vertebrae
Clavicle
Coccyx
Costal cartilage
Cranium
Femur
Fibula
Greater trochanter
Humerus
Ilium
Innominate bone

Ischium
Lesser trochanter
Lumbar vertebrae
Mandible
Maxilla
Metacarpals
Metatarsals
Occipital bone
Olecranon process of ulna
Orbit
Patella
Parietal bone

Phalanges
Pubis
Radius
Sacrum
Scapula
Sternum
Tarsals
Thoracic vertebrae
Tibia
Ulna
Vertebral column
Xiphoid process

1. _____

2. _____

3. _____

4. _____

5. _____

6. _____

7. _____

8. _____

9. _____

10. _____

11. _____

12. _____

13. _____

14. _____

15. _____

16. _____

17. _____

18. _____

19. _____

20. _____

21. _____

22. _____

23. _____

24. _____

25. _____

26. _____

27. _____

28. _____

29. _____

30. _____

31. _____

32. _____

33. _____

34. _____

35. _____

36. _____

37. _____

38. _____

39. _____

40. _____

41. _____

42. _____

43. _____

44. _____

45. _____

46. _____

47. _____

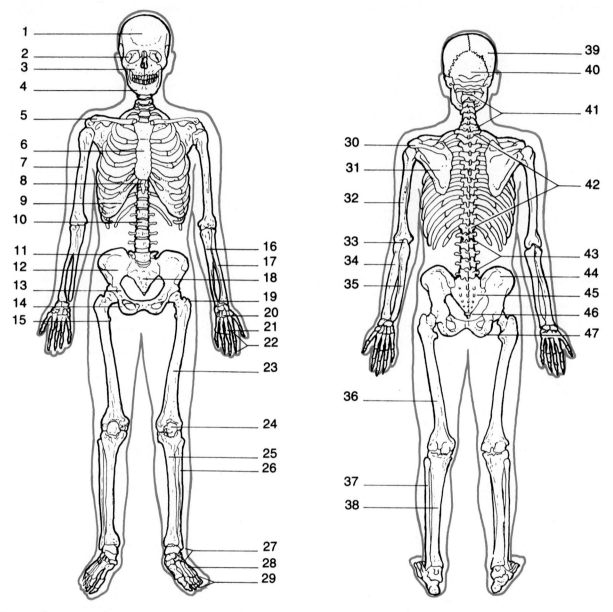

Figure 6-9.   **Skeleton, anterior view (anatomic position).**

Figure 6-10.   **Skeleton, posterior view (anatomic position).**

Exercise 7: Matching:

____ **1.** sacrum	**A.**	extreme tip of vertebral column
____ **2.** clavicle	**B.**	jawbone
____ **3.** femur	**C.**	smaller bone of lower leg
____ **4.** humerus	**D.**	large weight-bearing bone of lower leg
____ **5.** sternum	**E.**	collar bone
____ **6.** zygomatic (or malar)	**F.**	a nasal bone
____ **7.** patella	**G.**	shoulder blade
____ **8.** coccyx	**H.**	next to last vertebral bone
____ **9.** scapula	**I.**	thigh bone
____ **10.** vomer	**J.**	kneecap
____ **11.** tibia	**K.**	medial long bone of the forearm
____ **12.** mandible	**L.**	breastbone
____ **13.** fibula	**M.**	lateral long bone of forearm
____ **14.** pubis	**N.**	small, lower, strongest portion of pelvic bone
____ **15.** ischium	**O.**	broad upper portion of pelvic girdle
____ **16.** carpals	**P.**	ankle bones
____ **17.** ilium	**Q.**	most anterior part of pelvic girdle
____ **18.** tarsals	**R.**	wrist bones
____ **19.** radius	**S.**	upper arm bone
____ **20.** ulna	**T.**	a cheek bone

Exercise 8: Using the list of terms below, identify each bone in Fig. 6-11 by writing its name in the corresponding blank.

Capitate bone
Trapezoid bone
Hamate bone
Olecranon process
Trapezium bone
Head

Navicular bone
Radial tuberosity
Phalanges
Ulna
Coronoid process

Lunate bone
Radius
Pisiform bone
Triquetrum bone
Metacarpal bones

1. _____
2. _____
3. _____
4. _____
5. _____
6. _____
7. _____
8. _____
9. _____
10. _____
11. _____
12. _____
13. _____
14. _____
15. _____
16. _____

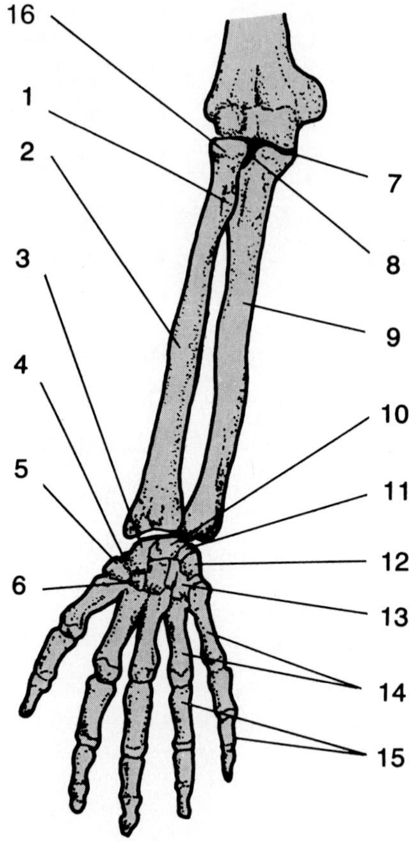

Figure 6-11. Bones of the forearm and hand.

Exercise 9: Using the list of terms below, identify each bone in Fig. 6-12 by writing its name in the corresponding blank.

Cuboid bone   Middle phalanx   Talus
Fibula   Metatarsal bones   Intermediate cuneiform
Proximal phalanx   Lateral cuneiform   Distal phalanx
Medial cuneiform   Tibia   Calcaneus
Navicular bone

1. _____
2. _____
3. _____
4. _____
5. _____
6. _____
7. _____
8. _____
9. _____
10. _____
11. _____
12. _____
13. _____

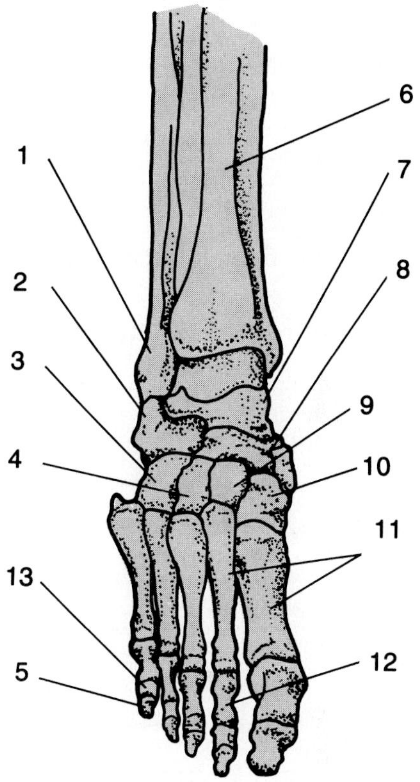

Figure 6-12. **Bones of the ankle and foot.**

Exercise 10: Complete the following:

1. Freely movable joints are classified as _____.

2. Slightly movable joints are classified as _____.

3. Immovable joints are classified as _____.

4. The bones that enter into the formation of the foot articulating with the tarsals and the phalanges are called

   _____.

5. A _____ joint permits movement in different directions.

6. A _____ joint is one in which the adjacent bone surfaces glide upon each other to permit movement.

7. Joints are described according to tissue structure as three types: _____, _____, and

   _____.

8. The cartilages attaching the first seven pairs of ribs to the sternum are _____ cartilages.

9. When movement is permitted in only one direction, the joint is called a _____ joint.

10. The sacs that contain synovial fluid, relieving pressure on moving parts, are called _____.

Exercise 11: Define each of the following different types of motion.

1. flexion _____.

2. extension _____.

3. abduction _____.

4. adduction _____.

5. rotation _____.

6. pronation _____.

7. supination _____.

8. circumduction _____.

9. eversion _____.

10. inversion _____.

Exercise 12: Give the meaning of the components of the following words and then define the word as a whole. Suffixes meaning *pertaining to* or *state or condition,* shown following a slash mark (/), are not to be defined separately. Before reaching for your medical dictionary, check the glossary at the end of the chapter.

1. Carpometacarpal:

    carpo_____

    metacarp/al_____

    _____

2. Costosternal:

    costo_____

    stern/al_____

    _____

3. Interphalangeal:

    inter_____

    phalange/al_____

    _____

4. Radiocarpal:

    radio_____

    carp/al_____

    _____

5. Talonavicular:

    talo_____

    navicul/ar_____

    _____

6. Temporomandibular:

    temporo_____

    mandibul/ar_____

    _____

7. Sacroiliac:

    sacro_____

    iliac_____

    _____

8. cuneocuboid:

    cuneo_____

    cuboid_____

    _____

9. Osteomyelitis:

    osteo_____

    myel_____

    itis_____

    _____

10. Spondylarthritis:

    spondlyl_____

    arthr_____

    itis_____

    _____

11. Amelia:

    a_____

    mel/ia_____

    _____

12. Anencephalia:

    an_____

    encephal/ia_____

    _____

13. Osteoarthritis:

    osteo_____

    arthr_____

    itis_____

    _____

14. Osteodystrophy:

    osteo_____

    dys_____

    troph/y_____

    _____

15. Osteolysis:

    osteo_____

    lysis_____

    _____

Chapter 6 Crossword Puzzle

Across
6. fluid-filled sacs
7. shoulder blades
8. upper arm bone
9. U-shaped bone in neck
10. hip socket
12. hollow within skull or face bones
15. chest vertebrae
17. membrane covering bone
18. long, lateral bone of lower leg
20. referring to backbone
22. an opening or hole in bone
25. one of two forearm bones
26. crescent-shaped carpal bone
27. kneecap
28. lower back vertebrae

Down
1. posterior portion of a vertebra
2. thigh bone
3. one of the seven tarsal bones
4. contained in medullary cavities
5. ankle bones
6. anterior portion of a vertebra
7. breastbone
10. study of joints
11. neck vertebrae
12. triangular bone of spine
13. one main part of skeleton
14. 206 bones
16. collarbone
19. shinbone
21. hook-like carpal bone
23. other main part of skeleton
24. tunnel

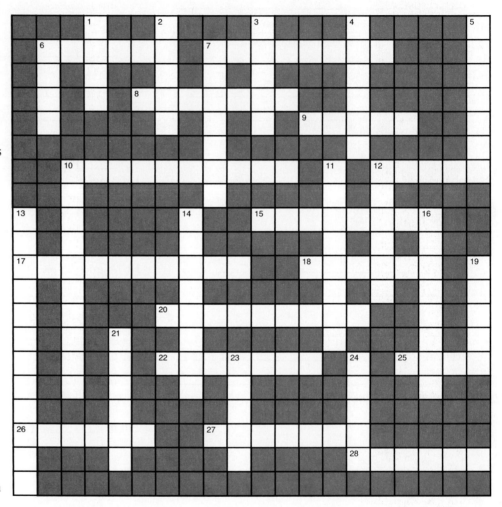

Chapter 6 Hidden Words Puzzle

```
S  L  L  A  R  O  Z  S  R  O  X  P  H  A  C  B  N  B  E  O
D  I  A  P  H  Y  S  I  S  B  R  V  O  W  V  M  T  F  F  Q
Y  B  S  G  V  M  S  T  E  R  N  U  M  E  U  K  C  Y  C  D
N  D  P  X  C  A  N  C  E  L  L  O  U  S  K  T  U  Z  O  R
I  Y  G  Z  M  M  Y  J  X  O  B  U  S  E  J  G  U  P  Y  B
E  O  H  Q  U  O  X  H  T  P  B  F  A  K  F  K  J  A  Y  D
V  M  E  D  U  L  L  A  R  Y  U  L  O  K  E  W  H  Q  V  W
Q  E  P  I  P  H  Y  S  E  S  R  M  A  X  I  L  L  A  R  Y
F  P  R  P  J  O  E  R  M  E  S  A  F  S  J  Y  E  G  H  P
M  R  T  T  E  O  R  L  I  R  A  K  X  K  T  S  T  T  Y  W
H  M  O  R  E  R  U  R  T  P  E  L  V  I  S  S  C  Q  O  S
R  V  C  N  I  B  I  E  I  W  Y  Y  V  K  A  Y  L  A  I  N
D  J  F  H  T  P  R  O  E  W  R  P  K  V  Z  L  K  U  D  J
I  T  X  U  E  A  N  A  S  T  O  M  O  S  E  S  F  Y  V  M
X  C  W  T  N  R  L  L  E  T  T  S  C  A  P  U  L  A  L  P
W  P  Q  B  P  I  I  X  H  H  E  Q  T  K  T  D  G  I  Z  Q
H  O  K  H  C  E  N  V  J  Z  I  U  Y  E  O  T  E  I  G  V
X  F  G  E  E  T  C  A  B  F  D  S  M  M  O  K  E  W  N  B
N  D  W  Z  R  A  C  F  Y  M  T  V  V  H  D  L  T  L  V  R
U  H  Q  R  Z  L  S  P  E  N  K  V  R  I  X  S  O  B  S  R
D  F  J  X  G  O  L  I  E  O  G  N  C  M  R  Z  Q  G  G  J
F  K  X  T  C  U  B  R  N  D  P  Y  J  V  T  J  N  J  Y  L
```

Can you find the 20 words hidden in this puzzle? All hidden word puzzles will
have words running from top to bottom, left to right, and diagonally downward.

ANASTOMOSES	EXTREMITIES	OSTEOBLASTS	CANCELLOUS
PERIOSTEUM	DIAPHYSIS	EPIPHYSES	MAXILLARY
MEDULLARY	OSTEOLOGY	VERTEBRAE	PARIETAL
SKELETON	FRONTAL	SCAPULA	STERNUM
BURSAE	PELVIS	AXIAL	HYOID

CHAPTER 6 ANSWERS

Exercise 1
1. compact bone tissue
2. cancellated or cancellous bone
3. diaphysis
4. epiphyses
5. appendicular, axial

Exercise 2
1. long
2. short
3. short
4. flat
5. flat

Exercise 3
1. mandible
2. temporal
3. sphenoid
4. palatines
5. parietals

Exercise 4
1. B   6. J
2. H   7. E
3. D   8. G
4. C   9. A
5. F   10. I

Exercise 5
1. coronal suture   10. frontal bone
2. parietal bone   11. sphenoid bone
3. temporal bone   12. ethmoid bone
4. squamous suture   13. lacrimal bone
5. lambdoidal suture   14. nasal bone
6. occipital bone   15. zygomatic or malar bone
7. external auditory meatus 16. zygomatic arch
8. mastoid process   17. maxilla
9. styloid process   18. mandible

Exercise 6
1. cranium
2. orbit
3. maxilla
4. mandible
5. clavicle
6. sternum
7. humerus
8. xiphoid process
9. costal cartilage
10. vertebral column
11. innominate bone
12. ilium
13. pubis
14. ischium
15. lesser trochanter
16. ulna
17. radius
18. sacrum
19. greater trochanter
20. carpals
21. metacarpals
22. phalanges
23. femur
24. patella
25. tibia
26. fibula
27. tarsals
28. metatarsals
29. phalanges
30. acromion
31. scapula
32. humerus
33. olecranon process of ulna
34. radius
35. ulna
36. femur
37. fibula
38. tibia
39. parietal bone
40. occipital bone
41. cervical vertebrae
42. thoracic vertebrae
43. lumbar vertebrae
44. ilium
45. sacrum
46. coccyx
47. ischium

Exercise 7
1. H
2. E
3. I
4. S
5. L
6. T
7. J
8. A
9. G
10. F
11. D
12. B
13. C
14. Q
15. N
16. R
17. O
18. P
19. M
20. K

Exercise 8
1. radial tuberosity
2. radius
3. navicular bone
4. capitate bone
5. trapezium bone
6. trapezoid bone
7. olecranon process
8. coronoid process
9. ulna
10. lunate bone
11. pisiform bone
12. triquetrum bone
13. hamate bone
14. metacarpal bones
15. phalanges
16. head

Exercise 9

1. fibula
2. calcaneus
3. cuboid bone
4. lateral cuneiform
5. distal phalanx
6. tibia
7. talus
8. navicular bone
9. intermediate cuneiform
10. medial cuneiform
11. metatarsal bones
12. proximal phalanx
13. middle phalanx

Exercise 10

1. diarthroses
2. amphiarthroses
3. synarthroses
4. metatarsals
5. ball-and-socket
6. gliding
7. synovial, fibrous, cartilaginous
8. costal
9. hinge
10. bursae

Exercise 11

1. bending of joint (such as an elbow)
2. straightening, or unbending (a joint)
3. drawing of a body part away from the midline (of the body)
4. drawing of a displaced body part toward midline (of the body)
5. turning of a body part on its own axis
6. turning down or downward
7. turning upward
8. movement describing a circle (as with an outstretched arm)
9. turning outward
10. turning inward

Exercise 12

1. carpometacarpal: wrist; between wrist and fingers—junction between wrist and bones, forming the palm of hand
2. costosternal: ribs; sternum—junction of ribs with sternum
3. interphalangeal: between; fingers or toes (phalanges)—articulation between phalanges
4. radiocarpal: radius; wrist—articulation between wrist and radius, or forearm bone
5. talonavicular: talus, astragalus, or ankle bone; navicular bone—articulation between talus (ankle bone) and navicular bone
6. temporomandibular: temporal; mandible—articulation between temporal bone and mandible, or jawbone
7. sacroiliac: sacrum; ilium—joint between sacrum and ilium
8. cuneocuboid: cuneiform; cuboid—junction between cuneiform and cuboid bones
9. osteomyelitis: bone; marrow; inflammation or infection—inflammation or infection of bone; it may spread through bone to involve the marrow
10. spondylarthritis: vertebrae or spine; joint; inflammation—arthritis of spine or inflammation of vertebrae
11. amelia: no or not; limbs—absence of a limb or limbs
12. anencephalia: no or not; brain—developmental anomaly with absence of cranial vault and cerebral hemispheres
13. osteoarthritis: bone; joint; inflammation—degenerative joint disease; inflammation of bone joint
14. osteodystrophy: bone; bad, difficult, disordered; nutrition or nourishment—defective bone formation
15. osteolysis: bone; dissolution—dissolution of bone

Answers: Chapter 6 Crossword Puzzle

			(1) A			(2) F				(3) T				(4) M					(5) T
	(6) B	U	R	S	A	E		(7) S	C	A	P	U	L	A	E				A
	O		C			M		T		L				R					R
	D		H		(8) H	U	M	E	R	U	S			R					S
	Y					R		R		S		(9) H	Y	O	I	D			A
								N						W					L
		(10) A	C	E	T	A	B	U	L	U	M		(11) C		(12) S	I	N	U	S
		R						M					E		A				
(13) A		T					(14) S			(15) T	H	O	R	A	C	I	(16) C		
P		H					K						V		R		L		
(17) P	E	R	I	O	S	T	E	U	M			(18) F	I	B	U	L	A		(19) T
E		O					L						C		M		V		I
N		L				(20) V	E	R	T	E	B	R	A	L			I		B
D		O		(21) H			T						L				C		I
I		G		A		(22) F	O	R	(23) A	M	E	N		(24) C		(25) U	L	N	A
C		Y		M			N		X					A			E		
U				A					I					N					
(26) L	U	N	A	T	E			(27) P	A	T	E	L	L	A					
A				E					L					(28) L	U	M	B	A	R
R																			

Answers: Chapter 6 Hidden Words Puzzle

```
.    .    .    .    .    O    .    .    .    .    .    .    .    .    .    .    .    .
D    I    A    P    H    Y    S    I    S    .    .    .    .    .    .    .    .    .
.    .    .    .    .    .    S    T    E    R    N    U    M    .    .    .    .    .
.    .    .    .    C    A    N    C    E    L    L    O    U    S    .    .    .    .
.    .    .    .    .    .    .    .    X    O    .    .    S    .    .    .    .    .
.    .    .    .    .    .    .    .    T    .    B    .    .    .    K    .    .    .
V    M    E    D    U    L    L    A    R    Y    U    L    .    .    E    .    .    .
.    E    P    I    P    H    Y    S    E    S    R    M    A    X    I    L    L    A    R    Y
F    .    R    P    .    .    .    .    M    .    S    A    .    S    .    .    E    .    H    .
.    R    .    T    E    .    .    .    I    .    A    .    X    .    T    .    .    T    Y    .
.    .    O    .    E    R    .    .    T    P    E    L    V    I    S    S    .    .    O    .
.    .    .    N    .    B    I    .    I    .    .    .    .    .    A    .    .    .    I    N
.    .    .    .    T    P    R    O    E    .    .    .    M    O    S    E    S    .    D    .
.    .    .    .    .    A    N    A    S    T    O    M    O    S    E    S    .    .    .    .
.    .    .    .    .    R    L    .    E    T    .    S    C    A    P    U    L    A    .    .
.    .    .    .    .    I    .    .    .    .    E    .    T    .    .    .    .    .    .    .
.    .    .    .    .    E    .    .    .    .    .    U    .    E    .    .    .    .    .    .
.    .    .    .    .    T    .    .    .    .    .    M    .    O    .    .    .    .    .    .
.    .    .    .    .    A    .    .    .    .    .    .    .    .    .    .    L    .    .    .
.    .    .    .    .    L    .    .    .    .    .    .    .    .    .    O    .    .    .    .
.    .    .    .    .    .    .    .    .    .    .    .    .    .    .    .    G    .    .    .
.    .    .    .    .    .    .    .    .    .    .    .    .    .    .    Y    .    .    .    .
```

Words:

> ANASTOMOSES	∨ EXTREMITIES	\ OSTEOBLASTS	> AXIAL
\ PERIOSTEUM	> DIAPHYSIS	> EPIPHYSES	> MAXILLARY
> MEDULLARY	\ OSTEOLOGY	\ VERTEBRAE	∨ PARIETAL
\ SKELETON	\ FRONTAL	> SCAPULA	> STERNUM
∨ BURSAE	> PELVIS	> CANCELLOUS	∨ HYOID

CHAPTER 6 GLOSSARY

Bones and Related Anatomic Terms

acetabulum (as″e-tab′ul-um): a cup-shaped socket in the hip joint (plural—*acetabula*).

acromion (ak-kro′me-on): outward extension of the spine of the shoulder blade forming the point of the shoulder (also called *acromial process*).

anastomosis (ah-nas″to-mo′sis): joining of blood vessels or other tubular structures (plural—*anastomoses*).

astragalus (as-trag′ah-lus): ankle bone (also called *talus*).

atlanto-: combining form referring to the *atlas*.

atlas (at′las): first cervical vertebra.

axis: second cervical vertebra.

calcaneus (kal-ka′ne-us): heel bone (also called *calcaneum*).

calvaria (kal-va′re-ah): skullcap.

capitate (kap′i-tate): a bone of the wrist.

carpus (kar′pus): any wrist bone.

clavicle (klav′i-k′l): collar bone.

coccyx (kok′siks): tailbone of the spinal column.

condyle (kon′dile): a rounded projection at the end of an articulating bone (such as the tibia or humerus).

coronal suture: suture formed by the frontal bone with the two parietal bones.

cubitus (ku′bi-tus): the forearm.

cuboid: cube-shaped bone on the outer side of the tarsus, between the calcaneus and the metatarsals.

cuneiforms (ku-ne′i-formz): three wedge-shaped bones in the foot.

diaphysis (di-af′i-sis): central part of the bone shaft.

epiphysis (e-pif′i-sis): end part of developing bone.

epicondyle (ep″i-kon′dile): a projection on a bone above its condyle.

ethmoid: bone of the skull behind the nose and between the orbits.

femur (fe′mur): thigh bone.

fibula (fib′u-lah): outer and smaller of the two lower leg bones.

fontanel, fontanelle (fon-tah-nel′): unossified areas (soft spots) of the cranium of an infant.

foramen magnum (fo-ra′men): large opening in the occipital bone at the base of the skull connecting the cranial cavity to the vertebral canal.

frontal bone: bone forming forepart of the cranium.

hamate (hah′mate): a bone of the wrist (also called *unciform*).

haversian canals (ha-ver′shan): network of canals in compact bone that contain blood and lymph vessels, nerves, and connective tissue (named after their discoverer).

humerus (hu′mer-us): upper arm bone.

hyoid (hi′oid): U-shaped bone located at the base of the tongue just above the thyroid cartilage.

ilium (il′e-um): pelvic bone.

incus (ing′kus): middle ossicle of the ear (resembling an anvil).

innominate (i-nom′i-nate): hip bone, including the ilium, ischium, and pubic bones (pelvic bones).

ischium (is′ki-um): pelvic bone.

lacuna (lah-ku′nah): a space (plural—*lacunae*).

lacrimal (lak′ri-mal): bone lying within medial angle of the orbit.

lambdoid suture (lam′doid): suture separating the occipital and parietal bones of the cranium.

lamella (lah-mel′ah): thin plate of bone (plural—*lamellae*).

lamina (lam′i-nah): thin plate or layer.

lentiform (len′ti-form): pea-shaped bone of the wrist (also called *pisiform*).

lunate (lu′nate): crescent-shaped bone of the wrist (also called *semilunar*).

malar (ma′lar): cheek bone (also called *zygomatic*).

malleolus (mal-le′o-lus): medial and lateral prominences on either side of the ankle joint.

malleus (mal′e-us): largest, hammer-shaped bone of the ossicles of the ear, attached to the tympanic membrane (eardrum).

mandible (man′di-b′l): lower jawbone.

manubrium (mah-nu′bre-um): uppermost portion of the sternum (plural—*manubria*).

mastoid process (mas′toid): process of the temporal bone located behind the ear (sometimes referred to as the *mastoid bone*).

metacarpal (met″ah-kar′pal): one of five bones of the hand.

metaphysis (me-taf′i-sis): area of spongy bone between the epiphyseal plate and diaphysis of long bone.

metatarsal (met″ah-tar′sal): foot bones between ankles and toes.

navicular (nah-vik′u-lar): boat-shaped bone of wrist or foot.

occipital (ok-sip′i-tal): bone forming back of skull.

olecranon (o-lek′rah-non): curved process of the ulna at the elbow.

ossein (os′e-in): organic content of bone.

ossicle (os′ik-ul): any small bone.

osteoblast (os′te-o-blast): bone-forming cell.

osteoclast (os′te-o-klast): remodeling cell of bone.

osteocyte (os′te-o-sit): bone cell (also called *osseous cell*).

osteogenesis (os″te-o-jen′e-sis): production of bone.

palate (pal′at): irregular bones forming a separation between the oral and nasal cavities.

parietal (pah-ri′e-tal): two bones forming the lateral surfaces of the cranium.

patella (pah-tel′ah): kneecap.

pelvic girdle: arch formed by the innominate bones.

periosteum (per″e-os′te-um): membrane covering bone.

phalanges (fa-lan′jez): bones of toes or fingers (singular—***phalanx***).

pisiform (pi′si-form): pea-shaped bone of the wrist (see ***lentiform***).

pubis: pubic bone (also called ***os pubis***).

pyramidale (pi-ram″i-da′le): wedge-shaped bone at the inner side of the wrist (also called ***os triquetrum***).

radius (ra′de-us): forearm bone.

sacrum (sa′krum): wedge-shaped bone of spinal column, just above the coccyx.

sagittal suture (saj′i-tal): suture between the parietal bones.

scaphoid (skaf′oid): boat-shaped bone of wrist or foot (see ***navicular***).

scapula (skap′u-lah): shoulder blade (plural—***scapulae***).

semilunar: crescent-shaped, carpal bone (also called ***lunate***).

sesamoid (ses′ah-moid): any small flat bone embedded in a tendon or joint capsule. (The patella is the largest sesamoid in the body.)

shoulder girdle: formed by clavicle and scapula.

sphenoid (sfe′noid): wedge-shaped bone at the base of the skull.

squamous suture (skwa′mus): suture between the parietal and temporal bones on the lateral side of the cranium and between the lower lateral portions of the occipital and temporal bones.

stapes (sta′pez): stirrup-shaped, innermost auditory ossicles.

sternum (ster′num): breastbone. The body of the sternum is called the ***gladiolus*** (glah-di′o-lus); the process at the lower end is called the ***xyphoid*** (zif′oid) ***process***; and the uppermost portion is called the ***manubrium***.

styloid process (sti′loid): projection on the distal end of the radius and the ulna.

substantia spongiosa ossium (sub-stan′she-ah spon″je-o′sah): inner spongy layer of bone.

symphysis pubis (sim′fi-sis): cartilaginous joint between pubic bones.

talus (ta′lus): ankle bone (see ***astragalus***).

tarsals (tar′salz): seven short bones of the ankle.

temporal: two irregular bones forming the sides and base of the skull.

tibia (tib′e-ah): larger of the two lower leg bones (shinbone).

trapezium (trah-pe′ze-um): wrist bone on the radial side.

trapezoid (trap′e-zoid): bone of the wrist.

triquetrum (tri-kwe′trum): wedge-shaped bone of the wrist (also called ***pyramidale***).

trochanter (tro-kan′ter): greater and lesser processes for attachment of muscles of the femur.

turbinate (tur′bi-nate): bone on lower side of nasal cavity (also called ***concha nasalis***).

ulna (ul′nah): forearm bone.

unciform (in′si-form): see ***hamate*** bone.

vertebra (ver′ta-brah): spinal column bone. (plural—***vertebrae***).

vomer (vo′mer): thin, flat bone forming lower part of nasal septum.

zygomatic (zi′go-mat′ik): cheek bone, or ***malar*** bone.

Cartilage and Related Anatomic Terms

alar (a′lar): winglike; greater and lesser cartilages of the nose.

articular: thin layer of hyaline cartilage on joint surfaces.

bursae: synovial fluid-filled connective tissue sacs.

calcified: cartilage containing calcium or calcareous matter.

costal: cartilage attaching ribs to the sternum and other ribs.

elastic: cartilage that is more flexible and elastic than hyaline cartilage.

epiphysial (ep′i-fiz′e-al): cartilage between epiphysis and diaphysis.

hyaline (hi′a-lin): flexible, glassy, translucent cartilage

nasal: cartilage of the nose.

semilunar: interarticular cartilage of the knee joint.

septal: cartilage of the nose.

sternal: cartilage connecting ribs to the sternum.

Joints and Related Anatomic Terms

acromioclavicular: junction between acromion and clavicle.

amphiarthroses (am″fe-ar-thro′sez): slightly movable joints.

arthrology: study of joints.

articulation (ar-tik″u-la′shun): junction between bones.

atlantoaxial: joint between atlas and axis.

ball-and-socket joint: round head of one bone fits into cavity of another, permitting movement in different directions.

calcaneo-astragaloid (kal-ka″ne-o-ah-strag′ah-loid): junction between calcaneus and astragalus.

calcaneocuboid (kal-ka″ne-o-ku′boid): junction between calcaneus and cuboid bone.

calcaneofibular (kal-ka″ne-o-fib′u-lar): junction between calcaneus and fibula.

calcaneonavicular (kal-ka″ne-o-nah-vik′u-lar): junction between calcaneus and navicular bone (also called ***calcaneoscaphoid***).

calcaneotibial (kal-ka″ne-o-tib′e-al): junction between calcaneus and tibia.

carpometacarpal (kar″po-met″ah-kar′pal): junction between carpus and metacarpal bone.

costosternal: junction of ribs with sternum.

costovertebral: junction of ribs with vertebrae.

coxal: referring to the hip joint.

cubital: referring to elbow joint.

cuboidonavicular: junction between cuboid and navicular.

cuneocuboid (ku″ne-o-ku′boid): junction between cuneiform and cuboid.

cuneoscaphoid (ku″ne-o-skaf′oid): junction between cuneiform and scaphoid (also called ***cuneonavicular***).

diarthroses (di″ar-thro′sez): freely movable joints.

hinge joint: movement permitted in only one plane, as in the elbow.

hip joint: articulation of femur with pelvic bones.

humeroradial (hu″mer-o-ra′de-al): junction between humerus and radius.

humeroscapular (hu″mer-o-skap′u-lar): articulation between humerus and scapula (also called ***scapulohumeral***).

humeroulnar (hu″mer-o-ul′nar): articulation between humerus and ulna.

intercarpal: articulation between carpal bones.

interphalangeal (in″ter-fah-lan′je-al): articulation between phalanges.

intertarsal: articulation between tarsal bones.

knee joint: articulation between upper and lower leg bones at knee.

lumbosacral: junction between sacrum and lumbar vertebrae.

metacarpophalangeal: junction between metacarpus and phalanges.

metatarsophalangeal: junction between metatarsus and phalanges.

pivot joint: one bone rotates over another.

radiocarpal: articulation between carpus and radius.

radioulnar: articulation between radius and ulna.

sacrococcygeal: junction between sacrum and coccyx.

sacroiliac (sa″kro-il′e-ak): joint between sacrum and ilium.

scapuloclavicular (skap″u-lo-klah-vik′u-lar): junction between scapula and clavicle.

sternoclavicular (ster″no-klah-vik′u-lar): junction between sternum and clavicle (also called ***sternocleidal***).

sternocostal: junction between sternum and ribs.

synarthroses (sin″ar-thro′sez): immovable joints.

synovial (si-no-ve-al): pertaining to the lubricating fluid secreted by the synovial membrane and contained in joint cavities, bursae, and tendon sheaths.

talocalcaneal: articulation between the talus (astragalus) and the calcaneus.

talofibular: articulation between the talus and fibula.

talonavicular (ta″lo-nah-vik′u-lar): articulation between talus and navicular (scaphoid) bone (also called ***taloscaphoid***).

tarsometatarsal: articulation between tarsals and metatarsals.

temporomandibular (tem″po-ro-man-dib′u-lar): articulation between mandible and temporal bone.

tibiofibular: articulation between tibia and fibula at ankle and knee.

tibiotarsal: articulation between tibia and tarsal bones.

Pathologic Conditions

Inflammation and Infections

Inflammations are characterized by pain, heat, redness, and swelling and may be accompanied by exudations. Inflammation is a condition resulting from injury to tissues, but not all inflammations are infections. *Infection* is an invasion of the body by pathogenic microorganisms to which tissues react. The term infection is generally applied to invasion by bacteria, viruses, protozoa, and helminths. These terms will be used in this sense throughout the book.

arthritis (ar-thri′tis): acute or chronic inflammation of one or more joints, characterized by pain and stiffness.

Brodie's abscess (bro′dez): chronic and latent infection in cancellous bone, with a small inflammatory focus.

bursitis (ber-si′tis): inflammation of a bursa.

caries (ka′re-ez): decay or death of bone, with chronic inflammation of the periosteum.

chondritis (kon-dri′tis): inflammation of a cartilage.

coxitis: inflammation of a hip joint (also called ***coxarthritis***).

epiphysitis (e-pif′i-si′tis): inflammation of the epiphysis of a bone, or of the cartilage separating it from the bone.

metatarsalgia (met″ah-tar-sal′je-ah): a neuralgia in the region of the metatarsal due to a foot abnormality, or an osteochondrosis of the heads of the metatarsal bones (also called ***Morton's disease***, ***Morton's toe***, ***Morton's neuralgia***, or ***Morton's foot***).

osteitis (os″te-i′tis): inflammation of bone.

osteoarthritis (os″te-o-ar-thri′tis): degenerative joint disease affecting articular cartilages and the synovial membranes.

osteochondritis (os″te-o-kon-dri′tis): inflammation of bone and cartilage.

osteomyelitis (os″te-o-mi″e-li′tis): inflammation of bone that may involve the periosteum, cancellous tissue, and marrow.

periosteomyelitis (per″e-os″te-o-mi″e-li′tis): inflammation of entire bone.

periostitis (per″e-os-ti′tis): inflammation of the periosteum.

Pott's disease: osteitis or caries of the vertebrae, usually tuberculous (also called **tuberculous spondylitis**).

spondylarthritis (spon″dil-ar-thri′tis): arthritis of spine.

spondylitis (spon″di-li′tis): inflammation of spinal column (**ankylosing spondylitis**, a form of arthritis, is also called **Marie-Strumpell disease**).

synovitis (sin″o-vi′tis): inflammation of the synovial membrane of a joint.

tenosynovitis (ten″o-sin″o-vi′tis): inflammation of a tendon and its synovial membrane.

tuberculosis, osseous: in the bones and joints, producing arthritis and cold abscess.

Hereditary, Congenital and Developmental Disorders

achondroplasia (ah-kon″dro-pla′ze-ah): hereditary, congenital disorder involving inadequate formation and growth of long bones and causing a particular form of dwarfism.

acrocephaly (ak″ro-sef′ah-le): malformation of skull due to early closure of sutures, causing a pointed, conical shape (also called **oxycephaly**).

acromegaly (ak″ro-meg′ah-le): enlargement of bones of extremities, fingers, toes, and soft tissue parts of the face, caused by excessive pituitary growth hormone.

amelia (ah-me′le-ah): anomaly characterized by absence of a limb or limbs.

amyoplasia congenita (ah-mi″o-pla′se-ah kon-jen′i-tah): lack of muscle growth and development in the neonate with deformity of most of the joints.

anencephalia (an″en-se-fa′le-ah): developmental anomaly in which the vault of the skull is missing and cerebral hemispheres may be missing or reduced to small masses.

arachnodactyly (ah′rak″no-dak′ti-le): abnormality in length of fingers and toes (also called **dolichostenomelia** or **arachnodactylia**).

arthroonychodysplasia (ar″thro-on″e-ko-dis-pla′ze-ah): hereditary malformation of head of radius, absence or hypoplasia of patella, and dystrophy of nails (also called **nail-patella syndrome, Fong's disease, onychoosteodysplasia**, or **onychoosteodystrophy**).

cleidocranial dysostosis (kli″do-kra′ne-al dis″os-to′sis): rare hereditary condition characterized by defective ossification of cranial bones, complete or partial absence of clavicles, and other anomalies.

clubfoot: congenitally deformed foot (see **talipes**).

clubhand: congenitally deformed hand.

coxa valga: hip deformity, involving an increase in the angle formed by the axis of the head and neck of the femur, and the axis of the shaft.

coxa vara: hip deformity, involving a decrease in the angle formed by the axis of the head and neck of the femur, and the axis of the shaft.

craniofacial dysostosis: premature fusion of skull bones, and other anomalies (also called **Crouzon's disease**).

craniorachischisis (kra″ne-o-rah-kis′ki-sis): fissure of skull and spinal column.

craniostosis (kra″ne-os-to′sis): ossification of cranial sutures.

dysostosis (dis″os-to′sis): defective ossification of fetal cartilages.

eccentrochondroplasia (ek-sen″tro-kon″dro-pla′se-ah): disorder of epiphysial development (also called **Morquio's syndrome**).

enchondromatosis (en′kon-dro-mat-osis): abnormal growth of cartilage in long bones causing distortion in length and thinness, producing fractures (also called **dyschondroplasia** and **Ollier's disease**).

exostosis (ek″sos-to′sis): abnormal bony growth projection.

fibrous dysplasia: painful, disabling bone development disorder producing thinning of bone cortex and replacement of marrow with fibrous tissue (either *monostotic*, involving only one bone, or *polyostotic*, involving many bones).

genu recurvatum (je′nu re-kur-va′tum): hyperextensive knee joint.

genu valgum: the knees are abnormally close together (knock-knee).

genu varum: lower extremities are bent outward (bowleg).

giantism: abnormal increase of growth in size and stature (also called **gigantism**).

hallux valgus (hal′uks): big toe bends toward the other toes.

hallux varus: big toe displaced away from other toes.

hemimelia (hem″e-me′le-ah): shortening or absence of all or part of the distal half of a limb.

Hurler's syndrome: hereditary condition involving deformities of bone and cartilage, and producing dwarfism (also called **gargoylism, chondro-osteodystrophy**, or **lipochondrodystrophy**).

infantile cortical hyperostosis: overgrowth of bones (also called **Caffey's disease**).

Klippel-Feil syndrome: reduction in number, or fusion of cervical vertebrae, producing short, thick neck, with limited neck motion.

macrobrachia (mak″ro-bra′ke-ah): abnormally large arms.

macrocephaly (mak″ro-sef′ah-le): abnormally large head.

macrognathia (mak″ro-na′the-ah): abnormally large jaws.

macropodia (mak″ro-po′de-ah): abnormally large feet.

Marfan's syndrome: hereditary connective tissue disorder characterized by abnormal length of phalanges and extremities (arachnodactyly), looseness of joints, and also affecting other systems. (Some medical authorities believe that Abraham Lincoln had this condition.)

opisthognathism (o″pis-tho′nah-thizm): receding jaws.

osteogenesis imperfecta: disorder in which the bones are extremely brittle and fracture easily (also called *fragilitas ossium*).

osteopetrosis (os″te-o-pe-tro′sis): hereditary disorder resulting in abnormally dense bone that fractures easily (also called *marble bones* or *Albers-Schonberg disease*).

osteopoikilosis (os″te-o-poi″ki-lo′sis): hereditary condition characterized by numerous dense calcified areas in bone that appear as mottled bone on x-rays.

prognathism (prog′nah-thizm): projecting jaws.

pyknodysostosis (pik″no-dis-os-to′sis): syndrome characterized by dwarfism, late or no closure of fontanels, underdevelopment of lower jaw and phalanges, and bone fragility. (Toulouse Lautrec is believed to have had this condition.)

scaphocephaly (ska″fo-sef′ah-le): long, narrow skull deformity caused by premature closing of the sagittal suture.

syndactylia (sin″dak-til′e-ah): webbed fingers or toes.

talipes (tal′i-pez): twisted foot (*clubfoot*).

Fractures

closed: simple fracture, no open wound on the skin.

Colles': fracture of lower end of radius with the lower fragment displaced posteriorly.

comminuted: bone crushed or splintered.

compound: open wound caused by the fracture.

double: fracture in two places (also called *segmental fracture*).

greenstick: one side of the bone broken and the other part bent (also called *hickory-stick fracture*).

impacted: one fragment driven into the other.

incomplete: continuity of the bone not completely destroyed.

silver-fork: fracture of lower end of radius.

splintered: bone is splintered into fragments.

transverse: bone fractured at right angles to its axis.

Metabolic and Deficiency Diseases

chondromalacia (kon″dro-mah-la′she-ah): softening of cartilage.

osteomalacia (os′te-o-mah-la′she-ah): softening of bone.

osteoporosis (os″te-o-po-ro′sis): abnormal loss of bone density.

renal osteodystrophy: bone changes caused by chronic kidney disease in childhood (also called *renal rickets* or *pseudorickets*).

rickets (rik′ets): condition in which bending and distortion of bone takes place, caused by deficiency of vitamin D in childhood.

scurvy: vitamin C deficiency condition producing abnormal formation of bones and teeth, and other clinical symptoms.

Oncology**

chondroblastoma: a tumor in a bone epiphysis (also called *Codman's tumor*).

chondrofibroma (kon″dro-fibro′mah): tumor with fibrous and cartilaginous tissue.

chondroma: tumor of cartilage cells.

chondromatosis (kon″dro-mah-to′sis): multiple chondromas.

chondromyoma: myoma containing cartilaginous elements.

chondromyxoma (kon″dro-mik-so′mah): myxoma containing cartilaginous elements (also called *chondromyxoid fibroma*).

chondromyxosarcoma*: malignancy with fibrous, mucous cartilaginous elements.

chondrosarcoma*: malignancy made up of cartilaginous elements.

osteoblastoma (os″te-o-blas-to′mah): benign tumor of osteoblasts.

osteochondroma (os″te-o-kon-dro′mah): benign tumor made up of bone and cartilage.

osteoma (os″te-o′mah): a bone tissue tumor.

osteosarcoma* (os″te-o-sar-ko′-mah): malignant bone tumor.

osteospongioma (os″te-o-spon″je-o′mah): neoplasm in bone cortex.

synovioma (sin-o″ve-o′mah): synovial membrane tumor involving joint or tendon.

Surgical Procedures

allograft: surgical removal of cancerous bone and replacement with donor bone.

arthrectomy (ar-threk′to-me): excision of a joint.

arthrocentesis (ar″thro-sen-te′sis): puncture of a joint.

arthrodesis (ar″thro-de′sis): surgical fixation of a joint by fusion of the joint surfaces (also called *artificial ankylosis*).

* Indicates a malignant condition.
** Oncology is the study of tumors (*neoplasms*), which may be benign or malignant.

arthroplasty (ar'thro-plas"te): plastic surgery to reconstruct joints.

arthrotomy (ar-throt'o-me): incision of a joint.

bursectomy (ber-sek'to-me): excision of a bursa.

bursotomy (ber-sot'o-me): incision of a bursa.

capsulorrhaphy (kap'su-lor'ah-fe): suturing of a joint capsule.

capsulotomy : incision of a joint capsule.

carpectomy (kar-pek'to-me): excision of all or part of a carpal bone.

chondrectomy (kon-drek'to-me): excision of cartilage.

chondrotomy (kon-drot'o-me): division or dissection of cartilage.

clavicotomy (klav"i-kot'o-me): dividing or cutting of a clavicle.

coccygectomy (kok"se-jek'to-me): excising of the coccyx.

condylectomy (kon"dil-ek'to-me): excising of a condyle (knuckle).

costectomy (kos-tek'to-me): excision or resection of a rib.

coxotomy (kok-sot'o-me): opening the hip joint.

cranioclasis (kra"ne-ok'lah-sis): crushing of the fetal head.

cranioplasty: plastic surgery on the skull.

craniotomy : any surgical procedure on the cranium.

craniotrypesis (kra"ne-o-tri-pe'sis): trephination of the skull.

laminectomy (lam"i-nek'toe-me): cutting out posterior arch of a vertebra (also called *rachiotomy* or *rachitomy*).

laminotomy (lam"i-not'o-me): division of lamina of a vertebra.

metatarsectomy (met"ah-tar-sek'tome): excision of metatarsus.

ostearthrotomy (os'te-ar-throt'o-me): excision of articular end of a bone.

ostectomy (os-tek'to-me): excision of all or part of a bone.

osteoclasis (os-te-ok'lah-sis): surgical fracture of a bone for reconstructive purposes.

osteoplasty (os'te-o-plas"te): plastic surgery of bone.

osteorrhaphy: suturing or wiring of a bone.

osteotomy (os"te-ot'o-me): cutting of a bone.

pubiotomy (pu"be-ot'o-me): cutting of the pubic bone.

scapulopexy (skap'u-lo-pek"se): fixing of scapula to chest wall or vertebrae.

spondylodesis (spon"di-lod'e-sis): short bone graft to fuse vertebrae.

spondylosyndesis (spon"di-lo-sin'de-sis): spinal fusion.

sternotomy (ster-not'o-me): cutting through the sternum.

synchondrotomy (sin"kon-drot'o-me): cartilaginous joint division.

syndesmopexy (sin-des'mo-pek"se): fixation of a dislocation by using the ligaments of the joint.

synosteotomy (sin"os-te-ot'o-me): dissection of the joints.

synovectomy (sin"o-vek'to-me): excision of synovial membrane of a joint.

Descriptive and Diagnostic Terms

ankylosis (ang"ki-lo'sis): immobility and consolidation of a joint.

arthralgia (ar-thral'je-ah): pain in a joint or joints (also called *arthrodynia*).

arthrocele (ar'thro-seal): swollen joint.

arthrolithiasis (ar"thro-li'thi-ah-sis): gout.

arthroneuralgia (ar"thro-nu-ral'je-ah): pain of a joint.

arthropathy (ar-throp'ah-the): any joint disease.

arthrosclerosis (ar'thro-skle-ro'sis): hardening or stiffening of a joint.

arthrosis (ar-thro'sis): articulation or disease of a joint.

chondralgia (kon-dral'je-ah): pain in a cartilage (also called *chondrodynia*).

chondroid (kon'droid): resembling cartilage.

chondronecrosis: death of cartilage.

chondroporosis (kon"dro-po-ro'sis): formation of spaces in cartilage occurring normally during ossification.

coccygodynia (kok"se-go-din'e-ah): pain of the coccyx (also called *coccyalgia* or *coccyodynia*).

coxodynia (kok"so-din'e-ah): pain of the hip (also called *coxalgia*).

hemarthrosis (hem"ar-thro'sis): seepage of blood into a joint.

hydrarthrosis (hi"drar-thro'sis): fluid in a joint cavity.

kyphosis (ki-fo'sis): humpback.

lordosis (lor-do'sis): curvature of the spine (swayback).

lumbago (lum-ba'go): lumbo-sacral pain.

ostealgia (os"te-al'je-ah): pain in a bone (also called *ostalgia* or *osteodynia*).

osteoclasia (os"te-o-kla'ze-ah): destruction and absorption of bony tissue.

osteodiastasis: separation of two bones.

osteodystrophy (os"te-o-dis'tro-fe): defective bone formation.

osteogenetic (os"te-o-je-net'ik): forming bone.

osteoid (os'te-oid): resembling bone.

osteolysis (os"te-ol'i-sis): bone dissolution caused by calcium loss.

osteomalacia (os"te-o-mah-la'she-ah): softening of bones.

osteonecrosis (os"te-o-ne-kro'sis): death of bone.

osteoneuralgia (os″te-o-nu-ral′je-ah): neuralgia of bone.

osteopathy (os″te-op′ah-the): any bone disease.

osteorrhagia (os″te-o-ra′je-ah): bone hemorrhage.

osteosclerosis (os″te-o-skle-ro′sis): abnormal hardening of bone.

scoliosis (sko″le-o′sis): abnormal lateral curvature of spine.

Laboratory Tests

arthrography: radiography (X-ray), using contrast media to outline soft tissue structures in a joint.

arthroscopy: examination of a joint interior using an arthroscope.

bone marrow biopsy: removal of bone marrow from sternum, iliac crest, vertebral column, or tibia for detection of leukemias, anemias, multiple myelomas, or any diseases affecting bone marrow. Red or white blood cells are evaluated for appearance, number, development, and infection (also called ***bone marrow aspiration***).

bone scan: injection of radioactive material into a vein. As seen by x-ray, the concentration of injected material in any specific area reveals an abnormal condition of bone, particularly metastatic bone cancer.

bone x-ray: radiographic examination of bone for presence of disease or fractures.

computerized tomography (CT): imaging device using x-rays at multiple angles through specific sections of the body, analyzed by computer to provide a total picture of the part being examined (also called ***computerized axial tomography [CAT]***).

discogram: x-ray of vertebral disc for diagnostic purposes.

dual energy radiography (DER): a low level radiation method of measuring bone mass to diagnose osteoporosis.

endoscopy: use of an endoscope to examine the interior of a joint, particularly the knee, for presence of torn cartilage.

hydroxyproline: urine test to detect bone diseases.

long bone x-ray: to determine growth patterns, joint deterioration, and growth of bone spurs.

lumbar puncture: needle aspiration of spinal canal fluid in lumbar area, to diagnose traumatic head, neck, or back injury.

magnetic resonance imaging (MRI): non-invasive method of scanning the body by use of an electromagnetic field and radio waves, which provides visual images on a computer screen and magnetic tape recordings (also called ***nuclear magnetic resonance [NMR]***). Used to examine tendons, ligaments, and bone marrow.

nuclear magnetic resonance (NMR): see ***magnetic resonance imaging***.

rheumatoid factor: blood test to detect rheumatoid arthritis.

skull x-ray: examination of bones and sinuses of the skull to detect pathologic conditions.

spinal x-ray: for detection of diverse abnormalities.

synovial fluid: tests of blood and synovial fluid to diagnose infections, inflammations, septic, and other conditions.

Chapter 7

The Muscular System

The Moving Force

CHAPTER OVERVIEW

This chapter presents the different muscles of the body, their composition, classification and relationship to other structures that aid in movement.

MUSCLES

The study of muscles is called *myology*. All human activity is carried on by muscles in conjunction with the skeleton to achieve movement. Although the skeleton provides attachment points and support for the muscles, it is the muscle tissue and its ability to extend and contract that effects movement.

There are over 600 muscles in the human body. Muscles constitute the major part of the fleshy portions of the body and one half of its weight, varying in proportion to the size of the individual. The form of the body is largely determined by the muscles covering the bones.

In addition to movement, the muscles have other roles, such as supporting and maintaining posture and producing body heat. They help form many of the internal organs (heart, uterus, lungs, and intestines). There is never a time when all the muscles are in a quiescent state, because the muscles of the heart, intestines, arteries, and stomach are at work, even though we are not aware of it.

ALLIED MUSCULAR STRUCTURES

Tendon

Tendons are the strong, fibrous, white bands that attach muscles to bones, enabling the movement of a part located some distance from the contracting muscle. For example, the muscles of the calf of the leg, by means of their tendons, control the movement of the ankles and toes. If the ankle's movement depended on its own muscles, it would need to be many times its present size. Similarly, the wrists and fingers are controlled by the muscles of the upper forearm by means of their tendons. One type of tendon, called an *aponeurosis*, is flat and ribbonlike.

Fascia

Fascia is a sheet of fibrous membrane that encloses muscles and separates them into groups.

Ligament

Ligaments are strong bands of fibrous tissue connecting bones or cartilage that aid or restrict movement and support organs.

Origin

The origin is the bone attached to a muscle, which remains relatively immovable when that particular muscle is contracted.

Insertion

The insertion is the bone attached to a muscle, which moves when that particular muscle is contracted.

Motor Nerve

A motor nerve causes muscle to move by stimulating a definite group of muscle fibers. The combination of the nerve cell and its group of muscle cells is called a *motor*, or *neuromotor* unit.

Tone

The tone of a muscle is the state of tension that is present when one is awake.

Review A

Complete the following:

1. The study of muscles is called _____.

2. Movement is produced by the ability of muscle to _____ and _____.

3. The relatively immovable bone to which a muscle is attached is known as its _____.

4. The movable bone to which a muscle is attached is known as its _____.

5. The state of tension present in a muscle while one is awake is known as _____.

COMPOSITION OF MUSCLE

Like other tissues of the body, muscle tissue is composed of cells. Muscle cells are long and slender and, because of their shape, called *fibers*. These fibers vary greatly in size, depending on their function, but they are always gigantic when compared to other body cells. The plasma membrane of a muscle cell is called a *sarcolemma*, and its cytoplasm is called *sarcoplasm*. The muscle fibers are held together by connective tissue and enclosed in fascia (fibrous membrane sheath). The fibers are able to contract, producing movement of the body or its organs. The speed of muscle contraction varies with individual muscles and the size of the structure to be moved. The smaller the structure to be moved, the more rapid is the muscle action. For example, the muscles that move the eyeball contract much more rapidly than those that move a large muscle such as the gluteus maximus of the hip.

Many movements of the body are carried out by several muscles or muscle groups acting together. The muscles have a rich vascular (blood) supply. Exercise increases muscle fiber thickness, but does not produce new fibers.

CLASSIFICATION OF MUSCLES

Muscles are divided into three types according to their function, shape and structure. These three types are *skeletal*, *visceral*, and *cardiac* (see Fig. 5-4).

Skeletal (Voluntary, Striated) Muscle

Skeletal muscles, which are attached to the skeleton, are called voluntary because they are controlled at will. They are called striated because, under a microscope, they have a cross-striated (striped) appearance. Other voluntary muscles, not attached to the skeleton, are those that move the eyeballs, tongue, pharynx, and some portions of the skin.

A typical voluntary muscle is made up of a fleshy mass of elongated muscle fibers held together in a casing of white fibrous tissue and supplied with a nerve that makes it contract and extend. When muscles contract, the fibers become shorter and thicker. An example of the contraction of a voluntary muscle is flexing the forearm and squeezing it tightly, so that the biceps muscle becomes thick and hard. Skeletal muscle is supplied by both the central and peripheral nervous systems (Chapter 14).

Visceral (Nonstriated or Smooth, Involuntary) Muscle

Visceral muscles, which are found in parts of the body such as the stomach, intestines, blood vessels, and iris of the eye, are made up of smooth, nonstriated, spindle-shaped fibers. These muscles are involuntary (not controllable at will), and are supplied by the autonomic nervous system (Chapter 14).

Cardiac (Striated, Involuntary) Muscle

The cardiac (heart) muscle, although involuntary, shows fine transverse striations under the microscope. Its appearance is an exception to other involuntary muscle tissue. The cardiac muscle is controlled by the autonomic nervous system (Chapters 9 and 14).

ATTACHMENT OF MUSCLES

The attachment of muscles to tendons, which extend to the fingers and toes, results in graceful movement and reduction of bulk that would be necessary for muscles to extend to the digits. Voluntary muscles usually attach to bone, but an exception is the larynx and thorax, where muscle is attached to cartilage. Usually, muscle is attached to the capsule of joints over which its tendon passes; other muscles may be attached to the skin, as in the cheeks, or to mucous membrane, as in the tongue. Muscles may also be attached to fascia of other muscles, like the flat muscles of the abdomen, or to body structures, like the eyeball.

MOVEMENT OF MUSCLES

A muscle does not act alone, but is dependent upon other muscles to assist in executing a desired movement. For this reason, muscles are referred to as ***prime movers***, ***antagonists***, and ***synergists*** (***syn-*** means together; ***-erg-*** refers to work).

The ***prime movers*** are those that actively produce a movement.

The ***antagonists*** are those in opposition to the prime movers, relaxing as the prime movers contract.

The ***synergists*** contract simultaneously with the prime mover to help execute a movement or steady a part.

The muscles, in conjunction with the skeleton, move the body. The different types of movements have been listed and described in a box in Chapter 6 on p. 75.

Review B

Complete the following:

1. Muscle cells are _____ and _____.

2. _____ is the plasma membrane of a muscle cell.

3. _____ is the cytoplasm of a muscle cell.

4. Three types of muscle tissue are _____, _____, and _____.

5. Muscles are classified according to how they produce movement, and are called _____,

_____, and _____.

HOW MUSCLES ARE NAMED

Muscle names are based on six points of identification:

1. Muscles may be named for their **action**.

   Example: ulnar flexor muscle of wrist (flexes wrist)

2. Muscles may be named for their **origin** *and* **insertion**.

   Example: occipitofrontal (between occipital and frontal skull bones)

3. Muscles may be named for their **location**.

   Example: external oblique muscle of abdomen (abdomen)

4. Muscles may be named for their **shape** or **use**.

   Examples: pyramidal (shaped like a pyramid); buccinator (cheek muscle used in blowing a trumpet)

5. Muscles may be named for the **direction** of fibers.

   Example: orbicular muscle of eye (around eye)

6. Muscles may be named according to the **number** *of sections*.

   Example: biceps (***bi-*** means two, ***-cep*** means head)

ADJECTIVES FOR MUSCLES

The following are some important adjectives that
    aid in the description of muscles.

azygous—not paired

bi-, tri-, and **quadri-**—two, three, and four

externus—external, or outer

gracilis—slender

latissimus—wide

longissimus—long

longus—long

medius—intermediate

orbicularis—surrounding

quadratus—square

rectus—straight

rhomboideus—diamond- or kite-shaped

scalenus—unequally triangular

serratus—sawtoothed

teres—round or cylindrical

transversus—crosswise

vastus—great

Review C

Complete the following:

1. There are six points of identification in naming muscles: _____, _____,

_____, _____, _____, and _____.

2. Orbicularis, in relation to muscle, means _____.

3. Quadratus, in relation to muscle, means _____.

4. Rhomboideus, in relation to muscle, means _____.

5. Teres, in relation to muscle, means _____.

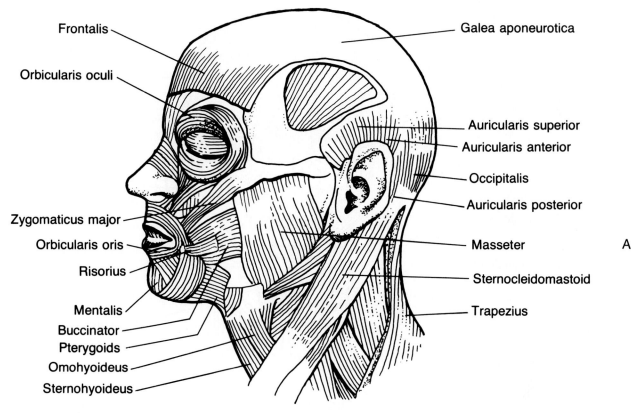

Figure 7-1.   A, Lateral view of facial and cranial muscles and several muscles of mastication.

MUSCLE GROUPS

The following paragraphs name and describe various muscles and their actions, according to their location in the body. Only a few muscles will be covered to provide the student with a basic understanding of this system. However, a more complete listing of the muscles and their related anatomic terms can be found in the glossary.

Muscles of the Scalp

There are no muscles over the top of the skull, only skin covering a broad, flat tendon called the *galea aponeurotica* (Fig. 7-1, A). This tendon connects to three muscle groups:

Occipitofrontal group: the *occipitalis* muscle pulls the scalp backward. The *frontalis* muscle raises the eyebrows, creates horizontal wrinkles on the forehead, and pulls the scalp forward;

Temporoparietal group: tightens scalp and moves ears upward;

Auricular group: three muscles (anterior, superior, posterior) that move the ear forward, upward and backward.

Facial Muscles

There are many facial muscles that produce a variety of movements (Fig. 7-1, B). Some of these are:

Orbicularis oculi (*ocul-* eye): muscle that moves the eyelids;

Orbicularis oris (*or-* mouth): muscle that draws the lips into a pucker;

Buccinator: muscle that compresses the cheek for smiling and blowing (also called *trumpeter* muscle);

Platysma: muscle (origin is in fascia of chest wall) that pulls down the corners of the mouth;

Risorius: muscle that draws out the angle of the mouth;

Masseters: muscles of mastication (chewing), which raise the mandible (and close the jaw);

Pterygoids: muscles that raise and move the mandible from side to side (opens and closes mouth).

Muscles of the Neck and Shoulder

Although there are a number of muscles in the neck, one of the most important is:

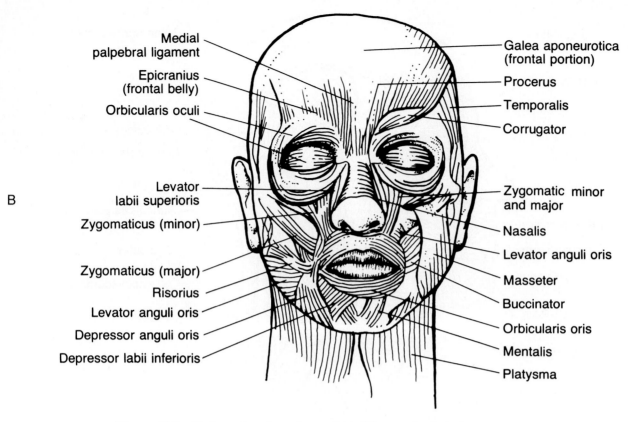

Figure 7-1. B, Anterior view of muscles of face and cranium.

The ***sternocleidomastoid***: muscle that tilts the head forward or to one side, and rotates it. This muscle is named for its origin in the sternum and clavicle, and its insertion in the mastoid process of the temporal bone (Figs. 7-2 and 7-3).

Other muscles in the neck and upper thorax assist in rotation of the head, flexing the head upon the neck, and breathing.

The ***trapezius*** muscle: superficial (surface) muscle of the back of the neck and upper trunk. Broad and flat, it raises, lowers, and shrugs the shoulder;

The ***pectoralis major*** muscle: adducts, and flexes the upper arm, drawing the arms across the chest;

The ***latissimus dorsi*** muscle: the broadest muscle in the back, extends and adducts the upper arm;

The ***teres major*** muscle: extends and adducts the upper arm and rotates it medially;

The ***deltoid*** muscle: abducts, flexes, and extends the upper arm.

Muscles of the Arms and Hands

In addition to the action of the muscles of the shoulder, back, and upper thorax, the muscles of the arms also contribute to the movement of the arms (Figs. 7-2 and 7-3).

The ***triceps brachii***: extends the lower arm;
The ***brachialis***: flexes the lower arm;
The ***biceps brachii***: flexes lower arm and suppinates lower arm and hand;
The ***pronator teres***: flexes and pronates the lower arm.

A group of ***flexor*** and ***extensor*** muscles, in conjunction with other muscles of the radius, ulna and phalanges, control the movements of the wrists, hands, and fingers. Each of the fingers has long flexor and extensor tendons leading from the forearm muscles. The flexors bend the fingers and aid in flexing the wrist and other finger joints. The extensors abduct and adduct the wrist, and extend the wrist and fingers. The thumb also has abductors, adductors, extensors and flexors.

Muscles of the Back

Some of the major muscles in the upper part of the back have already been discussed under shoulder movements. Small muscles deep in the back control the joints between the vertebrae, steadying the vertebral column so that it can be used as a lever by long muscles. Specific muscles steady the vertebral column, maintain posture, abduct and rotate the trunk, and aid in movement of the head (Figs. 7-2 and 7-3).

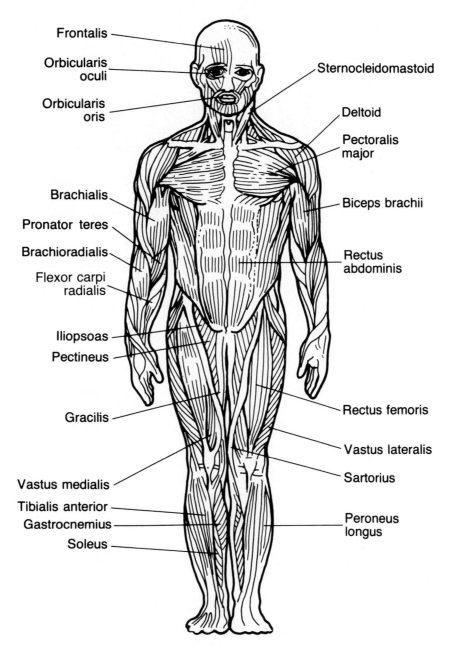

Frontalis

Orbicularis oculi

Orbicularis oris

Sternocleidomastoid

Deltoid

Pectoralis major

Brachialis

Pronator teres

Brachioradialis

Flexor carpi radialis

Biceps brachii

Rectus abdominis

Iliopsoas

Pectineus

Gracilis

Rectus femoris

Vastus lateralis

Sartorius

Vastus medialis

Tibialis anterior

Gastrocnemius

Soleus

Peroneus longus

Figure 7-2.   Anterior superficial muscles of the body.

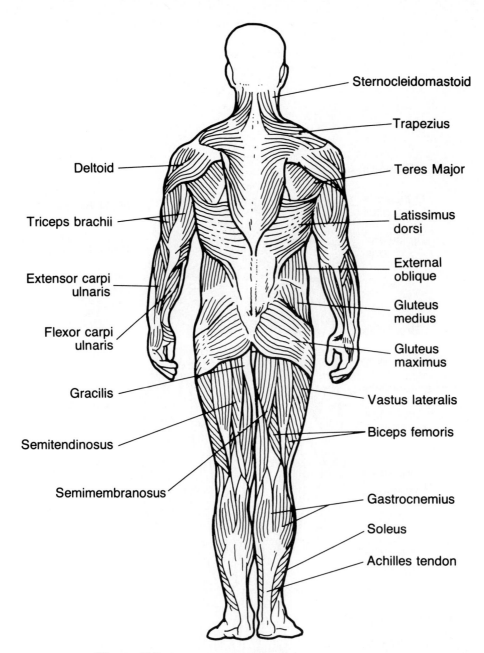

Deltoid

Triceps brachii

Extensor carpi
ulnaris

Flexor carpi
ulnaris

Gracilis

Semitendinosus

Semimembranosus

Sternocleidomastoid

Trapezius

Teres Major

Latissimus
dorsi

External
oblique

Gluteus
medius

Gluteus
maximus

Vastus lateralis

Biceps femoris

Gastrocnemius

Soleus

Achilles tendon

Figure 7-3   Posterior superficial muscles of the body.

Muscles of the Thorax

The muscles of the thorax are:

The ***external intercostals***;
The ***internal intercostals***;
The ***diaphragm***.

During respiration, the external intercostals lift the ribs, the internal intercostals lower them, and the diaphragm contracts and flattens out, causing the thorax to enlarge, and creating more room for the lungs to expand.

Abdominal Muscles

The abdominal muscles (Figs. 7-2 and 7-3) are:

The ***external oblique;***
The ***internal oblique***;
The ***rectus abdominis***;
The ***transversus abdominis***.

These muscles keep the viscera in place, support and compress the abdomen, help to maintain posture, and contract during childbirth, defecation, coughing, and

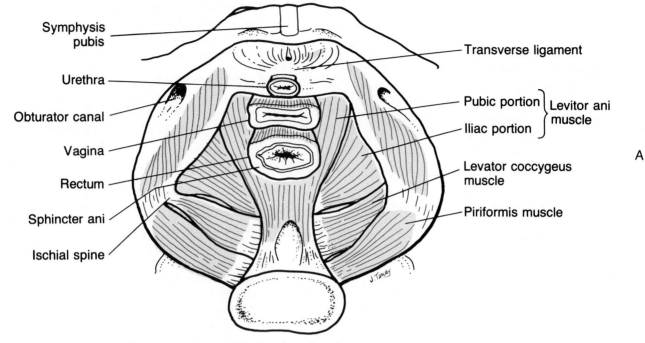

Symphysis pubis
Urethra
Obturator canal
Vagina
Rectum
Sphincter ani
Ischial spine

Transverse ligament
Pubic portion
Iliac portion
} Levitor ani muscle
Levator coccygeus muscle
Piriformis muscle

A

Figure 7.4.   **A, Muscles of the female pelvic floor.**

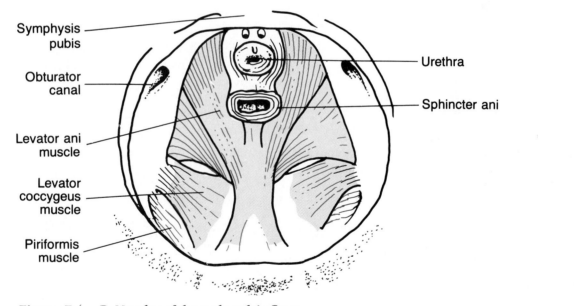

Symphysis pubis
Obturator canal
Levator ani muscle
Levator coccygeus muscle
Piriformis muscle

Urethra
Sphincter ani

B

Figure 7.4.   **B, Muscles of the male pelvic floor.**

sneezing. Additionally, they assist in flexing and rotating the vertebral column.

Muscles of the Pelvic Floor

The chief muscles of the pelvic floor (Fig. 7-4, A and B) are:

The ***perineum***: (region between anus and vagina in the female, and anus and scrotum in the male); forms part of the supporting pelvic floor;

The ***levator coccygeus*** muscle and the ***levator ani*** muscle: two muscles that are important in supporting the pelvic organs, and take part in defecation and childbirth;

The ***sphincter ani***: keeps the anus closed.

Muscles of the Thigh and Leg

The muscles of the thigh and leg (Figs. 7-2 and 7-3) have several functions in movement. The most important of these muscles are:

The **obturator internus**: laterally rotates the thigh;

The **obturator externus**: laterally rotates the thigh;

The **gemellus superior**: laterally rotates the thigh;

The **gemellus inferior**: laterally rotates the thigh;

The **piriformis**: laterally rotates, abducts, and extends the thigh;

The **quadratus femoris**: flexes and extends the leg and laterally rotates the thigh.

The **gluteal group** includes:

The **gluteus minimus**: abducts and rotates the thigh;

The **gluteus medius**: abducts and rotates the thigh;

The **gluteus maximus**: extends and rotates the thigh.

The **tensor fasciae latae**: abducts the thigh.

The **iliopsoas**: flexes the thigh and trunk.

The **adductor** group includes:

The **longus**, **brevis**, and **magnus**: powerful adductors;

The **gracilis**: flexes the leg and adducts the leg and thigh.

The **quadriceps femoris group** includes:

The **rectus femoris**: flexes thigh and extends the leg;

The **vastus lateralis**: extends the leg;

The **vastus medialis**: extends the leg;

The **vastus intermedius**: extends the leg.

The **sartorius**: flexes and adducts the leg.

The **hamstring group** of muscles descends in the back of the thigh, their tendons forming the *hamstrings*. They include:

The **semimembranosus**: extends the thigh;

The **semitendinosus**: extends the thigh;

The **biceps femoris**: extends the thigh and flexes the leg.

The **gastrocnemius**: flexes the leg and extends the foot. This muscle and the soleus (see Muscles of the Foot, below) are commonly called the calf muscles, and their tendon is the **Achilles** tendon.

Muscles of the Foot

The chief muscles of the foot (Figs. 7-2 and 7-3) include:

The **soleus**: extends the foot;

The **tibialis anterior**: turns the foot in and flexes it;

The **tibialis posterior**: turns the foot in and extends it;

The **peroneus longus**: turns the foot outward and extends it;

The **peroneus brevis**: turns the foot outward and flexes it;

The **peroneus tertius**: turns the foot outward and flexes it.

Like the muscles in the fingers, those of the toes have flexor, abductor, adductor, and extensor tendons. In the foot they move the phalangeal joints, keep the foot and toes firmly on the ground, and aid in walking, dancing, running, jumping, dorsiflexion of the ankle, and eversion and inversion of the foot.

Review D

Complete the following:

1. The broad, flat tendon over the top of the skull is called the _____.

2. The auricular group of muscles moves the _____.

3. The buccinator muscle is also called the _____.

4. The _____ muscle is named for its origin in the sternum and clavicle, and its insertion in the mastoid process.

5. The diaphragm is a muscle of respiration located in the _____.

6. _____ muscles contract when we cough or sneeze.

7. The gluteal group of muscles is divided into _____ sections.

8. The muscle that pulls down the corner of the mouth is the _____.

9. A broad, flat, superficial muscle of the back of the neck and trunk is the _____.

10. Muscles for chewing are the _____.

Answers to Review Questions: The Muscular System

Review A
1. myology
2. extend, contract
3. origin
4. insertion
5. tone

Review B
1. long, slender
2. sarcolemma
3. sarcoplasm
4. skeletal, visceral, cardiac
5. prime movers, antagonists, synergists

Review C
1. action, origin and insertion, location, shape or use, fiber direction, number of sections or divisions
2. surrounding
3. square
4. diamond- , or kite-shaped
5. round

Review D
1. galea aponeurotica
2. ear
3. trumpeter (muscle)
4. sternocleidomastoid
5. thorax
6. abdominal
7. three
8. platysma
9. trapezius
10. masseters

CHAPTER 7 EXERCISES

MUSCULAR SYSTEM: THE MOVING FORCE

Exercise 1: Complete the following:

1. The strong fibrous white bands that attach muscles to bones are called _____.

2. The strong bands of tissue that hold bones together and support organs are called _____.

3. A particular type of tendon that is flat and ribbonlike is called a(n) _____.

4. The immovable attachment of a muscle, or the point at which it is anchored by a tendon to a bone, is called its _____.

5. The nerve that causes a muscle to move is called a(n) _____.

Exercise 2: Matching:

____ 1. skeletal
____ 2. visceral muscle
____ 3. cardiac muscle
____ 4. prime mover
____ 5. antagonist
____ 6. sarcolemma
____ 7. synergist
____ 8. insertion
____ 9. striated
____10. nonstriated

A. muscles that work together

B. muscle that actively produces a movement

C. striped

D. muscle that can be moved voluntarily

E. smooth

F. muscle that cannot be moved at will

G. muscle acting in opposition to another

H. heart muscle

I. movable bone attached to muscle

J. plasma membrane of a muscle cell

Exercise 3: Multiple choice:

1. Unpaired muscles are described as:
   a. azygous
   b. gracilis
   c. serratus
2. Long muscles are referred to as:
   a. longissimus
   b. latissimus
   c. medius
3. Muscles surrounding a part are described as:
   a. orbicularis
   b. externus
   c. transversus
4. Muscles that have four insertions may include the term:
   a. bi-
   b. tri-
   c. quadri-
5. A round or cylindrical muscle may include the term:
   a. teres
   b. orbicularis
   c. azygous

Exercise 4: Muscles may be named in six ways. Study the statements below and identify the manner in which the following muscles are named by placing the correct letter in the space provided.

A. Action: has a verb-based root with a suffix, followed by the name of the structure affected.
B. Joining the names of the points of origin and attachment, with an adjective suffix.
C. Location: usually includes an adjective, followed by the location of the muscle.
D. For their shape or for the way the muscle is used.
E. According to the direction of the muscle fibers.
F. According to the number of sections or divisions forming them.

____ **1.** brachioradialis

____ **2.** buccinator

____ **3.** extensor carpi

____ **4.** external oblique abdominal

____ **5.** biceps brachii

____ **6.** orbicularis

____ **7.** platysma

____ **8.** levator scapulae

____ **9.** flexor carpi radialis

____**10.** tibialis anterior

Exercise 5: Using the list of terms below, identify each muscle in Fig. 7-5 by writing its name in the corresponding blank.

Frontalis
Sternocleidomastoid
Biceps brachii
Flexor carpi radialis
Gastrocnemius
Gracilis
Rectus femoris
Sartorius

Orbicularis oculi
Deltoid
Brachialis
Peroneus longus
Tibialis anterior
Iliopsoas
Vastus lateralis
Pronator teres

Orbicularis oris
Pectoralis major
Brachioradialis
Soleus
Vastus medialis
Rectus abdominis
Pectineus

1. _____
2. _____
3. _____
4. _____
5. _____
6. _____
7. _____
8. _____
9. _____
10. _____
11. _____
12. _____
13. _____
14. _____
15. _____
16. _____
17. _____
18. _____
19. _____
20. _____
21. _____
22. _____
23. _____

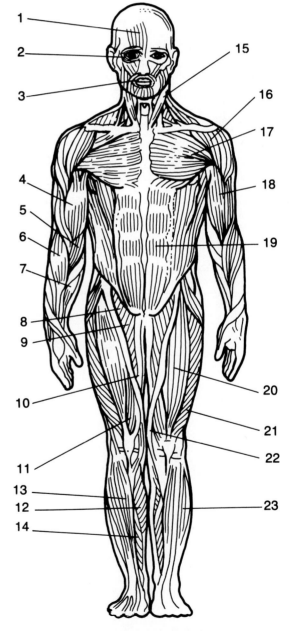

Figure 7-5. Anterior superficial muscles of the body.

Exercise 6: Using the list of terms below, identify each muscle or tendon in Fig. 7-6 by writing its name in the corresponding blank.

Sternocleidomastoid
Triceps brachii
Extensor carpi ulnaris
External oblique
Vastus lateralis
Semitendinosus
Achilles tendon

Trapezius
Teres major
Gracilis
Gluteus medius
Biceps femoris
Gastrocnemius

Deltoid
Latissimus dorsi
Flexor carpi ulnaris
Gluteus maximus
Semimembranosus
Soleus

1. _____
2. _____
3. _____
4. _____
5. _____
6. _____
7. _____
8. _____
9. _____
10. _____
11. _____
12. _____
13. _____
14. _____
15. _____
16. _____
17. _____
18. _____
19. _____

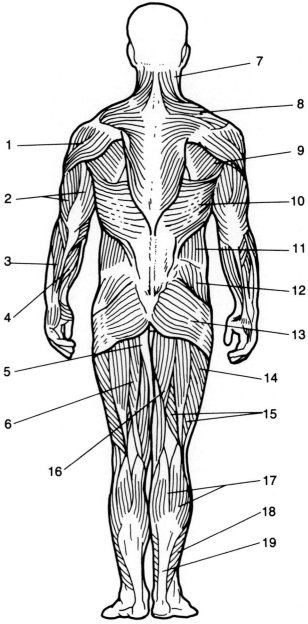

Figure 7-6.   Posterior superficial muscles of the body.

Exercise 7: Matching:

____ **1.** orbicularis oculi   **A.** surrounding the mouth

____ **4.** masseters   **B.** surrounding eyes

____ **3.** sternocleidomastoid   **C.** back of neck and upper trunk controlling shoulder movements

____ **4.** trapezius   **D.** sternum and clavicle to mastoid process

____ **5.** buccinator   **E.** frontal abdominal muscle

____ **6.** pronator teres   **F.** flexes and pronates lower arm

____ **7.** serratus   **G.** cheek muscle

____ **8.** gluteus maximus   **H.** hip muscle

____ **9.** latissimus dorsi   **I.** sawtooth muscle

____ **10.** rectus abdominis   **J.** broad muscle of back

____ **11.** orbicularis oris   **K.** facial muscle for chewing

Exercise 8: Give the meaning of the components of the following words and then define the word as a whole. Suffixes meaning *pertaining to* or *state or condition,* shown following a slash mark (/), are not to be defined separately. Before reaching for your medical dictionary, check the glossary at the end of the chapter.

1. Amyotrophia:

   a _____

   myo _____

   troph/ia _____

   _____

2. Myofibrosis:

   myo _____

   fibr/osis _____

   _____

3. Fasciodesis:

   fascio _____

   desis _____

   _____

4. Myotenotomy:

   myo _____

   teno _____

   tomy _____

   _____

5. Myalgia:

   my _____

   algia _____

6. Myoedema:

   myo _____

   edema _____

   _____

7. Tenostosis:

   ten _____

   ost/osis _____

   _____

8. Myoma:

   my _____

   oma _____

   _____

9. Myorrhaphy:

   myo _____

   rrhaphy _____

   _____

10. Myosclerosis:

   myo _____

   scler/osis _____

   _____

11. Tenosynovectomy:

   teno _____

   synov _____

   ectomy _____

   _____

12. Myomelanosis:

   myo _____

   melan/osis _____

   _____

Chapter 7 Crossword Puzzle

Across

2. the study of muscles
4. flat, ribbon-like type of tendon
10. plasma membrane of a muscle cell
12. contracts with a prime mover to move or steady a part
14. name this "tailor" muscle
15. the meaning of latissimus
16. location of the brachialis
17. waking state muscle tension
23. muscle group and tendons descending back of thigh
24. one of three gluteal muscles
25. second of three gluteal muscles
27. fibrous membrane sheet
28. nerve type causing muscle to move
29. tendon of calf muscles

Down

1. root meaning "head"
3. orbicularis of eyelid
4. muscle that opposes prime mover
5. immovable attachment of muscle
6. movable attachment of muscle
7. muscle cell cytoplasm
8. one of two calf muscles
9. bands attaching muscles to bones
11. third of gluteal muscle group
13. diaphragm location
18. supporting and connecting band
19. muscle of neck and upper back
20. supports part of pelvic floor
21. orbicularis of the lips
22. 3 groups moving forehead and ears
26. term for muscle cells

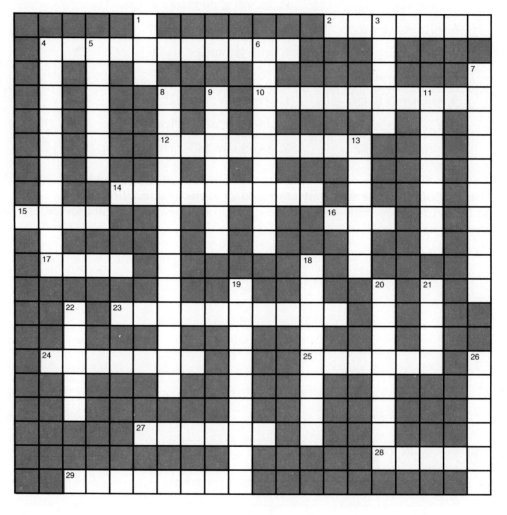

Chapter 7 Hidden Words Puzzle

```
E  C  F  G  Q  S  A  B  B  S  R  D  L  P  X  C  W  S  Q  X  U  V
T  P  V  L  T  O  H  I  S  K  E  L  E  T  A  L  Y  F  N  Q  N  U
F  H  V  M  E  O  J  N  Y  C  H  Q  B  T  J  H  Q  R  V  M  H  G
B  R  S  Y  N  X  U  S  N  L  K  E  J  M  G  W  S  O  T  E  N  E
D  F  W  B  D  O  O  E  E  F  T  X  B  U  J  Y  N  A  W  K  S  L
U  E  A  E  O  R  G  R  R  K  Q  T  T  L  B  J  C  E  V  C  X  X
C  F  E  S  N  I  V  T  G  S  J  E  T  T  U  M  G  D  U  S  C  D
M  Z  S  M  C  G  C  I  I  J  O  N  M  L  R  H  S  Y  X  L  N  S
M  R  N  O  W  I  L  O  S  V  I  S  C  E  R  A  L  O  S  T  L  F
F  E  P  O  M  N  A  N  T  A  G  O  N  I  S  T  S  L  A  P  U  O
V  I  S  T  O  U  S  P  S  Z  B  R  L  D  G  R  Q  P  A  E  A  K
H  O  B  H  R  T  S  L  O  J  W  S  G  C  F  C  G  P  V  C  T  T
E  V  L  E  H  V  I  C  I  N  V  O  L  U  N  T  A  R  Y  K  X  U
M  C  F  U  R  N  F  W  L  G  E  K  C  H  L  N  R  R  Y  I  M  C
I  X  U  Y  N  S  I  G  N  E  A  U  E  R  X  J  J  F  D  K  Y  L
O  Q  O  H  P  T  C  G  W  D  S  M  R  C  G  T  B  S  R  I  M  W
I  P  S  J  Q  R  A  M  Q  G  M  W  E  O  D  D  D  Q  B  S  A  F
P  Q  U  X  F  I  T  R  E  Q  D  L  B  N  S  O  D  I  U  C  K  C
I  T  R  Q  B  A  I  P  Y  N  E  H  J  V  T  I  N  L  Q  F  E  T
B  A  S  J  X  T  O  R  D  C  F  P  I  V  T  M  S  E  D  U  D  I
R  M  H  Q  R  E  N  Y  S  U  V  Q  R  F  Y  M  O  U  W  U  Q  R
F  G  K  N  T  D  W  U  J  B  U  C  W  Z  R  I  M  B  V  A  E  J
```

Can you find the 20 words hidden in this puzzle? All hidden word puzzles will have words running from top to bottom, left to right, and diagonally downward.

CLASSIFICATION	ANTAGONISTS	APONEUROSIS	INVOLUNTARY
SYNERGISTS	INSERTION	VOLUNTARY	EXTENSOR
LIGAMENT	SKELETAL	STRIATED	VISCERAL
CARDIAC	FASCIA	FIBERS	FLEXOR
MUSCLE	ORIGIN	SMOOTH	TENDON

CHAPTER 7 ANSWERS

Exercise 1
1. tendons
2. ligaments
3. aponeurosis
4. origin
5. motor nerve

Exercise 2
1. D   6. J
2. F   7. A
3. H   8. I
4. B   9. C
5. G   10. E

Exercise 3
1. azygous
2. longissimus
3. orbicularis
4. quadri-
5. teres

Exercise 4
1. brachioradialis—B
2. buccinator—D
3. extensor carpi—A
4. external oblique abdominal—C
5. biceps brachii—F

6. orbicularis—E
7. platysma—D
8. levator scapulae—A
9. flexor carpi radialis—A
10. tibialis anterior—C

Exercise 5

1. frontalis
2. orbicularis oculi
3. orbicularis oris
4. brachialis
5. pronator teres
6. brachioradialis
7. flexor carpi radialis
8. iliopsoas
9. pectineus
10. gracilis
11. vastus medialis
12. gastrocnemius
13. tibialis anterior
14. soleus
15. sternocleidomastoid
16. deltoid
17. pectoralis major
18. biceps brachii
19. rectus abdominis
20. rectus femoris
21. vastus lateralis
22. sartorius
23. peroneus longus

Exercise 6

1. deltoid
2. triceps
3. extensor carpi ulnaris
4. flexor carpi ulnaris
5. gracilis
6. semitendinosus
7. sternocleidomastoid
8. trapezius
9. teres major
10. latissimus dorsi
11. external oblique
12. gluteus medius
13. gluteus maximus
14. vastus lateralis
15. biceps femoris
16. semimembranosus
17. gastrocnemius
18. soleus
19. Achilles tendon

Exercise 7

1. B
2. K
3. D
4. C
5. G
6. F
7. I
8. H
9. J
10. E
11. A

Exercise 8

1. amyotrophia: no; muscle; nourishment—atrophy of muscle
2. myofibrosis: muscle; fibrous tissue—muscle tissue replaced by fibrous tissue
3. fasciodesis: fascia; binding—suturing of fascia to skeletal attachment
4. myotenotomy: muscle; tendon—surgical incision of tendon of a muscle
5. myalgia: muscle; pain—painful muscle
6. myoedema: muscle; swelling—swelling of muscle
7. tenostosis: tendon; bone—ossification of tendon
8. myoma: muscle; tumor—tumor of muscle
9. myorrhaphy: muscle; suturing—suturing of muscle
10. myosclereosis: muscle; hardening—hardening of muscle
11. tenosynovectomy: tendon; synovial sheath; excision—surgical excision of tendon sheath
12. myomelanosis: muscle; melanin pigment—area of black pigment in a muscle

Answers: Chapter 7 Crossword Puzzle

					1 C								2 M	Y	3 O	L	O	G	Y
	4 A	P	5 O	N	E	U	R	O	S	6 I	S				C				
	N		R		P					N					U				7 S
	T		I			8 G		9 T		10 S	A	R	C	O	L	E	11 M	M	A
	A		G			A		E		E					I		I		R
	G		I			12 S	Y	N	E	R	G	I	S	13 T			N		C
	O		N			T		D		T				H			I		O
	N			14 S	A	R	T	O	R	I	U	S		O			M		P
15 W	I	D	E			O		N		O			16 A	R	M		U		L
	S					C		S		N				A			S		A
	17 T	O	N	E		N						18 L		X					S
						E			19 T			I			20 P		21 O		M
		22 S		23 H	A	M	S	T	R	I	N	G	S		E		R		
		C				I			A			A			R		I		
	24 M	A	X	I	M	U	S		P			25 M	E	D	I	U	S		26 F
		L				S			E			E			N				I
		P							Z			N			E				B
					27 F	A	S	C	I	A		T			U				E
									U						28 M	O	T	O	R
		29 A	C	H	I	L	L	E	S										S

Answers: Chapter 7 Hidden Words Puzzle

```
. .  F  .  .  .  .  .  .  .  .  .  .  .  .  .  .  .  .  .  .
. .  .  L  T  .  .  I  S  K  E  L  E  T  A  L  .  .  .  .  .
. .  .  .  E  .  .  N  Y  .  .  .  .  .  .  .  .  .  .  .
. .  .  .  N  X  .  S  N  .  .  E  .  .  .  .  .  .  .  .
.  F  .  .  D  O  O  E  E  .  .  X  .  .  .  .  .  .  .  .
. .  A  .  O  R  .  R  R  .  T  .  .  .  .  .  .  .  .  .
. .  .  S  N  I  .  T  G  .  E  .  .  .  .  .  .  .  .  .
. .  .  M  C  G  C  I  I  .  .  N  .  .  .  .  .  .  .  .
. .  .  O  .  I  L  O  S  V  I  S  C  E  R  A  L  .  .  .  .
F  .  .  O  M  N  A  N  T  A  G  O  N  I  S  T  S  .  .  .  .  .
V  I  .  T  .  U  S  P  S  .  .  R  .  .  .  .  .  .  .  .
.  O  B  H  .  .  S  L  O  .  .  .  .  .  C  .  .  .  .  .
. .  L  E' .  .  I  C  I  N  V  O  L  U  N  T  A  R  Y  .  .  .
. .  .  U  R  .  F  .  L  G  E  .  .  .  .  R  .  .  .  .
. .  .  .  N  S  I  .  .  E  A  U  .  .  .  .  .  D  .  .  .
. .  .  .  .  T  C  .  .  .  M  R  .  .  .  .  .  I  .  .
. .  .  .  .  R  A  .  .  .  E  O  .  .  .  .  A  .
. .  .  .  .  I  T  R  .  .  .  .  N  S  .  .  .  .  .  C
. .  .  .  .  A  I  .  Y  .  .  .  T  I  .  .  .  .
. .  .  .  .  T  O  .  .  .  .  .  .  S  .  .  .  .
. .  .  .  .  E  N  .  .  .  .  .  .  .  .  .  .  .
. .  .  .  .  D  .  .  .  .  .  .  .  .  .  .  .  .
```

Words:

\/ CLASSIFICATION	> ANTAGONISTS	\ APONEUROSIS	> INVOLUNTARY
\/ SYNERGISTS	\/ INSERTION	\ VOLUNTARY	\/ EXTENSOR
\ LIGAMENT	> SKELETAL	\/ STRIATED	> VISCERAL
\ CARDIAC	\ FASCIA	\ FIBERS	\ FLEXOR
\ MUSCLE	\/ ORIGIN	\/ SMOOTH	\/ TENDON

CHAPTER 7 GLOSSARY

Muscles and Related Anatomic Terms

abduction (ab-duk'shun): movement that draws a body part away from the mid-line of the body.

abductor muscles: muscles that abduct.

Achilles tendon (ah-kil'ez): a powerful tendon of the gastrocnemius and soleus at the back of the heel (also called *calcaneal tendon*), named for a Greek hero whose only vulnerable spot was his heel.

adduction (ad-duk'shun): movement that draws a body part toward the mid-line of the body.

adductor muscles: muscles that adduct.

adductor longus, magnus, and **brevis:** a group of adductor muscles of the thigh that also assist in flexion, extension and rotation.

antagonist: a muscle acting in opposition to another.

aponeurosis (ap"o-nu-ro'sis): a flattened, ribbonlike, white tendon that connects a muscle to the part it moves (plural—*aponeuroses*).

auriculares (aw"rik-u-la'rez): group of muscles of the ear; **anterior, posterior,** and **superior.**

biceps (bi'seps): indicates two origins (or heads) of a muscle.

brachialis (bra-ke-a'lis): arm muscle that flexes the forearm.

brachioradialis: lower arm muscle that flexes the forearm.

buccinator (buk'si-na"tor): a cheek muscle (also called *trumpeter*).

cardiac: muscle of the heart.

coccygeus (kok-sij'e-us): muscle supporting and raising the coccyx.

constrictor pharyngis: muscle group that constricts the pharynx; **inferior, medius,** and **superior.**

deltoid (del'toid): muscle that abducts, flexes, and extends upper arm.

diaphragm (di'ah-fram): musculomembranous wall between abdominal and thoracic cavities.

erector spinae: deep muscle of the back that aids in maintaining balance (also called *sacrospinalis*).

extensors: muscles that extend a part.

fascia (fash'e-ah): sheet of fibrous membrane that encloses muscles and separates them into groups (plural—*fasciae*).

fascia lata femoris: broad external fascia enveloping muscles of the thigh.

fasciculus (fah-sik'u-lus): a small bundle or cluster (referring to muscle, tendon, or nerve fibers; plural—*fasciculi*).

fibromuscular: composed of muscular and fibrous tissue.

fixator muscles: muscles that steady a part while other muscles execute movement.

flexor: muscle that flexes or bends a joint.

galea aponeurotica (ga'le-ah): the broad, flat tendon over the top of the skull.

gastrocnemius (gas"trok-ne'me-us): muscle of the lower leg (calf), resembling the shape of the stomach, that flexes the leg and extends the foot.

gemellus (je-mel'us): twin thigh muscles, inferior and superior, that aid in lateral rotation of the thigh (plural—*gemelli*).

gluteal (gloo'te-al): referring to the buttock, a group of muscles, **gluteus maximus, medius,** and **minimus,** which abduct, rotate, and extend the thigh.

gracilis (gras'i-lis): flexes leg and adducts leg and thigh.

hamstring group: three large muscles that descend in the back of the thigh, their tendons forming the "hamstrings," are the **semimembranosus** and the **semitendinosus,** which extend the thigh, and the **biceps femoris,** which extends the thigh and flexes the leg.

iliacus (il-i'ah-kus): muscle that flexes thigh and trunk.

iliocostalis: muscle group including the **iliocostalis dorsi,** which keeps the thoracic spine erect; the **iliocostalis lumborum,** which extends the lumbar spine; and the **iliocostalis cervicis,** which extends the cervical spine.

iliopsoas (il"e-o-so'as): **iliacus** and **psoas major** muscles combined and referred to as one muscle, which flexes the thigh and trunk.

infrahyoid muscles: small, flat, ribbonlike muscles of the neck, including the **sternothyroid, sternohyoid, thyrohyoid,** and **omohyoid** muscles, which hold the hyoid bone to the sternum, scapula, and clavicle.

infraspinatus (in"frah-spi-na'tus): muscle that rotates the humerus laterally.

inspiratory muscles: muscles that aid in inspiration, such as the **diaphragm** and the **interocostals.**

intercostals: respiratory muscles, situated between the ribs.

interossei (in"ter-os'e-i): muscles of the hand and foot that flex, abduct and adduct fingers and toes.

interspinales (in"ter-spi-nal'ez): muscle group that extends the vertebral column in the cervical, thoracic and lumbar regions.

involuntary muscle: muscle that cannot be moved at will.

latissimus dorsi (lah-tis'i-mus dor'si): the broadest muscle of the back, which extends and adducts the upper arm.

levator ani (le-va'tor): muscle of the pelvic floor.

levator scapulae: muscle that raises the scapula.

ligaments: strong bands of fibrous tissue connecting bones or cartilage, which aid or restrict movement and support organs.

longissimus muscles (lon-jis'i-mus): group of muscles, including the **capitas,** which draws the head backward and rotates it, the **cervicis**, which extends the cervical vertebrae, and the **thoracis**, which extends the thoracic vertebrae.

lumbricales (lum′bri-ka′les): phalangeal muscles of the foot and hand.

masseter (mas-se′ter): chewing muscles.

multifidus spinae (mul-tif′i-dus): muscles that extend and rotate the vertebral column.

oblique external abdominal: muscle that compresses and supports the abdominal viscera.

oblique internal abdominal: muscle that compresses and supports the abdominal viscera.

obturator externus and **internus** (ob′tu-ra″tor): muscles that rotate the thigh laterally.

occipitofrontal (ok-sip″i-to-fron-t′al): a group of flat muscles of the forehead and scalp.

orbicularis oculi (or-bik″u-la′ris): muscle that moves the eyelids.

orbicularis oris: muscle that draws lips into a pucker.

orbitalis: muscle that makes eye protrude.

palatoglossus (pal″ah-to-glos′us): muscle for elevating the tongue and constricting the passage from mouth to throat.

palatopharyngeus: muscle that aids in swallowing.

pectineus: muscle that flexes and adducts the thigh.

pectoralis major and **minor** (pek″to-ra′lis): muscles that adduct and flex upper arms (**major**), and draw shoulder forward and down (**minor**).

peroneus longus, brevis, and **tertius** (per″o-ne′us): lower leg muscles aiding in movement of the feet.

piriformis (pir″i-for′mis): pear-shaped muscle that laterally rotates, abducts and extends the thigh.

platysma (plah-tiz′mah): facial muscle of expression that pulls down the corners of the mouth.

popliteal (pop″li-te′al): muscle that flexes and rotates the leg medially.

pronator teres and **quadratus:** muscles that flex and pronate the lower arm.

psoas major and **minor** (so′as): muscles that flex the trunk and thigh, medially rotating the thigh.

pyramidal (pi-ram″id′al): muscle that tenses the abdominal wall.

quadratus femoris (kwod-ra′tus): thigh muscle for adduction and lateral rotation.

quadratus lumborum: muscle that laterally flexes the trunk.

quadriceps femoris (kwod′ri-seps): muscle (four-headed) that extends the leg.

rectus abdominis (rek′tus ab′dom′i-nus): muscle supporting abdomen and flexing lumbar vertebrae.

rectus capitis: muscles of head, anterior, lateral, and posterior major and minor muscles that support, flex, and extend the head.

rectus femoris: muscle that extends the leg and flexes the thigh.

rhomboideus major and **minor** (rom-boi′de-us): rhomboid muscles (kite-shaped) that elevate, adduct, and retract the scapulae.

risorius (ri-so′re-us): facial muscle that draws out the angle of the mouth.

sarcolemma: plasma membrane of muscle cells.

sarcoplasm: the cytoplasm of muscle cells.

sartorius (sar-to′re-us): muscle of the thigh, deriving its name from its ability to flex and adduct the leg to that position assumed by a tailor sitting cross-legged at work (**sartorius** means tailor).

scalenus: group of muscles that raise the first and second ribs.

semimembranosus: muscle that extends the thigh.

semispinalis (sem″e-spi-na′lis): group of muscles for movement of the vertebral column and head.

semitendinosus (sem″e-ten″di-no′sus): muscle that extends the thigh.

serratus (ser-ra′tus): muscle group; **anterior**, **posterior superior**, and **posterior inferior** rotates scapula, raises shoulder, abducts arm, and raises and lowers ribs during respiration.

soleus (so′le-us): muscle that extends the foot.

sphincters (sfingk′ters): circular muscles that constrict an orifice, such as the anus, urethra, and pyloris.

splenius (sple′ne-us): muscle group (**capitis** and **cervicis**) that extends and rotates the head and neck.

sternocleidomastoid (ster″no-kli″do-mas′toid): muscle that tilts the head forward or to one side, and rotates it.

subclavius (sub-kla′ve-us): muscle that moves the clavicle.

subcostals: muscles that raise the ribs in inspiration.

subscapularis (sub″skap-u-la′ris): muscle that rotates the arm medially.

supinator (su″pi-na′tor): muscle that turns the forearm upward.

supraspinatus (su″prah-spi-na′tus): muscle that abducts the arm.

synergists (sin′er-jists): muscles that work together.

tensor fasciae latae: muscle that abducts the thigh.

teres major and **minor** (te′rez): extends and adducts the upper arm and rotates it medially.

tibialis anterior and **posterior** (tib″e-a′lis): muscles that extend, flex, and turn the foot in.

tone: state of tension, present to a degree in muscles at all times.

transversus abdominis: the transverse abdominal muscles that compress and support the viscera of the abdomen.

trapezius (trah-pe′ze-us): a trapezoid-shaped muscle of the back of the neck and upper trunk that controls shoulder movements.

triceps brachii (tri′seps): muscle that extends the forearm.

vastus intermedius, lateralis, and **medialis** (vas′tus): muscle group that extends the leg.

voluntary muscle: muscle that can be moved at will.

Pathologic Conditions

Inflammations and Infections

dermatomyositis (der″mah-to-mi″o-si′tis): connective tissue disease characterized by inflammation of the skin, underlying tissues, and muscles, with necrosis of muscle fibers.

fasciitis (fas″e-i′tis): inflammation of the fascia (also called **fascitis**).

myocellulitis (mi″o-sel″u-li′tis): myositis with cellulitis (inflammation of cellular tissue).

myochorditis (mi″o-kor-di′tis): inflammation of the muscles of the vocal cords.

myofascitis (mi″o-fas-i′tis): inflammation of a muscle and its fascia.

myositis (mi″o-si′tis): inflammation of voluntary muscle.

myositis ossificans (o-sif′i-kans): a myositis characterized by bony deposits in muscle tissue.

myotenositis (mi″o-ten″o-si′tis): inflammation of a muscle and its tendon.

polymyalgia rheumatica (pol′i-mi-al′j-ah): pain caused by inflammation in more than one muscle group.

shin splints: swelling and pain caused by strain of pretibial muscle following overexertion.

tenositis: inflammation of a tendon (also called **tenontitis** or **tenonitis**).

tenostosis (ten″os-to′sis): conversion of tendon tissue into bone or bony substance.

tenosynovitis (ten″o-sin″o-vi′tis): inflammation of a tendon sheath (also called **tenovaginitis** or **tendovaginitis**).

torticollis (tor″ti-kol′is): an acute myositis of the cervical muscles (also called **wryneck**).

trichiniasis or **trichinosis** (trik″i-ni′ah-sis; trik″i-no′sis): disease caused by eating undercooked, parasite-infected meat with symptoms of nausea, diarrhea, colic and fever, followed by stiffness, pain, and swelling of muscles.

Degenerative and Innervative Disorders

amyotrophy or **amyotrophia:** atrophy of muscles.

Dupuytren's contracture (du-pwe′trahnz): disease affecting the palmar fascia of the hand, causing the ring and little finger to contract toward the palm (named for its discoverer).

muscular atrophy: wasting away of muscle tissue (types and causes are multiple).

myasthenia gravis (mi″as-the′ne-ah): debilitating, muscular disease, with progressive paralysis of the muscles, especially affecting muscles of the face, lips, tongue, throat, and neck.

myofibrosis (mi″o-fi-bro′sis): overgrowth of fibrous tissue, replacing muscle tissue.

myoparalysis: paralysis of a muscle or muscles.

myotonia (mi″o-to′ne-ah): increased muscular irritability and contractility (tonic spasm), with delayed relaxation.

myotonia acquisita: myotonia caused by injury or disease.

spastic paralysis: paralysis marked by spasticity of muscles of the affected part and heightened tendon reflexes.

Volkmann's contracture (folk′mahnz): contracture of the fingers and sometimes the wrists (named for its discoverer), with loss of muscle power, caused by vascular (blood flow) blockage (also called **ischemic muscular atrophy**).

Hereditary, Congenital and Developmental Disorders

congenital amyotonia (ah-mi″o-to′ne-ah): term used to describe several rare congenital diseases of infants and children, characterized by lack of muscular development (also called **atonic pseudoparalysis**, **myatonia congenita**, and **Oppenheim's disease**).

muscular dystrophy: a group of hereditary diseases characterized by progressive weakness and atrophy of muscles without nervous system involvement (also called **Erb's** or **Erb-Landouzy disease**, **idiopathic muscular atrophy**, and **myodystrophia**).

myotonia congenita: hereditary, congenital disease, characterized by spasm and rigidity of muscles when moved after rest or when mechanically stimulated, with stiffness disappearing as muscles are used (also called **paramyotonia congenita**, **myotonia hereditaria**, **Eulenburg's disease**, and **Thomsen's disease**).

pseudohypertrophic muscular dystrophy: progressive dystrophy of the muscles of the shoulder and pelvic girdles, beginning in childhood, with hypertrophy progressing to atrophy of the muscles (also called **Duchenne's muscular dystrophy**, **Erb's paralysis**, **Zimmerlin's dystrophy**, and **pseudohypertrophic muscular atrophy**).

Werdnig-Hoffman syndrome: hereditary, progressive, muscular atrophy, beginning in infancy and followed by early death (also called **Hoffmann-Werdnig's syndrome**, **familial spinal muscular atrophy**, and **progressive spinal muscular atrophy of infants**).

Oncology

desmoid tumor: very hard fibroma, most frequently in abdominal muscles, especially in women who have borne children.

leiomyoma (li″o-mi-o′mah): benign tumor of smooth muscle, usually found in the uterus (commonly known as fibroid tumor).

leiomyosarcoma* (li″o-mi″o-sar-ko′mah): malignant tumor of smooth muscle usually found in uterus or retroperitoneal region.

myoblastoma (mi″o-blas-to′mah): a benign lesion of soft tissue (also called *myoblastomyoma*).

myofibroma: tumor with muscular and fibrous elements.

myoma (mi-o′mah): tumor composed of muscle tissue.

myosarcoma*: malignant tumor of muscular tissue.

rhabdomyoma: benign tumor arising from striated muscle.

rhabdomyochondroma (rab″do-mi″o-kon-dro′mah): benign tumor composed of two or more types of cells (also called *rhabdomyomyxoma*).

rhabdomyosarcoma* (rab″do-mi″o-sar-ko′mah): very malignant tumor of striated muscle (also called *rhabdomyoblastoma*).

Surgical Procedures

fasciectomy (fash″e-ek′to-me): excision of fascia.

fasciodesis (fash″e-od′e-sis): suturing of fascia to tendon or other facia.

fascioplasty (fash′e-o-plas″te): plastic repair of fascia.

fasciorrhaphy (fash″e-or′ah-fe): repair of torn fascia.

fasciotomy (fash″e-to′o-me): incision of a fascia.

myectomy (mi-ek′to-me): excision of a part of a muscle.

myoplasty (mi′o-plas″te): plastic repair of muscle.

myorrhaphy (mi-or′ah-fe): repair of a divided muscle (also called *myosuture*).

myotenotomy (mi″o-ten-ot′o-me): cutting of muscle and tendon (also called *tenomyotomy* or *tenontomyotomy*).

myotomy: incision or dissection of a muscle.

tenodesis (ten-od′e-sis): suturing of a tendon to a bone.

tenoplasty (ten′o-plas″te): plastic repair of a tendon.

tenorrhaphy (ten-or′ah-fe): suturing of a divided tendon (also called *tenosuture*).

tenosynovectomy (ten″o-sin″o-vek′to-me): excision of the sheath of a tendon.

tenotomy: cutting of a tendon.

Descriptive and Diagnostic Terms

myalgia (mi-al′je-ah): pain in a muscle (also called *myodynia*).

myoclonus (mi-ok′lo-nus): spasm of a muscle or muscles.

myodiastasis (mi″o-di-as′tah-sis): muscle separation.

myodystonia (mi″o-dis-to′ne-ah): muscle tone disorder.

myoedema (mi″o-e-de′mah): fluid accumulation in muscle.

myogelosis (mi″o-je-lo′sis): hardening of muscle in a specific area, especially in the gluteal region.

myokinesis (mi″o-ki-ne′sis): movement of a muscle or its fibers, especially during a surgical procedure.

myology: study of muscles.

myolysis: disintegration of muscle tissue.

myomalacia (mi″o-mah-la′she-ah): softening of a muscle.

myomelanosis (mi″o-mel″ah-no′sis): area of black pigment in a muscle.

myonecrosis (mi″o-ne-kro′sis): death of muscle fibers.

myopathy (mi-op′ah-the): any disease of the muscles.

myosclerosis (mi″o-skle-ro′sis): hardening of muscle tissue.

myospasm (mi′o-spazm): spasm of a muscle.

myotasis (mi-ot′ah-sis): stretching of a muscle.

tenodynia (ten″o-din′e-ah): pain in a tendon (also called *tenalgia*).

tetany: paroxysmal spasms.

tic: twitch or spasm of a muscle.

Laboratory Tests

biopsy: removal of tissue for microscopic examination.

computerized tomography (CT): imaging device using x-rays at multiple angles through specific sections of the body, analyzed by computer to provide a total picture of the part being examined to detect tumors in muscle tissue (also called *computerized axial tomography [CAT]*).

creatine phosphokinase: blood serum test to detect enzyme elevations found in patients with muscular dystrophy and other muscle conditions.

electromyography: electrical recording of the changes in skeletal muscle resulting from electrical stimulation.

inulin clearance: a urine test to evaluate the rate at which inulin is excreted, to diagnose muscle diseases.

magnetic resonance imaging (MRI): non-invasive method of scanning the body by use of an electromagnetic field and radio waves, which provides visual images on a computer screen, and magnetic tape recordings, to detect muscle disease (also called *nuclear magnetic resonance [NMR]*).

3-methoxy-hydroxymandelic acid: a urine test in which elevated levels of adrenaline and noradrenaline indicate muscle conditions such as muscular dystrophy and myasthenia gravis.

myoglobin: test for protein found in normal muscle tissue, which, when present in urine, indicates extensive muscle destruction.

myokinesimeter: testing device to measure muscular contractions by stimulation with electrical current.

nuclear magnetic resonance (NMR): see **magnetic resonance imaging**.

trichina agglutinin: test of blood serum that reveals the presence of trichinosis.

* Indicates a malignant condition.

Chapter 8

The Integumentary System

The Skin and Its Accessory Structures

It's a Fact:
The average adult changes his or her outer skin about every 27 days, making a total of about 1000 skins in a 70-year period.

CHAPTER OVERVIEW

This chapter describes the skin, the largest and one of the most remarkable organs of the body, and its accessory organs—hair, sweat glands, sebaceous glands, and nails—which form the integumentary system.

SKIN

The study of skin is called ***dermatology***. The skin, which covers the body, has a variety of functions necessary to survival. It acts as a barrier against the invasion of microorganisms, protects underlying structures from injury, helps to maintain and regulate body temperature, and acts as a receptor for the sensations of touch, heat, cold, pressure, and pain. Along with the kidneys, intestines, and lungs, the skin plays a crucial role in disposing of waste products.

Under normal conditions the temperature of the body is maintained through a heat-regulating mechanism that keeps a balance between heat production and heat loss. The body produces heat by metabolism of the food ingested, and the amount of heat produced is directly connected to the amount of work done by the muscles.

Most body heat loss occurs through the skin by:

1. transfer from the skin to a cooler surface without direct contact—called ***radiation***
2. transfer from the skin to objects in direct contact—called ***conduction***
3. transfer from the skin by movement of fluid or air—called ***convection***
4. perspiration—called ***evaporation***

The remainder of heat loss occurs through the mucous membranes of the respiratory, digestive, and urinary tracts.

Review A

Complete the following:

1. The accessory organs of the skin are the _____, _____, _____, and

    _____.

2. The study of skin is called _____.

3. The body produces heat by _____ of food taken in.

4. Heat loss due to perspiration is called _____.

5. Transfer of heat from skin to a cooler surface without direct contact is called _____.

Composition of the Skin

The skin is composed of two principal layers, the *epidermis*, the outer, thinner layer visible to the naked eye, and the *dermis* (or *corium*), the inner, thicker layer (Fig. 8-1).

Epidermis

The epidermis is made up of stratified squamous epithelial tissue. The layers of the epidermis, from the dermis outward, are:

The *stratum germinativum* (basal layer)—the cells in this innermost layer multiply continuously to compensate for the constant loss of cells from the surface of the epidermis. These new cells push upward into each succeeding layer, eventually die, and are sloughed off. The process is continuous.

The *stratum granulosum* (granular layer)—so-called because it contains granules visible in the cytoplasm of the cells, which begin to die in this layer. The stratum granulosum may not be present in some areas of thin skin.

The *stratum lucidum* (clear layer)—so-called because of its closely packed, clear cells, and found only in the thicker skin of the soles of the feet and the palms of the hands.

The *stratum corneum* (horny layer)—composed of flat, lifeless, *keratinized* (*kerat-* means horny tissue) cells, which appear as overlapping dry scales making up the outer skin layer. If these scales are unbroken, they can prevent the entrance of microorganisms. Dead cells are continuously sloughed off this layer and replaced by new ones from the stratum germinativum.

Skin color is determined by the amount of *melanin* (skin pigment) in the stratum germinativum layer of the epidermis. Melanin serves as protection by screening ultraviolet rays from harming the underlying tissue. Heredity is the chief factor influencing the lightness or darkness of a person's skin color, in conjunction with sunlight and some hormones.

Dermis

The dermis (corium) is made up of a dense, fibrous connective tissue containing blood vessels and nerves. A subcutaneous layer under the dermis consists of *areolar* (loose, ordinary) and *adipose* (fatty) tissue. In the dermis are the hair shafts, with small bundles of involuntary muscle called the *arrector pili* attached to the hair follicles. When one is frightened, or exposed to cold, these muscles contract, the hair "stands up," and the skin forms what is known as "gooseflesh." *Sebaceous* (oil-producing, to lubricate the hair) glands, sweat glands, and receptors for the sensations of touch, heat, cold, and pain, are also found in the dermis.

Structure of the Skin

The structure of the skin differs throughout the body. It is tough and stretchable, and varies in thickness. It is thick on the palms of the hands and soles of the feet, and thin on the eyelids. There are differences in moistness, roughness, dryness, and smoothness, according to the presence of sebaceous and sweat glands. The skin is firm and elastic in youth, but with age it becomes wrinkled, dry, loose and saggy, particularly in the regions of the neck, hands, and around the eyes and mouth.

The structure of the skin over the palms of the hands and soles of the feet is different from that of the rest of the body. It has ridges, unique to each individual, particularly on the fingers and toes, that do not change throughout life. Each individual pattern differs from all others, providing a basis for the use of fingerprints as a means of positive identification.

Review B

Complete the following:

1. Skin is composed of two principal layers: _____ and _____ .

2. Skin contains receptors for the sensations of _____ , _____ , _____ ,

and_____ .

3. Thick skin is found on the _____ and_____ .

4. Thin skin is found on the_____ .

5. Keratinized cells are found on the stratum_____ .

Hair

Almost all parts of the body are covered by hair, although in many areas it is so fine that it is scarcely discernible. There is no hair on the palms of the hands, the soles of the feet, and the palmar and plantar surfaces of the fingers and toes. Hair first appears on the fetus, and, at puberty, there is an added growth of body hair, especially in the areas of the pubes and axillae in both sexes, with males developing facial hair.

Hair develops from a structure in the dermis called the ***hair papilla***, located at the base of a tube, the ***hair follicle***, extending to the outside of the epidermis. Cells at the base of the follicle increase, push upward, and keratinize, forming the visible ***hair shaft*** at the surface.

The texture, amount, distribution and color of hair vary, with hereditary factors playing a major role. Hair loses pigment with increasing age.

There seems to be no known function for body hair. Head and facial hair affords some protection against cold and sunlight. The ***cilia*** (eyelashes), ***supercilia*** (eyebrows), and the hair in the ears and nose provide some protection against entry by insects and dust, and the eyelashes and brows also provide shade.

Sweat Glands

The ***sudoriferous*** (sweat) glands are excretory organs of the skin, and serve a function in the cooling of the body. They are the most numerous of the skin glands, and there are more on the palms, soles, forehead, and axillae. An ***eccrine*** (ordinary) sweat gland is a coiled, tubular structure, in the form of a ball, embedded in the dermis, with its duct emerging on the skin surface as a sweat pore (Fig. 8-1).

Perspiration is constantly secreted, and usually evaporates as fast as it is formed, except during muscular exercise or exposure to heat, when it increases more rapidly than it can evaporate. ***Apocrine*** glands, located in the axillae, around the anus, and in the genital area, are larger sweat glands, with a strong smelling secretion stimulated by excitement and emotion.

Sebaceous Glands

The sebaceous glands are sac-like structures, secreting a substance called ***sebum***, which lubricates the skin and hair. Sebaceous glands are far more numerous on the scalp, forehead, face, and chin than in other parts of the body, and are mainly associated with hair follicles. However, some open on the surface independently of hairs, on the eyelids, labia minora (vaginal lips), prepuce (sheath of the clitoris or penis), and areola (area around the nipple). When sebaceous gland ducts become blocked with sebum, a pimple or blackhead may develop.

Ceruminous Glands

Ceruminous glands are classified as modified sweat glands, located in the external ear canal, secreting a yellowish, waxy substance called ***cerumen*** (ear wax).

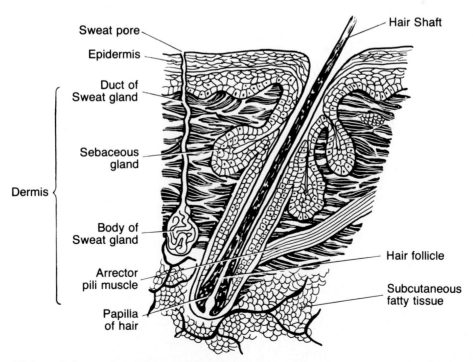

Figure 8-1 Composition of skin.

Nails

The nails are a modified form of epidermis that grow from epithelial cells located at the base of each nail under the **lunula** (half-moon shaped white portion). The nails are keratinized, flat, translucent, resilient plates that derive their pink appearance from the underlying blood vessels.

Review C

Complete the following:

1. Cells at the base of the _____ increase, push upward, keratinize, and form the visible hair shaft.

2. The word _____ means eyebrows.

3. Another word for sweat gland is _____.

4. Sebaceous glands secrete _____.

5. The yellowish, waxy secretion in the ears is called _____.

Answers to Review Questions: The Integumentary System

Review A
1. hair, sweat glands, sebaceous glands, nails
2. dermatology
3. metabolism
4. evaporation
5. radiation

Review B
1. epidermis, dermis
2. touch, heat, cold, pain

3. palms of hands, soles of feet
4. eyelid(s)
5. corneum

Review C
1. hair follicle
2. supercilia
3. sudoriferous
4. sebum
5. cerumen

CHAPTER 8 EXERCISES

INTEGUMENTARY SYSTEM: THE SKIN AND ITS ACCESSORY STRUCTURES

Exercise 1: Complete the following:

1. The epidermis is composed of four layers of cells. They are:

a. _____   c. _____

b. _____   d. _____

2. Body heat is lost through the skin by _____, _____, _____, and

_____.

3. Hair covers almost all parts of the body except the _____ of the hands and the _____ of the feet.

4. The _____ and _____ serve as a protection to shade the eyes and keep out harmful objects and dust.

5. Another term for dermis is _____.

Exercise 2: Using the list of terms below, identify each part in Fig. 8-2 by placing its name in the corresponding blank.

Hair shaft   Epidermis   Dermis
Subcutaneous fatty tissue   Papilla of hair   Duct of sweat gland
Sebaceous gland   Body of sweat gland   Arrector pili muscle
Hair follicle   Sweat pore

1. _____
2. _____
3. _____
4. _____
5. _____
6. _____
7. _____
8. _____
9. _____
10. _____
11. _____

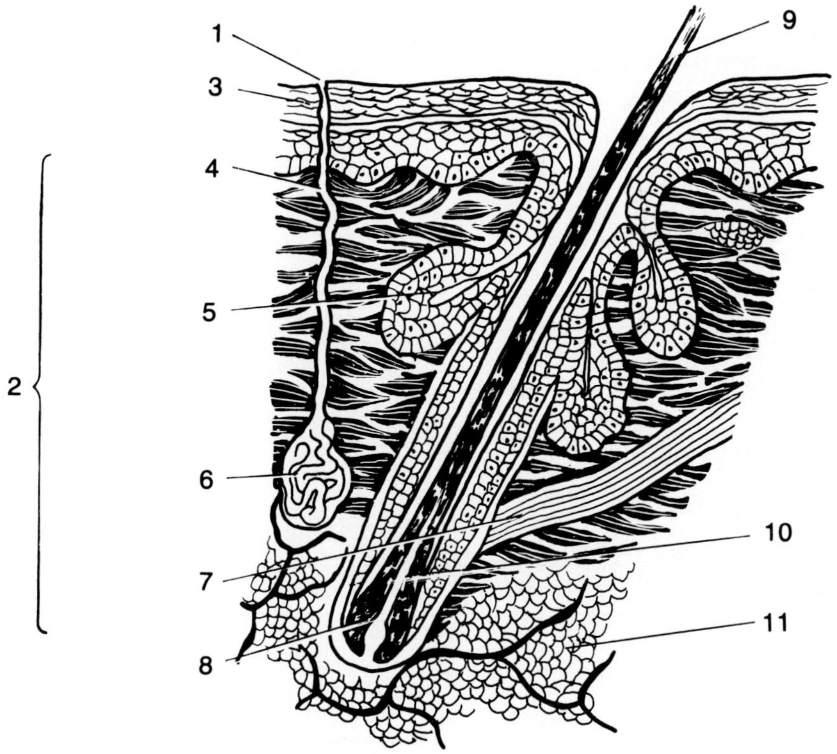

Figure 8-2.   Composition of skin.

Exercise 3: Matching:

____ **1.** sebaceous glands   **A.** barrier, receptor, waste disposal

____ **2.** apocrine glands   **B.** glands with ducts opening around hair follicles

____ **3.** ceruminous glands   **C.** large sweat glands with strong-smelling secretion

____ **4.** dermis   **D.** pigment of skin or hair

____ **5.** lunula   **E.** secretions of sebaceous glands

____ **6.** arrector pili   **F.** dense, fibrous connective tissue

____ **7.** areola   **G.** area around the nipple

____ **8.** melanin pigment   **H.** crescent-shaped portion at nail base

____ **9.** sebum   **I.** modified sweat glands located in the external ear canal

____ **10.** skin   **J.** small muscles of the skin that produce "gooseflesh"

Exercise 4: Give the meaning of the components in the following words and then define the word as a whole. Suffixes meaning *pertaining to* or *state or condition,* shown following a slash mark (/), are not to be defined separately. Before reaching for your medical dictionary, check the glossary at the end of the chapter.

1. Dermatosclerosis:

   derm/ato _____

   scler/osis _____

   _____

2. Tinea barbae:

   tinea _____

   barb/ae _____

   _____

3. Cutis hyperelastica:

   cutis _____

   hyper _____

   elastic/a _____

   _____

4. Ichthyosis congenita:

   ichthy/osis _____

   congenita _____

   _____

5. Neurofibroma:

   neuro _____

   fibr _____

   oma _____

   _____

6. Anhidrosis:

   an _____

   hidr/osis _____

   _____

7. Dyskeratosis:

   dys _____

   kerat/osis _____

   _____

8. Purpura:

   purpura _____

   _____

9. Exfoliative dermatitis:

   exfolia/tive _____

   derm/at _____

   itis _____

   _____

10. Actinic dermatitis:

   actin/ic _____

   derm/at _____

   itis _____

   _____

Chapter 8 Crossword Puzzle

Across

1. term for sweat gland
4. study of the skin
6. one of 4 epidermal layers
8. form fingerprints
9. an accessory organ gland
10. number of principal skin layers
11. one of the skin layers
15. heat loss by direct contact
17. a type of sweat gland
20. one of 4 epidermal layers
21. one of 4 epidermal layers
23. skin pigment
24. a skin accessory organ
25. skin color is due to _____

Down

2. heat loss by perspiration
3. heat loss by fluid/air movement
5. heat loss without direct contact
7. sebaceous gland secretion
12. a type of sweat gland
13. outer layer of skin
14. largest organ of body
16. another word for inner skin layer
18. yellow ear secretion
19. tube from which hair grows
22. half-moon portion of nail

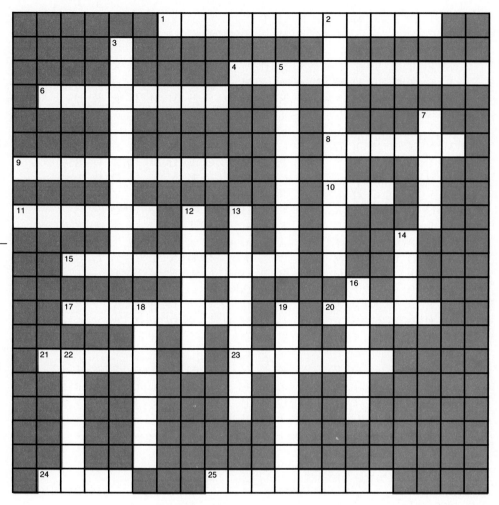

Chapter 8 Hidden Words Puzzle

```
L U N U L A R G S U F W H Y P H O W V A E Y J
B K M Y D E R M I S U C T F Y E F F E E J L T
A P O C R I N E T R E M V F O I G O I X V P T
S C D M O Q M P O X O B T A I V U I B T C U Y
A G K E R A T I N L X K U V R R G I Q V X F H
L I P L A Q I D W R A J A M F Q V U N B D R W
H Q U A U T R E N K A R X M J S B M M P E B N
R I Q N X H O R N Y D I N A A E M W S S W I T
U N U I D P U M M B I Y H L G B O L K F F D X
H O M N N L H I D O P Q X M U A K R L O L W H
D T A T G X Z S N A O P M V V C E U H Y X N B
T H E H X H E U U C S G G W F E U Y C M D Q E
D S Q F J D C H U D E R M A T O L O G Y Y L K
O S M Q G U L C K G O R K D W U L Y D B C S Z
I R U L K U E W C R R U H K S T L M U O I R
S I Y H P P A P I L L A I M W U N Y I X N T Y
Y P L R U G R F M M G J N F I P H N T C D C G
K B Y A A R A M G I H B T U E N L F K W L S L
W F X P B T I J D R F F E Q L R O K S T T E Y
J B L N E H F F N O R W G C E A O U E T A Y S
G P M U D S F U V T P D U V H U R U S N U Y G
B U M J V M R K G U M W M H S V S H S J E F S
J L W K I O R W U T J Z E G M J U K F Q V Y X
W J D N X Z B O P S W K N N X L H K W C B K I
R R Y H E P R I T P L Z T E P B H I L U O A R
L Y H A K J G T I J I Q A P Z K U K Y L A Z Y
L F Y J J J E C M I M T R B G C B B Z Z J H W
P T S X T A C S X B Q I Y P P H V E B W K P P
```

Can you find the 20 words hidden in this puzzle?

INTEGUMENTARY	SUDORIFEROUS	DERMATOLOGY	CERUMINOUS
EPIDERMIS	FOLLICLES	SEBACEOUS	APOCRINE
GRANULAR	ADIPOSE	AREOLAR	KERATIN
MELANIN	PAPILLA	DERMIS	LUNULA
BASAL	CLEAR	HORNY	SEBUM

CHAPTER 8 ANSWERS

Exercise 1

1. a. stratum germinativum or basal layer
   b. stratum granulosum or granular layer
   c. stratum lucidum or clear layer
   d. stratum corneum or horny layer
2. radiation, conduction, convection, evaporation
3. palms, soles
4. cilia (eyelashes), supercilia (eyebrows)
5. corium

Exercise 2

1. sweat pore
2. dermis
3. epidermis
4. duct of sweat gland .
5. sebaceous gland
6. body of sweat gland
7. arrector pili muscle
8. papilla of hair
9. hair shaft
10. hair follicle
11. subcutaneous fatty tissue

Exercise 3

1. B	**6.** J
2. C	**7.** G
3. I	**8.** D
4. F	**9.** E
5. H	**10.** A

Exercise 4

1. dermatosclerosis: skin; hardening—hardening of the skin
2. tinea barbae: ringworm; beard—ringworm of bearded area of face
3. cutis hyperelastica: skin; increase; elastic tissue—looseness, or hyperelasticity, of skin
4. ichthyosis congenita: fish (scales); congenital—skin resembling fish scales
5. neurofibroma: nerve; fibrous; tumor—tumor composed of fibrous and nervous elements
6. anhidrosis: no sweat; condition—inability to perspire or sweat
7. dyskeratosis: disordered; keratin—faulty development of epidermis with abnormal, premature, or imperfect keratinization
8. purpura: purple petechiae (pinhead-size hemorrhage spots)—cluster of petechiae, with purplish appearance
9. exfoliative dermatitis: shedding; skin; inflammation—an inflammatory scaling (shedding) or redness of skin
10. actinic dermatitis: ultraviolet light; skin; inflammation—inflammation of skin caused by exposure to ultraviolet light

Answers: Chapter 8 Crossword Puzzle

Across

1. SUDORIFEROUS
4. DERMATOLOGY
6. GRANULAR
8. RIDGES
9. SEBACEOUS
10. TWO
11. DERMIS
15. CONDUCTION
17. APOCRINE
20. HORNY
21. CLEAR
23. MELANIN
24. HAIR
25. HEREDITY

Down (letters as shown in grid)

- 2. E V A D I A T I O N (column)
- 3. C O V E T ...
- 5. A D I P O S E ...
- 7. S U B U M ...
- 12. E C R D E R E N ...
- 13. E P R O R I S S ...
- 14. S K I ...
- 16. C I ...
- 18. O N R E N ...
- 19. F O R ...
- 22. L U N U L ...

Answers: Chapter 8 Hidden Words Puzzle

```
L U N U L A . . . . . . . . . . . . .
B . . . D E R M I S . . . . . . . . .
A P O C R I N E . . E . . . . . . . .
S . . M . . . P O . . B . . . . . . .
A . K E R A T I N L . . U . . . . . .
L . L . . D . A . M . . . . . . . . .
. . . A . . E . A R . . . S . . . . .
. . . N . H O R N Y D . . . . E . . .
. . . I . . M . I . . . B . . . . . .
. . . N . . I . P . . . A . . . . . .
. . . . . . S . O . . . C . . . . . .
. . . . . . U C S . . . F E . . . . .
. . . . . C . . D E R M A T O L O G Y . . .
. . . . . L . . G O R . . . U L . . . .
. . . . . E . . R R U . . S . L . . . .
. . . . P A P I L L A I M . . . . I . .
. . . . . R . . . . N F I . . . . C . . .
. . . . . . . . . . T U E N . . . . L . .
. . . . . . . . . . E . L R O . . . . E .
. . . . . . . . . . G . A O U . . . . S
. . . . . . . . . . U . . R U S . . . .
. . . . . . . . . . M . . . . S . . .
. . . . . . . . . . E . . . . . . . .
. . . . . . . . . . N . . . . . . . .
. . . . . . . . . . T . . . . . . . .
. . . . . . . . . . A . . . . . . . .
. . . . . . . . . . R . . . . . . . .
. . . . . . . . . . Y . . . . . . . .
```

Words:

\/ INTEGUMENTARY	\ SUDORIFEROUS	> DERMATOLOGY	\ CERUMINOUS
\/ EPIDERMIS	\ FOLLICLES	\/ SEBACEOUS	> APOCRINE
\ GRANULAR	\/ ADIPOSE	\ AREOLAR	> KERATIN
\/ MELANIN	> PAPILLA	> DERMIS	> LUNULA
\/ BASAL	\/ CLEAR	> HORNY	\ SEBUM

CHAPTER 8 GLOSSARY

Skin and Related Anatomic Terms

apocrine glands (ap'o-krin): sweat glands, larger than the eccrines, with a strong-smelling secretion, located in the regions of the axillae, anus, and genitalia.

areola (ah-re'o-lah): a circular, pigmented area, surrounding another area of a different color (as around the nipple).

arrector pili (pe'le): small muscle of the skin that raises the skin surface, creating gooseflesh.

cilia (sil'e-ah): eyelashes (singular—*cilium*).

corium (ko're-um): another term for dermis.

derma (der'mah): skin.

dermis: inner, thicker layer of skin.

duct (dukt): tubelike passage, especially for excretions or secretions (also called *ductus*).

ductule (dukt'ule): tiny duct.

eccrine glands (ek'rin): ordinary sweat glands (also called *exocrine glands*).

epidermis (ep''i-der'mis): outer layer of skin.

exocrine glands (ek-so'krin): duct glands that empty secretions on skin surface (e.g.: sweat glands).

hair bulb: the expansion at the proximal (root) end of the hair.

hair follicle (fol'i-k'l): the tube in which the hair grows.

hair shaft: the portion extending beyond the surface of the skin.

keratin (ker'ah-tin): hard, protein constituent of hair, nails, epidermis, horny tissues, and tooth enamel.

lunula (lu'nu-lah): whitish, half-moon shaped, base of the nail.

melanin (mel'ah-nin): dark pigment of skin, hair, and other areas of the body.

sebaceous gland (se-ba'shus): secretes sebum that lubricates skin and hair.

sebum (se'bum): oily secretion of the sebaceous glands.

stratum corneum: outer (horny) layer of the epidermis.

stratum germinativum (jer''mi-na''-te'vum): innermost layer of epidermis (also called *basal layer*).

stratum granulosum: grainy layer of epidermis above the basal layer, which may not be present in thin skin (also called *granular layer*).

stratum lucidum (lu'sid-sum): translucent layer of epidermis found only on the palms and soles, above the granular layer (also called *clear layer*).

subcutaneous: located under the skin.

sudoriferous glands (su''dor-if'er-us): sweat glands.

supercilia (su''per-sil'e-ah): eyebrows. (singular—*supercilium*).

supernumerary (su''per-nu'mer-ar''e): occurring in more than the usual number.

Descriptive Terms

anhidrosis (an''hi-dro'sis): abnormal reduction of sweating.

bulla (bul'ah): a large lesion filled with fluid (also called a *blister*, *bleb*, or *vesicle*).

cicatrix (sik-a'triks): scar (plural—*cicatrices*).

cyanosis (si''ah-no'sis): bluish skin color due to an excess of oxygen-starved hemoglobin in the blood.

dyskeratosis: an abnormal alteration in keratinization.

ecchymosis (ek'i-mo'sis): minute, flat, circumscribed, reddish-purple spot caused by intradermal or submucous hemorrhages (also called *petechia*).

erythema: term referring to redness of the skin, caused by congestion of the capillaries, usually followed by name of specific condition or cause.

exanthema (ek-san'the'mah): any rash due to fever or disease (also called *exanthem*).

exfoliation: shedding or desquamation of the horny layer of the epidermis.

fissure: crack or groove.

hirsutism (her'sut-izm): abnormal hairiness.

hyperhidrosis: excessive sweating.

hyperkeratosis: overgrowth of the horny layer of the epidermis (also called *acanthokeratodermia*).

keloid (ke'loid): scar tissue.

macula (mak'u-lah): small, discolored spot on skin, that can be seen but not felt.

nodule (nod'ul): a small, visible knot protruding above the skin.

pallor: paleness of skin.

papule (pap'ul): small, rounded, solid elevation of the skin.

purpura (pur'pu-rah): group of conditions with purple-red or brown-red discolorations on the epidermis, caused by hemorrhage into the tissues (small ones are **petechiae**, large ones are **ecchymoses**).

pustule (pus'tul): pus collected in a hair follicle or pore.

scale: horny epithelial cells on epidermis, or shed from it.

spongiosis (spon''je-o-sis): edematous swelling within the cells of the epidermis.

Pathologic Conditions

Many eruptive diseases of the skin are symptoms of specific, multiple-system diseases (see Chapter 17).

Inflammations and allergies

acne: inflammation of the skin, caused by plugging of sebaceous glands, with development of papules and pustules.

actinic dermatitis: inflammation of the skin produced by exposure to ultraviolet and other radiation.

allergic dermatitis (der″mah-tit′is): skin inflammation caused by allergy.

angioneurotic edema: condition in which there is sudden onset of swollen (edematous) areas of skin, mucous membranes or other tissues due to allergy or unknown causes (also called *giant urticaria*).

aphthous stomatitis (af′thus sto-mah-ti′tis): inflammation of mucous membranes of the mouth, characterized by small, white, ulcerlike lesions (also called *canker sores*).

chilblain: localized, painful erythema, due to frostbite, with itching and swelling of ears, fingers, and toes (also called *erythema pernio*).

contact dermatitis: caused by contact with various allergy-producing substances (also called *dermatitis venenata*).

decubitus ulcer: skin surface lesion resulting from pressure on affected areas that results in defective circulation (also called *bedsore*).

dermatitis (der″mah-ti′tis): inflammation of the skin.

dermatitis herpetiformis (her-pet″i-form′is): chronic, recurrent, inflammatory dermatitis with grouped skin eruptions and severe itching and burning (also called *Duhring's disease* and *dermatitis multiformis*).

dermatitis medicamentosa (med″i-kah-men-to′sah): caused by sensitivity to drugs.

dermatocellulitis (der″mah-to-sel″u-li′tis): inflammation of the skin and underlying connective tissue.

dermatoconiosis (der″mah-to-ko″ne-o′sis): dermatitis caused by dust.

dermatographia (der″mah-to-graf′e-ah): a type of urticaria in which wheals or welts appear with very slight pressure or scratching.

dermatosis (der″mah-to′sis): any skin disease, especially those not usually associated with inflammation.

discoid lupus erythematosus (DLE): a limited form of lupus (see Chapter 17), a systemic disease, with cutaneous lesions of the face appearing as erythema, overgrowth of horny tissue, plugging of follicles, and usual butterfly pattern over nose and cheeks.

eczema (ek′ze-mah): general term for acute or chronic dermatitis.

exfoliative dermatitis: dermatitis, with scaling, itching, loss of hair, and redness of skin, resulting from any of several abnormal skin conditions.

frostbite: tissue damage caused by exposure to extreme cold, or by contact with chemicals that have a rapid freezing action.

occupational dermatitis: produced by exposure to materials in the workplace (also called *industrial dermatitis*).

parakeratosis: scaly dermatosis caused by overabundance of keratinocyte nuclei in the horny layer of the epidermis.

rosacea (row-zay′-shuh): reddening of the nose and adjoining areas produced by dilation of inflamed surface blood vessels, accompanied by an acne condition caused by plugged oil glands (also called *acne rosacea*).

seborrheic dermatitis (seb″o-re′ik): chronic, inflammatory dermatitis with yellowish, greasy scaling of the skin, especially the scalp, face, ears, and forehead, accompanied by pruritus (itching).

urticaria (ur″ti-ka′re-ah): skin reaction, usually allergic, with wheals appearing on skin, accompanied by pruritus (also called *hives*).

wheal (wheel): round, smooth, slightly elevated lesion on the skin, whiter or redder than surrounding area, that itches severely and is usually evidence of an allergy.

Bacterial, Fungal, Viral, and Parasitic Infections

carbuncle (kar′bung-k′l): infection of the skin and underlying tissues in the form of **furuncles** (boils), usually caused by *Staphylococcus aureus*.

cellulitis: inflammation, usually bacterial, possibly purulent, involving loose subcutaneous tissue.

chiggers: infestation by larvae of mites, causing severe itching and dermatitis.

dermatophytosis (der″mah-to-fi-to′sis): fungal infection of the skin, especially the feet (also called *dermomycosis* and *epidermomycosis*).

ecthyma (ek-thi′mah): form of impetigo or skin infection with shallow lesions and crusting, caused by streptococci and staphylococci.

erysipelas (er″i-sep′e-las): acute, contagious infections of the skin and subcutaneous tissue with swelling and redness of affected regions, caused by hemolytic streptococci.

erythema infectiosum: childhood illness caused by parvovirus B19 (not related to dog parvovirus). The contagious stage is a four to fourteen day incubation period preceding the breakout of a facial rash signalling the end of the contagious stage (also called *fifth disease*).

felon: abscess of distal end of finger, usually around the nail.

furunculosis (fu-rung″ku-lo′sis): persistent, consecutive occurrence of boils over a period of time.

herpes (her′pez): recurrent, infectious, inflammatory disease of the skin or other epithelial tissue, characterized by clusters of small vesicles, caused by herpesvirus (usually followed by a modifying term to identify the particular condition).

herpes febrilis: herpes simplex (type 1) virus-produced condition (also called cold sore or fever blister).

herpes genitalis: herpes simplex (type 2) virus-produced condition of the genital areas of both sexes.

impetigo: streptococcal-caused skin infection, with groups of minute vesicles that rupture and spread (also called *impetigo contagiosa*).

onychomycosis (on"i-ko-mi-ko'sis): a disease of the nails in which they become opaque, white, thick, brittle, and easily crumble (also called *ringworm* of the nails).

paronychia (par"o-nik'e-ah): bacterial or viral inflammation of the skin around the fingernail.

pediculosis: infestation by head, body or pubic lice, causing intense itching.

scabies: contagious skin disease caused by invasive mites, producing intense itching and eczema.

tinea (tin'e-ah): general name for a variety of superficial fungal skin infections (ringworm), with a modifier to identify the type: (e.g.: **tinea pedis**—of foot (athlete's foot), **tinea capitis**—of scalp, **tinea cruris**—jock itch, etc.).

toxic epidermal necrolysis (TEN): staphylococcus infection, usually affecting children under 10, causing outer layers of skin to split, separate, and peel, resembling skin after scalding (also called *scalded skin syndrome*).

wart: virus caused, benign, small, tumorlike epidermal growth (also called *verruca*).

Hereditary, Congenital and Developmental Disorders

albinism: congenital defect in melanin development, causing lack of pigment in skin, hair, and eyes.

cutis hyperelastica (hy'per-e-las'ti-kah): hereditary disorder marked by hyperextensibility of the joints with fragile and hyperelastic skin (also called *Ehlers-Danlos syndrome*).

ectodermal dysplasia: genetic condition with poorly functioning or no sweat glands, sparse hair follicles, missing or abnormal finger or toe nails, and a rash-prone skin, in addition to other systemic abnormalities.

epidermolysis bullosa (EB) (ep"i-der-mol'i-sis bul-lo-sah): a group of grave, inherited, noncontagious skin disorders characterized by soft, peeling epidermis, with formation of bullae and vesicles at sites exposed to trauma.

ichthyosis congenita (ik"the-o'sis kon-jen'i-tah): rare hereditary condition in which infant is covered with a "fish-scale" membrane, which peels off within 24 hours of birth, followed by healing or recurrence of the condition.

keratosis follicularis (fo-lik"u-lah'ris): rare, hereditary skin disorder marked by areas of crusting, itching, and rough papules on the scalp, face, neck, and trunk (also called *Darier's disease*).

pachyonychia congenita (pak"e-o-nik'e-ah): rare inherited condition with thickening of nails, thickening of skin on soles of feet and palms of hands, and leukoplakia of mouth mucous membranes (also called *Jadassohn-Lewandowsky syndrome*).

psoriasis: hereditary, chronic dermatosis, with bright red macules covered by scales, most commonly involving the scalp, elbows, knees and shins.

xeroderma pigmentosum (ze"ro-der'mah pig-men-to'sum): rare, inherited, frequently fatal disease in which skin and eyes are unusually sensitive to light; the condition can progress to malignancy.

Other Skin Conditions

alopecia (al-o-pe'shi-ah): hair loss.

Beau's lines: horizontal depressions across nail plate, possibly due to illness or malnutrition.

calcinosis cutis (kal"si-no'sis): condition characterized by calcium salts being deposited in the skin.

callosities (kah-los'i-tez): localized overgrowths of the outer (horny) layer of the epidermis.

koilonychia (koy-lo-nik'ee-ah): nail plates become depressed and spoonlike, possibly due to thyroid disease or anemia (also called *spoon nails*).

necrobiosis lipoidica (nek"ro-bi-o'sis li-poi'di-kah): skin condition marked by degeneration of the connective and elastic tissues especially in the upper dermis, with lesions usually occurring on the shins; commonly found in diabetics (also known as *necrobiosis lipoidica diabeticorum*).

pemphigus: formerly fatal, debilitating skin and mucus membrane disease, etiology unknown; characterized by weeping bullae (blisters) that rupture and leave raw spots, leading to possible infection; treated with corticosteroids and other immunosuppressive medications.

skin tag: small outgrowth of skin, most commonly on the neck (also called *cutaneous papilloma*).

vitiligo (vit-i-li'go): loss of pigment-producing cells, resulting in irregularly shaped lighter, or white, patches on the surface of the skin. Authorities theorize it may be hereditary, acquired, or possibly an auto-immune disease (the pop star Michael Jackson is reported to have this condition).

xanthoma (zan-tho'mah): lipid deposits in the skin forming yellow papules or nodules.

yellow nail syndrome: nails become thick and yellow; related to chronic respiratory disease, as well as lymph and thyroid diseases.

Oncology

actinic keratosis*: flat or raised, reddish or skin color growth affecting middle-aged or elderly people, caused by exposure to the sun's rays; it may develop into squamous cell carcinoma.

basal cell carcinoma*: malignant tumor of the epithelium that seldom metastasizes or spreads (also called ***hair-matrix carcinoma***).

carcinoma cutaneum*: malignant tumor of the epithelium.

dermatofibroma (der″mah-to-fi-bro′mah): fibrous tumor of the skin.

epithelial carcinoma*: malignant epithelioma.

epithelioma: tumor of epithelial tissue.

hidradenoma (hi″drad-e-no′mah): benign skin tumor composed of epithelial elements of sweat glands (also called ***syringocystadenoma***).

intraepidermal carcinoma*: confined to the epidermis, without penetration of basal layer.

intraepidermal epithelioma* (ep″i-the″le-o′mah): precancerous tumor of the epidermis.

leiomyoma cutis (li″o-mi-o′mah): benign smooth muscle tumor of arrector pili muscles.

lenticular carcinoma*: skin cancer with flattened nodules and papules running together into surface masses.

melanocytic nevus: pigmented nevus (see **nevus**).

melanoma*: malignant, pigmented, skin tumor that can develop from a melanocytic nevus.

nevus: circular overgrowth on skin (also called ***mole***).

sebaceous cyst: cyst of a sebaceous gland plugged with sebum.

seborrheic keratosis: benign tumor of the epidermis with many yellow or brown raised lesions on the skin (also called ***seborrheic wart***).

squamous cell carcinoma*: type of carcinoma from squamous epithelium (also called ***epidermoid carcinoma***).

syringocystadenoma: see **hidradenoma**.

tuberous carcinoma*: skin cancer with nodular projections.

verrucous carcinoma*: epidermoid cancer usually in mucosa of cheek, but can affect other soft tissues such as larynx and genitals.

Surgical Procedures

dermabrasion: surgical removal of epidermis and some dermis as needed to remove scar tissue,

* Indicates a malignant condition.

tattoos, moles, and other skin irregularities (also called ***planing***).

excisional biopsy: surgical incision to remove tissue of all or part of a lesion and surrounding normal-appearing tissue.

punch biopsy: sample of tissue obtained by use of a punch.

skin graft: surgical procedure to replace non-regenerative skin.

accordion graft: graft skin with multiple slits to permit stretching over large area.

artificial skin graft: graft derived from laboratory-grown epidermis sheets started from a postage stamp size sample of skin taken from individual for autograft or other donor sources; appears to minimize rejection.

autodermic graft: skin graft taken from patient's own body

cutis graft: grafting of skin after removal of epidermis and subcutaneous fat to replace fascia in plastic procedures.

delayed graft: original graft shifted to new area.

heterodermic graft: skin graft from donor of another species (also called ***dermatoheteroplasty***).

Laboratory Tests

biopsy: removal of tissue for microscopic examination.

buccal smear: scraping of cells from inner surface of cheek for detection of hereditary abnormalities.

computerized tomography (CT): imaging device using x-rays at multiple angles through specific sections of the body, analyzed by computer to provide a total picture of the part being examined (also called ***computerized axial tomography [CAT]***). Used to detect tumors in epithelial tissue.

intradermal tests: several tests using injection of substances subcutaneously to observe reaction.

 PPD (purified protein derivative): test for tuberculosis (also called ***Mantoux test***).

 Schick: test for diphtheria.

 Dick: test for scarlet fever.

patch test: skin test for sensitivity to particular allergens, by placing small amount of substance in solution on skin and covering for several days to note skin allergic response.

scratch test: a test for allergy by inserting suspected substances into scratches on skin surface to observe allergic reaction.

tissue culture: epithelial cells, taken from body, grown in a medium for diagnostic or research purposes.

Section Three

The Internal Mechanisms of the Body

This is the third of the five sections of **LEARNING MEDICAL TERMINOLOGY.** This section contains four chapters that describe the internal workings of the body.

Chapter 9 presents the **Cardiovascular System** and its relation to the production and circulation of blood throughout the body.

Chapter 10 discusses the **Respiratory System** and its importance in providing the body with oxygen and eliminating waste gases from cell metabolism.

Chapter 11 describes how the **Gastrointestinal System** functions, from digestion of food through the elimination of solid wastes.

Chapter 12 presents the **Genitourinary System,** beginning with the system's role in eliminating liquid waste and ending with the reproductive functions of both sexes.

As in the previous section, there are drawings within the chapters illustrating the principal parts of the anatomy in that particular chapter. In addition, there are colored plates at the front of the text that provide more vivid detail.

CHAPTER 9

The Cardiovascular System

The Transports of the Body

It's a Fact:
The blood in the average adult body travels 168 million miles every 24 hours.

CHAPTER OVERVIEW

This chapter explains the structures and functions of the heart, the various types of blood vessels, the characteristics of blood, and the mechanism of circulation.

THE CARDIOVASCULAR SYSTEM

The cardiovascular system includes the heart, blood vessels, blood, and its circulation.

THE HEART

The **cardiac muscle** (heart) is a hollow muscular organ, divided into four chambers and about the size and shape of a large clenched fist (Figs. 9-1 and 9-2). It lies between the lungs, in the middle of the chest, behind the sternum, with about two thirds to the left and one third to the right. The **base**, or upper border, of the heart is just below the second rib, and the **apex**, or lower border, of the heart points downward and to the left, separated from the anterior chest wall by the lungs and pleura. The heart is a pump that circulates the blood in the body, to nourish and to remove waste products from the tissues.

Structure of the Heart

The heart is covered by a saclike membrane, which has three layers:

The **pericardium**—tough, fibrous external layer; and two internal serous layers:

The **parietal** layer—lining the pericardium, and
The **visceral** layer (**epicardium**)—covering the surface of the heart.

There is a space between the two layers of serous membrane called the **pericardial space**, which contains several drops of pericardial fluid.

The heart wall is composed of three layers. The outer layer is the **epicardium** (visceral layer) described above. The middle layer, the **myocardium**, is the **cardiac** (heart) muscle itself, and the innermost layer, the **endocardium**, lines the chambers of the heart and covers its valves.

Chambers of the Heart

The hollow of the heart is divided into four chambers. Each of the upper two chambers is called an **atrium** (plural—**atria**) and each of the lower two chambers is called a **ventricle**. A wall called the **interatrial septum** divides the atria into right and left sides, and a similar wall, the **interventricular septum**, divides the ventricles into right and left sides. There is no communication between the two sides (Fig. 9-1).

The atria have thin walls and are the receiving chambers. The ventricles, which do the pumping, have thick walls. The right side of the heart receives blood from the body tissues and sends it to the lungs to be oxygenated. The left side of the heart receives blood from the lungs and sends it to the tissues. The walls of the left ventricle are thicker than the walls of the right ventricle because it pumps blood to all the blood vessels of the body; the right ventricle pumps blood only to the lungs.

Valves

Between the atria and ventricles are valves. These valves close to ensure that the blood flows in one direction and to prevent a backflow of blood into the atria. The left atrium and the left ventricle are separated by the **mitral** or **bicuspid** (two flaps) **valve**. The right atrium and the right ventricle are separated by the **tricuspid** (three flaps) *valve*. The *semilunar* (half-moon-shaped) *valves*, which prevent a backflow of blood from the arteries into the ventricles, are located at the bases of the *pulmonary artery* and the *aorta* (Fig. 9-1).

Conduction System

The heart begins its pumping action in utero. This action is dependent on a conduction system that includes:

The *sinoatrial node (SA node)*—also called the *pacemaker*, consists of cells in which electrical impulses originate, producing atrial contractions, and forcing blood into the ventricles;

The *atrioventricular node (AV node)*—consists of conductile cells through which the electrical impulses continue down to

The *atrioventricular bundle* (or *bundle of His*)—and on to

The *Purkinje fibers*—that move the impulses on to stimulate the contraction of the ventricles.

After a brief rest period, the entire process repeats itself (Fig. 9-2).

Nerve Function in Heart Action

The *autonomic* nervous system has two divisions with opposite actions on the heart:

The *parasympathetic* division, mainly supplying the SA and AV nodes, slows the heart rate, reduces impulse conduction, and constricts the coronary arteries;

The *sympathetic* division, through the cardiac nerves, also acts on the SA and AV nodes to increase the heart rate and impulse conduction, and dilate the coronary arteries (see Chapter 14).

Cardiac Cycle

The cardiac cycle includes the *systole* (contraction) and *diastole* (relaxation) of the atria and the ventricles. The heart chambers do not contract all at one time. The two atria contract in unison and as they relax, the two ventricles contract. Similarly, as the ventricles relax, the atria contract and the cycle is repeated.

When the atria contract, the blood is forced into the ventricles through the bicuspid and tricuspid valves, which open to allow the blood to pass from the atria to the ventricles, while the semilunar valves close to prevent

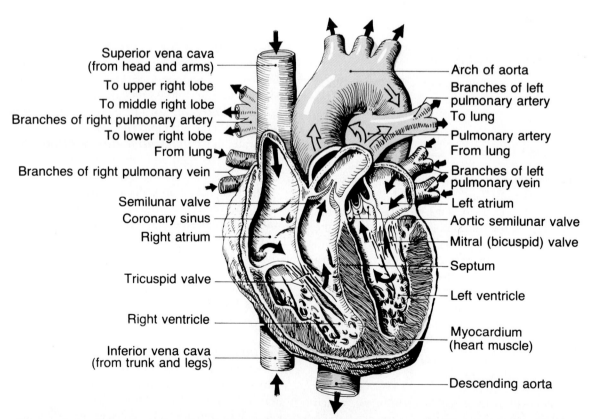

Figure 9-1. **Frontal section showing the four chambers of the heart and the valves, openings, and major blood vessels. Arrows indicate direction of the blood flow. (The branches of the right pulmonary vein continue from the right lung, behind the heart, to enter the left atrium.)**

blood from entering the aorta or the pulmonary artery.

When the atria relax, blood enters the atrial chambers from the pulmonary veins and venae cavae, and the ventricles contract. When the ventricles contract, the bicuspid and tricuspid valves close to prevent backflow to the atria, and the semilunar valves open to permit the blood to flow from the ventricles into the aorta and pulmonary artery.

When the ventricles relax, the semilunar valves close, the bicuspid and tricuspid valves open, the atria contract, and blood from the atria again starts to fill the ventricles, repeating the cycle.

TYPES OF BLOOD VESSELS

The human body has three major types of blood vessels: *arteries*, *capillaries*, and *veins*.

Arteries

Oxygenated blood is carried from the heart to all structures of the body by the arteries, which are elastic tubes with thick walls composed of three layers:

The *tunica intima* (or *intimal layer*): a lining of endothelium;

The *tunica media* (or *medial layer*): a muscle layer;

The *tunica adventitia* (or *tunica externa*): a fibrous outer coat.

Arterioles, Capillaries, and Venules

Arteries become smaller and smaller, branching and rebranching throughout the body, finally becoming *arterioles* (small arteries). The arterioles feed the blood into *capillaries*, which are billions of minute, very thin-walled vessels that communicate with other capillaries. The capillaries distribute the blood to the tissues, and other capillaries pick up the blood from the tissues and return it to *venules* (small veins), which pass the blood to the veins, and the veins return the blood to the heart.

Veins

The veins are hollow tubes, similar to the arteries, that have thinner and less elastic walls and transport blood back to the heart. The venules (smallest veins) collect blood from the capillaries, connect to larger veins, and finally join the *venae cavae* (singular—*vena cava*) to return the blood to the heart. Within the venous channels are valves that help to prevent backflow of blood and allow it to be propelled forward, with some assistance from alternate contraction and relaxation of the muscles of the limbs.

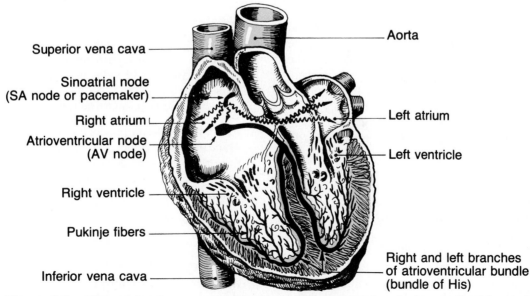

Figure 9-2.   The conduction system of the heart. The sinoatrial node (pacemaker) located in the wall of the right atrium sets the basic heart rhythm.

Review A

Complete the following:

1. The cardiovascular system includes the _____, _____, _____, and

   _____.

2. The heart is called the _____ muscle.

3. The hollow of the heart is divided into _____ chambers.

4. The external layer of the saclike membrane covering the heart is called the _____.

5. The valves of the heart prevent a _____ of blood into the atria.

6. The conduction system of the heart consists of the _____, _____,

   _____, and _____.

7. The _____ nervous system has two divisions with opposite actions on the heart.

8. The cardiac cycle includes the systole or _____ and the diastole or _____ of the atria

   and ventricles.

9. The three major types of blood vessels are _____, _____, and _____.

10. Arteries carry _____ blood from the heart throughout the body, and _____ transport

    it back to the heart.

BLOOD

Blood is made up of about 55% *plasma* (liquid) and 45% formed elements, which consist of *erythrocytes* (red cells), *leukocytes* (white cells), and *platelets* (*thrombocytes*). Blood transports oxygen from the lungs to the body tissues, collects carbon dioxide waste from the tissues, and brings it back to the lungs to be expelled. It distributes nutrients throughout the body, collects waste products of metabolism (urea, uric acid, creatinine, etc.), and delivers them to the excretory organs for disposal. It carries hormones of the different ductless glands (such as the thyroid and parathyroid glands) to the cells, maintains the fluid content of the tissues, and serves as a temperature regulator for the body. The average adult body contains about 6 quarts of blood, which may vary with the size and health of the individual.

Among the nutrients carried by the blood are *lipids* (fats and oils) such as *cholesterol* and *triglicerides*, which are needed for energy, and for manufacturing important hormones and salts. The lipids combine with proteins to form molecules that circulate in the blood as *lipoproteins*. Two of the major lipoproteins are *low-density lipoprotein (LDL)* and *high-density lipoprotein (HDL)*. LDL is commonly called "the bad cholesterol" because it is responsible for the deposit of cholesterol into the walls of the arteries, resulting in atherosclerosis (see Glossary). HDL is commonly called "the good cholesterol" because it has a role in metabolizing and eliminating excess cholesterol. Triglicerides function to provide energy for the tissues.

Plasma

The clear, straw-colored, liquid portion of blood, approximately 90% water and 10% solutes, with protein making up the major portion of solutes, is called *plasma*. Other solutes present in plasma, in much smaller amounts, include nutrients (lipids, glucose, and amino acids), end products of metabolism (urea, creatinine, uric and lactic acids), gases (oxygen and carbon dioxide), and hormones, enzymes, and antibodies.

Blood Cells

All blood cells have their origin in undifferentiated *stem cells*, the *hemocytoblasts*, which develop in the embryo. In children, blood cells are produced in almost all bone marrow, whereas in the adult, blood cells are produced in red bone marrow only.

> *Proerythroblasts* produce *erythrocytes*;
> *Myeloblasts* produce *granulocytes*;
> *Lymphoblasts* produce *lymphocytes*;
> *Monoblasts* produce *monocytes*;
> *Megakaryoblasts* produce *platelets*.

The logical progression through which the immature cells mature is given in Fig. 9-3.

Erythrocytes

At maturity, *erythrocytes* are extremely small, non-nucleated, biconcave (indented on both sides) disks (Figs. 9-3 and 9-4). They contain *hemoglobin* (*heme*—iron; *globin*—protein), an iron-containing pigment that,

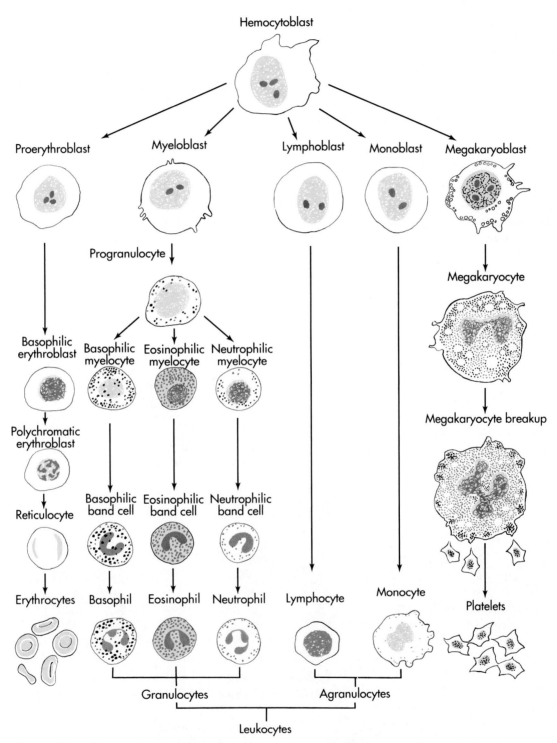

Figure 9-3.   Hematopoiesis. All cells are derived from a single progenitor cell, the hemocytoblast, which gives rise to the progenitors of each cell type. (From Seeley and others: *Anatomy and Physiology*, St. Louis, 1989, Mosby-Year Book, Inc.)

in combination with oxygen, gives the blood its red color. Hemoglobin combines with oxygen in the lungs and distributes it to body cells; there the hemoglobin combines with carbon dioxide, which it carries to the lungs for disposal. The average life span of erythrocytes is estimated to be about 120 days. If iron is lacking in erythrocytes, there is a reduction of hemoglobin and the number of red cells, resulting in an anemia.

Leukocytes

Much less numerous than erythrocytes, **leukocytes** are colorless and have nuclei (Figs. 9-3 and 9-4). Although leukocytes are considered constituents of blood, they are also included in the Lymphatic and Immune Systems (Chapter 16). They are divided into two groups:

Granulocytes—originating in bone marrow, have lobed nuclei, cytoplasm that contains fine granules, and are classified according to staining characteristics:
  neutrophils—the most numerous, make up about 70% of all leukocytes, have red and blue staining granules, and mainly function in

phagocytosis (digesting invading micro-organisms);
eosinophils—make up about 2% to 5% of all leukocytes, have orange or yellow acid dye staining granules, and function to detoxify foreign proteins from allergens or parasitic infections;
basophils—make up about 1% of all leukocytes, and have purple, basic dye staining granules, and mainly function in allergies and prevent coagulation in blood vessels.

Agranulocytes—originating in lymphatic organs, with clear, nongranular cytoplasm and either a round, or horseshoe-shaped, single nucleus:
  lymphocytes—make up about 20% to 25% of all leukocytes, have a rounded nucleus, and function in phagocytosis and in antibody formation;
  monocytes—make up about 3% to 8% of all leukocytes, have a horseshoe-shaped nucleus, and mainly function in phagocytosis.

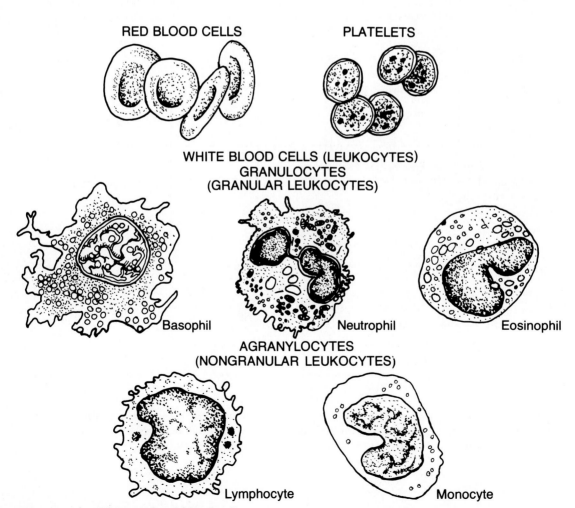

Figure 9-4. White and red blood cells.

Platelets (Thrombocytes) and Clotting Mechanism

Platelets (**thrombocytes**) originate in red bone marrow from **megakaryocyte** cells (Fig. 9-3). Small pieces of the cell break off and become platelets, which function in the clotting mechanism.

Clotting is the result of a chemical reaction. The thrombocytes attach to the injured blood vessel and begin to release several substances that constrict blood vessels and hasten clotting. **Prothrombin** and **fibrinogen** are proteins, made in the liver and present in blood plasma, that are necessary for clotting. Prothrombin is converted to **thrombin**, and thrombin changes fibrinogen to **fibrin**, which enmeshes the red blood cells, platelets, and plasma to form a clot, and close the wound.

ABO Blood Group

Blood for transfusion, under normal conditions, is carefully matched to the recipient. Blood is grouped into four types or groups, named for the **antigens** (substances that stimulate the immune system to form antibodies) found on the membranes of red blood cells. (For a fuller discussion of antigens and antibodies, see Chapter 16.)

The four blood types are:

- **A**: antigen A and anti-B antibodies are present—can receive only type A or O blood in transfusion;
- **B**: antigen B and anti-A antibodies are present—can receive only type B or O blood in transfusion;
- **AB**: both A and B antigens present with no antibodies—generally referred to as a **universal recipient**, who in extreme emergency, can receive any blood type in transfusion;
- **O**: neither A nor B antigens, with both anti-A and anti-B antibodies present—generally can receive only type O blood in transfusion but is referred to as a **universal donor**, who in an emergency, can give to any other blood type, in transfusion.

Rh Factor

In addition to blood being typed in the ABO blood group, blood is classified according to the presence of one or more of a number of **Rh** antigens. Blood is identified as either Rh positive or Rh negative, depending on whether or not an Rh antigen is present on the membranes of the red blood cells.

BLOOD PRESSURE

Blood pressure is the force exerted by the heart in pumping blood through the vessels of the body. **Systolic pressure** is produced by the blood pressing against the walls of the arteries during contraction of the ventricles of the heart. **Diastolic pressure** is produced by the blood pressing against the walls of the arteries during relaxation of the ventricles. Normal blood pressure in the average adult is about 120 (systolic) over 80 (diastolic). The difference between the systolic and diastolic pressures is called **pulse pressure**. Diastolic pressure is considered more important medically because it shows the least amount of pressure to which the arterial walls are subjected. The condition in which the blood pressure is elevated is called **hypertension**, and low blood pressure is called **hypotension**.

THE PULSE

The **pulse** is produced by the blood pumping out of the heart and into the aorta. This action rhythmically increases and decreases the pressure on the walls of the aorta, which, because of their elasticity, expand as the blood enters and relax as it leaves. This rhythm is then transmitted from the aorta to surface arteries, where it is felt as the pulse.

Review B

Complete the following:

1. There are about _____ quarts of blood in the average adult.

2. The clear, straw-colored, liquid portion of blood is called _____.

3. Erythrocytes contain an iron-containing pigment called _____.

4. A lack of iron in erythrocytes results in _____.

5. Small, nonnucleated, biconcave, disklike blood cells are called _____.

6. Leukocytes are divided into two groups, _____, and _____.

7. _____ originate in red bone marrow, and function in the clotting mechanism.

8. The four blood types are _____, _____, _____, and _____.

9. The difference between systolic and diastolic pressure is called _____.

10. The pumping of blood from the heart into the aorta produces the _____.

CIRCULATION OF THE BLOOD

The blood circulates throughout the body in a closed vascular system. One circuit of the blood, taking it through most of the body, is known as **systemic circulation**, which includes a segment called **hepatic portal circulation**. A second circuit, **pulmonary circulation**, takes the blood through the lungs.

Systemic Circulation

Blood circulates from the left ventricle to the aorta, arteries, arterioles, capillaries, venules, and veins of the body, and returns to the right atrium. This **systemic circulation** includes a circuit through the abdominal digestive organs known as **hepatic portal circulation**.

Hepatic Portal Circulation

Blood from veins in the visceral walls and organs (gallbladder, pancreas, spleen, stomach, and intestines) is carried to the liver by the hepatic portal vein. From the liver, the hepatic veins carry the blood to the inferior vena cava, which drains into the right atrium, where pulmonary circulation begins.

Pulmonary Circulation

Blood passes from the right atrium into the right ventricle, which contracts, forcing blood into the pulmonary artery, which has two branches, one going to each lung. In the lung the blood discharges carbon dioxide, is oxygenated, and then drains into the pulmonary veins, which empty into the left atrium, and finally into the left ventricle, where another systemic circuit begins.

Pulmonary veins are the only veins that carry oxygenated blood, which is a bright crimson color. All other veins carry waste products in the blood, making it a darker red color.

Tracing the Circulation

It takes about 1 minute for the blood to make a complete circuit of the body and return, always following the same pattern:

Left ventricle → arteries → arterioles → capillaries of body tissues → venules → veins → right atrium → right ventricle → pulmonary artery → arterioles of lung → lung capillaries → lung venules → pulmonary veins → left atrium → left ventricle (Fig. 9-5).

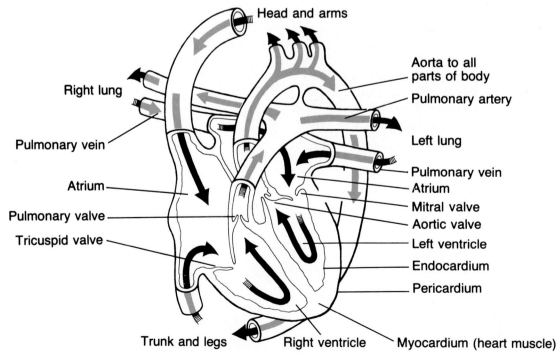

Figure 9-5. Circulation of blood through the heart.

THE MAJOR BLOOD VESSELS OF CIRCULATION

The Arteries

The **aorta**, the largest artery in the body, originating from the left ventricle of the heart, arches up around the left lung, and passes down along the spinal column, through the diaphragm. It branches into other arteries that supply the head, neck, arms, chest, and abdomen (abdominal aorta), finally dividing into arteries that supply the lower extremities (Fig. 9-6).

The branches from the **aorta** include the:

ascending aorta—branches into the

right coronary
and   arteries that supply the right
left coronary   and
                                left sides of the myocardial muscle

aortic arch—branches into three large arteries:

the **brachiocephalic (innominate)** divides into
the **right subclavian** artery, supplying the
right arm, and the
right common carotid, supplying the right
side of the head, branches into the
right internal carotid, supplying the
cranial cavity, and the
right external carotid, supplying the
neck and head outside the cranial cavity.

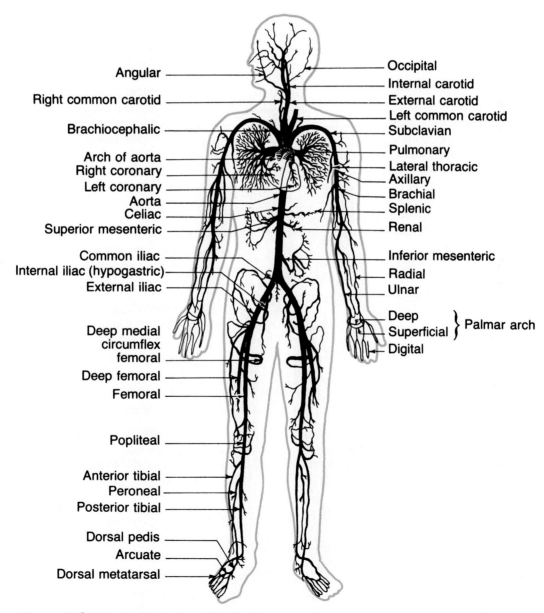

Angular
Right common carotid
Brachiocephalic
Arch of aorta
Right coronary
Left coronary
Aorta
Celiac
Superior mesenteric
Common iliac
Internal iliac (hypogastric)
External iliac
Deep medial circumflex femoral
Deep femoral
Femoral
Popliteal
Anterior tibial
Peroneal
Posterior tibial
Dorsal pedis
Arcuate
Dorsal metatarsal

Occipital
Internal carotid
External carotid
Left common carotid
Subclavian
Pulmonary
Lateral thoracic
Axillary
Brachial
Splenic
Renal
Inferior mesenteric
Radial
Ulnar
Deep
Superficial } Palmar arch
Digital

Figure 9-6. Principal arteries of the body.

the **left common carotid**—the second large artery, supplying the left side of the head, branches into
internal and **external** divisions, which function similar to those of the right common carotid.
the **left subclavian**—the third large artery, supplying the left arm with blood.

The right and left subclavian arteries branch into:
the **vertebral**—supplying the neck and brain, and
the **axillary**—the largest artery of the arm, passing from the armpit down the inner side of the arm, continuing into
the **brachial**—in the upper arm, branching at the elbow into

the **radial** and **ulnar** (named for lower arm bones)—branching into smaller arteries supplying the hands. (The radial artery can be felt at the wrist where the pulse is taken).

descending aorta—which divides into two segments:

descending thoracic aorta—divides into branches,
the **visceral**—supplying pericardium, bronchi, mediastinum, and esophagus;
the **parietal**—supplying diaphragm, mammaries, and chest muscles.
descending abdominal aorta—has four branches;

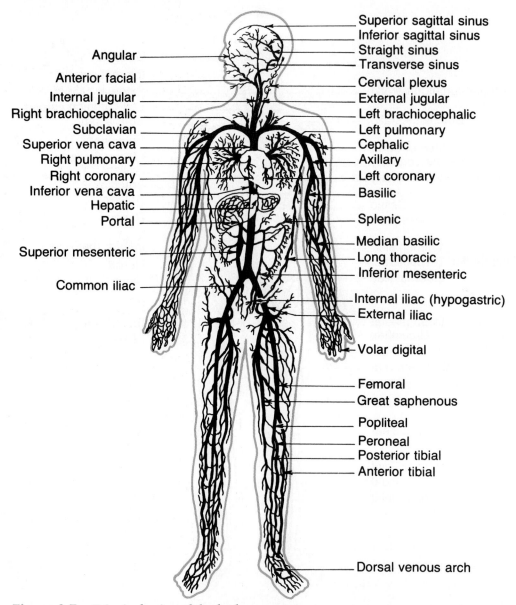

Figure 9-7.   **Principal veins of the body.**

the *visceral*
and
the *parietal* } supplying abdominal and pelvic organs

the *right common iliac*
the *left common iliac* } divides into

right and *left internal iliacs*, supplying the pelvic wall and viscera, and the *right* and *left external iliacs*, supplying the legs and continuing into the *femoral*, *popliteal*, and *anterior* and *posterior tibials* into the toes.

The Veins

The previous section traced the blood from the heart, through the arteries, to the extremities. This section will describe the return of the blood, through the veins, to the heart (Figs. 9-1 and 9-7).

The *pulmonary* veins are four veins that return the blood from the lungs to the *left atrium* of the heart, and are the only veins that carry freshly oxygenated blood.

Veins lying deep within the tissues are called *deep* veins; those close to the surface, and sometimes visible through the skin, are called *superficial* veins. The large veins of the cranium are called *sinuses*, but bear no relation to the sinuses of bony tissue (Fig. 9-7).

The *internal jugular veins* are deep veins draining the skull and brain. The superficial *external jugular veins* drain the scalp, face, and neck. Both jugulars empty into the *subclavian veins*.

The *axillary*, *scapular* and *thoracic* deep veins and the *cephalic* and *basilic* superficial veins also empty into the *subclavian veins*.

The *subclavian veins* empty into the *brachiocephalic* (also called *innominate*) veins. The *brachiocephalic* veins empty into the *superior vena cava* to the *right atrium*.

The veins draining the lower extremities are both superficial and deep. The veins of the feet and lower leg drain into two superficial veins, the *small saphenous* and the *great saphenous*.

The *small saphenous veins* drain into the *popliteals*, deep veins draining into the *femorals*.

The *great saphenous veins* drain into the *femorals*.

The *femorals* are deep veins of the thigh that drain into the *external iliacs*.

The *external iliacs* are deep veins of the groin that join

The *internal iliacs* (or *hypogastrics*), deep veins draining the pelvic viscera. The *external* and *internal iliacs* join to form the *common iliacs*.

The *common iliacs* join to become the *inferior vena cava*.

The *inferior vena cava* empties into the *right atrium*.

Specific veins drain the blood from the stomach, intestines, spleen, pancreas, gallbladder, and liver and empty into the *inferior vena cava* for return to the *right atrium*, as described in *hepatic portal circulation*.

The veins of the stomach are the *right* and *left gastroepiploic*, the *pyloric*, and the *gastric* (also called *coronary*).

The veins of the intestines are the *superior* and *inferior mesenteric*, *right* and *left colic*, *ileocolic*, and *sigmoid*.

The veins of the spleen are the *splenic*.

The veins of the pancreas are the *pancreatic*.

The veins of the gallbladder are the *cystic*.

All of these veins connect with, and drain into, the *hepatic portal vein*, which enters the liver. From there the blood leaves through the *hepatic vein*, which drains into the *inferior vena cava*, finally emptying into the *right atrium*.

Review C

Complete the following:

1. Blood circulation consists of two circuits: _____ circulation, which includes a segment called _____ circulation; and a second circuit called _____ circulation.

2. _____ veins are the only veins carrying oxygenated blood.

3. The blood makes a complete circuit of the body in about _____ minute(s).

4. The _____ is the largest artery in the body.

5. The _____ arteries supply the myocardial muscle.

6. The pulse of the _____ artery can be felt at the wrist.

7. The three branches of the aorta are the _____, _____, and _____.

8. Veins lying close to the surface are called _____ veins, and those within the tissues are called _____ veins.

9. The internal and external _____ veins drain regions of the head and neck.

10. The _____ drains into the right atrium.

Answers to Review Questions: The Cardiovascular System

Review A
1. heart, blood vessels, blood, circulation
2. cardiac
3. four
4. pericardium
5. backflow
6. sinoatrial node or pacemaker, atrioventricular node, bundle of His or atrioventricular bundle, Purkinje fibers
7. autonomic
8. contraction, relaxation
9. arteries, capillaries, veins
10. oxygenated, veins

Review B
1. 6
2. plasma
3. hemoglobin
4. anemia
5. erythrocytes or red blood cells
6. granulocytes, agranulocytes
7. platelets or thrombocytes
8. A, B, AB, O
9. pulse pressure
10. pulse

Review C
1. systemic, portal, pulmonary
2. pulmonary
3. 1 minute
4. aorta
5. coronary

6. radial
7. ascending aorta, aortic arch, descending aorta
8. superficial, deep
9. jugular
10. inferior vena cava

CHAPTER 9 EXERCISES

THE CARDIOVASCULAR SYSTEM: THE TRANSPORTS OF THE BODY

Exercise 1: Complete the following:

1. Blood carries _____ from the lungs to body tissues and collects _____ from tissues to take back to the lungs to be expelled.

2. Two components made in the liver that are necessary for clotting blood are _____ and _____.

3. Blood is made up of _____, _____, _____ and _____.

4. The iron-containing pigment in red blood cells is _____.

5. The two groups of white blood cells, or _____, are those with a lobed nucleus and cytoplasm with fine granules called _____, and those with a single nucleus and clear, nongranular cytoplasm called _____.

6. In the first group in the above statement, there is a further classification, according to staining characteristics, as follows: _____ (red and blue staining granules), _____ (orange or yellow acid dye staining granules), and _____ (purple basic dye staining granules).

7. The white blood cells constitute an important element in protection of the body against invasion by microorganisms through their power to attack bacteria, called _____.

8. The force the heart exerts in pushing blood through the vessels of the body is _____.

9. The contraction of the heart in measurement of the above force is called _____.

10. The _____ pressure is the lowest because it is present during relaxation of the heart.

Exercise 2: Matching:

____ **1.** cardiosclerosis   **A.** decrease in lymphocytes

____ **2.** angiosclerosis   **B.** decrease in granulocytes

____ **3.** erythropoiesis   **C.** inner coat of blood vessel

____ **4.** granulocytopoiesis   **D.** decrease of erythrocytes

____ **5.** granulocytopenia   **E.** production of erythrocytes

____ **6.** erythropenia   **F.** hardening of walls of a vessel

____ **7.** leukocytopenia   **G.** production of granulocytes

____ **8.** lymphocytopenia   **H.** relaxation of heart

____ **9.** tunica adventitia   **I.** an upper chamber of the heart

____**10.** tunica intima   **J.** decrease of leukocytes

____**11.** atrium   **K.** contraction of heart

____**12.** systole   **L.** a lower heart chamber

____**13.** sinoatrial node   **M.** pacemaker

____**14.** diastole   **N.** external coat of blood vessel

____**15.** ventricle   **O.** hardening of heart tissues and vessels

Exercise 3: Complete the following:

1. The blood vessel that carries blood from the heart to the lungs is called the _____ artery.

2. The large artery that carries blood from the heart to all parts of the body is the _____.

3. The three large arteries branching from the aortic arch are the _____, _____, and _____.

4. The circulation from the abdominal digestive organs through the liver into the inferior vena cava is called _____ circulation.

5. The arteries supplying right and left sides of myocardial muscle are the _____.

6. The heart is divided into four chambers; two _____ and two _____.

7. The Rh factor may be _____ or _____.

8. Blood circulating from the left ventricle and returning to the right atrium is known as _____ circulation.

9. Blood passing from the right atrium into the right ventricle, to the lungs and back to the left atrium is known as

_____ circulation.

10. _____ is commonly called "the bad cholesterol."

Exercise 4: The arrows in Fig. 9-8 trace the flow of blood through the heart. The heart valves are labeled with numbers; the heart chambers, membranes, and vessels are labeled with letters. In the blanks provided below, place the name of the structure opposite the appropriate letter or number.

A. _____   G. _____

B. _____   H. _____

C. _____   I. _____

D. _____   J. _____

E. _____   K. _____

F. _____

1. _____   3. _____

2. _____   4. _____

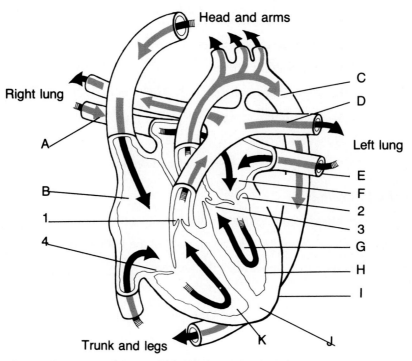

Figure 9-8.   Circulation of blood through the heart.

Exercise 5: Using the list of terms below, identify each structure in Fig. 9-9 by writing its name in the corresponding blank.

Aortic semilunar valve
Branches of right pulmonary vein
Left ventricle
Septum
Right atrium
Branches of left pulmonary artery
Coronary sinus
Mitral (bicuspid) valve
Superior vena cava
Arch of aorta

Branches of left pulmonary vein
Descending aorta
Myocardium
Tricuspid valve
Pulmonary artery
Branches of right pulmonary artery
Inferior vena cava
Right ventricle
Semilunar valve
Left atrium

1. _____

2. _____

3. _____

4. _____

5. _____

6. _____

7. _____

8. _____

9. _____

10. _____

11. _____

12. _____

13. _____

14. _____

15. _____

16. _____

17. _____

18. _____

19. _____

20. _____

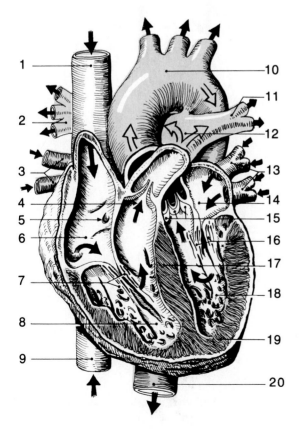

Figure 9-9. **Frontal section showing the four chambers of the heart and the valves, openings, and major blood vessels. Arrows indicate direction of the blood flow. (The two branches of the right pulmonary vein continue from the right lung, behind the heart, to enter the left atrium.)**

Exercise 6: Using the list of terms below, identify each artery in Fig. 9-10 by writing its name in the corresponding blank.

Angular	Digital	Peroneal
Anterior tibial	Dorsal metatarsal	Popliteal
Aorta	Dorsal pedis	Posterior tibial
Arch of aorta	External carotid	Pulmonary
Arcuate	External iliac	Radial
Axillary	Femoral	Renal
Brachial	Inferior mesenteric	Right common carotid
Brachiocephalic	Internal carotid	Right coronary
Celiac	Internal iliac	Splenic
Common iliac	Lateral thoracic	Subclavian
Deep femoral	Left common carotid	Superficial palmar arch
Deep medial	Left coronary	Superior mesenteric
Circumflex femoral	Occipital	Ulnar
Deep palmar arch		

1. _____
2. _____
3. _____
4. _____
5. _____
6. _____
7. _____
8. _____
9. _____
10. _____
11. _____
12. _____
13. _____
14. _____
15. _____
16. _____
17. _____
18. _____
19. _____
20. _____

21. _____
22. _____
23. _____
24. _____
25. _____
26. _____
27. _____
28. _____
29. _____
30. _____
31. _____
32. _____
33. _____
34. _____
35. _____
36. _____
37. _____
38. _____
39. _____

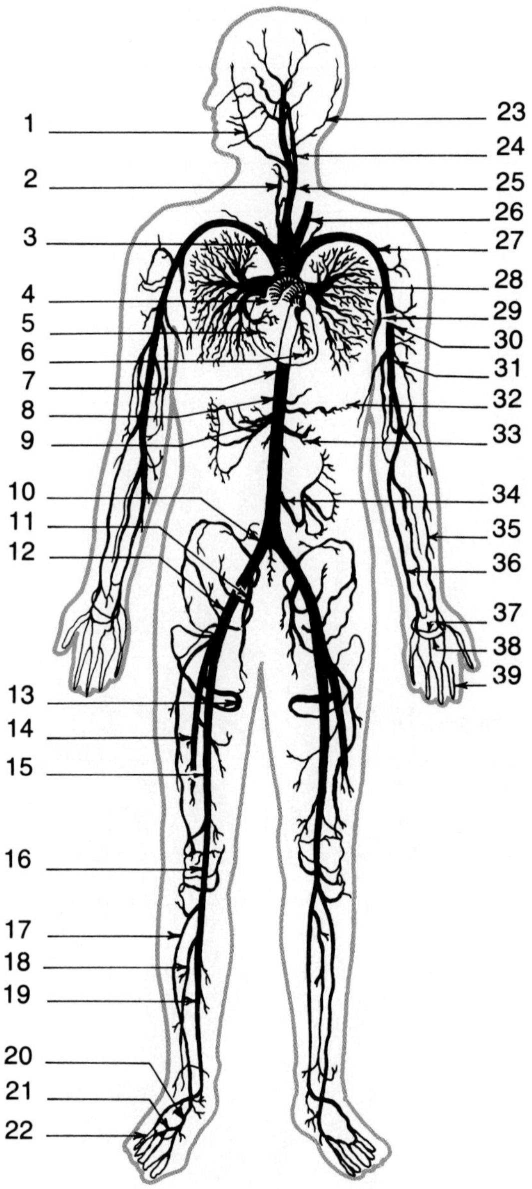

Figure 9-10. Principal arteries of the body.

Exercise 7: Using the list of terms below, identify each vein in Fig. 9-11 by writing its name in the corresponding blank.

Angular	Hepatic	Portal
Anterior facial	Inferior mesenteric	Posterior tibial
Anterior tibial	Inferior vena cava	Right brachiocephalic
Axillary	Inferior sagittal sinus	Right coronary
Basilic	Internal iliac	Right pulmonary
Cephalic	Internal jugular	Splenic
Cervical plexus	Left brachiocephalic	Straight sinus
Common iliac	Left coronary	Subclavian
Dorsal venous arch	Left pulmonary	Superior mesenteric
External iliac	Long thoracic	Superior sagittal sinus
External jugular	Median basilic	Superior vena cava
Femoral	Peroneal	Transverse sinus
Great saphenous	Popliteal	Volar digital

1. _____   21. _____

2. _____   22. _____

3. _____   23. _____

4. _____   24. _____

5. _____   25. _____

6. _____   26. _____

7. _____   27. _____

8. _____   28. _____

9. _____   29. _____

10. _____   30. _____

11. _____   31. _____

12. _____   32. _____

13. _____   33. _____

14. _____   34. _____

15. _____   35. _____

16. _____   36. _____

17. _____   37. _____

18. _____   38. _____

19. _____   39. _____

20. _____

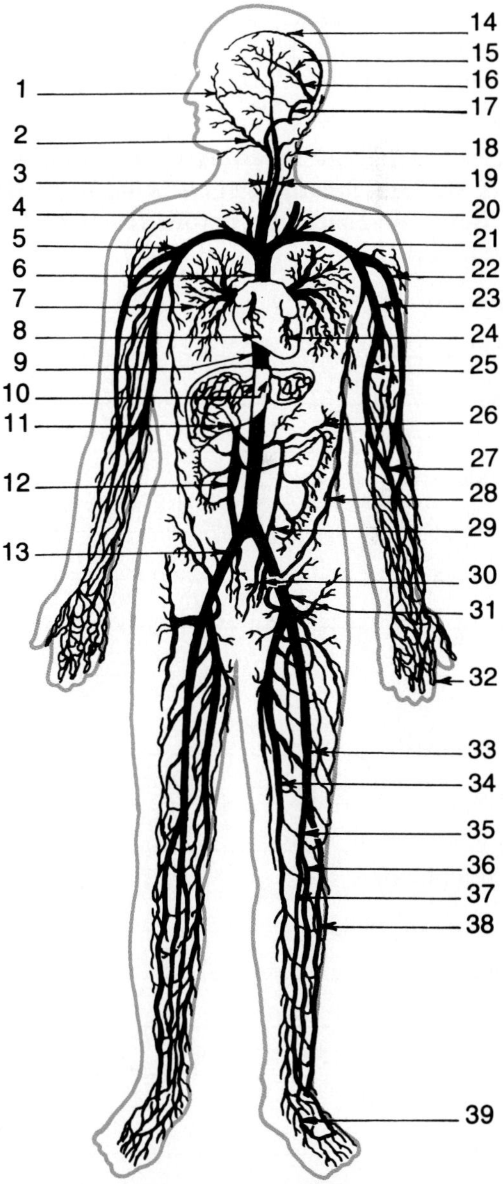

Figure 9-11.   **Principal veins of the body.**

Exercise 8: Multiple choice:
1. An excessive amount of blood in the body is called:
   a. erythremia   b. polyemia   c. hemophilia
2. Inflammation of serous membranes with serous effusion is called:
   a. polyarteritis   b. thromboangiitis   c. polyserositis
3. Effusion of blood into a cavity, such as the testis, is called:
   a. hematocele   b. hematocolpos   c. hematomyelia
4. Inflammation of an artery is called:
   a. aortitis   b. arteritis   c. phlebitis
5. Excision of a portion of an artery is called:
   a. angiotomy   b. arteriectomy   c. arteriotomy
6. Convulsive movements of the heart atrium or ventricle are called:
   a. congestive heart failure   b. cardiac arrest   c. fibrillations
7. Disease of lungs or their blood vessels produces heart disease called:
   a. aortic insufficiency   b. cor pulmonale   c. mitral insufficiency
8. Galloping rhythm of the heart might be described as:
   a. arrhythmia   b. bradycardia   c. blowing heart murmur
9. Stoppage of heartbeat might be described as:
   a. cardiac arrest   b. fibrillation   c. atrioventricular block
10. Paroxysmal thoracic pain characterized by feelings of suffocation and radiation of pain down the arm is specifically called:
    a. angina pectoris   b. coronary heart disease   c. congestive heart failure

Exercise 9: Give the meaning of the components in the following words and then define the word as a whole. Suffixes meaning *pertaining to* or *state or condition*, shown following a slash mark (/), are not to be defined separately. Before reaching for your medical dictionary, check the glossary at the end of the chapter.

1. Aortitis:

   aort _____

   itis _____

   _____

2. Endocarditis:

   endo _____

   card _____

   itis _____

   _____

3. Pericarditis:

   pericard _____

   itis _____

   _____

4. Pyelophlebitis:

   pyelo _____

   phleb _____

   itis _____

   _____

5. Hematemesis:

   hemat _____

   emesis _____

   _____

6. Hematoperitoneum:

   hemato _____

   peritoneum _____

   _____

7. Hemophthalmia:

   hem _____

   ophthalm/ia _____

   _____

8. Metrorrhagia:

   metro _____

   rrhag/ia _____

9. Arteriosclerosis:

   arterio _____

   scler/osis _____

   _____

10. Leukemia:

    leuk _____

    emia _____

    _____

Chapter 9 Crossword Puzzle

Across

1. innermost membrane covering heart
3. "good" cholesterol
5. upper border of heart
7. minute blood vessels
9. conduction node in heart
11. external covering of heart
12. membrane lining pericardium
16. undifferentiated stem cell
21. wall between heart chambers
24. red blood cells
25. bicuspid valve
26. this term means iron
27. major type of blood vessel
28. valve separating right atrium and ventricle

Down

1. very small veins
2. positive or negative antigen
4. "bad" cholesterol
6. lower border of heart
8. veins carrying oxygenated blood
9. aortic _____
10. relaxation part of cardiac cycle
12. thrombocytes
13. largest artery
14. number of heart wall layers
15. blood group
17. heart muscle
18. lower heart chambers
19. upper heart chamber
20. the sinoatrial node
22. liquid portion of blood
23. a leukocyte
26. the atrioventricular bundle

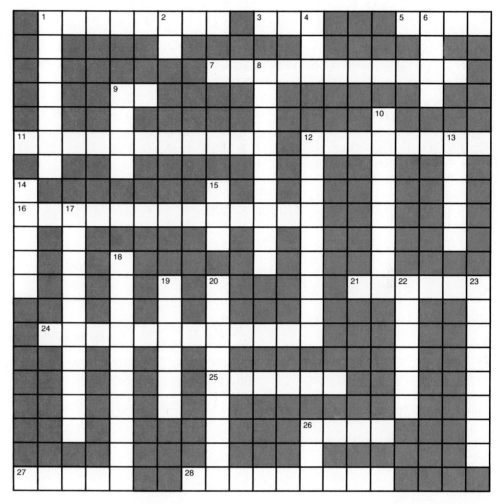

Chapter 9 Hidden Words Puzzle

```
F  J  H  R  K  S  J  L  Y  U  V  H  N  X  J  L  M  Y  Q  L  Z  D
O  Y  X  F  L  Y  T  A  Y  S  V  Y  P  V  J  F  Q  U  O  P  V  M
E  E  D  U  E  S  X  B  H  E  H  T  T  R  Q  G  Z  K  L  F  J  P
C  V  S  A  U  T  O  N  O  M  I  C  Y  H  W  H  Q  H  W  N  J  W
D  A  P  H  K  O  L  K  K  I  M  P  Y  V  R  M  H  O  C  Y  W  R
V  Y  W  S  O  L  Q  W  D  L  I  X  D  H  M  E  R  B  E  L  B  L
R  A  X  P  C  E  W  B  Q  U  D  T  R  O  L  W  D  X  Q  T  J  V
E  O  L  E  Y  D  K  Q  R  N  K  L  J  J  G  D  T  E  C  F  B  U
S  Y  Y  V  T  M  O  A  L  A  U  Y  D  M  U  S  R  O  N  Y  D  Y
L  F  R  L  E  P  I  C  A  R  D  I  U  M  M  S  N  I  E  Y  T  M
Z  R  P  I  S  S  E  I  C  S  A  S  I  Y  T  M  L  W  L  K  Y  N
G  B  I  E  C  B  N  R  A  E  T  Y  T  G  L  H  B  Y  U  W  P  K
H  D  A  W  R  H  D  C  Y  P  M  G  X  W  T  C  Q  W  L  D  N  W
B  A  B  R  V  I  O  U  S  T  G  T  Q  K  D  L  U  U  Q  B  T  V
C  M  K  G  T  F  C  L  I  U  H  Q  O  N  T  K  F  A  Y  X  Z  T
O  S  N  O  D  E  A  A  E  M  H  R  H  V  T  R  P  T  U  L  B  O
Z  T  Y  U  L  B  R  T  R  S  U  V  O  K  M  N  M  R  U  C  P  Z
J  V  J  S  X  C  D  I  Q  D  T  B  I  C  U  S  P  I  D  I  D  J
D  G  Q  M  T  B  I  O  E  F  I  E  X  S  Y  F  A  A  T  C  F  U
F  Q  B  U  C  E  U  N  X  S  B  U  R  Q  C  T  F  S  E  R  U  I
W  Q  W  R  H  G  M  N  Y  A  O  P  M  O  J  E  E  P  V  C  A  K
M  P  P  N  F  E  W  I  D  X  O  B  Y  V  L  O  R  S  U  T  U  L
A  X  E  K  W  I  E  B  C  L  G  Q  I  J  G  E  M  A  D  O  R  R
L  X  W  M  E  W  V  F  L  A  E  T  U  S  D  Z  V  T  L  V  I  N
```

Can you find the 20 words hidden in this puzzle?

ERYTHROCYTES	CIRCULATION	ENDOCARDIUM	PERICARDIUM
CHOLESTEROL	EPICARDIUM	LEUKOCYTES	AUTONOMIC
SEMILUNAR	ARTERIES	BICUSPID	SYSTEMIC
VISCERAL	SYSTOLE	BUNDLE	MITRAL
SEPTUM	VALVES	ATRIA	NODE

CHAPTER 9 ANSWERS

Exercise 1
 1. oxygen, carbon dioxide waste
 2. prothrombin, fibrinogen
 3. plasma, white cells (leukocytes), red cells (erythrocytes), and platelets
 4. hemoglobin
 5. leukocytes, granulocytes, agranulocytes (lymphocytes or monocytes)
 6. neutrophils, eosinophils, basophils
 7. phagocytosis
 8. blood pressure
 9. systolic pressure
10. diastolic

Exercise 2
1. O	6. D	11. I
2. F	7. J	12. K
3. E	8. A	13. M
4. G	9. N	14. H
5. B	10. C	15. L

Exercise 3
 1. pulmonary artery
 2. aorta
 3. brachiocephalic or innominate, left common carotid, and left subclavian arteries
 4. hepatic portal circulation
 5. right and left coronaries
 6. atria, ventricles
 7. positive, negative
 8. systemic
 9. pulmonary
10. LDL (low-density lipoprotein)

Exercise 4
1. pulmonary valve   3. aortic valve
2. mitral valve   4. tricuspid valve

A. pulmonary vein   G. left ventricle
B. atrium   H. endocardium
C. aorta   I. pericardium
D. pulmonary artery   J. myocardium
E. pulmonary vein   K. right ventricle
F. atrium

Exercise 5
 1. superior vena cava   11. branches of left pulmonary artery
 2. branches of right pulmonary artery 12. pulmonary artery
 3. branches of right pulmonary vein 13. branches of left pulmonary vein
 4. semilunar valve   14. left atrium
 5. coronary sinus   15. aortic semilunar valve
 6. right atrium   16. mitral (bicuspid) valve
 7. tricuspid valve   17. septum
 8. right ventricle   18. left ventricle
 9. inferior vena cava   19. myocardium
10. arch of aorta   20. descending aorta

Exercise 6

1. angular
2. right common carotid
3. brachiocephalic
4. arch of aorta
5. right coronary
6. left coronary
7. aorta
8. celiac
9. superior mesenteric
10. common iliac
11. internal iliac
12. external iliac
13. deep medial circumflex femoral
14. deep femoral
15. femoral
16. popliteal
17. anterior tibial
18. peroneal
19. posterior tibial
20. dorsal pedis
21. arcuate
22. dorsal metatarsal
23. occipital
24. internal carotid
25. external carotid
26. left common carotid
27. subclavian
28. pulmonary
29. lateral thoracic
30. axillary
31. brachial
32. splenic
33. renal
34. inferior mesenteric
35. radial
36. ulnar
37. deep palmar arch
38. superficial palmar arch
39. digital

Exercise 7

1. angular
2. anterior facial
3. internal jugular
4. right brachiocephalic
5. subclavian
6. superior vena cava
7. right pulmonary
8. right coronary
9. inferior vena cava
10. hepatic
11. portal
12. superior mesenteric
13. common iliac
14. superior sagittal sinus
15. inferior sagittal sinus
16. straight sinus
17. transverse sinus
18. cervical plexus
19. external jugular
20. left brachiocephalic
21. left pulmonary
22. cephalic
23. axillary
24. left coronary
25. basilic
26. splenic
27. median basilic
28. long thoracic
29. inferior mesenteric
30. internal iliac
31. external iliac
32. volar digital
33. femoral
34. great saphenous
35. popliteal
36. peroneal
37. posterior tibial
38. anterior tibial
39. dorsal venous arch

Exercise 8

1. polyemia
2. polyserositis
3. hematocele
4. arteritis
5. arteriectomy
6. fibrillations
7. cor pulmonale
8. arrhythmia
9. cardiac arrest
10. angina pectoris

Exercise 9

1. aortitis: aorta; inflammation—inflammation of aorta
2. endocarditis: endocardium; inflammation—inflammation of endocardium
3. pericarditis: pericardium; inflammation—inflammation of pericardium
4. pyelophlebitis: kidney pelvis; vein; inflammation—inflammation of veins of kidney pelvis
5. hematemesis: blood; vomiting—vomiting of blood
6. hematoperitoneum: blood; peritoneum—accumulation of blood in the peritoneum
7. hemophthalmia: blood; eye—accumulation of blood in the eye
8. metrorrhagia: uterus; hemorrhage or profuse bleeding—abnormal uterine bleeding, especially between menses
9. arteriosclerosis: artery; hardening—hardening of the arteries or an artery
10. leukemia: white cells; blood—malignant disease of the blood

Answers: Chapter 9 Crossword Puzzle

	1 V	I	S	C	E	2 R	A	L		3 H	D	4 L				5 B	6 A	S	E
	E					H						D					P		
	N							7 C	A	8 P	I	L	L	A	R	I	E	S	
	U			9 A	V					U							X		
	L			R						L					10 D				
11 P	E	R	I	C	A	R	D	I	U	M		12 P	A	R	I	E	T	13 A	L
	S			H						O		L			A			O	
14 T								15 A		N		A			S			R	
16 H	E	17 M	O	C	Y	T	O	B	L	A	S	T			T			T	
R		Y						O		R		E			O			A	
E		O		18 V						Y		L			L				
E		C		E		19 A		20 P				E		21 S	E	22 P	T	U	23 M
		A		N		T		A				T				L			O
	24 E	R	Y	T	H	R	O	C	Y	T	E	S				A			N
		D		R		I		E								S			O
		I		I		U		25 M	I	T	R	A	L			M			C
		U		C		M		A								A			Y
		M		L				K				26 H	E	M	E				T
				E				E				I							E
27 V	E	I	N	S			28 T	R	I	C	U	S	P	I	D				

Answers: Chapter 9 Hidden Words Puzzle

```
. . . . . S . . . . . . . . . . . . . . . .
. . . . L Y . . . S . . . . . . . . . . . .
. . . . E S . . . E . . . . . . . . . . . .
. . . A U T O N O M I C . . . . . . . . . .
. . . . K O . . . I . . . . . . . . . . . .
V . . . O L . . . L . . . . . . . . . . . .
. A . C E . . . U . . . . . . . . . . . . .
. . L . Y . . . . N . . . . . . . . . . . .
. . . V T . . . . A . . . . . . . . . . . .
. . . . E P I C A R D I U M . . . . . . . .
. . P . S S E I . S . . . . . . . . . . . .
. . . E C . N R . E . . . . . . . . . . . .
. . A . R H D C Y P . . . . . . . . . . . .
. . . R . I O U . T . . . . . . . . . . . .
. . . . T . C L . U H . . . . . A . . . . .
. S N O D E A A E M . R . . . . T . . . . .
. . Y . . . R T R S . V O . . . M R . . . .
. . . S . . D I . D T B I C U S P I D . . .
. . . . . T B I O E . I E . S Y . A T . . .
. . . . . . E U N . S . U R . C T . . . R . .
. . . . . . . M N . . . M O . E E . . . A .
. . . . . . . . I D . . . . L . R S . . . L
. . . . . . . . . C L . . . . . . . A . . .
. . . . . . . . . . E . . . . . . . . L . . .
```

Words:

\ ERYTHROCYTES	\/ CIRCULATION	\/ ENDOCARDIUM	PERICARDIUM
\ CHOLESTEROL	> EPICARDIUM	\/ LEUKOCYTES	> AUTONOMIC
\/ SEMILUNAR	\ ARTERIES	> BICUSPID	\ SYSTEMIC
\ VISCERAL	\/ SYSTOLE	\ BUNDLE	\ MITRAL
\/ SEPTUM	\ VALVES	\/ ATRIA	> NODE

CHAPTER 9 GLOSSARY

Cardiovascular System Related Anatomic Terms

Heart

aortic valve: semilunar valve that prevents backflow of blood from the aorta to the heart.

apex (a′peks): rounded tip of heart, pointing left and downward.

atrial appendage: ear-shaped continuation of the left and right upper part of the atria.

atrioventricular node: located in the right atrium near the lower portion of the interatrial septum, and composed of a small mass of atypical cardiac muscle tissue (also called *AV node*, *Aschoff's node*, and *Tawara's node*).

atrioventricular valves: valves between atria and ventricles of the heart (the left valve is the **bicuspid**, or **mitral**, and the right valve is the **tricuspid**).

atrium (a′tre-um): left or right upper chamber of the heart.

bundle of His: a band of specialized cardiac muscle fibers that arise in the atrioventricular node and branch down on both sides of the interventricular septum, transmitting the atrial contraction rhythm to the ventricles (also called *atrioventricular bundle*).

chordae tendineae (kor′de ten″din′e-e): tendinous strings resembling cords that extend from the cusps of the atrioventricular valves to the papillary muscles of the heart, which prevent valve inversion.

conus arteriosus (ko′nus ar-te″re-o′sus): upper, anterior angle of the right ventricle where the pulmonary artery begins (also called *infundibulum of the heart*).

cor: another name for the heart.

coronary arteries and **veins:** blood vessels of the heart.

cusp: leafletlike segment of the cardiac valve.

diastole (di-as′to-le): relaxation stage of the heart action.

ductus arteriosus: blood vessel in fetal circulation connecting pulmonary artery to descending aorta.

endocardium: endothelial membrane lining the chambers of the heart.

epicardium: outermost serous layer covering the heart.

foramen ovale cordis (fo-ra′men o″vah′le): opening between the atria in the fetal heart, normally closed after birth.

interventricular: between ventricles.

myocardium: thick middle muscle layer of the heart wall.

pacemaker: sinoatrial node, which initiates the heartbeat and regulates its rate.

pericardium: external layer of the membrane covering the heart.

pulmonary valve: valve at the base of the pulmonary artery (also called *semilunar valve*).

Purkinje fibers: specialized cardiac muscle fibers that are involved in the impulse-conducting system of the heart.

semilunar valves: refers to the half-moon shape of the valves at the base of the pulmonary artery and aorta.

sinoatrial node: see **pacemaker**.

systole (sis′to-le): contraction stage of heart action.

valves: membranous structures in passages, that close to prevent the reflux of contents.

Blood and Blood Vessels

basophil (ba′so-fil): granular leukocyte cell that stains with basic dyes.

capillary: small blood vessel that connects arterioles with venules, forming a vast network throughout the body.

eosinophil (e″o-sin′o-fil): granular leukocyte cell that stains readily with orange or yellow acid eosin dyes.

erythrocyte (e-rith′ro-sit): red blood cell.

erythropoiesis (e-rith″ro-poi-e′sis): red blood cell production.

granulocyte (gran′u-lo-sit): cell containing granules (leukocytes with cytoplasmic granules of neutrophils, basophils, or eosinophils).

granulocytopoiesis (gran″u-lo-si″to-poi-e′sis): production of granulocytes.

hematopoiesis (hem″ah-to-poi-e′sis): production of red blood cells (also called *hemopoiesis*).

heme: insoluble, nonprotein, iron-containing portion of hemoglobin.

hemoglobin: iron-containing red pigment (heme) that combines with a protein substance (globin), giving blood its red color.

heparin (hep′ah-rin): anti-coagulant substance.

leukocyte (lu″ko-sit): white blood cell.

leukocytopoiesis: leukocyte production (also called *leukopoiesis*).

lymphocyte (lim′fo-sit): clear, nongranular leukocyte with single, round nucleus that functions in phagocytosis and antibody formation.

lymphopoiesis (lim″fo-poi-e′sis): production of lymphocytes.

macrocyte (mak′ro-sit): abnormally large erythrocyte.

megakaryocyte (meg″ah-kar′e-o-sit): giant cell of bone marrow that produces mature blood platelets.

megalocyte (meg′ah-lo-sit): large nonnucleated erythrocyte.

monocyte: phagocytic, mononuclear white blood cell (leukocyte).

monocytopoiesis (mon″o-si″to-poi-e′sis): formation of monocytes.

neutrophil (nu′tro-fil): neutral dye staining granular leukocyte containing lobed nucleus (also called ***polymorphonuclear leukocyte***).

phagocytosis (fag″o-si-to′sis):the ingestion and destruction of microorganisms, cells, and foreign matter.

plasma: liquid portion of blood.

plasmocyte: plasma cell.

platelet: disklike, nonnucleated element in the blood, originating in the red bone marrow and necessary for coagulation of blood (also called ***thrombocyte***).

prothrombin: factor in the blood plasma that converts to thrombin and is part of the blood clotting mechanism.

reticulocyte (re-tik′u-lo-sit″): immature red blood cell, which shows basophilic reticulum (network) under vital staining.

sinusoid (si′nus-oid): large, variable, anastomosing, terminal blood vessel, with reticuloendothelium lining, found in organs such as the liver, suprarenals, and heart (also called ***sinusoidal capillary***).

thrombin: enzyme of prothrombin, that changes fibrinogen to fibrin.

thrombocyte: blood platelet.

thromboplastin (throm″bo-plas′tin): substance in blood and body tissue that aids in converting prothrombin to thrombin.

tunica: term for a coat or covering of a blood vessel, organ or body part.

tunica adventitia or **tunica externa vasorum:** the fibrous elastic outer covering of blood vessels.

tunica intima vasorum: inner coat of blood vessel.

tunica media vasorum: middle coat of blood vessel.

vas: vessel.

Arteries

Most of the arteries in this glossary are frequently encountered arteries and their branches, appearing in records of procedures and disorders.

aorta (a-or′tah): largest artery in the body and main trunk of the entire arterial system.

aortic arch: continuation of the ascending portion of the aorta.

arteriole (ar-te′re-ol): tiny arterial branch.

ascending pharyngeal: branch of the external carotid artery that distributes to the pharynx, soft palate, ear, and meninges.

auricular posterior (aw-rik′u-lar): branch of the external carotid artery that serves the middle ear, mastoid cells, parotid gland, auricle of the ear and various muscles.

axillary (ak′si-lar″e): branch of the subclavian artery that distributes to the axilla, chest, shoulder, and upper extremity.

basilar (basi-lar): branch of the vertebral artery distributing to the brainstem, cerebellum, posterior cerebrum, and internal ear.

brachial (bra′ke-al): axillary artery branch distributing to the shoulder, arm, and hand.

brachiocephalic (innominate) (brak″e-o-se-fal′ik): aortic arch branch distributing to the right side of the head, neck, and arm.

carotids (kah-rot′ids): right and left common carotids, originating from the brachiocephalic artery and the aortic arch respectively, distributing to the right and left sides of the head.

celiac trunk: branch of the abdominal aorta distributing to the stomach, liver, pancreas, spleen, and duodenum.

cerebellar (ser″e-bel′ar): three cerebellar arteries distributing to the cerebellum, and/or medulla, pineal body and mid-brain.

cerebral (ser′e-bral): distributes to cerebrum and its structures.

colic: distributes to the colon.

coronary: left and right arteries distributing to the left and right sides of the myocardial muscle (atria and ventricles).

cystic: distributes to the gallbladder.

deferential: distributes to the ureter, ductus deferens, testes, and seminal vesicles.

dorsalis pedis: distributes to the foot and toes.

epigastric: three arteries serving respectively the abdominal muscles and peritoneum; the abdominal muscles, skin, and diaphragm; and the skin of the abdomen, the inguinal lymph nodes, and superficial fascia.

esophageal: thoracic aorta branch that distributes to the esophagus.

femoral: branch of the external iliac artery that distributes to the external genitalia, lower leg, and lower abdominal wall.

gastric: three arteries distributing to the esophagus and curvatures of the stomach.

gastroduodenal: branch of the hepatic artery that distributes to the stomach, duodenum, pancreas, and greater omentum.

gastroepiploic (gas″tro-ep″i-plo′ik): two arteries distributing to the stomach and greater omentum.

gluteal: two arteries that distribute to the buttocks and thighs.

hemorrhoidal (hem″o-roi′dal): three arteries distributing to the anal canal and rectum.

hepatic: distributes to the stomach, pancreas, duodenum, liver, gallbladder, and greater omentum.

ileal (il′e-al): branch of the superior mesenteric artery that distributes to the ileum.

ileocolic: branch of the superior mesenteric artery distributing to the cecum, appendix, ascending colon, and ileum.

iliac (il′e-ak): the common iliac artery and its branches distribute to the pelvis, abdominal wall, lower limbs, external genitalia, pelvic visceral wall, buttocks, reproductive organs, and the mid-thigh.

iliolumbar: branch of the internal iliac artery that distributes to the pelvic bones and muscles, fifth lumbar vertebra, and sacrum.

intercostal: thoracic aorta branch distributing to thoracic wall.

internal spermatic: branch of the abdominal aorta that distributes to the ureter, epididymis, and testis (also called *testicular artery*).

intestinal: branch of the superior mesenteric artery that distributes to the jejunum, ileum, duodenum, and colon.

laryngeal (lah-rin′je-al): inferior and superior branches of the thyroid arteries, which distribute respectively to the larynx (superior), esophagus, and trachea (inferior).

lingual: branch of the external carotid artery that distributes to the tongue, sublingual gland, tonsil, and epiglottis.

lumbar: branch of the abdominal aorta that distributes to the abdominal walls and the renal capsule.

malleolar: two arteries distributing to the ankle joint.

mammary: distributes to the anterior thoracic wall, diaphragm, and mediastinal structures (also called *internal thoracic artery*).

maxillary: two arteries distributing to the jaws, teeth, chewing muscles, ear, nose, nasal sinuses, palate, and meninges.

mesenteric: inferior and superior branches of the abdominal aorta distributing respectively to the lower half of the colon and rectum and the small intestine and proximal half of the colon.

nutrient: any artery that supplies blood to the bone marrow (also called *medullary artery*).

obturator: branch of the internal iliac artery that distributes to the pelvic muscles and hip joint.

occipital: branch of the external carotid artery that distributes to the muscles of the neck, scalp, meninges, and mastoid cells.

ophthalmic: branch of the internal carotid artery that distributes to the eyes, orbits, and adjacent facial structures.

ovarian: branch of the abdominal aorta that distributes to the ovaries, uterine tubes, and ureters.

pancreaticoduodenal (pan″kre-at″i-ko-du″o-de′nal): two arteries that distribute to the pancreas and duodenum.

peroneal: branch of the posterior tibial artery that distributes to the ankle and deep calf muscles.

phrenic: two pairs of arteries, inferior and superior, distributing to the diaphragm and suprarenal glands.

popliteal: femoral artery branch distributing to the knee and calf.

pudendal: external and internal branches of the femoral and internal iliac arteries, respectively, distributing to the external genitalia.

pulmonary: the only arteries in the body that carry nonoxygenated blood, which is delivered to the lungs for oxygenation.

radial: brachial artery branch distributing to forearm and hand.

renal: branch of the abdominal aorta that distributes to the kidneys, suprarenals, and ureters.

sacral: two arteries distributing respectively to adjacent structures of the coccyx and sacrum, and to the sacrum, coccyx, and rectum.

sigmoid: branch of the inferior mesenteric artery that distributes to the sigmoid colon.

splenic: branch of the celiac trunk that distributes to the spleen, stomach, pancreas, and greater omentum.

subclavian: two arteries distributing to the neck, upper limbs, thoracic wall, spinal cord, brain, and meninges.

subcostal: branch of the thoracic aorta that distributes to the upper posterior abdominal wall.

subscapular: branch of the axillary artery that distributes to the shoulder and scapular areas.

temporal: three pairs of arteries, superficial, middle, and deep, distributing to the head.

thoracic: three arteries, lateral, superior and internal, distributing respectively to the pectoral muscles and mammary glands; the axillary area of the chest wall; and the diaphragm, structures of the mediastinum, and the anterior thoracic wall.

thyrocervical trunk: branch of the subclavian artery distributing to the scapular area, deep neck, and thyroid.

thyroid: two arteries distributing to the thyroid gland and neighboring structures.

tibial: two arteries that distribute to the leg, ankle, and foot.

transverse cervical: branch of subclavian artery distributing to the neck and scapular muscles.

ulnar: brachial artery branch distributing to forearm and hand.

uterine: branch of the internal iliac artery that distributes to the uterus, uterine tubes, vagina, and ovaries.

vertebral: subclavian artery branch distributing to the neck, vertebral column, cerebellum, internal cerebrum, and spinal cord.

Veins

Most of the veins in this glossary are frequently encountered veins and their branches, appearing in records of procedures and disorders.

auricular: two veins that are anterior and posterior to the ear.

axillary: basilic and brachial vein continuation to subclavians.

azygos (az′i-gos): three veins of the trunk that empty into the superior vena cava.

basalis: veins of the cerebral area.

basilic: (bah-sil′ik): veins of the forearm and hand.

brachiocephalic (innominate) (brak″e-o-se-fal′ik): left and right branches unite to form the superior vena cava.

bronchial: veins that bring blood back from the lung.

cardiac: veins of the heart, including coronary veins (also called ***venae cordis***).

cephalic: (se-fal′ik): veins of the forearm and arm.

cerebellar: veins of the cerebellum.

cerebral: numerous veins that drain blood from the brain (also called ***venae cerebri***).

cervical: deep vein of the neck.

choroid (ko′roid): veins of choroid plexus and other brain areas.

circumflex: a group of veins serving femoral and iliac areas.

colic: right, medial, and left veins of intestines.

comitans (kom′i-tans): veins accompanying arteries or nerves.

common iliac: large veins draining blood from pelvis and leg, joining to form inferior vena cava.

cutaneous: small subcutaneous veins draining into deep veins.

cystic: vein of the gallbladder.

digital: group of veins serving the palms, fingers, soles and toes.

dorsal veins of clitoris: deep and superficial veins of the clitoris.

dorsal veins of penis: deep and superficial veins of the penis.

epigastric: comitans veins of the epigastric arteries.

esophageal: veins of the esophagus.

facial: superficial and deep veins of the facial structures.

femoral: comitans veins of the femoral artery of the thigh.

gastric: group of veins serving the stomach, including the pyloric and the coronary vein of the stomach.

gastroepiploic: comitans right and left veins of the stomach and omentum.

gluteal: comitans veins of the thighs and buttocks.

hemorrhoidal: group of veins of the rectal area.

hepatic: veins that drain the liver.

hepatic portal: carries blood from the digestive system to the liver.

hypogastric: veins of the lower and middle abdomen, joining the external iliac to form the common iliac vein.

ileocolic: veins draining the ileum, cecum, appendix, and part of the ascending colon.

iliac: external and internal, join with the saphenous to form the common iliac vein.

iliolumbar: comitans vein of the iliolumbar artery, serving the iliac and lumbar regions.

intercostal: comitans veins that accompany intercostal arteries.

interlobular: renal and hepatic veins.

intervertebral: numerous veins comitans with spinal nerves.

jejunal and ileal: veins draining the jejunum and ileum and joining the superior mesenteric vein.

jugular: two pairs of veins, internal and external, serving the head and neck.

labyrinthine (lab″i-rin′thin): comitans veins of the ear.

laryngeal: inferior and superior veins of the larynx.

lateral thoracic: veins draining the side of the thoracic wall.

lingual: veins serving the tongue, area below the tongue and mandibular glands, and floor of the mouth.

lumbar: comitans veins of the lumbar region.

mammary: thoracic artery comitans vein (also called ***internal thoracic***).

median antebrachial: veins of the forearms.

median cubital: veins of the elbow and forearm, most commonly used for venipuncture site (also called ***intermediate basilic***).

mediastinal: veins of the mediastinum.

mesenteric: intestinal comitans veins emptying into hepatic portal vein.

nasal: vein of the nose.

obturator: veins of the hip joint and thigh muscles.

occipital: veins of the head.

ophthalmic: inferior and superior veins of the orbital area.

ovarian: veins of the ovary.

palatine: veins of the area of the palate.

pancreatic: veins of the pancreas.

pancreaticoduodenal: comitans veins of the pancreas and duodenum.

parotid: veins of the parotid gland.

pericardiac: small veins of the pericardium of the heart.

peroneal: comitans veins of the lower leg.

pharyngeal: veins of the pharyngeal area.

phrenic: veins of the diaphragm.

plexus: network of nerves, lymph, or blood vessels.

popliteal: veins from the knee area into the femoral vein.

pudendal: comitans veins draining perineum and external genitalia.

pulmonary: four veins returning oxygenated blood from the lungs to the left atrium of the heart.

renal: comitans veins of the kidney.

sacral: comitans veins emptying into the iliac veins.

saphenous (sah-fe′nus): **great**, the longest vein in the body running from foot to thigh, and **small**, running from foot to knee.

sigmoid: veins of the sigmoid colon.

spermatic: veins that drain the testes and epididymis.

spinal: veins draining the blood from the spinal cord.

splenic: vein draining the spleen (also called ***lienal vein***).

subclavian: main veins of the upper extremity, joining the internal jugulars to form the two brachiocephalic veins.

supraorbital: veins of the anterior scalp.

suprarenal: veins of the adrenal glands.

temporal: veins draining the temporal region of the head.

thoracoepigastric: veins of the trunk.

thyroid: veins of the thyroid gland.

tibial: comitans veins of the leg emptying into the popliteal.

tracheal: veins of the trachea.

ulnar: comitans veins of the forearm.

uterine: veins of the uterus.

venae cavae: two large veins that return blood to the heart, the **superior** from the head, neck, chest, and upper extremities, and the **inferior** from the abdominal viscera, pelvis, and lower extremities.

venae vasorum (va-so′rum): small veins that return blood from the walls of blood vessels.

venules: minute veins.

vertebral: veins of the vertebrae.

vesical: veins of the bladder (usually the urinary bladder).

volar: veins of the palm of the hand and sole of the foot.

Pathologic Conditions

Inflammations and infections

aortitis: inflammation of the aorta.

arteritis (ar″te-ri′tis): inflammation of an artery.

bacteremia: bacteria in the blood.

carditis: inflammation of the heart.

endarteritis: inflammation of the tunica intima of an artery.

endarteritis deformans: persistent endarteritis characterized by fatty degeneration of the tissue of the arteries and forming of deposits of lime salts.

endarteritis obliterans: endarteritis with narrowing and closure of the arterial lumen (space within a tube).

endocarditis (en″do-kar-di′tis): inflammation of the endocardium (lining) membrane of the heart.

erythrocytosis: abnormal increase in red blood cells, usually caused by infection.

leukocytosis: temporary increase in number of leukocytes in the blood, caused by inflammation, infection, or hemmorhage.

myocarditis (mi″o-kar-di′tis): inflammation of the heart muscle.

panarteritis: inflammatory arterial disease, involving all layers of the arterial wall.

periarteritis: inflammation of the adventitia (outer layer) of an artery.

pericarditis (per″i-kar′dit′is): inflammation of the pericardium.

perisplenitis: inflammation of the outer covering of the spleen and the surrounding structures.

phlebitis (fle-bi′tis): inflammation of a vein, with formation of a thrombus, accompanied by pain, stiffness, and edema.

polyarteritis: inflammatory condition of the arterial system with many destructive lesions.

polyserositis (pol″e-se-ro-si′tis): general inflammatory condition of the serous membranes, accompanied by serous effusion.

pyelophlebitis (pi″e-lo-fel-bi′tis): inflammatory condition of the renal pelvis veins.

septicemia (sep″ta-se′me-ah): general systemic blood infection caused by the presence of pathogenic microorganisms or their toxins (also called **blood poisoning**).

thromboangiitis (throm″bo-an″je-i′tis): thrombi (blood clots) accompanying inflammation of the intima (inner coat) of a blood vessel.

thrombophlebitis: inflammation of a vein with clot formation.

Hemorrhages and related conditions

disseminated intravascular coagulation (DIC): simultaneous hemorrhage and thrombosis caused by overstimulation of blood clotting mechanisms, due to disease or injury.

epistaxis (ep″i-stak′sis): nosebleed.

hemarthrosis (hem″ar-thro′sis): presence of blood in a joint.

hematemesis (hem″at-em′e-sis): vomiting of blood.

hematencephalon (hem″at-en-sef′ah-lon): cerebral hemmorhage.

hematocele (hem′ah-to-sel″): blood in a cavity or cyst.

hematocoelia (hem″ah-to-se′le-ah): escape of blood into the peritoneal cavity (**coel** means cavity).

hematocolpos (hem″ah-to-kol′pos): menstrual blood accumulated in the vagina (**colpo** means vagina).

hematoma (hem″ah-to″mah): blood, usually clotted, accumulated in a tissue, organ, or space due to a blood vessel wall break.

hematometra (hem″ah-to-me′trah): accumulation of blood in the cavity of the uterus.

hematomphalocele (hem″at-om′fal′o-sel): umbilical hernia filled with blood (**cele** means protrusion).

hematomyelia (hem″ah-to-mi-e′le-ah): bleeding into the spinal cord.

hematopericardium (hem″ah-to-per″i-kar′de-um): escape of blood into the pericardium (also called **hemopericardium**).

hematoperitoneum (hem″ah-to-per″it-to-ne′um): escape of blood into the peritoneum.

hematorrhachis (hem-ah-tor′ah-kis): bleeding into the spinal column (**rhachis** means spine).

hematorrhea (hem′ah-to-re′ah): profuse hemorrhage.

hematosalpinx (hem″ah-to-sal′pinks): accumulation of blood in a tube, most frequently a uterine tube (also called **hemosalpinx**).

hematospermatocele (hem″ah-to-spermat′o-sel): sperm-filled cyst containing blood.

hematotympanum (hem″ah-to-tim′pah-num): bleeding into the middle ear.

hematuria: blood in the urine.

hemophthalmia (he″mof-thal′me-ah): bleeding into the eyeball (also called *hemophthalmos* or *hemophthalmus*.)

hemoptysis (he-mop′ti-sis): spitting of blood, or bloody sputum (*ptysis* means spitting).

hemothorax: accumulation of blood in the pleural cavity.

melena: passing of tarry stools due to presence of digested blood.

menorrhagia (men″o-ra′je-ah): abnormally heavy menstrual flow.

metrorrhagia (me″tro-ra′je-ah): abnormal uterine bleeding, especially between menstrual periods.

petechial hemorrhages (pe-te′ke-al): small pinpoint hemorrhages in the skin or the mucous membranes.

postpartum hemorrhage: hemorrhage following childbirth.

Anemias

anemia: reduction in red blood cells.

aplastic anemia: anemia resulting from bone marrow disease or destruction.

deficiency anemia: anemia caused by lack of necessary nutritional substances.

hemolytic anemia: anemia resulting from the destruction of erythrocytes.

hypochromic microcytic anemia: iron-deficiency anemia.

macrocytic anemia: anemia in which erythrocytes are enlarged.

myelophthisic anemia (mi″e-lof′thi-sik): anemia caused by dissolution or crowding out of the blood-forming tissues by lesions (also called *leukoerythroblastosis*).

pernicious anemia: megaloblastic anemia resulting from failure of the gastric mucosa to secrete a factor necessary to form erythrocytes and absorb vitamin B_{12}.

Leukemias

This is a limited listing of leukemias. Refer to a medical dictionary for a more detailed listing with definitions.

leukemia (lu-ke′me-ah): malignant progressive disease, marked by an abnormal increase in the production of leukocytes and a decrease in erythrocytes and platelets, causing an anemia and vulnerability to infection and hemorrhage. Classified as (1) acute or chronic; (2) cell involved (myeloid, lymphoid, or monocytic); and (3) increase or nonincrease of abnormal cells.

aleukemic leukemia: leukemia in which the peripheral white blood cell count is normal or below normal.

leukemia cutis: leukemia with general or localized skin involvement, having nodular lesions with accumulation of leukemic cells in the skin.

monocytic leukemia: leukemia in which monocytes are the predominant white blood cells.

myeloblastic leukemia: leukemia in which myeloblasts are the predominant white blood cells.

stem cell leukemia: leukemia that is difficult to type because the prevailing cells are too immature and may be lymphoblasts, myeloblasts, or monoblasts.

Hereditary, congenital and developmental disorders

coarctation of aorta (ko″ark-ta′shun): deformity of the aorta causing narrowing of its lumen.

Cooley's anemia: one of a group of familial hemolytic anemias occurring in neonates (also called *thalassemia*).

dextrocardia: heart is displaced to the right side of the thoracic cavity.

dextroposition of the aorta: aorta is displaced to the right (see **tetralogy of Fallot**).

Eisenmenger's complex: interventricular septal defect with pulmonary hypertension and hypertrophy of the ventricle on the right side, accompanied by cyanosis.

hemophilia (he″mo-fil′e-ah): hereditary disease in which there is a deficiency in the clotting of blood.

hereditary hemorrhagic telangiectasia (tel-an″je-ek-ta′ze-ah): familial condition marked by many small angiomas of the mucous membranes and skin frequently accompanied by gastrointestinal bleeding or epistaxis.

patent ductus arteriosus: open duct between the left pulmonary artery and descending aorta in the fetus that normally closes at birth.

pulmonary stenosis: narrowing of the passage between the pulmonary artery and the right ventricle.

sickle cell anemia: hemolytic anemia caused by a hereditary genetic defect, occurring most frequently in blacks.

tetralogy of Fallot (fal-o′): group of four cardiac anomalies, including pulmonary stenosis, dextroposition of the aorta, interventricular septal defect, and marked hypertrophy of the right ventricle (also called *Fallot's tetrad*).

thalassemia: see **Cooley's anemia**.

transposition of aorta and pulmonary artery: aorta originates from the right ventricle and the pulmonary artery originates from the left ventricle, causing cyanosis due to lack of oxygen in the blood (also called *transposition of great vessels*).

Other abnormalities

agranulocytosis (ah-gran″u-lo-si-to′sis): disease characterized by a sudden decrease in granulocytes and the appearance of lesions of the mucous membranes, especially in the gastrointestinal tract and on the skin.

altitude alkalosis: increased alkalinity in the blood and body tissues caused by high altitude.

aneurysm: blood-filled, saclike formation, caused by localized dilation of a blood vessel wall (usually an artery) or the heart.

angialgia: pain in a vessel (also called *angiodynia*).

angina: refers to any condition with attacks of suffocating, paroxysmal pain.

angina pectoris (an-ji′nah pec′tor-is): severe, paroxysmal chest pain, usually radiating from the cardiac area of the chest to the left shoulder and down the left arm.

angiomegaly (an″je-o-meg′ah-le): enlargment of a blood vessel.

angionecrosis (an′je-o-nekro′sis): necrosis (death) of blood vessel walls.

angioparalysis: paralysis affecting a blood vessel.

angiosclerosis: sclerosis (hardening) of blood vessel walls.

angiostenosis: narrowing of vessels.

aortic insufficiency: blood from the aorta flows back to the left ventricle because of malfunctioning of the semilunar valve of the aorta.

arrhythmia (ah-rith′me-ah): abnormal rhythm of the heartbeat.

arteriolonecrosis (ar-te″re-o″lo-ne-kro′sis): necrosis of cells forming arteriole walls.

arteriolosclerosis (ar-te″re-o″lo-skle-ro′sis): thickening and hardening of the walls of arterioles.

arteriomalacia (ar-te″re-o-mah-la′she-ah): softening of arterial coats.

arterionecrosis (ar-te″re-o-ne-kro′sis): necrosis of walls of an artery.

arteriosclerosis (ar-te″re-o-skle-ro′sis): classification of diseases of the arteries, marked by a thickening of the walls of the arteries and loss of their elasticity.

arteriospasm (ar-te′re-o-spazm): spasm of an artery.

arteriostenosis (ar-te″re-o-ste-no′sis): narrowing of the lumen of an artery.

atherosclerosis (ath″er-o″skle-ro′sis): type of arteriosclerosis marked by the formation of plaques containing cholesterol and lipids within the intima of large- and medium- sized arteries.

bradycardia: slow heart beat.

cardiac arrest: abrupt stopping of cardiac function and absence of arterial blood pressure.

cardiac edema: edema symptomatic of congestive heart failure.

cardiac hypertrophy: enlargement of the heart.

cardiac murmur: abnormal sound heard between the normal heart sound of lub-dub.

cardialgia: pain in the upper anterior chest or abdomen (also called *cardiodynia*).

cardiectasis (kar″de-ek′tah-sis): expansion of the heart.

cardiohepatomegaly (kar″de-o-hep″ah-to-meg′ah-le): swelling of the heart and liver.

cardiomalacia (kar″de-o-mah-la′she-ah): abnormal softening of the heart muscle.

cardiomegaly (kar″de-o-meg′ah-le): enlargement of the heart.

cardiomyoliposis (kar″de-o-mi″o-li-po′sis): fatty deterioration of the muscles of the heart.

cardionecrosis (kar″de-o-ne-kro′sis): death of heart tissue.

cardioptosis (kar″de-o-to′sis): downward displacement of the heart.

carotenemia: presence of carotene in the blood, sometimes producing a jaundicelike skin coloring.

congestive heart failure: prolonged inability of the heart to pump and maintain the blood flow adequately, resulting in impaired circulation, edema throughout the body, and blood backed up in the veins leading to the heart.

cor pulmonale: cardiac condition caused by pulmonary hypertension resulting from disease of the lungs or their blood vessels.

cyanosis: bluish skin color caused by reduced amounts of hemoglobin in the blood.

embolism (em′bo-lizm): blocking of a blood vessel by an obstruction, such as a blood clot, air bubble, fat globule, tissue, bacteria clump, or amniotic debris, carried by the flow of blood.

erythremia (er″i-thre′me-ah): chronic polycythemia (excessive formation of red blood cells) with hyperplasia (overgrowth) of bone marrow, and increase of blood volume.

erythrocytosis (e-rith″ro-si-to′sis): increase of red blood cells in circulation.

erythropenia: deficiency of erythrocytes (also called *erythrocytopenia*).

fibrillation: arrhythmia with uncoordinated, irregular contractions of the heart muscle affecting the atria and/or ventricles.

granulocytopenia (gran″u-lo-si″to-pe′ne-ah): decrease of granulocytes in the blood (also called *granulopenia*).

granulocytosis: unusually large number of granulocytes in the blood.

heart block: partial or complete interference with the conduction of the cardiac electrical impulses.

hemangiectasis (hem″an-je-ek′tah-sis): dilation of blood vessels (also called *angiectasis*).

hematocytopenia (hem″ah-to-si″to-pe′ne-ah): deficiency in the elements of the blood cells.

hematocytosis: increase in the elements of the blood.

hematopenia: decrease in blood.

hemoglobinemia (he″mo-glo′bi-ne′meah): abnormally large amounts of hemoglobin in blood plasma.

hemolith: stone in the wall of a blood vessel.

hypertension: high blood pressure.

hypotension: low blood pressure.

infarct: area of tissue that is damaged or necrotic because of an insufficient blood supply resulting from an obstruction to circulation.

ischemia: local, temporary deficiency of blood supply to an area of the body caused by an obstruction in the blood vessel supplying the area.

leukopenia: reduction in the amount of white blood cells (also called *leukocytopenia*).

lymphocytopenia: decrease of lymphocytes in the blood.

lymphocytosis: excess of lymphocytes in the blood (also called *lymphocythemia*).

mitral valve prolapse (MVP): protrusion of the mitral valve into the left atrium, causing backflow of blood due to incomplete closure.

Monckeberg's (menk′e-bergz) **arteriosclerosis:** type of arteriosclerosis affecting the medial arterial coat with calcium deposits, destroying elastic and muscle fibers (also called *medial arteriosclerosis*).

monocytopenia: decrease of monocytes in the blood.

monocytosis: increase of monocytes in the blood.

myocardial infarction: occlusion (blockage) of a coronary artery, resulting in heart muscle damage.

neutropenia: decrease of neutrophils in the blood (also called *neutrocytopenia*).

occlusion: obstruction of a blood vessel that may be caused by a thrombus or an embolus.

palpitation: rapid action, or tachycardia, of the heart.

paroxysmal tachycardia (par″ok-siz′mal): sudden onset of rapid heartbeat, beginning and ending abruptly.

phlebangioma: aneurysm of a vein.

phlebectasia (fleb″ek-ta′ze-ah): swelling of a vein or veins, or a varicosity (also called *phlebectasis*).

phlebemphraxis (phleb″em-frak′sis): obstruction of a vein by a clot or plug (*emphraxis* means stoppage).

phlebolithiasis: condition marked by the development of calculi in the veins.

phlebosclerosis : hardening of the walls of a vein (also called *venosclerosis*).

phlebostenosis: narrowing of the walls of a vein.

polycythemia: increase of erythrocytes in the blood.

polycythemia vera (pol″e-si-the′me-ah ver′ah): excess of red blood cells with blood volume increase, along with splenomegaly, leukocytosis, and thrombocythemia.

polyemia: excessive amount of blood in the body.

purpura fulminans: extremely rare, severe, and often fatal blood disorder, usually occurring after an infectious disease in children, producing clotting and bleeding simultaneously.

Raynaud's disease: idiopathic (cause unknown) disorder of arterial circulation, resulting in cyanosis of digits, nose and/or ears.

Raynaud's phenomenon: blanching or cyanosis of digits due to arterial spasm, caused by cold or emotion.

reticulocytopenia (re-tik″u-lo-si″to-pe′ne-ah): decrease in the amount of reticulocytes in the blood (also called *reticulopenia*).

Stokes-Adams syndrome: sudden loss of consciousness (often with convulsions); may accompany heart block.

superior vena cava syndrome (SVCS): edema of the neck, face, or upper arms caused by excessive venous pressure in the superior vena cava.

tachycardia: rapid heart beat.

thrombocytopenic purpura (throm″bo-si″to-pe′nik pur′pu-rah): progressive, systemic condition, which may be fatal, with hemorrhages of mucous membranes, decrease in platelets, and anemia.

thrombosis: development, or presence, of a blood clot or thrombus.

thrombus: blood clot obstructing a blood vessel.

transient ischemic attack (TIA): temporary blockage of blood supply to the brain, causing loss of brain function for about 24 hours.

varicose (var′i-kos): lasting , abnormal swelling, as in varicose vein (*varico* means twisted and swollen).

vascular abnormalities: abnormal arteries are described as beaded, dilated, obstructed, sclerosed, or tortuous, and abnormal veins are described as dilated, distended, inflamed, varicosed, or thrombosed.

vasoconstriction (vas″o-kon-strik′shun): narrowing of blood vessels.

vasodilation: the expansion of blood vessels.

vasospasm: blood vessel spasm causing a narrowing in its diameter.

*Oncology**

atrial myxoma: benign tumor composed of primary connective tissue cells that originate in the interatrial septum.

carotid body tumor: benign, encapsulated, spherical mass at the bifurcation (branching) of the common carotid artery.

hemangioma: benign tumor caused by a cluster of newly formed blood vessels.

plasmacytoma*: plasma cell neoplasm in or outside of bone marrow.

Surgical Procedures

anastomosis (ah-nas″to-mo′sis): creation of a passage between two vessels.

aneurysmectomy (an″u-riz-mek′to-me): completely removing an aneurysm by excising the sac.

aneurysmoplasty (an″u-riz′mo-plas″te): repairing of an aneurysm by plastic surgery.

*Indicates a malignant condition.

aneurysmorrhaphy (an″u-riz-mor′ah-fe): suturing of an aneurysm.

aneurysmotomy (an″u-riz-mot′o-me): incision of an aneurysmal sac.

angiectomy (an″je-ek′to-me): excision of a vessel.

angioneurectomy (an″je-o-nu-rek′to-me): excision of vessel and nerve.

angioneurotomy (an″je-o-nu-rot′o-me): cutting of vessels and nerves.

angioplasty (an′je-o-plas″te): repair of a vessel.

angiorrhaphy (an″je-or′ah-fe): suture of a vessel.

angiostomy (an″je-os′to-me): opening of a blood vessel for insertion of a tube.

angiotomy: incision of a blood vessel.

aortotomy: cutting of the aorta.

arteriectomy: excision of a section of an artery.

arterioplasty (ar-te″re-o-plas′te): repair of an artery.

arteriorrhaphy (ar-te″re-or′ah-fe): suture of an artery.

arteriotomy: incision of an artery.

artificial cardiac pacemaker: device (implanted or external), used in place of a defective sinoatrial node to supply electrical impulses to the heart.

atriotomy: incision of the heart atrium.

bone marrow transplantation (BMT): bone marrow is harvested from a compatible donor and transplanted in the recipient for the treatment of anemias, leukemias, and other conditions.

cardiac prosthesis: artificial replacement of cardiac tissue, such as plastic valves and patches or plastic tubular grafts for diseased arteries.

cardiocentesis (kar″de-o-sen-te′sis): surgical puncture or incision of the heart.

cardiotomy (kar″de-ot′o-me): incision of the heart.

coronary artery bypass graft (CABG): a section of a mammary artery or a saphenous vein is sutured to either side of an obstructed coronary artery to improve the flow of blood to the heart muscle.

directional coronary atherectomy (DCA): a method of shaving and removing plaque from clogged arteries in the heart by a motor-driven catheter equipped with a balloon, cutter, and storage chamber.

embolectomy (em″bo-lek′to-me): excision of an embolus.

excimer laser angioplasty: a catheter equipped with a laser is guided into a blocked artery having extended plaque segments difficult to treat conventionally (see **percutaneous transluminal coronary angioplasty**). Ultraviolet energy pulses vaporize the plaque into gas that dissolves in the blood.

hemorrhoidectomy (hem″o-roid-ek′to-me): excision of hemorrhoids (varicose veins of the rectal area).

homograft replacement of heart: transplant of a healthy human donor heart as a replacement for an irreparably damaged human heart.

open heart surgery: surgical procedures requiring prolonged manipulation inside the heart, with the heart detached from systemic circulation and a heart-lung machine replacing its function.

percutaneous transluminal coronary angioplasty (PTCA): commonly called **balloon angioplasty**, because a catheter with a balloon tip is inserted in the coronary artery and inflated, pushing obstructing plaque against the vessel walls to allow free flow of blood.

pericardiectomy: excision of the pericardium.

pericardiocentesis: puncture of the pericardial cavity (also called *pericardicentesis*).

pericardiotomy: incision of the pericardium.

phlebophlebostomy (fleb″o-fle-bos′to-me): anastomosis of two veins.

phleboplasty (fleb′o-plast″te): repair of a vein.

phleborrhaphy (fleb-or′ah-fe): suture of a vein.

thrombectomy (throm-bek′to-me): excision of a thrombus from a blood vessel.

valvuloplasty (val′vu-lo-plas″te): repair of a valve.

valvulotomy (val″vu-lot′o-me): incision of a valve, like those of the heart (also called *valvotomy*).

venipuncture: puncture of a vein, to draw blood.

ventriculotomy (ven-trik″u-lot-o-me): incision of a heart ventricle.

Vineberg coronary artery procedure: surgical technique to implant a healthy artery into the heart muscle in the area of coronary disease.

Laboratory Tests and Procedures

abdominal aortography: x-ray studies of the abdominal aorta and other vessels, using contrast medium.

activated partial thromboplastin time: blood test to screen coagulation disorders and clotting factors.

angiocardiogram: contrast medium is injected in order to study the heart and its vessels by use of x-ray.

angiogram: a contrast medium is injected into the blood vessels and an x-ray is taken (used to study vessels throughout the body).

apolipoprotein test: measures blood content of apolipoprotein, which breaks down cholesterol.

arterial plethysmography: noninvasive procedure to rule out occlusion in lower extremities.

aspartate aminotransferase (AST): a blood test to detect myocardial infarction (formerly called *serum glutamic-oxaloacetic transaminase—SGOT*).

ballistocardiogram: test that records motion transmitted to the body by the heart pumping.

blood culture: sample of blood is incubated in a growth medium to determine the type of organism causing infection.

bone marrow aspiration: insertion of a needle into the sternum or iliac crest to obtain samples of bone marrow for analysis, to diagnose disorders involving red and white blood cells, by evaluating them as to appearance, numbers, development, and presence of infection.

capillary fragility test: use of a blood pressure cuff to determine the fragility of small blood vessels, which is indicative of various diseases of blood vessels.

cardiac catheterization: passage of a small catheter into the heart via a vein in the neck, arm, groin, or leg to inject dye for x-ray purposes, to record pressure, and to discover anomalies of the heart.

cholesterol test: a test to determine the level of cholesterol, a necessary blood lipid which, if too high, is considered a risk factor in coronary heart disease (see **lipoprotein tests**).

citrate agar hemoglobin electrophoresis: laboratory procedure that identifies various forms of hemoglobin, which may indicate various hereditary anemias such as sickle cell.

coagulation tests: tests of blood plasma and serum to determine clotting ability.

complete blood count (CBC): tests to determine the number of red cells (RBC), white cells (WBC), hematocrit (HCT), and hemoglobin (Hgb) percent in the blood.

computerized tomography (CT): imaging device using x-rays at multiple angles through specific sections of the body, analyzed by computer to provide a total picture of the part being examined (also called ***computerized axial tomography [CAT]***).

Coombs' test: test to determine the various types of anemia and blood incompatibility in pregnant women and their fetuses.

differential blood count: percentages of leukocytes in a blood sample.

echocardiography (cardiac ultrasound examination): use of high-frequency sound waves to visualize the heart for assessment of valvular heart disease, and overall heart function.

electrocardiograph (EKG or ECG): instrument producing a graphic record of the electrical currents of the heart.

erythrocyte sedimentation rate (ESR): measurement of the rate at which red blood cells settle in unclotted blood, as an indication of the presence of inflammatory diseases and infections.

functional magnetic resonance imaging (FMRI): detects blood flow, metabolism, gas and water diffusion and movement in functioning systems (also see **magnetic resonance imaging**).

glucose tolerance test: measurement of blood sugar levels at specific intervals following a fasting patient's intake of a quantity of glucose, used to determine effectiveness of metabolism of sugar.

hematocrit (HCT): method to determine erythrocytic volume in whole blood.

hemogram: written record of the differential blood count

hemolysis: procedure to separate hemoglobin from red blood cells.

lipoprotein tests: evaluates amounts and types of fatty substances in the blood (also see **cholesterol**). High levels of **high density lipoproteins (HDL)** are related to decreased risk of heart disease; whereas high levels of **low density lipoproteins (LDL)** and **triglycerides** are risk factors in heart disease.

magnetic resonance imaging (MRI): noninvasive method of scanning the body by use of an electromagnetic field and radio waves, which provides visual images on a computer screen and magnetic tape recordings (also called ***nuclear magnetic resonance [NMR]***).

nuclear magnetic resonance (NMR): see **magnetic resonance imaging**.

positron emission tomography (PET): noninvasive method of scanning using computer-analyzed radionuclides to detect abnormalities in heart and blood vessel function (also called ***positron emission computerized tomography [PECT]***).

prothrombin time: test to determine the time necessary for clot formation in plasma, which provides a measure of the activity of various coagulation factors.

radionuclide angiocardiography: noninvasive method of imaging the chest as a large volume of a blood-labeling agent (radionuclides like thallium or technetium), circulates through the heart and major blood vessels in order to assess ventricular function (also called ***blood pool imaging***).

reticulocyte count: measure of bone marrow activity, which decreases in hemolytic diseases, and elevates after an anemic attack or hemorrhage.

rubacell test: blood test to determine immunity to German measles.

serum enzyme tests: series of tests measuring enzymes released into the blood after a heart attack.

spatial vectorcardiogram: electrocardiogram projected in three planes (three-dimensional), showing electrical activity of the heart muscle and its contraction and relaxation.

thallium stress test: use of radioactive thallium salts injected in minute amounts to mimic the effect of potassium on heart muscle, used in conjunction with an imaging machine to visualize the action of the heart under resting and stress conditions.

thrombolysis: dissolving of a blood clot, particularly by injection of the chemicals streptokinase and urokinase, which appear to spur the body's own mechanisms for dissolution and removal.

trans-esophageal echocardiography: method of visualizing the heart from behind by passing a probe through the mouth and down the esophagus (also see **echocardiography**).

venography: x-ray procedure using contrast dye to determine the presence of blood clots.

venous plethysmography: noninvasive test to evaluate vein function in the lower extremities.

CHAPTER 10

The Respiratory System

The Breath of Life

It's a Fact:
Some snoring reaches a volume of 69 decibels, just slightly below the noise level of a pneumatic drill.

CHAPTER OVERVIEW

In this chapter the various parts of the respiratory system are presented, the system's interaction with the circulatory system is described, and the process of respiration is reviewed and illustrated.

STRUCTURES AND FUNCTIONS

The organs of the respiratory system include the *nose*, *pharynx*, *larynx*, *trachea*, *bronchi*, and *lungs*, and the *thorax* and *diaphragm*, which are accessory structures.

The process of respiration generally involves the *inspiration* (inhalation) of air that contains oxygen (O_2) for use by the cells of the body, and the *expiration* (exhalation) of carbon dioxide (CO_2), which has been removed as a waste product from the cells of the body.

The respiratory system depends on the circulatory system to complete the respiratory cycle, because oxygen inhaled by the lungs is transported via the blood to all parts of the body, and carbon dioxide is collected by the blood and brought back to the lungs to be exhaled.

ORGANS OF THE UPPER RESPIRATORY TRACT

The Nose

The *nose* (Fig. 10-1) is that part of the respiratory system serving as an entry for air and an exit for carbon dioxide. A ciliated, epithelial, mucous membrane (*mu-*

cosa), lines the nose and much of the respiratory tract, serving as a filter for dust and other foreign matter. The nose warms and moistens entering air and has *olfactory* (sense of smell) receptors located in the nasal mucosa (the combining forms for nose are *naso* and *rhino*).

The Pharynx

The *pharynx* (throat) is a musculomembranous, sac-like structure, about 5 inches (12 cm) in length, attached to the base of the skull above and continuous with the *esophagus* below, lined with a mucous membrane (Fig. 10-1). It communicates with the nasal chambers, mouth, larynx, and *eustachian tubes*, and is divided into three parts: the *nasopharynx* (opening into the back of the nasal chambers and into the eustachian tubes), the *oropharynx* (opening into the back of the mouth), and the *laryngopharynx* (opening into the larynx and esophagus).

The pharynx is used by the respiratory and digestive tracts as a passageway for air and food, and has a role in the speech process.

The pharyngeal tonsils (adenoids) are located on the posterior wall of the nasopharynx, and the palatine and lingual tonsils are in the oropharynx. The tonsils and their functions are described in detail in Chapter 16.

The Larynx

The *larynx* (Fig. 10-1) is commonly called the voice box and is located just below the pharynx. The larynx also serves as a passageway for air, and protects the airway against foods entering during swallowing. It plays an important role as the main organ of speech, since air, passing through the *glottis* during expiration, causes a vibration producing the sound of the voice. Other structures also play a part in this process.

The larynx is a musculocartilaginous structure lined with mucous membrane and moved by muscles of the hyoid group (named for the hyoid bone), which suspend

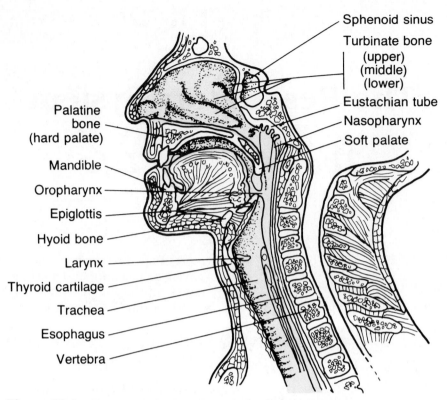

Figure 10-1.   Upper respiratory tract, including some bones.

the larynx from the hyoid, the base of the skull, and the mandible, anchoring it to the sternum. The movement of the larynx as a whole changes its size and shape to produce the complete range of sound between high and low notes. Other muscles of the larynx connect cartilages important to respiration, speech, and swallowing.

The larynx is made up of nine cartilages. The three largest are the ***thyroid***, the ***epiglottis***, and the ***cricoid*** (Fig. 10-2), all of which are separate structures, and there are three pairs of accessory cartilages, the ***arytenoid***, ***corniculate***, and ***cuneiform***.

The thyroid cartilage, largest of the three single cartilages, is shield-shaped, forming the projection called "Adam's apple." The epiglottis cartilage, a leaf-shaped flap attached to the thyroid cartilage at one side, closes the trachea during swallowing to prevent food from entering it. The cricoid cartilage is ring-shaped and is the lowest of the cartilages of the larynx.

The mucous membrane lining the larynx forms two pairs of folds, one pair above the other. The upper pair are called ***false vocal cords***, which have no part in speech, while the lower pair, the ***true vocal cords***, vibrate to create sounds as air passes out of the lungs. Three factors in determining the voice pitch are tension, elasticity, and rigidity of the vocal cords. Between the true vocal cords is a slit called the ***glottis***, the most constricted area of the air passage of the larynx.

Review A

Complete the following:

1. The _____ and _____ are accessory structures of the respiratory system.

2. The main functions of the nose are to _____ and _____ entering air.

3. The pharynx is divided into _____ parts.

4. The larynx is commonly called the _____ .

5. The "Adam's apple" is formed by the _____ cartilage.

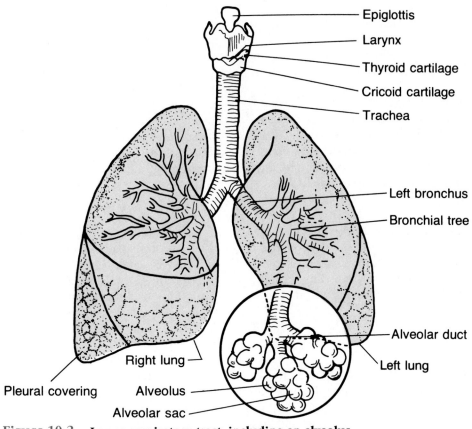

Epiglottis
Larynx
Thyroid cartilage
Cricoid cartilage
Trachea

Left bronchus
Bronchial tree

Alveolar duct
Left lung

Right lung

Pleural covering   Alveolus

Alveolar sac

Figure 10-2.   Lower respiratory tract, including an alveolus.

ORGANS OF THE LOWER RESPIRATORY TRACT

The Trachea

The ***trachea*** (windpipe) is a tube formed of smooth muscle with 16 to 20 C-shaped rings of cartilage embedded in the muscle tissue (Fig. 10-2). It is approximately 4 inches (10 cm) long and 1 inch (2.5 cm) wide, stretching from the larynx to the bronchi and lined with mucous membrane. The main function of the trachea is to maintain its part of the airway.

The Bronchi

At its lower end the trachea separates into smaller airways called the right and left ***primary bronchi*** (singular—***bronchus***), with the right bronchus being slightly larger than the left. The bronchi, like the trachea, are lined with a ciliated mucous membrane, and have C-shaped, cartilaginous rings in their walls, until entering the lungs when the rings become complete (O-shaped). The two primary bronchi enter the lungs, one to the right

lung and one to the left, dividing into smaller branches called ***secondary bronchi***, which branch into ***bronchioles***, which continually branch into smaller and smaller bronchioles, finally becoming ***alveolar ducts***, which have ***alveolar sacs*** at their termination. The walls of the alveolar sacs are composed of many ***alveoli***, which are minute, squamous epithelial lined spaces, allowing the lungs to achieve their main function, the exchange of oxygen and carbon dioxide.

As the bronchioles get smaller, the cartilage rings begin to disappear, until there are no rings in the alveolar ducts, sacs, or alveoli. The structure of the bronchi and their bronchioles resembles an upside-down tree, which is referred to as the ***bronchial tree***.

The Lungs

The ***lungs***, two large, cone-shaped, closed membranous sacs in the pleural cavity, are the organs of respiration (Fig. 10-2). Each sac contains millions of minute alveoli and blood capillaries lining its membranes. (It has been estimated that there are more than 300 million alveoli in a pair of lungs.) The lungs are encased in a serous membranous sac called the ***visceral pleura***, and the ***thoracic cavity***, in which the lungs are located, is lined with another serous membrane called the ***parietal pleura***. These pleural membranes reduce friction during respiration. The space between the two membranes is called the ***pleural cavity*** or ***potential space***.

Each lung occupies half of the thoracic cavity, extending from a point slightly above the clavicles down to the diaphragm, and separated from the other by the space between the two pleural cavities, the ***mediastinum***. Because of the position of the heart, the right lung is larger than the left, with three lobes, ***superior***, ***middle***, and ***inferior***, while the left has only two lobes, ***superior*** and ***inferior***.

The functions of the lungs are distributing air to the alveoli and exchanging gases, produced by a cooperative effort of the alveoli and their blood capillaries. Early in life the lungs are pink in color, but over time become mottled and dark gray because of the inhalation of dust, soot, nicotine, and tar.

The Thorax

The ***thoracic*** (chest) ***cavity*** is lined with a layer of serous membrane, similar to that covering the lungs, allowing for lubrication of both surfaces during respiration. It is divided into three parts: the ***right*** and ***left*** ***pleural cavities***, and the ***mediastinum***, which contains the heart, thymus, esophagus, trachea, bronchi, nerves, various arteries, veins, lymphatic vessels and nodes.

The shape and slant of the ribs and their attachment to the spine allow them to be raised and lowered as the lungs expand and contract, creating a significant role for the thorax in the respiratory process. On inspiration, particular muscles raise the thorax, making it larger and allowing the lungs to expand, and on expiration, the lungs empty, the thorax is lowered and becomes smaller.

The Diaphragm

The ***diaphragm***, a dome-shaped, musculomembranous partition separating the thoracic and abdominal cavities, and attached to the lumbar vertebrae, lower ribs, and sternum, is the chief muscle of respiration. (The action of the diaphragm is regulated by cranial nerves III, IV, and V, a point remembered by some medical students with the rhyme "three, four, five, keep the diaphragm alive.")

During inspiration the diaphragm contracts, flattens, and lowers, increasing the capacity of the thoracic cavity, and allowing the lungs to fill with air and expand. On expiration the diaphragm relaxes and returns to its original position.

Review B

Complete the following:

1. The trachea is also known as the _____ .

2. There are _____ primary bronchi.

3. The sac encasing the lungs is called the _____ .

4. The thoracic cavity is divided into three parts, the _____, _____, and

   _____ .

5. The diaphragm separates the _____, and _____ cavities.

THE PROCESS OF RESPIRATION

The respiratory cycle is divided into three parts: ***inspiration***, inhalation of air; ***expiration***, exhalation of air; and ***rest***, the interval between inspiration and expiration. Normally, the adult cycle is completed about 12 to 18 times per minute.

Respiration involves oxygen being passed throughout the body by the circulation, and carbon dioxide wastes returning via the blood to the lungs to be exhaled. The bright red color of arterial blood results from the mix of oxygen and hemoglobin being carried to the tissues, while the dark red color of venous blood indicates that very little oxygen is present in the blood returning from the tissues.

The amount of oxygen retained by the tissues depends on need, since tissues do not store oxygen, and they will not take more oxygen than is needed. Increased activity of any tissue calls for more oxygen. During strenuous exercise, the use of oxygen may be more than doubled, with a significant increase in the amount of blood supplied to the muscles, consequently increasing the amounts of oxygen consumed and carbon dioxide discharged.

The flow of air into and out of the lungs depends entirely on changes in the capacity of the thoracic cavity. Inspiration and expiration are strictly in accordance with the pressure differences between the atmosphere and the air in the lungs caused by expansion or contraction of the thoracic boundaries. Approximate amounts indicated are for the average adult male (Table 10-1).

Tidal volume (TV)—the volume of air inspired or expired during ordinary respiration (amounting to about 500 ml).

Inspiratory reserve volume (IRV)—the maximum volume of air that can be forcibly inspired in addition to tidal volume (about 3000 ml). The same principle applies to expiration.

Expiratory reserve volume (ERV)—the volume of air that can be forcibly expelled in addition to the tidal volume (about 1100 ml). No matter how forcibly one exhales, some air will always remain trapped in the alveoli because the intrathoracic pressure is below the atmospheric (normal air) pressure.

Residual volume (RV)—the volume of trapped air in the alveoli (about 1200 ml).

Vital capacity (VC)—the largest volume of air that can be moved in and out of the lungs. It is the sum of the inspiratory and expiratory reserve volumes plus the tidal volume (about 4600 ml).

The respiratory center in the brain controls the movements of respiration. The nerves from the brain that pass down to the chest wall and diaphragm to control respiration are:

the **vagus** nerve—originating in the brain, sends branches to the larynx, heart, bronchi, esophagus, stomach, liver, and abdomen

the **phrenic** nerve—originating in the cervical spine, passing to the diaphragm

the **thoracic** nerves—originating in the thoracic spinal cord, are the nerves of the muscles of the thorax

In summary, during inspiration, the thoracic cavity enlarges in all directions, the diaphragm contracts and descends, the ribs elevate, and air is drawn into the lungs. During expiration there is relaxation of the inspiratory muscles, and the thoracic framework resumes its original position. As the lungs contract, the diaphragm relaxes upward toward the thoracic cavity.

Table 10-1   RESPIRATORY VOLUMES

Term	Meaning	Volume
Tidal volume (TV)	Air breathed during ordinary respiration	500 ml
Inspiratory reserve volume (IRV)	Air forcibly inspired in addition to tidal volume	3000 ml
Expiratory reserve volume (ERV)	Air forcibly expired in addition to tidal volume	1100 ml
Residual volume (RV)	Air trapped in the lungs at all times	1200 ml
Vital capacity (VC)	TV + IRV + ERV	4600 ml

Review C

Complete the following:

1. The cycle of respiration is divided into three parts, _____, _____, and

_____.

2. The volume of inhaled air during ordinary respiration is called _____ volume.

3. The trapped air in the alveoli is called _____.

4. The respiratory center is in the _____.

5. The three nerves that control respiration are the _____, _____, and

_____.

Answers to Review Questions: The Respiratory System

Review A
1. thorax, diaphragm
2. warm, moisten
3. three
4. voice box
5. thyroid

Review B
1. windpipe
2. two
3. visceral pleura
4. right pleural cavity, left pleural cavity, mediastinum
5. thoracic, abdominal

Review C
1. inspiration (inhalation), expiration (exhalation), rest
2. tidal
3. residual volume
4. brain
5. vagus, phrenic, thoracic

CHAPTER 10 EXERCISES

THE RESPIRATORY SYSTEM: THE BREATH OF LIFE

Exercise 1: Complete the following:

1. The process of respiration generally involves _____ and _____ .

2. The organs of the respiratory system are _____ , _____ , _____ ,

   _____ , _____ , and _____ .

3. The function(s) of the pharynx is (are)_____

   _____

   _____ .

4. In respiration, the functions of the larynx are_____

   _____ .

5. The three large cartilages of the larynx are _____ , _____ , and _____ .

6. The two pairs of vocal cords are named _____ and _____ .

7. The function of the trachea is to _____ .

8. The _____ lung is composed of three lobes.

9. The structure that separates the lungs from each other and divides the thoracic cavity into two parts is the

   _____ .

10. The diaphragm descends during the _____ phase of respiration.

Exercise 2: Matching:

____	**1.** air sac of the lung	**A.** diaphragm
____	**2.** branch of the trachea going to each lobe of the lung	**B.** oxygen
____	**3.** warms and moistens entering air	**C.** carbon dioxide
____	**4.** odorless, colorless gas formed in tissues and excreted by the lungs	**D.** mucous membrane
____	**5.** has a role in respiration, digestion, and speech	**E.** bronchiole
____	**6.** potential space between the parietal and visceral pleural membranes	**F.** pleural cavity
____	**7.** muscular and membranous partition that separates the thoracic cavity from the abdominal cavity	**G.** bronchus
____	**8.** epithelial lining of the nose	**H.** alveoli
____	**9.** small branch of the bronchial tree extending from secondary bronchi	**I.** nose
____	**10.** gas present in air, necessary for survival	**J.** pharynx

Exercise 3: Using the list of terms below, identify each part in Fig. 10-3 by writing its name in the corresponding blank.

Oropharynx

Nasopharynx

Larynx

Vertebra

Thyroid cartilage

Sphenoid sinus

Epiglottis

Trachea

Mandible

Turbinate bones

Hyoid bone

Esophagus

1. _____

2. _____

3. _____

4. _____

5. _____

6. _____

7. _____

8. _____

9. _____

10. _____

11. _____

12. _____

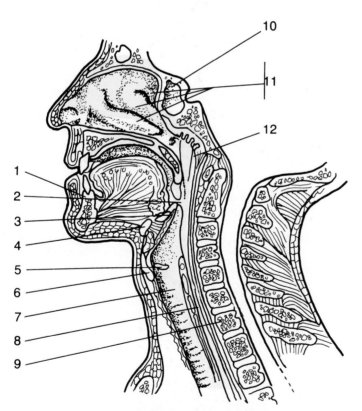

Figure 10-3.   Upper respiratory tract, including some bones.

Exercise 4: Name the structures in Fig. 10-4 identified by the following numbers.

1. _____

2. _____

3. _____

4. _____

5. _____

6. _____

7. _____

8. _____

9. _____

10. _____

11. _____

12. _____

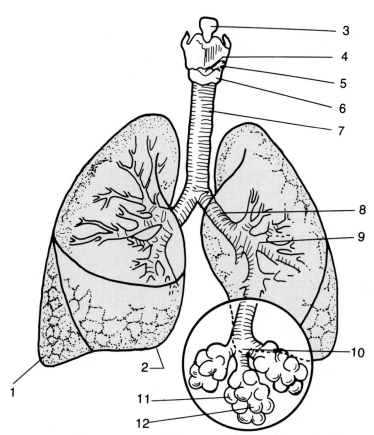

Figure 10-4.   **Lower respiratory tract, including an alveolus.**

Exercise 5: In the blank following each pair of words, indicate whether their meaning is the same or opposite.

1. expiration
   inspiration_____

2. visceral pleura
   pulmonary pleura_____

3. trachea
   windpipe_____

4. pharynx
   throat_____

5. tidal volume
   residual volume_____

Exercise 6: Give the meaning of the components in the following words and then define the word as a whole. Suffixes meaning *pertaining to* or *state or condition* are not to be defined separately, and are shown following a slash (/) mark. Before reaching for your medical dictionary, check the glossary at the end of the chapter.

1. Nasopharyngitis:

   naso_____

   pharyng_____

   itis_____

   _____

2. Rhinitis:

   rhin_____

   itis_____

   _____

3. Anthracosilicosis:

   anthraco_____

   silic/osis_____

   _____

4. Tracheobronchitis:

   tracheo_____

   bronch_____

   itis_____

   _____

5. Bronchostenosis:

   broncho_____

   sten/osis_____

   _____

6. Laryngoptosis:

   laryngo_____

   ptosis_____

   _____

7. Tracheostenosis:

   tracheo_____

   sten/osis_____

   _____

8. Bronchorrhagia

   broncho_____

   rrhag/ia_____

   _____

9. Mediastinitis:

   mediastin_____

   itis_____

   _____

10. Pharyngosalpingitis:

   pharyngo_____

   salping_____

   itis_____

   _____

Chapter 10 Crossword Puzzle

Across

2. leaf-shaped lid-like cartilage
5. musculomembranous partition
6. a nerve controlling respiration
8. upside-down tree structure
10. upper vocal cords
12. pharyngeal tonsils
15. small bronchi branches
16. combining form for nose
18. intake part of respiration cycle
22. part of respiration cycle
24. windpipe
25. pleura lining thoracic cavity
26. a nerve controlling respiration
27. volume of trapped air in alveoli

Down

1. normal air breathed in and out
2. exhalation
3. pleural sac encasing lungs
4. combining form for nose
7. minute air spaces in lungs
9. the lung with two lobes
11. membrane lining respiratory tract
13. a nerve controlling respiration
14. space between pleural cavities
17. number of cartilages in voice box
19. space between lining of lungs and thoracic cavity
20. the largest bronchus
21. throat
23. shield-shaped cartilage

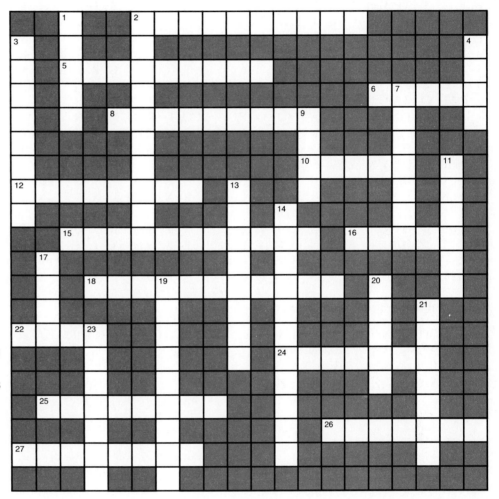

Chapter 10 Hidden Words Puzzle

```
C C R V G B A P J S H F R R Y W T I O Q X U O R W Y
D C R E U D U T Z J V M R G S O O J E E I P B X C L
V A G U S P K H H Y Q S O S F Y I X D W X J K L F X
S U M I E P R K D M X I T M H T O I N M G U Q R E L
M Y G U U B I X D C Q D E L L H R B S M A S P W K Y
P T K R S B S R I P Q H E I W O O L E U K G Z E U B
V F J T X M R F A N L M K Z T Q P P N C X I K U J K
F J C E V K S O F T H R P D K B H T Q O P E I M H S
Y V V S L O H E N U I A D R Q N A O R S R F T Q M V
V K C N Q X L L C C D O L H G N R V E A K N J L P G
S Y E G T V X U X Y H L N A T Z Y V E N C P T P D F
G U O Z U K G V M E D I A S T I N U M U C H O Y R F
E Q L Q X P D D D E G Q S R C I X T A E G R E T W I
R S V K E X H A L A T I O N Y Y O U K U M E H A U P
P G G R Q L W G U W B T P L G N C N Q S V N B P H W
I V P D M E N T F H K V H L N B G L O T T I S J O T
C B M D U Q M Z V Y L V A O E L X O E A H C S N C J
I F V W U I J Z R E M T R G R U D Z P C J Y G V R B
G Y N L S T G V B N D B Y C O A R X I H L A R Y N X
N X G L D G X J N W Z T N Y A L X A A I A N M O S M
N L C W D N L B E E K T X L E K F Y K A K R D R I E
O R J H D L R S A N Q M Y B G R P S J N T I Y E V D
F L Q Z H Z W B E G N H H U H X V X Y T P Y D N R C
E O L W S J B E W F Y N Q O W B N R L T L J P Z X Y
```

Can you find the 20 words hidden in this puzzle?

LARYNGOPHARYNX	MEDIASTINUM	NASOPHARYNX	RESPIRATION
EUSTACHIAN	EXHALATION	INHALATION	OROPHARYNX
BRONCHI	GLOTTIS	PHRENIC	THYROID
TRACHEA	LARYNX	MUCOSA	PLEURA
THORAX	VOLUME	CYCLE	VAGUS

CHAPTER 10 ANSWERS

Exercise 1
1. inspiration (inhalation), and expiration (exhalation)
2. nose, pharynx, larynx, trachea, bronchi, lungs
3. to communicate between the nasal chambers, mouth, larynx, and eustachian tubes; as a passageway for food and air; also has a role in the speech process
4. provide an air passage and protect the airway against food entering during swallowing
5. thyroid, epiglottis, cricoid
6. true, false
7. maintain its part of airway
8. right
9. mediastinum
10. inspiration (or inhalation)

Exercise 2
1. H   5. J   9. E
2. G   6. F   10. B
3. I   7. A
4. C   8. D

Exercise 3
1. mandible
2. oropharynx
3. epiglottis
4. hyoid bone
5. larynx
6. thyroid cartilage
7. trachea
8. esophagus
9. vertebra
10. sphenoid sinus
11. turbinate bones
12. nasopharynx

Exercise 4
1. pleural covering
2. right lung
3. epiglottis
4. larynx
5. thyroid cartilage
6. cricoid cartilage
7. trachea
8. left bronchus
9. bronchial tree
10. alveolar duct
11. alveolus
12. alveolar sac

Exercise 5
1. opposite
2. same
3. same
4. same
5. opposite

Exercise 6
1. nasopharyngitis: nose; pharynx; inflammation—inflammation of nose and pharynx
2. rhinitis: nose; inflammation—inflammation of nose or nasal passages
3. anthracosilicosis: coal; silica—a form of pneumoconiosis caused by inhalation of coal dust
4. tracheobronchitis: trachea; bronchi; inflammation—inflammation of trachea and bronchi
5. bronchostenosis: bronchi; narrowing—narrowing of bronchi
6. laryngoptosis: larynx; falling—falling or displacement of the larynx from normal position
7. tracheostenosis: trachea; narrowing—narrowing of the trachea
8. bronchorrhagia: bronchi; hemorrhage—bronchial hemorrhage
9. mediastinitis: mediastinum; inflammation—inflammation of the mediastinum
10. pharyngosalpingitis: pharynx; eustachian tube; inflammation—inflammation of the pharynx and eustachian tube

Answers: Chapter 10 Crossword Puzzle

		¹T		²E	P	I	G	L	O	T	T	I	S				
³V		I		X													⁴N
I		⁵D	I	A	P	H	R	A	G	M							A
S		A		I							⁶V	⁷A	G	U	S		O
C		L		⁸B	R	O	N	C	H	I	A	L	⁹L		L		O
E				A						E		V				
R				T					¹⁰F	A	L	S	E		¹¹M	
¹²A	D	E	N	O	I	D	S		¹³T		T			O		U
L				O				H		¹⁴M			L		C
		¹⁵B	R	O	N	C	H	O	L	E	S		¹⁶R	H	I	N	O
	¹⁷N					R		D						S	
	I		¹⁸I	N	¹⁹S	P	I	R	A	T	I	O	N	²⁰R		A
	N			O		C	A				I		²¹P	
²²R	E	S	²³T		T		I	S			G		H	
		H		E		C	²⁴T	R	A	C	H	E	A	
		Y		N		I			T		R	
²⁵P	A	R	I	E	T	A	L		N			Y	
	O		I			U	²⁶P	H	R	E	N	I	C
²⁷R	E	S	I	D	U	A	L		M			X	
	D			L							

Answers: Chapter 10 Hidden Words Puzzle

```
. .  R  .  .  .  .  .  .  .  .  .  .  .  .  .  .  .  .  .  .  .  .
. .  .  E  .  .  .  .  .  .  .  .  .  .  .  .  .  .  .  .  .  .  .
V A  G  U  S  .  .  .  .  .  .  .  .  .  .  .  .  .  .  .  .  .  .
. .  .  .  .  P  .  .  .  .  .  O  .  .  .  .  .  .  .  .  .  .  .
. .  .  .  .  I  .  .  .  .  .  R  .  M  .  .  .  .  .  .  .  .  .
. .  .  .  B  .  R  I  .  .  .  .  O  .  U  .  .  .  .  .  .  .  .
. .  .  .  .  R  .  A  N  .  .  .  P  .  C  .  .  .  .  .  .  .  .
. .  .  V  .  O  .  T  H  .  .  .  H  T  .  O  .  .  .  .  .  .  .
. .  .  .  O  .  N  .  I  A  .  .  A  .  R  S  .  .  .  .  .  .  .
. .  .  .  .  L  .  C  .  O  L  .  .  R  .  A  .  .  .  .  .  .  .
. .  .  .  .  .  U  .  .  H  L  N  A  .  .  Y  .  .  .  C  P  .  .
. .  .  .  .  .  .  M  E  D  I  A  S  T  I  N  U  M  .  .  H  .  .
. .  .  .  .  .  .  E  .  .  S  R  C  I  X  .  .  E  .  R  E  .  .
. .  .  .  E  X  H  A  L  A  T  I  O  N  Y  Y  O  .  .  U  .  E  .  A  .  .
. .  .  .  .  .  .  .  .  T  P  .  N  C  N  .  S  .  N  .  .  .  .
. .  .  .  .  .  .  .  .  H  L  .  G  L  O  T  T  I  S  .  .  .  .
. .  .  .  .  .  .  .  .  A  O  E  .  .  O  E  A  H  C  .  .  .  .
. .  .  .  .  .  .  .  .  R  .  R  U  .  .  P  C  .  Y  .  .  .  .
. .  .  .  .  .  .  .  .  Y  .  A  R  .  .  H  L  A  R  Y  N  X  .
. .  .  .  .  .  .  .  .  N  .  .  X  A  .  I  A  .  .  O  .  .  .
. .  .  .  .  .  .  .  .  X  .  .  .  .  A  .  R  .  I  .  .  .  .
. .  .  .  .  .  .  .  .  .  .  .  .  .  N  .  Y  .  D  .  .  .  .
. .  .  .  .  .  .  .  .  .  .  .  .  .  .  N  .  .  .  .  .  .  .
. .  .  .  .  .  .  .  .  .  .  .  .  .  X  .  .  .  .  .  .  .  .
```

Words:

\ LARYNGOPHARYNX	> MEDIASTINUM	∨ NASOPHARYNX	\ RESPIRATION
∨ EUSTACHIAN	> EXHALATION	\ INHALATION	∨ OROPHARYNX
\ BRONCHI	> GLOTTIS	∨ PHRENIC	\ THYROID
\ TRACHEA	> LARYNX	∨ MUCOSA	\ PLEURA
\ THORAX	\ VOLUME	\ CYCLE	> VAGUS

CHAPTER 10 GLOSSARY

Respiratory System Related Anatomic Terms

ala nasi: winglike flare forming the outer side of each nostril.

alveolar ducts: connecting passages between the bronchioles and the alveolar sacs.

alveoli (al-ve′o-lie): air cells of the lungs (singular— *alveolus*).

apex nasi: tip of nose.

apex pulmonis: pointed upper extremity of the lung.

arytenoid cartilage (ar″e-te′noid): small, jug-shaped cartilage of the larynx.

bridge: upper portion of external nose, formed by nasal bones.

bronchial tree: trachea, bronchi, and bronchioles.

bronchiole (brong′ke-ol): a small branch of the bronchi (plural—*bronchioli*).

bronchus (brong′kus): branch of the trachea going to each lobe of the lung (plural—*bronchi*).

carbon dioxide (CO$_2$): odorless, colorless gas formed in the tissues as a waste product, and expelled by the lungs.

choanae osseae (ko-a′ne): the openings between the nasopharynx and the nasal cavity (*choana* means funnel-shaped cavity).

cilia (sil′e-ah): tiny hairlike processes on epithelial tissue that filter out foreign matter (singular— *cilium*).

concha nasalis (kong′kah): shell-shaped structures of the nasal cavity and paranasal chambers (*concha* means shell).

cricoid cartilage: cartilage of the larynx.

diaphragm (di′ah-fram): musculomembranous partition that separates the thoracic cavity from the abdominal cavity (commonly called *muscle of inspiration*).

ductus arteriosus (duk′tus ar-te″re-o′sus): fetal blood channel from the pulmonary artery to the aorta.

epiglottis (ep″i-glot′is): leaf-shaped, lidlike cartilage that covers the entrance to the larynx.

ethmoid sinus: air spaces within the ethmoid bone that open into the nasal cavity (also called *ethmoidal air cells*).

expiration or **exhalation:** breathing out; expelling air from the lungs.

expiratory reserve volume: amount of air that can be forcibly expelled, beyond that exhaled during ordinary respiration.

frontal sinuses: two air spaces in the frontal bone communicating with the nasal cavity by the nasofrontal duct.

glottis (glot′is): slit between the true vocal cords, helping to produce vocal sound.

hilus of lung: depression on the mediastinal surface of each lung for entry of bronchi, blood vessels, and nerves.

inspiration or **inhalation:** breathing of air into the lungs.

inspiratory reserve volume: amount of air that can be forcibly inhaled, beyond that inhaled during ordinary respiration.

laryngopharynx: that part of the pharynx below the upper edge of the epiglottis, opening into the larynx and esophagus (also called *hypopharynx*).

larynx (lar′inks): musculocartilaginous structure, at the top of the trachea and below the root of the tongue and hyoid bone, housing the vocal cords (also called *voicebox*).

maxillary sinuses: two air spaces in the maxilla, communicating with the middle opening of the nasal cavity on each side.

mediastinum: space in the thorax between the two pleural sacs, containing the heart, blood vessels, etc.

mucous membrane: epithelial lining of the respiratory tract.

nares (na′rez): the nostrils (singular—*naris*).

nasal septum: membranous, skeletal partition between nasal cavities.

nasopharynx (na″zo-fahr′inks): that part of the pharynx, above the soft palate of the mouth, opening into the nose.

oropharynx (o″ro-fahr′inks): that part of the pharynx, between the soft palate and the upper edge of the epiglottis.

oxygen (O$_2$): an element in air necessary for life, used by all cells of the body.

parietal pleura: the lining of the thoracic cavity.

pharynx: airway between the nasal chambers, the mouth, and the larynx; also a passageway for food.

phrenic nerve (fren′ik): nerve of the diaphragm.

pleura (ploor′ah): serous membrane, encasing the lungs, lining the thoracic cavity, and enclosing the pleural cavity (potential space).

pleural cavity: *potential space* between the parietal and visceral layers of the pleura.

residual volume: air remaining in the lungs after forced expiration.

respiration: process involving inspiration and expiration, distribution of oxygen to the cells of the body, and the removal of carbon dioxide from these cells.

retropharynx: back part of pharynx.

sphenoid sinuses: two spaces in the anterior portion of the sphenoid bone, opening into the nasal cavity.

tidal volume: air inhaled or exhaled in ordinary respiration.

trachea: cartilaginous, muscular tube, extending from the larynx to the bronchi (also called the *windpipe*).

tracheal rings: C-shaped rings of cartilage embedded in the muscle tissue of the trachea.

vagus nerve (va′gus): nerve extending from the brain to the pharynx, larynx, thoracic and abdominal viscera (*vagus* means wandering).

vestibule: front part of the nostrils and nasal cavity.

visceral pleura: serous sac covering the lungs.

vital capacity: largest amount of air that can be moved in and out of the lungs, the sum total of inspiratory and expiratory reserves plus tidal air.

vocal cords: two pairs of membranous bands in the larynx, with the superior pair (false vocal cords), not having any part in speech, and the inferior pair (the true vocal cords), vibrating to produce sound.

windpipe: trachea.

Pathologic Conditions

Inflammations and Infections

The infections below primarily affect the lungs. Other infections that involve the lungs and other organs are described in Chapter 17, Multiple System Diseases.

arytenoiditis (ar-it″e-noi-di′tis): inflammation of a laryngeal arytenoid cartilage.

aspergilloma (as″per-jil-o′mah): granulomatous mass of the *Aspergillus* fungus in a pulmonary cavity or bronchus.

bronchiectasis (brong″ke-ek′tah-sis): chronic dilation of bronchi or bronchioles, as a consequence of an obstruction or an inflammation.

bronchiolitis (brong″ke-o-li′tis): inflammation of the bronchioles.

bronchitis (brong-ki′tis): inflammation of the bronchial membranes.

bronchopneumonia (brong″ko-nu-mo′neah): inflammation of the lungs originating in the terminal bronchioles.

bronchosinusitis (brong″ko-si″nus-i′tis): simultaneous inflammation of the bronchi and sinuses.

chorditis (kor-di′tis): inflammation of a vocal cord.

coccidioidomycosis (kok-sid″e-oi″do-mi-ko′sis): several forms of respiratory fungal infection, of which the primary type is an acute, benign disease caused by the *Coccidioides immitus fungus* (also known as *valley fever*, *desert fever*, and *San Joaquin Valley fever*).

diphtheria (dif-the′re-ah): acute, infectious, contagious disease affecting the mucous membranes of the nose, throat, and/or bronchial tree, and marked by formation of a thin, gray-white, false membrane.

epiglottitis (ep″i-glot-ti′tis): inflammation of the epiglottis (also called *epiglottiditis*).

histoplasmosis (his′to-plaz-mo′sis): systemic fungal respiratory infection caused by the inhalation of spores of *Histoplasma capsulatum*.

influenza: acute, contagious, respiratory disease transmitted by airborne viral droplet infection, occurring in epidemics (attacking many people in an area at the same time), with symptoms of headache, weakness, sore throat, and myalgia. Three general types of influenza are designated A, B, and C, with new strains emerging periodically and named for the geographic location first noted (Asian, Hong Kong, Chile, Panama, etc.) or the animal source (swine, equine, etc.), with only A and B types causing epidemics.

laryngitis (lar″in-ji′tis): inflammation of the larynx.

laryngopharyngitis (lah-ring″go-far″in-ji′tis): inflammation of the larynx and pharynx.

laryngophthisis (lar″ing-gof′thi-sis): tuberculosis of the larynx.

laryngotracheitis (lah-ring″go-trak″ke-i′tis): inflammation of larynx and trachea.

laryngotracheobronchitis (lah-ring″go-tra″ke-o-brong-ki′tis): inflammation of the larynx, trachea, and bronchi.

laryngovestibulitis (lah-ring″go-ves-tib″ul-i′tis): inflammation of the laryngeal vestibule.

Legionnaires' disease: acute form of bacterial pneumonia, with influenza-like symptoms, and a mortality rate of about 15%, caused by the *Legionella pneumophilia bacterium*, which is believed to be water-borne; moist soil and air-conditioning cooling towers have been suspect (also called *legionellosis*).

mediastinitis (me″de-as″ti-ni′tis): inflammation of the tissues of the mediastinum.

nasopharyngitis (na″zo-far″in-ji′tis): inflammation of the nose and pharynx.

nasosinusitis: inflammation of the nose and the paranasal sinuses.

pansinusitis (pan″si-nus-i′tis): inflammation of all the nasal sinuses.

pertussis: whooping cough (also called *broncho-cephalitis*).

pharyngitis: inflammation of the mucous membranes of the pharynx.

pharyngolaryngitis (fah-ring″go-lar″inji′tis): inflammation of the membranes of the pharynx and larynx.

pharyngorhinitis: inflammation of the mucous membranes of the pharynx and nose.

pleurisy: inflammation of the pleura.

pleuropericarditis: inflammation of the pleura and pericardium.

pleuropneumonia (ploor′o-nu-mo′ne-ah): pleurisy with pneumonia.

pneumocystis carinii pneumonia (PCP): rare pneumonia condition usually seen in conjunction with AIDS (Chapters 16 and 17).

pneumonia (nu-mo′ne-ah): inflammation and congestion of the lungs (also called **pneumonitis**).

pneumopleuritis (nu″mo-ploo-ri′tis): pleurisy with presence of air in the pleural cavity.

psittacosis (sit-ah-ko′sis): respiratory viral infection (usually a pneumonia) transmitted to humans through contact with infected birds (also called **parrot fever**).

Q fever: febrile rickettsial respiratory infection caused by *Coxiella burnetii*.

rhinitis: inflammation of the nasal mucous membranes.

rhinolaryngitis: inflammation of the membranes of the nose and larynx.

rhinopharyngitis: inflammation of the nasal and pharyngeal mucous membranes.

rhinosalpingitis: inflammation of the mucous membranes of the nose and eustachian tubes.

sinusitis (sin″nus-i′tis): inflammation of the membrane lining a sinus.

tracheitis (tra″ke-i′tis): inflammation of the membrane lining the trachea.

tracheobronchitis: inflammation of the membranes lining the trachea and bronchi.

tuberculosis: infectious disease caused by the *Mycobacterium tuberculosis organism*, characterized by formation of tubercles in the lung tissues, with possible dissemination throughout the body.

Other Conditions and Diseases

allergic rhinitis: any allergic response of the nasal mucosa.

aphonia: loss of ability to speak.

apnea: cessation of breathing.

asphyxia: condition resulting from lack of oxygen.

asthma (az′mah): disease marked by recurring attacks of paroxysmal shortness of breath, wheezing, and coughing.

atelectasis (at′e-lek′tah-sis): collapse of the lung, or incomplete expansion of the lung at birth.

berylliosis (ber″il-le-o′sis): disease, marked by formation of granulomas, usually in the lungs, caused chiefly by inhalation of beryllium salts fumes.

broncholithiasis (brong″ko-li-thi′ah-sis): stone in a part of the tracheobronchial tree.

bronchoplegia (brong″ko-ple′je-ah): paralysis of the bronchial tube walls.

bronchorrhagia (brong″ko-ra′je-ah): bronchial hemorrhage.

bronchorrhea (brong″ko-re′ah): excessive discharge of mucus from the lung air passages.

bronchospasm (brong′ko-spazm): spasm of the muscles of the walls of the bronchi.

bronchostenosis: narrowing of a bronchial tube.

chronic obstructive pulmonary disease (COPD): general term for pulmonary obstructive diseases, with breathing difficulties, such as *chronic bronchitis* and *emphysema*.

croup (kroop): condition occurring in young children marked by a laryngeal obstruction with a characteristic barking cough (also called **laryngostasis**).

deviated septum of nose: nasal septum shifted to right or left, due to a congenital defect, disease, or trauma.

dysphonia (dis-fo′ne-ah): difficulty in speaking.

dyspnea (disp-ne′ah): difficulty in breathing.

emphysema (em″fi-se′mah): chronic pulmonary condition marked by abnormal increases in the size of the air spaces in the lungs, due to alveolar dilation or destructive changes to alveoli walls.

epistaxis (ep″i-stak′sis): nosebleed.

hemopneumothorax: blood and air in the pleural cavity.

hemoptysis (he-mop′ti-sis): spitting of blood.

hemothorax: blood in the pleural cavity.

hiccup: involuntary, spasmodic contraction of the diaphragm causing characteristic sounds in breathing (also called **hiccough**).

hyaline membrane disease: respiratory distress condition affecting premature neonates, characterized by *atelectasis* (collapse of lung tissue).

hyperpnea (hi″perp-ne′ah): abnormal increased respiration.

hyperventilation: abnormally prolonged, rapid, deep breathing.

hydropneumothorax: collection of fluid and air in the pleural cavity.

hydrothorax: fluid in the pleural cavity.

laryngalgia (lar″in-gal′je-ah): pain in the larynx.

laryngoplegia (lar″ing-go-ple′je-ah): paralysis of the larynx.

laryngoptosis (lah-ring″go-to′sis): dropping or displacement of the larynx from its normal position.

laryngorrhagia (lar″ing-go-ra′je-ah): hemorrhage from the larynx.

laryngospasm (lah-ring′go-spazm): spasmodic closing of the larynx.

laryngostenosis (lah-ring″go-ste-no′sis): narrowing of the larynx.

nasopharyngeal cyst: sac-like growth between the nose and pharynx.

orthopnea (or″thop-ne′ah): inability to breathe unless in an upright position.

pleuralgia (ploor-al′je-ah): pain in the chest (also called **pleurodynia** or **costalgia**).

pneumoconiosis (nu″mo-ko″ne-o′sis): chronic condition caused by inhalation of particulate substances into the lungs, such as *asbestosis—*

asbestos fibers; *bagassosis*—sugar cane waste; *baritosis*—barium dust; *byssinosis*—cotton dust; *coal worker's (CWP)*, including *anthracosis*—coal dust; *silicosis*—stone, sand or flint containing silicon dioxide; and *siderosis*—iron dust; *farmer's lung*—dust from moldy hay; and *stannosis*—tin dust, all of which are considered occupational and environmental diseases.

pneumohemothorax: air and blood in the pleural cavity.

pneumohydrothorax: air and fluid in the pleural cavity.

pneumolithiasis (nu″mo-li-thi′ah-sis): stone in the lungs.

pneumomalacia (nu″mo-mah-la′she-ah): softening of lung tissue.

pneumomediastinum: air in the mediastinum.

pneumomelanosis (nu″mo-mel″ah-no′sis): blackening of the lungs by inhalation of coal dust or smoke.

pneumonocirrhosis (nu-mo″no-si-ro′sis): hardening of the lungs.

pneumopyothorax: air and pus in the pleural cavity.

pneumorrhagia (nu″mo-ra′je-ah): hemorrhage from the lungs.

pneumothorax: air in the pleural cavity.

pulmonary edema: serous fluid accumulation in the air sacs and tissues of the lung.

pulmonary fibrosis: progressive, usually fatal, fibrosis of the walls of the alveoli of the lungs (also called ***diffuse interstitial pulmonary fibrosis***).

pyothorax: collection of pus in the pleural cavity (also called ***empyema***).

rales (rahlz): abnormal breathing sounds heard in the lungs.

rhinodynia (ri″no-din′e-ah): pain of the nose.

rhinolith: stone in the nasal cavity.

rhonchus (rong′kus): whistling or rattling sound in the throat or bronchi.

tracheorrhagia (tra″ke-o-ra′je-ah): tracheal hemorrhage.

tracheostenosis (tra″ke-o-ste-no′sis): narrowing of the trachea.

*Oncology**

adenocystic carcinoma*: malignancy of the mucous glands of the respiratory tract.

alveolar cell carcinoma*: malignancy originating in the bronchioles and metastasizing to the alveolar surfaces (also called ***bronchiolar carcinoma***).

bronchial adenoma*: benign or malignant, slow-growing tumor of the mucous membranes of the bronchi.

bronchogenic carcinoma*: malignancy that originates in the mucosa of the primary bronchi.

*Indicates a malignant condition.

epidermoid carcinoma*: malignancy in which the cells differentiate as they do in the epidermis, and become keratinized (also called ***squamous cell carcinoma***).

glioma of nose (gli-o′mah): tumorlike mass of glial tissue at the base of the nose.

laryngeal papillomatosis (pap″i-lo-mah-to′sis): benign tumor of laryngeal epithelial mucous membranes, including warts, polyps, and condylomas, which may also occur on the trachea and other respiratory structures.

oat cell carcinoma*: extremely malignant, bronchogenic, accounting for one-third of lung cancers (also called ***small cell carcinoma***).

polyp (pol′ip): tumor having a pedicle, commonly found in nose.

polyposis of nose: multiple polyps in nose.

Surgical Procedures

arytenoidectomy (ar″e-te″noid-ek′to-me): excision of an arytenoid cartilage of the larynx.

arytenoidopexy (ar″i-te-noi′do-pek″se): fixation of the arytenoid cartilage or muscle.

aspiration: use of suction to remove fluid or gas from a cavity (also means breathing in).

bronchoplasty (brong′ko-plas″te): plastic repair of a bronchus.

bronchorrhaphy (brong-kor′ah-fe): repair of a bronchus by suturing.

bronchostomy (brong-kos′to-me): surgical creation of an opening into a bronchus.

bronchotomy: incision of a bronchus.

cordectomy (kor-dek′to-me): excision of all or part of a vocal cord.

cordopexy (kor′do-pek″se): outward fixation of a vocal cord to relieve stenosis of the larynx.

cricoidectomy (kri″koi-dek′to-me): excision of the cricoid cartilage of the larynx.

cricotomy (kri-kot′o-me): incision to divide the cricoid cartilage of the larynx.

cricothyrotomy (kri″ko-thy″ro-to-me): emergency incision through the larynx and cricothyroid membrane to clear the airway.

epiglottidectomy (ep″i-glot′i-dek′to-me): excision of the epiglottis.

ethmoidectomy (eth″moi-dek′to-me): excision of all or part of the partition between the ethmoid sinuses.

intubation: insertion of a tube into the airway to clear it of obstruction, named for the location of insertion (e.g.: oral, nasal, endotracheal).

laryngectomy (lar″in-jek′to-me): excision of the larynx.

laryngopharyngectomy (lah-ring″go-far″in-jec′to-me): excision of the larynx and pharynx.

laryngoplasty (lah-ring′go-plas″te): plastic repair of the larynx.

laryngoscope (lah-ring'go-skop): instrument for the examination of the larynx.

laryngostomy (lar"ing-gos'to-me): creating a permanent opening in the larynx through the neck.

laryngotomy (lar"ing-got'o-me): incision of the larynx for repair of stenosis or removal of tumors (also called ***laryngofissure***).

laryngotracheotomy (lah-ring"go-tra"ke-ot'o-me): incision of trachea and larynx to clear airway.

phrenicectomy (fren"i-sek'to-me): excision of part of the phrenic nerve.

phrenicotomy (fren"i-kot'o-me): division of the phrenic nerve.

pleuracotomy (ploor"ah-kot'o-me): creation of an opening into the chest wall for drainage (also called ***thoracotomy*** or ***thoracostomy***).

pleurectomy (ploor-ek'to-me): excision of all or part of the pleura.

pleuracentesis (ploor'ah-sen-tee'sis): paracentesis (surgical puncture) of the thoracic cavity for drainage (also called ***pleurocentesis***, ***thoracentesis***, or ***thoracocentesis***).

pleuroparietopexy (ploor"o-pah-ri'e-to-pek"se): fixation of the visceral pleura to the chest wall.

pneumocentesis (nu"mo-cen-te'sis): puncture of lung for aspiration of fluid.

pneumonectomy: excision of a lung.

pneumonorrhaphy (nu"mo-nor'ah-fe): suture of lung.

pneumonotomy (nu"mo-not'o-me)": incision of lung.

pneumonopexy (nu'mo-no-pek"se): fixation of lung to the chest wall.

rhinoplasty (ri'no-plas"te): plastic repair of the nose.

septectomy (sep-tek'to-me): excision of nasal septum.

sinusotomy: incision into a sinus.

thoracentesis: see **pleuracentesis**.

thoracoplasty (tho"rah-ko-plas'te): removal of ribs for collapse of the lungs.

tracheoplasty (tra'ke-o-plas"te): plastic repair of trachea.

tracheorrhaphy (tra"ke-or'ah-fe): suture of the trachea.

tracheostomy (tra'ke-os'to-me): creation of an artifical opening into the trachea through the neck (also called ***tracheotomy***).

Laboratory and Examination Procedures

auscultation: use of a stethoscope, an instrument that magnifies sounds within the chest cavity.

bronchogram: x-ray of the bronchi and its branches, using a contrast medium.

bronchoscopy (brong'ko-sko-pee): examination of the bronchi by means of a bronchoscope (fiberoptic flexible tube or endoscope, inserted through mouth or trachea).

computerized tomography (CT): imaging device using x-rays at multiple angles through specific sections of the body, analyzed by computer to provide a total picture of the part being examined (also called ***computerized axial tomography [CAT]***).

chest x-ray: examination to determine presence of lung disease.

endoscopy: examination using an endoscope (flexible tube with a light and refracting mirrors) to examine the larynx and esophagus.

laryngoscopy: examination of the larynx and upper trachea using a laryngoscope (an endoscope) to detect tumors and other abnormalities.

lung scan: visualization procedures involving intravenous injection of radioactive material to diagnose pulmonary emboli and lung structure and function, and inhalation of radioactive gas to diagnose nonfunctioning lung areas and other abnormalities.

magnetic resonance imaging (MRI): noninvasive method of scanning the body by use of an electromagnetic field and radio waves, which provides visual images on a computer screen and magnetic tape recordings (also called ***nuclear magnetic resonance [NMR]***).

nuclear magnetic resonance (NMR): see **magnetic resonance imaging**.

percussion: the use of light, sharp taps to the anterior and posterior chest surfaces to detect abnormalities by the sound produced.

pulmonary function tests: group of tests, using a spirometer (instrument into which the patient breathes to provide measure of volume and rate of air inhaled and exhaled). Although not a comprehensive list, some of the tests are described below.

functional residual capacity (FRC): the volume remaining in lungs after ordinary exhalation.

inspiratory capacity (IC): maximum volume that can be inhaled after normal ordinary exhalation.

maximum expiratory pressure (MEP): pressure produced on exhalation.

maximum inspiratory pressure (MIP): pressure produced on inhalation.

residual volume (RV): volume remaining in lungs after maximal exhalation.

tidal volume (TV): volume of air in one inhalation or exhalation.

timed forced expiratory volume (FEV): volume of air that can be exhaled forcibly in one second, as a measure of total lung capacity.

total lung capacity (TLC): largest volume in lungs after maximal inhalation.

vital capacity (VC): maximum volume of air that can be expelled after maximal forced inhalation.

throat culture: incubation, in a growth medium, of material taken from throat surfaces, to determine presence and type of infection.

CHAPTER 11

The Gastrointestinal System

The Food Processor

It's a Fact:
The acid of the human stomach is so corrosive that it can eat through the metal of an automobile body.

CHAPTER OVERVIEW

In this chapter, the gastrointestinal system and its parts and functions are described and explained, with illustrations.

STRUCTURES AND FUNCTIONS

The organs of the gastrointestinal system, commonly called the **digestive** (or **alimentary**) tract, form a tube-like passage through the body cavities, extending from the **mouth** to the **anus** by way of the **pharynx, esophagus, stomach**, and **intestines**. The main functions of this system are to carry food for digestion, prepare it for absorption, and carry waste material for elimination. The accessory organs of digestion are the **teeth, salivary glands, liver, gallbladder**, and **pancreas**.

Food is chewed in the mouth and is swallowed by way of the pharynx and esophagus, passing through the neck and thorax into the abdomen, where it is received by the stomach. The stomach partially digests the food before it is passed on to the small intestine for further digestion and absorption, and the residue moves on to the large intestine, where it is retained until it is excreted through the anus. All the organs of the digestive tract except the pharynx and esophagus are in the abdominal cavity (Fig. 11-1).

The movement of contents through the digestive tract is aided by **peristalsis**, an involuntary wavelike movement produced by circular and longitudinal muscle fibers of the tubes of the body.

THE MOUTH
Lips

The **lips** (**labia** means lips) form the entrance to the mouth. They are covered on the outside by thin skin and on the inside by mucous membrane that extends to cover the surfaces of the oral cavity. In contrast to the surrounding thick skin, the thin skin covering the lips reveals the underlying red blood in the capillary bed.

Oral Cavity

The **oral cavity** is formed by the arch of the upper and lower jaws. It contains the gums (**gingivae** means gums) and teeth (**dento-** and **donto-** refer to teeth) and divides the cavity into a vestibule between the teeth and lips and a mouth cavity behind the teeth. The structure forming the roof of the mouth is the **palate**, which is divided into the **hard** and **soft** palates.

Palates and Arches

The **hard palate** is a rigid bony structure covered with mucous membrane. The **soft palate** is a partition between the mouth and nasopharynx composed of muscle tissue shaped like an arch and covered with mucous membrane.

At the posterior border of the mouth the soft palate hangs in two curved folds, forming the **palatine arches**, between which the **uvula**, a soft, conical process, projects.

The **fauces** is the constricted opening between the arches and the second part of the pharynx, the **oropharynx**.

Cheeks

The **cheeks** are formed by buccinator muscles and a subcutaneous pad of fat, the buccal pad. The muscles keep the food between the teeth during the act of chewing, and the elastic tissue of the mucous membrane of the

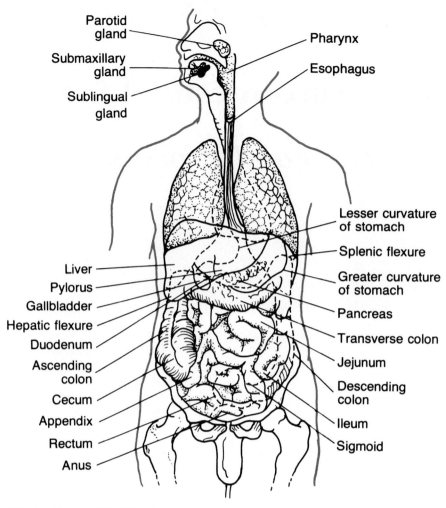

Figure 11-1.   Digestive tract.

cheeks keeps the lining from forming folds that otherwise could be bitten during chewing.

Floor of the Mouth

The *floor* of the mouth is formed by a series of structures under the mucous membrane, including the *sublingual gland*, the deep part of the *submaxillary gland*, and the *lingual nerve* and *vein*.

Tongue

The *tongue* is composed of skeletal muscle tissue covered by mucous membrane. It keeps food between the teeth during chewing and aids in swallowing by means of pressure against the hard palate. A thin mucous membrane, the *lingual frenulum*, anchors the underside of the tongue to the floor of the mouth.

The small elevations on the sides and upper surface of the tongue are called *papillae*, which are of three types: *filiform*, *fungiform*, and *vallate*, the latter two containing the taste buds (Fig. 11-2).

Gingivae (Gums)

The *gingivae* consist of mucous membranes with supporting fibrous tissue covering the surfaces of the maxilla and mandible (jawbones). Richly vascular but poorly innervated, the gums form a collar around each tooth.

Teeth

There are 32 permanent teeth at maturity (Fig. 11-3) including the two upper and two lower third molars (commonly called wisdom teeth). In each jaw are two *central* and two *lateral incisors*, which are chisel-shaped to aid in biting or cutting. On the outer side of each incisor is a pointed *canine* tooth, which aids in grasping and tearing food. Next to the canines are the *first* and *second premolars*, and the *first*, *second*, and *third molars*, all of which are broad and are used to crush and grind the food.

Each tooth has a *crown*, the part projecting from the gumline; a *neck*, located in the gumline; and a *root*, which firmly fixes the tooth in the *alveolus* (socket) in conjunction with *cementum*, a bonelike connective tissue that covers the root and neck. *Periodontium*, a

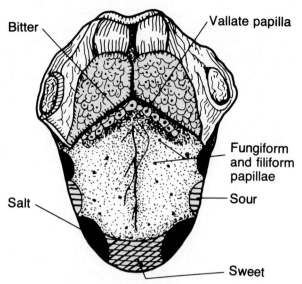

Figure 11-2.   Tongue: location of taste buds.

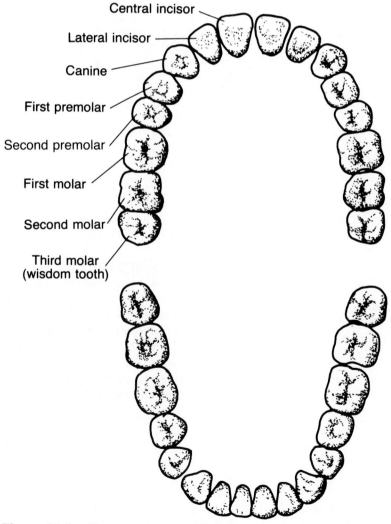

Figure 11-3.   The permanent teeth (32).

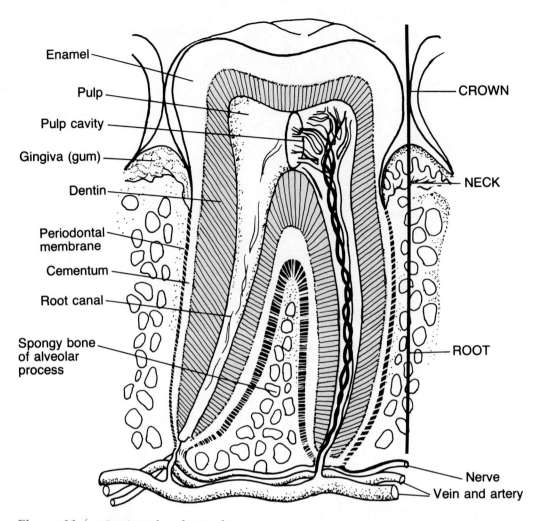

Figure 11-4.   Sectioned molar teeth.

fibrous type of connective tissue, covers the root of the tooth, is embedded in the cementum, and attaches to alveolus walls. This periodontal tissue assists in holding the tooth in place and helps to cushion and support it against pressure produced in chewing and biting.

Teeth have three layers (Fig. 11-4):

Enamel—the hardest substance in the body, covering the crown of the tooth.

Dentin—the bulk of the tooth, including the crown, neck, and root, and surrounding the pulp cavity.

Pulp cavity—space within the tooth containing connective tissue, sensory nerves, and lymph and blood vessels.

Salivary Glands

The mucous membranes of the mouth contain numerous small glands, the submandibular, sublingual, and parotid glands (Fig. 11-1), that secrete a thin, lubricating, serous fluid called *saliva*.

The chief functions of saliva are to dissolve or lubricate food to facilitate swallowing and to initiate digestion of some carbohydrates. The smell, sight, or thought of food causes the secretion of saliva.

Review A

Complete the following:

1. Another name for the gastrointestinal system is _____.

2. The wavelike movement of the tubes of the GI system is called _____.

3. The roof of the mouth is formed by the _____.

4. The taste buds are located on the _____.

5. The three parts of a tooth are the _____, _____, and _____.

THE PHARYNX

The **pharynx**, a musculomembranous, saclike structure, is described in Chapter 10 as part of the respiratory system, although it serves a dual purpose as an airway and as a passageway for food.

THE ESOPHAGUS

The **esophagus**, a narrow musculomembranous tube about 10 inches (25 cm) long and $\frac{1}{2}$ inch (1 cm) in diameter, leads from the pharynx and descends in front of the vertebral column to enter the stomach. The walls of the esophageal tube are thick but are collapsible because they lack supporting cartilaginous rings such as those found in the trachea.

THE PROCESS OF SWALLOWING

There are three phases to the act of swallowing. Only the first is voluntary; the other two are instinctive reflexes. The voluntary phase is the passing of food from the mouth into the pharynx. This is followed by a second, involuntary (reflex) phase, which passes the food into the esophagus from the pharynx, and a third, involuntary (reflex) phase, which passes the food into the stomach from the esophagus (Fig. 11-1).

Because it functions as an organ of both the respiratory and digestive systems, the pharynx communicates with the oral and nasal cavities above and the larynx and esophagus below. When food enters the pharynx, all other openings are blocked to ensure its passage to the esophagus. This blocking is achieved by the tongue pressing against the hard palate to close off the oral cavity, the soft palate rising to block the nasal cavity, and contraction of the laryngeal opening. In addition, as previously noted (Chapter 10), the epiglottis cartilage closes the trachea during swallowing to prevent food from entering it. Swallowing also stimulates a momentary respiratory suspension that helps to guard against the passage of food into the respiratory tract. This process is an involuntary reflex action, and is part of the second phase of swallowing.

The third phase of swallowing takes place in the esophagus, where the food is propelled by pharyngeal muscle contraction (**peristalsis**) through the sphincter muscle into the stomach.

THE STOMACH

The stomach (**gastro** refers to stomach), a musculomembranous, curved, pouchlike structure, is located toward the left side of the upper abdominal cavity, below the liver and diaphragm (Fig. 11-1), and is divided into three sections:

> **fundus**—the rounded section above the esophageal opening.
> **body**—the middle section.
> **pylorus**—the lower, small end.

Curvatures

The right upper margin of the stomach is the **lesser curvature**, and the lower left margin is the **greater curvature**.

Sphincter Muscles

The ringlike muscles that contract to close an opening are called **sphincter** muscles. The **cardiac sphincter** muscle is located between the esophagus and the stomach, relaxing to allow food to enter the stomach and contracting while digestion takes place, preventing the stomach contents from **reflux** (backward flow). The **pyloric sphincter** muscle is located between the **pylorus** of the stomach and the **duodenum**, contracting to prevent the stomach contents from escaping during digestion and then relaxing to allow the contents to enter the duodenum after the digestive process has been completed.

Gastric Coats and Glands

The stomach wall is made up of four coats: an outer **serous** coat, a **muscular** coat (consisting of **circular**, **longitudinal**, and **oblique fibers**), a **submucous** coat, and a **mucous lining** coat. The muscles of the stomach walls allow for expansion when food enters it and mix and churn these foods during the digestive process. Scattered throughout the mucosa of the stomach are innumerable microscopic, tubular, **gastric glands**. The gastric juice produced by these glands contains **enzymes**, **mucin**, **intrinsic factor** (necessary for absorption of vitamin B_{12}), and **hydrochloric acid**. The food in the stomach mixes with these secretions, forming a partially digested semiliquid called **chyme**, that is passed on to the **small intestine** for further digestion.

Review B

Complete the following:

1. The _____ serves a dual purpose in the respiratory and gastrointestinal systems.

2. The _____ tube is thick walled but collapsible.

3. There are _____ phases to the act of swallowing.

4. The stomach is divided into the _____, _____, and _____.

5. The curvatures of the stomach are the _____ and the _____ curvatures.

THE DIGESTIVE PROCESS

Food remains in the stomach from 1 to 4 hours after eating, and as the stomach contents liquefy, they pass into the **duodenum**. The chyme moves through the **jejunum** and **ileum** by means of the peristaltic waves and is further digested and absorbed. When the ileum empties into the **colon**, the contents contain water to be absorbed by the **large intestine** and waste to be eliminated from the body.

THE ABDOMINAL CAVITY

The stomach and the large and small intestines are enclosed in a space between the diaphragm and pelvis,

the **abdominal cavity**, which is lined with a serous membrane, the **parietal peritoneum** (Figs. 11-1 and 11-5). A membranous fold of this peritoneum, the **mesentery**, connects a portion of the intestines to the posterior abdominal wall, and an extension of the peritoneum, the **visceral peritoneum**, covers all or part of many visceral organs and helps to hold them in place.

A double fold of the peritoneum, the **omentum**, attaches to the stomach, connecting it with abdominal viscera. The **greater omentum** extends from the greater curvature of the stomach, covers the intestines, and is attached to the **transverse colon**. The **lesser omentum** extends from the lesser curvature of the stomach to the liver and the first part of the duodenum. Fat, distributed throughout the omentum, prevents abrasion and helps to keep the intestines warm.

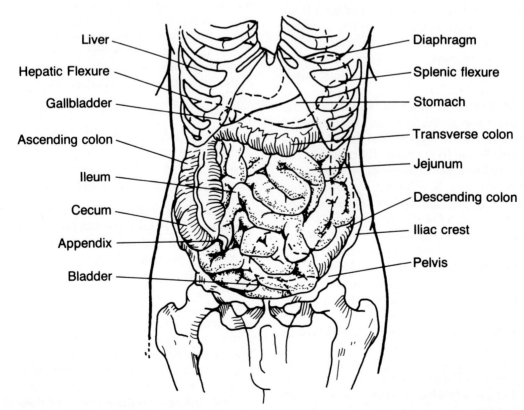

Figure 11-5. Subdiaphragmatic digestive tract organs. (Dotted lines show locations of hidden digestive organ structures.)

The Small Intestine

The ***small intestine*** (***entero*** refers to intestines) is the coiled 20-foot (about 6 m) muscular tube that occupies almost all of the abdomen (Figs. 11-1 and 11-5) and is divided into three parts:

Duodenum—attached to the pyloric end of the stomach, extending to the jejunum, approximately 10 inches (25 cm) long, crescent-shaped, with both the pancreatic and common bile ducts emptying into it.

Jejunum—the middle section of the small intestine, about 8 feet (2.5 m) in length, held in place by the mesentery and never very full because vigorous peristaltic waves rapidly move the fluid content into the ileum.

Ileum—the longest part of the small intestine, about 12 feet (3.5 m) in length, located in the lower abdomen and ending at the large intestine, and in which most of the absorption of food takes place.

The intestinal digestive juice, containing mucus and many enzymes of digestion, is stimulated to flow by a hormone, ***secretin***, which is produced by the intestinal glands when the chyme reaches the small intestine. The digestive process is completed in the small intestine, and the digested food is then absorbed through the intestinal walls into the blood by the ***villi***, countless threadlike projections in the mucous membrane lining the small intestine.

The Large Intestine

The ***large intestine*** is from 5 to 6 feet (1.5 to 1.8 m) in length and about $2\frac{1}{2}$ inches (6 cm) in diameter at its widest point, decreasing in diameter as it progresses to the anus. It is divided into the ***cecum*** (with its ***appendix***), ***colon***, and ***rectum*** (Figs. 11-1 and 11-5).

Cecum

The first part of the large intestine, the ***cecum***, located in the right lower quadrant of the abdomen, is 2 to 3 inches (5 to 8 cm) in length and forms a dilated, blind pouch that joins the ***colon*** just below the juncture of the ***ileum*** and the ***colon***.

The ***vermiform*** (means wormlike) ***appendix*** is a narrow, tubelike projection about the size and shape of a worm, attached to the ***cecum***, which can be surgically removed without any disturbance of body function.

Colon

The ***colon*** is divided into four sections:

ascending colon—lies vertically on the right side of the abdomen, reaches to the lower margin of the liver, and joins the ***ileum*** at the ***cecal***

junction (Fig. 11-5). The ***ileocecal valve*** allows matter to pass from the ileum into the colon but prevents a reversal of this process. The ascending colon turns and bends, becoming the

transverse colon—crosses the upper abdomen from right to left, below the stomach and liver, and above the small intestine.

descending colon—extends downward from below the stomach on the left side of the abdomen to the ***iliac crest***.

sigmoid colon—an S-shaped curve from the ***iliac crest*** down to the ***rectum***.

Rectum

The last segment of the large intestine, the ***rectum***, is 7 to 8 inches (18 to 20 cm) in length and is lined with a mucous membrane with multiple upright folds called ***rectal columns***, each of which is supplied with an artery and vein. The last section of the rectum, the ***anal canal***, about 1 inch (2.5 cm) in length, terminates in the ***anus***, which is protected by an ***internal*** (smooth muscle) ***sphincter*** muscle and an ***external*** (striated muscle) ***sphincter*** muscle.

THE PANCREAS

The ***pancreas***, a large, elongated, lobulated gland divided into four parts: ***head***, ***neck***, ***body***, and ***tail***. It is located behind the stomach, its head and neck in the duodenal curve, its body extending transversely, and its tail touching the spleen (Fig. 11-1).

The pancreas is both an ***exocrine gland*** (secreting into ducts) and a ductless secreting ***endocrine gland***. The exocrine cells secrete ***pancreatic juice***, which contains enzymes necessary for digestion and is collected within the pancreas and transferred into the duodenum. Groups of endocrine cells, the ***islands*** or ***islets of Langerhans***, secrete two major hormones, ***insulin*** and ***glucagon***, which have opposing roles in carbohydrate metabolism (Chapter 13).

THE LIVER

The largest gland in the body, the ***liver*** (***hepat*** refers to liver), classified as an exocrine gland, weighs about 3 to 4 pounds (1.4 kg) and is located in the upper right abdomen under the diaphragm (Fig. 11-1). It is very soft and pliable and is a reddish-brown color because it contains numerous blood vessels. The liver has four major functions:

1. Secretes bile for use in the digestive process.
2. Essential to the metabolism of proteins, fats, and carbohydrates.

3. Filters and destroys foreign matter and neutralizes toxins.

4. Stores iron, glycogen, and vitamins A, B$_{12}$, and D.

The Biliary System

The **bile ducts** within the liver join together, forming the larger **right** and **left hepatic ducts**, emerging from the liver, and uniting to form a single **hepatic duct**. This hepatic duct joins the **cystic duct** (emerging from the gallbladder), forming the **common bile duct**, which opens into the duodenum 3 to 4 inches (8 to 10 cm) below the pyloric opening of the stomach.

The Gallbladder

The **gallbladder** (**cholecyst** means gallbladder), a pear-shaped sac about 3 to 4 inches (8 to 10 cm) in length, the walls of which are composed of a serous, a muscular, and a mucous coat, is located on the inferior surface of the liver (Fig. 11-1).

The main function of the gallbladder is to store the concentrated bile deposited by the hepatic and cystic ducts and then to contract and expel the bile into the duodenum during digestion (**chol-** and **chole-** mean bile).

Review C

Complete the following:

1. The three divisions of the small intestine are the _____, _____, and

   _____.

2. The large intestine is divided into the _____, _____, and _____.

3. The pancreas is divided into _____, _____, _____, and

   _____.

4. The hepatic and cystic ducts join to form the _____.

5. The walls of the gallbladder have a _____, _____, and _____ coat.

Answers to Review Questions: The Gastrointestinal System

Review A
1. digestive or alimentary tract
2. peristalsis
3. hard and soft palates
4. tongue
5. crown, neck, root

Review B
1. pharynx
2. esophageal
3. three

4. fundus, body, pylorus
5. greater, lesser

Review C
1. duodenum, jejunum, ileum
2. cecum, colon, rectum
3. head, neck, body, tail
4. common bile duct
5. serous, muscular, mucous

CHAPTER 11 EXERCISES

THE GASTROINTESTINAL SYSTEM: THE FOOD PROCESSOR

Exercise 1: Complete the following:

1. The chief organs of the alimentary tract are _____, _____, _____, _____, and _____.

2. The accessory organs of the digestive tract are _____, _____, _____, _____, and _____.

3. The organs in the digestive tract through which food passes as it travels from the mouth to the anus are, in order, _____, _____, _____, _____, _____, and _____.

4. Five of the structures in the oral cavity are _____, _____, _____, _____, and _____.

5. The two main functions of the tongue in the digestive system are _____ and _____.

6. The four types of teeth are _____, _____, _____, and _____.

7. The thin, lubricating, serous fluid secreted by the salivary glands is called _____.

8. The two chief functions of the secretions of the salivary glands are _____ and _____.

9. The dual functions of the pharynx are _____ and _____.

10. The names of the curvatures of the stomach are _____ and _____.

11. The names, in order, of the divisions of the small intestine are _____, _____, and _____.

12. The process of digestion is completed in the _____.

13. The _____ is the serous membrane that lines the abdominal cavity.

14. Two hormones secreted by the islands of Langerhans are _____, and _____.

15. Four important functions of the liver are _____.

16. The main function of the gallbladder is to _____.

17. Most of the water absorption of the body take place in the _____.

18. The voluntary stage of swallowing is the _____ stage.

19. The peritoneal fold that attaches the intestine to the posterior abdominal wall is called the _____.

20. The double fold of peritoneum attached to the stomach, connecting it with the abdominal viscera, is called the _____.

Exercise 2: Using the list of terms below, identify the parts in Fig. 11-6 by writing the names in the corresponding blanks.

Parotid gland
Esophagus
Gallbladder
Liver
Hepatic flexure
Rectum
Descending colon
Transverse colon
Sublingual gland

Appendix
Submaxillary (or submandibular) gland
Pancreas
Pharynx
Duodenum
Ileum
Anus

Greater curvature of stomach
Cecum
Lesser curvature of stomach
Splenic flexure
Ascending colon
Pylorus
Jejunum
Sigmoid

1. _____

2. _____

3. _____

4. _____

5. _____

6. _____

7. _____

8. _____

9. _____

10. _____

11. _____

12. _____

13. _____

14. _____

15. _____

16. _____

17. _____

18. _____

19. _____

20. _____

21. _____

22. _____

23. _____

24. _____

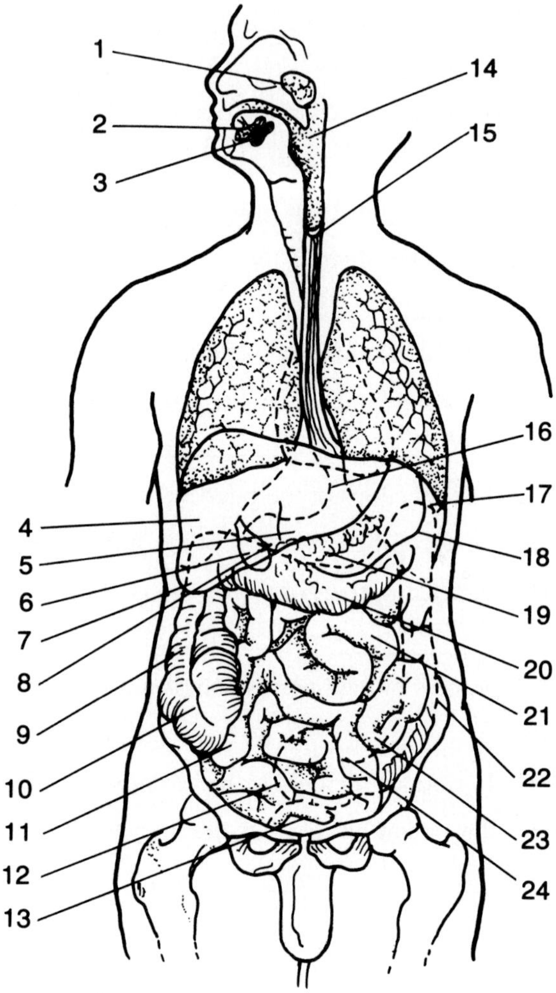

Figure 11-6.   Digestive tract.

Exercise 3: Matching:

____ **1.** rigid bony structure in the roof of the mouth

____ **2.** partition between the mouth and nasopharynx

____ **3.** constricted opening between arches and oropharynx

____ **4.** musculomembranous tube from pharynx to stomach

____ **5.** lower left margin of the surface of the stomach

____ **6.** upper right margin of the surface of the stomach

____ **7.** very hard substance that covers the exposed part of the tooth

____ **8.** chief substance of the tooth surrounding pulp

____ **9.** semifluid material produced by gastric digestion of food

____ **10.** threadlike projections covering the mucosa of the small intestine

____ **11.** any one of the four front teeth of either jaw

____ **12.** broad teeth used in grinding food

____ **13.** archlike structure formed by the soft palate at the posterior border of the mouth

____ **14.** pendulum of the soft palate

____ **15.** ringlike muscles that contract to close an opening

A. soft palate

B. hard palate

C. dentin

D. incisor

E. fauces

F. esophagus

G. sphincter

H. molars

I. palatine arch

J. chyme

K. lesser curvature

L. enamel

M. greater curvature

N. uvula

O. villi

Exercise 4: Multiple choice:

1. The peritoneal fold that attaches the intestine to the posterior abdominal wall is the:
   a. lesser curvature
   b. mesentery
   c. omentum
2. The part of the pancreas touching the spleen is the:
   a. neck
   b. tail
   c. head
3. The second part of the pharynx is called:
   a. nasopharynx
   b. fauces
   c. oropharynx
4. The dilated intestinal pouch that joins the colon below the juncture of the ileum and colon is the:
   a. appendix
   b. cecum
   c. anal canal
5. Vermiform is a name given to the:
   a. cecum
   b. appendix
   c. rectum
6. The number of coats in the stomach wall is:
   a. three
   b. four
   c. five
7. Another name for the gallbladder is:
   a. choledochus
   b. ductus choledochus
   c. cholecyst
8. The fluid secreted by the liver and poured into the intestines is called:
   a. chyle
   b. bile
   c. chyme
9. The involuntary, wavelike movement of the gastrointestinal tract is called:
   a. alimentary
   b. peristalsis
   c. gastritis
10. The bonelike connective tissue covering the root and neck of a tooth is called:
    a. periodontium
    b. enamel
    c. cementum

Exercise 5: Give the meaning of the components in the following words and then define the word as a whole. Suffixes meaning *pertaining to* or *state or condition* shown following a slash mark (/), are not to be defined separately. Before reaching for your medical dictionary, check the glossary at the end of the chapter.

1. Cholangitis:

chol _____

ang _____

itis _____

_____

2. Diverticulitis:

diverticul _____

itis _____

_____

3. Enterogastritis:

entero _____

gastr _____

itis _____

_____

4. Gastoenterocolitis:

gastr _____

entero _____

col _____

itis _____

_____

5. Hepatitis:

hepat _____

itis _____

_____

6. Ileitis:

ile _____

itis _____

_____

7. Ileocolitis:

ileo _____

col _____

itis _____

_____

8. Linguopapillitis:

linguo _____

papill _____

itis _____

_____

9. Proctitis:

proct _____

itis _____

_____

10. Gastroduodenitis:

gastro _____

duoden _____

itis _____

_____

11. Glossitis:

gloss _____

itis _____

_____

12. Gingivitis:

gingiv _____

itis _____

_____

Chapter 11 Crossword Puzzle

Across

3. a function of the GI system

4. tooth part above the gum line

5. chisel-shaped teeth

8. a function of the GI system

9. a part of the small intestine

11. connects intestines to abdominal wall

12. largest gland in body

16. small elevations on tongue

19. lower small end of stomach

21. peritoneum of abdominal cavity

22. hardest body substance

23. membrane attached to stomach

Down

1. involuntary wave-like movement

2. combining form meaning intestines

4. root meaning gallbladder

6. endocrine/exocrine gland

7. a function of the GI system

10. upper jaw bone

13. lower jaw bone

14. tooth socket

15. entrance sphincter of stomach

17. part of small intestine

18. third molar teeth

20. conical process between palatine arches

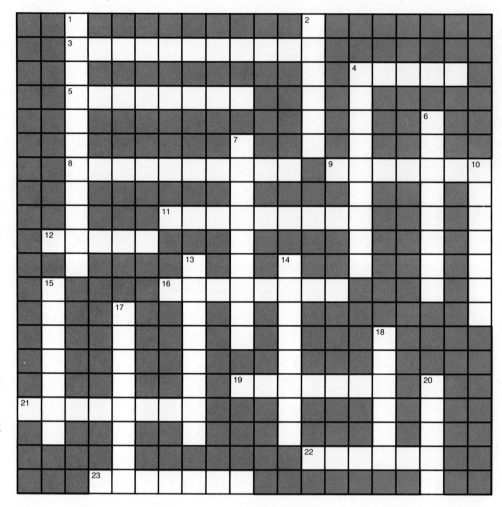

Chapter 11 Hidden Words Puzzle

```
H  C  N  T  O  F  X  Q  U  G  W  T  Q  P  I  D  T  B
C  X  O  I  I  A  S  O  O  I  T  O  Y  B  R  X  X  E
A  I  I  Y  L  O  L  F  F  N  D  H  Q  Q  H  B  U  L
Y  L  W  T  N  L  T  I  H  G  D  E  Y  D  V  O  L  O
H  J  V  X  S  F  N  B  A  I  P  P  U  W  P  X  T  M
M  K  C  E  C  U  M  N  C  V  K  A  P  D  C  N  H  A
N  P  V  N  O  X  Y  E  P  A  R  T  I  T  I  O  N  Y
G  A  L  L  B  L  A  D  D  E  R  I  T  G  F  K  X  T
C  P  L  F  V  Q  U  S  Y  W  R  C  P  J  X  M  N  T
M  I  U  I  U  I  S  S  U  B  L  I  N  G  U  A  L  W
I  L  E  H  M  N  S  P  H  I  N  C  T  E  R  G  J  Z
F  L  R  Q  M  E  D  C  A  R  P  A  R  O  T  I  D  K
F  A  C  O  L  O  N  U  E  L  C  T  F  D  N  N  Z  Z
R  E  C  T  U  M  G  T  S  R  A  S  I  U  P  E  S  P
M  T  Y  F  B  H  W  B  A  W  A  T  L  U  J  V  U  Z
H  X  J  C  G  R  O  J  L  R  V  L  E  N  A  I  Q  M
R  K  R  Z  H  Q  X  M  I  K  Y  W  U  S  V  G  W  U
T  M  R  B  I  E  E  O  V  U  J  O  M  B  L  L  K  K
G  Q  E  G  L  C  N  C  A  K  O  Z  T  E  Y  D  S  M
R  D  O  U  N  I  U  Z  R  V  M  T  V  R  C  N  D  L
L  D  P  M  F  J  K  Q  Y  Z  I  X  H  V  P  U  Q  D
X  N  M  P  U  G  Y  U  N  M  J  W  M  P  D  X  O  B
W  K  D  K  T  D  W  M  T  O  E  O  W  U  E  V  G  I
Z  L  H  V  T  L  Q  A  U  U  E  S  U  P  H  M  X  H
```

Can you find the 20 words hidden in this puzzle?

GALLBLADDER	ALIMENTARY	PERITONEUM	SUBLINGUAL
PARTITION	SPHINCTER	ALVEOLUS	GINGIVAE
PAPILLAE	SALIVARY	VISCERAL	ENZYMES
HEPATIC	PAROTID	FUNDUS	PALATE
RECTUM	CECUM	COLON	ILEUM

CHAPTER 11 ANSWERS

Exercise 1
1. mouth, pharynx, esophagus, stomach, intestines
2. teeth, salivary glands, liver, gallbladder, pancreas
3. mouth, pharynx, esophagus, stomach, small intestine, large intestine
4. gums, teeth, palatine arches, palates (soft and hard), salivary glands, tongue, uvula, and fauces
5. keeps food between teeth during chewing, aids in swallowing
6. incisors, canines, premolars, molars
7. saliva
8. dissolve or lubricate food to facilitate swallowing, initiate digestion of some carbohydrates
9. airway, passageway for food
10. lesser, greater
11. duodenum, jejunum, ileum
12. small intestine
13. peritoneum
14. insulin, glucagon
15. secretion of bile for digestion; fat, protein, and carbohydrate metabolism; filters and destroys foreign matter and neutralizes toxins; stores iron, glycogen and vitamins A, B_{12}, and D
16. store the concentrated bile
17. large intestine
18. first
19. mesentery
20. omentum

Exercise 2

1. parotid gland
2. submaxillary (or submandibular) gland
3. sublingual gland
4. liver
5. pylorus
6. gallbladder
7. hepatic flexure
8. duodenum
9. ascending colon
10. cecum
11. appendix
12. rectum
13. anus
14. pharynx
15. esophagus
16. lesser curvature of stomach
17. splenic flexure
18. greater curvature of stomach
19. pancreas
20. transverse colon
21. jejunum
22. descending colon
23. ileum
24. sigmoid

Exercise 3

1. B	**9.** J
2. A	**10.** O
3. E	**11.** D
4. F	**12.** H
5. M	**13.** I
6. K	**14.** N
7. L	**15.** G
8. C	

Exercise 4

1. mesentery
2. tail
3. oropharynx
4. cecum
5. appendix
6. four
7. cholecyst
8. bile
9. peristalsis
10. cementum

Exercise 5

1. cholangitis: bile; vessels; inflammation—inflammation of bile duct
2. enterogastritis: intestine; stomach; inflammation—inflammation of intestines and stomach
3. diverticulitis: diverticulum (or pouch); inflammation—inflammation of a diverticulum
4. gastroenterocolitis: stomach; small intestine; colon; inflammation—inflammation of stomach, small intestine, and colon
5. hepatitis: liver; inflammation—inflammation of the liver
6. ileitis: ileum; inflammation—inflammation of ileum
7. ileocolitis: ileum; colon; inflammation—inflammation of ileum and colon
8. linguopapillitis: tongue; papillae; inflammation—inflammation around papillae of the tongue
9. proctitis: rectum; inflammation—inflammation of rectum
10. gastroduodenitis: stomach; duodenum; inflammation—inflammation of stomach and duodenum
11. glossitis: tongue; inflammation—inflammation of tongue
12. gingivitis: gums; inflammation—inflammation of gums

Answers: Chapter 11 Crossword Puzzle

		1 P										2 E							
		3 E	L	I	M	I	N	A	T	I	O	N							
		R										T		4 C	R	O	W	N	
		5 I	N	C	I	S	O	R	S			E		H					
		S										R		O			6 P		
		T							7 D			O		L			A		
		8 A	B	S	O	R	P	T	I	O	N		9 J	E	J	U	N	U	10 M
		L							G					C			C		A
		S				11 M	E	S	E	N	T	E	R	Y			R		X
	12 L	I	V	E	R				S					S			E		I
		S					13 M		T		14 A			T			A		L
	15 C					16 P	A	P	I	L	L	A	E				S		L
	A			17 D			N		O		V								A
	R			U			D		N		E				18 W				
	D			O			I				O				I				
	I			D			B		19 P	Y	L	O	R	U	S		20 U		
21 P	A	R	I	E	T	A	L				U				D		V		
	C			N			E				S				O		U		
				U								22 E	N	A	M	E	L		
			23 O	M	E	N	T	U	M								A		

Answers: Chapter 11 Hidden Words Puzzle

```
.   .   .   .   .   .   .   .   .   G   .   .   .   .   .   .   .
.   .   .   .   .   .   .   .   .   I   .   .   .   .   .   .   .
A   .   .   .   .   .   .   .   .   N   .   H   .   .   .   .   .
.   L   .   .   .   .   .   .   .   G   .   E   .   .   .   .   .
.   .   V   .   .   .   .   .   .   I   .   P   .   .   .   .   .
.   .   C   E   C   U   M   .   .   V   .   A   .   .   .   .   .
.   P   .   .   O   .   .   .   P   A   R   T   I   T   I   O   N   .
G   A   L   L   B   L   A   D   D   E   R   R   I   .   .   .   .   .   .
.   P   L   F   V   .   U   .   .   .   R   C   .   .   .   .   .   .
.   I   .   I   U   I   .   S   U   B   L   I   N   G   U   A   L   .
.   L   .   .   M   N   S   P   H   I   N   C   T   E   R   .   .
.   L   .   .   .   E   D   C   A   .   P   A   R   O   T   I   D   .
.   A   C   O   L   O   N   U   E   L   A   .   .   N   .   .
R   E   C   T   U   M   .   T   S   R   A   .   I   .   .   E   .   U
.   .   .   .   .   .   .   .   A   .   A   T   L   .   .   .   .   M
.   .   .   .   .   .   .   .   L   R   .   L   E   .   .   .
.   .   .   .   .   .   .   .   I   .   Y   .   U   .
.   .   .   .   E   .   .   V   .   .   M   .
.   .   .   .   .   N   .   A   .   .
.   .   .   .   .   .   Z   R   .   .
.   .   .   .   .   .   .   Y   .   .
.   .   .   .   .   .   .   .   M   .
.   .   .   .   .   .   .   .   E   .
.   .   .   .   .   .   .   .   .   S
```

Words:

> GALLBLADDER   \ ALIMENTARY   \ PERITONEUM   > SUBLINGUAL
> PARTITION   > SPHINCTER   \ ALVEOLUS   ∨ GINGIVAE
∨ PAPILLAE   ∨ SALIVARY   \ VISCERAL   \ ENZYMES
∨ HEPATIC   > PAROTID   \ FUNDUS   \ PALATE
> RECTUM   > CECUM   > COLON   ∨ ILEUM

CHAPTER 11 GLOSSARY

Gastrointestinal System Related Anatomic Terms

alimentary or **digestive tract:** passage from mouth to anus.

alveolus (al-ve′o-lus): tooth socket in the maxilla and mandible (also refers to air sac of lung).

ampulla (am-pul′lah): sac-shaped dilation of a canal or tube.

anal canal: most distal portion of the alimentary tract.

antrum (an′trum): any partially closed cavity, and particularly the pyloric end of the stomach that is partly shut off, during digestion, by the sphincter.

anus (a′nus): distal opening of the alimentary canal.

appendix: any appendage, especially the vermiform appendix attached to the cecum.

bicuspid (bi-kus′pid): premolar tooth.

bile: secretion of the liver that aids in digestion.

biliary: pertaining to bile.

body of pancreas: part of pancreas extending from its neck to its tail.

buccal surface of tooth: surface of the tooth next to the cheek.

cecum (se′kum): blind pouch that joins the colon just below the juncture of the ileum and colon and has vermiform appendix attached.

celiac (se′le-ak): pertaining to the abdomen.

cholecyst (ko′le-sist): gallbladder.

choledochus (ko-led′o-kus): common bile duct.

chyle (kil): milky fluid conveyed by lymphatic vessels from the intestine, after digestion, into the circulation.

chyme (kim): semifluid contents of stomach after digestion.

colon: part of large intestine extending from cecum to rectum.

common bile duct: duct formed by the junction of the cystic and hepatic ducts.

cuspid (kus′pid): canine tooth.

cystic duct: duct extending from neck of gallbladder to join the hepatic duct to form the common bile duct.

dentin: type of connective tissue surrounding the tooth pulp that is covered by enamel on the exposed tooth and by cementum on the part implanted in the jaw.

duodenal glands: glands in the submucous layer of the duodenum (also called ***Brunner's glands***).

duodenum (du″o-de′num): first portion of small intestine, extending from the pylorus of the stomach to the jejunum.

enamel: hard, white substance (hardest in body) covering the dentin of the exposed part of the tooth.

epigastrium (ep″i-gas′tre-um): upper, middle portion of abdomen.

esophagus (e-sof′ah-gus): musculomembranous canal that extends from the pharynx to the stomach.

fauces (faw′sez): passage from the throat to the oropharynx.

flexure (flek′sher): bend, fold, or curved part of a structure.

gallbladder: pear-shaped organ on the undersurface of the liver, for the storage of bile.

gastric glands: glands of the stomach that secrete digestive chemicals.

gingivae (jin′ji-vie): gums of the mouth.

glossopalatine arch: anterior fold of mucous membrane on either side of the oral pharynx, connected with the soft palate and enclosing the glossopalatine muscle (also called ***palatine arch*** or ***pharyngopalatine arch***).

hypogastrium (hi″po-gas′tre-um): lowest, middle abdominal region.

ileocecal valve: mucous membrane folds between ileum and cecum, to prevent reflux from colon into ileum (also called ***ileocolic valve***).

ileum: distal portion of the small intestine, extending from the jejunum to the cecum.

incisor (in-si′zer): any one of the four front teeth of either jaw.

intestinal glands: tiny, tubular depressions in the intestinal mucous membrane (also called ***Lieberkuhn's glands***).

islands of Langerhans (lahng′er-hanz): irregular, microscopic formations of cells in the pancreas, secreting insulin and glucagon.

jejunum (je-joo′num): portion of the small intestine that extends from the duodenum to the ileum.

labia (la′be-ah): lips.

lingua (ling′gwah): tongue.

liver: large, dome-shaped gland in the upper part of the abdomen under the diaphragm on the right side.

mesentery (mes′en-ter″e): peritoneal fold that attaches the intestine to the posterior abdominal wall.

omentum: fold of peritoneum that connects the stomach with other visceral organs.

oropharynx: section of pharynx that lies between the soft palate and the epiglottis.

palate: roof of the mouth separating the oral cavity from the nasal cavity.

pancreas: large, elongated, lobed gland, located behind the stomach, divided into four parts: head, neck, body, and tail.

parotid salivary gland: large salivary gland located near the ear.

peptic glands: glands of the mucous membrane of the stomach, secreting acid and pepsin.

peristalsis (per″i-stal′sis): wavelike movement by which the alimentary tract propels its contents.

peritoneum (per″i-to′ne-um): serous membrane lining the abdominal cavity, with a part of it covering viscera and holding them in place.

pharynx: musculomembranous opening into the nasal cavities, mouth, larynx, and esophagus.

pylorus: distal opening of stomach through which stomach contents enter the duodenum.

rectosigmoid: lower portion of sigmoid and upper portion of rectum.

rugae (roo′guy): wrinkles, or folds, appearing on the surface of the mucous membrane of the stomach when the muscular coat contracts.

saliva (sah-li′vah): clear secretion of the salivary glands, containing the digestive enzyme ***ptyalin amylase***.

salivary glands: oral cavity glands that secrete saliva.

secretin: hormone produced by glands of the duodenum that stimulates secretion of pancreatic juice.

sigmoid: S-shaped flexure of colon, extending from the end of the descending colon to the upper part of the rectum.

sphincter (sfingk′ter): ringlike muscle that closes a natural opening.

stomach: ovoid, musculomembranous digestive pouch below the esophagus.

sublingual salivary glands: smallest of the salivary glands, located beneath the tongue on either side.

submandibular and **submaxillary salivary glands:** salivary glands below the angle of the lower jaw on either side.

tongue: freely moving, muscular organ of taste, located in floor of the mouth, that aids in mastication, swallowing, and articulation of sound.

uvula: soft, conical, pendulumlike process hanging between the palatine arches.

villi: threadlike projections covering the mucosa of the small intestine that aid in the absorption of digested matter.

Pathologic Conditions

Inflammations, Infections, and Toxic Conditions

ancylostomiasis (an-si-lo-sto-mi′ah-sis): infection with hookworm, a member of the genus *Ancylostoma*

anusitis: inflammation of the anus.

aphthous stomatitis (af′thus): ulcer of the mucous membranes of the mouth, commonly called ***canker sore***.

appendicitis: inflammation of the appendix.

ascariasis (as″kah-ri′ah-sis): infection with parasitic intestinal roundworms, of the genus *Ascaris*.

cheilitis (ki-li′tis): inflammation of the lip.

cholangiolitis (ko-lan″je-o-li′tis): inflammation of the bile duct tubules.

cholangitis (ko″lan-ji′tis): bile duct inflammation.

cholecystitis (ko″le-sis-ti′tis): inflammation of the gallbladder.

colitis: inflammation of the colon; may be episodic, as in *irritable bowel syndrome*, which includes *spastic colon* and *mucous colitis*, or chronic, as in *Crohn's disease* and *ulcerative colitis*.

Crohn's disease: a chronic inflammatory disease affecting the ileum, cecum and colon (also called ***regional enteritis***).

cysticercosis (sis″ti-ser-ko′sis): infection with tapeworm larvae, of the genus *Cysticercus*.

distomiasis (dis″to-mi′ah-sis): infection with a trematode worm of the genus *Fasciola*.

diverticulitis (di″ver-tik-u-li′tis): inflammation of a pocket (*diverticulum*) in the intestine.

duodenitis: inflammation of the duodenum.

dysentery (dis′en-ter″ee): any of a number of disorders that involve inflammation of the intestines, particularly the colon.

enteritis (en″ter-i′tis): inflammation of the intestines, particularly the small intestine.

enterobiasis (en″ter-o-bi′ah-sis): roundworm infection with nematodes of the genus *Enterobius vermicularis*, commonly called pinworm, seatworm, or threadworm (also called ***oxyuriasis***).

enterocolitis (en″ter-o-ko-li′tis): inflammation of the colon and small intestine.

enterogastritis (en″ter-o-gas-tri′tis): inflammation of the intestines and stomach (also called ***gastroenteritis***).

enterohepatitis (en″ter-o-hep-ah-ti′tis): inflammation of the intestines and liver.

esophagitis (e-sof″ah-ji′tis): inflammation of the esophagus.

food poisoning: sudden illness caused by eating food contaminated with any one of a large group of bacterial or other toxic substances, including bacterial food poisoning and shellfish poisoning.

gastritis: inflammation of the stomach.

gastroduodenitis: inflammation of the stomach and duodenum.

gastroenterocolitis (gas″tro-en″ter-o-ko-li′tis): inflammation of the stomach, small intestine, and colon.

gastrohepatitis (gas″tro-hep-ah-ti′tis): inflammation of the stomach and liver.

gastroileitis (gas″tro-il-e-i′tis): inflammation of the stomach and ileum.

Giardiasis (je″ar-di′ah-sis): a parasitic infection of the intestinal tract, caused by the protozoa *Giardia lamblia*.

gingivitis (jin″ji-vi′tis): inflammation of the gums.

glossitis (glos-si′tis): inflammation of the tongue.

hemorrhagic colitis: gastrointestinal infection caused by ingestion of undercooked meat contaminated by a rare form of *E. coli* bacteria.

hepatitis (hep″ah-ti′tis): inflammation of the liver due to toxic or viral causes, with symptoms of anorexia, nausea, jaundice, and enlargement and tenderness of the liver.

herpes simplex (her′pez): cold sore or fever blister of the mouth or nares caused by herpes virus.

ileitis (il″e-i′tis): inflammation of the ileum.

ileocolitis (il″e-o-ko-li′tis): inflammation of ileum and colon.

jejunitis (je″joo-ni′tis): inflammation of the jejunum.

jejunoileitis (je-joo″no-il″e-i′tis): inflammation of the jejunum and ileum.

linguopapillitis (ling″gwo-pap″i-li′tis): inflammation of the papillae of the tongue.

pancreatitis (pan″kre-ah-ti′tis): inflammation of the pancreas.

parotitis (par″o-ti′tis): inflammation of the parotid salivary gland (*mumps* is epidemic or infectious parotitis).

peptic ulcer disease: inflammation of the stomach and/or duodenum, caused by the bacteria *Helicobacter pylori*, which destroys cells of the mucus membrane lining, resulting in ulceration by acid and/or enzymes.

perihepatitis: inflammation of the serous covering of the liver.

periodontal disease: inflammation affecting the tissue around a tooth, caused by bacteria, the most common being *Porphyromonas gingivalis*, resulting in tooth loss.

peritonitis (per′i-to-ni′tis): inflammation of the peritoneum.

proctitis: inflammation of the rectum.

pulpitis: inflammation of the dental pulp.

Salmonellosis: acute gastroenteritis due to ingestion of food and or water contaminated with *Salmonella* bacteria, with symptoms of sudden onset of abdominal pain, nausea, vomiting, and fever (also called *Salmonella enteriditis*).

Shigellosis: infection caused by *Shigella* bacteria, with cramping, abdominal pain, watery diarrhea, high fever, and general muscle pain, transmitted by person-to-person contact and ingestion of contaminated food and water.

sialadenitis (si″al-ad″e-ni′tis): salivary gland inflammation.

strongyloidiasis (stron″ji-loi-di′ah-sis): infection with an intestinal roundworm of the genus *Strongyloides*.

trichuriasis (trik″u-ri′ah-sis): infection with an intestinal parasite of the genus *Trichuris*.

ulcerative colitis: chronic inflammatory disease, with watery diarrhea containing blood, mucus and pus, resulting in ulceration of the colon and rectum.

Vincent's stomatitis: ulcerative, necrotizing inflammation of the gums or oral mucosa (also called *trench mouth*)

Hereditary, Congenital, and Developmental Disorders

aglossia: absence of tongue.

annular pancreas: developmental defect in which the pancreas lies in the bend of the duodenum, forming a ring encircling the duodenum, sometimes causing an intestinal obstruction.

ankyloglossia (ang″ko-lo-glos′e-ah): tongue-tie.

atresia (ah-tre′ze-ah): occlusion or absence of a normal body opening or tubular formation; may occur in the anus, the bile ducts, or the esophagus.

cleft palate: incomplete closure in the midline of the palate.

congenital hypertrophic pyloric stenosis: abnormal enlargement of the pyloric sphincter muscle of the stomach, creating an obstruction to the passage of gastric contents to the duodenum.

congenital megacolon: developmental abnormality with loss of muscle function and hypertrophic dilation of the colon (also called *Hirschsprung's disease*).

glycogenosis: group of hereditary disorders of glycogen metabolism.

harelip: cleft in the upper lip.

Hutchinson's teeth: tooth deformity with narrow-edged, grooved permanent incisors, caused by congenital syphilis.

hyperbilirubinemia (hi″ber-bil″i-roo″bi-ne′me-ah): benign, familial disorders marked by excessive bilirubin in the blood (also called *Gilbert's disease*).

macrocheilia: excessively large lips.

macroglossia: excessively large tongue (also called *megaloglossia*).

macrostomia: abnormally wide mouth.

Meckel's diverticulum: residual pouch of the embryonic omphalomesenteric duct.

megalogastria (meg″ah-lo-gas′tre-ah): abnormally large stomach.

microgastria: unusually small stomach.

microstomia: unusually small mouth.

neonatal necrotizing enterocolitis (NEC): condition of a newborn in which the intestinal mucosa or submucosa becomes necrotic.

oligodontia: developmental anomaly in which there are fewer than the usual number of teeth.

transposition of abdominal viscera: reversal of normal position of the abdominal organs.

tyrosinemia: rare, hereditary disorder of the liver in which the metabolism of amino acids is disrupted, resulting in liver failure.

Other Abnormalities

achalasia (ak'ah-la'ze-ah): failure to relax, especially in relation to sphincter muscles.

achlorhydria (ak"klor-hi'dre-ah): absence of hydrochloric acid in gastric secretions.

acholia (ah-ko'le-ah): absence of bile secretion.

achylia (ah"ki-le'ah): absence of digestive juices in the stomach.

aerophagia (a"er-o-fa'je-ah): swallowing of air, with belching (*eructation*).

anorexia: lack of appetite.

ascites (ah-si'tez): accumulation of fluid in the abdominal cavity.

bulimia: gorging food, followed by self-induced vomiting (also called ***hyperorexia***).

cachexia (kah-kek'se-ah): generalized poor nutrition.

calculus: formation of a stone (plural—***calculi***).

cholelithiasis (ko"le-li-thi'ah-sis): gallstones.

cholesteroleresis (ko-les"ter-ol-er'e-sis): increase in elimination of cholesterol in bile.

cholesterosis (ko-les"ter-o'sis): excessive deposits of cholesterol in tissues (also called ***cholesterolosis***).

chylous ascites (ki'lus ah-si'tez): accumulation of chyle in the peritoneal cavity due to thoracic duct obstruction.

cirrhosis (sir-ro'sis): liver disease with progressive destruction of liver cells.

colic: acute, paroxysmal, abdominal pain.

constipation: sluggish bowel with difficult or incomplete evacuation.

crepitus (krep'i-tus): flatulent discharge from bowels.

dental caries: destruction of the enamel, dentin, or cementum of a tooth, resulting in tooth decay and cavities.

diabetes insipidus; diabetes mellitus: see Chapter 13 glossary.

diarrhea: frequent discharge of abnormally liquid feces.

dyspepsia: indigestion, caused by other disorder.

diverticulosis (di"ver-tik"u-lo'sis): presence of pouches within the intestines, protruding through the intestinal wall.

emesis: vomiting.

enterocystocele (en"ter-o-sis'to-sel): hernia involving both the bladder and intestinal walls.

enterolith (en'ter-o-lith): stone in the intestines.

enteroptosis (en"ter-op-to'sis): dislocation of the intestines.

eructation: belching.

fecalith (fe'kah-lith): stonelike fecal mass.

fistula: abnormal opening between two organs, or between a hollow organ and the body surface, commonly found in gastrointestinal system.

gastralgia: pain in the stomach.

gastroesophageal reflux disorder (GERD): regurgitation of stomach contents into the esophagus.

gastrolith: stone in the stomach.

gastroptosis (gas"tro-to'sis): downward dislocation of the stomach.

halitosis: bad breath.

hemochromatosis (he"mo-kro"mah-to'sis): metabolic disorder with abnormal accumulation of iron in the body tissues, cirrhosis of the liver, and diabetes mellitus.

hemoperitoneum (he"mo-per"i-to-ne'um): escape of blood into the peritoneal cavity.

hepatomalacia (hep"ah-to-mah-la'she-ah): softening of the liver.

hepatomegaly: enlarged liver.

hepatosplenomegaly: enlarged liver and spleen.

hernia: protrusion of an organ or part through its normal containing structures (also called ***rupture***).

hiatal hernia (hi-a'tal): protrusion of part of the stomach through the esophageal opening of the diaphragm.

hydrops (hi'drops): abnormal accumulation of fluid in tissues or a body cavity (formerly called *dropsy*).

hypercementosis (hi"per-se"men-to'sis): excessive development of cementum on the roots of the teeth.

hyperchlorhydria (hi"per-klor-hi'dre-ah): excessive hydrochloric acid in the gastric secretion.

hypercholesterolemia (hi"per-ko-les'ter-e'me-ah): abnormal increase of cholesterol in the blood.

hypercholia: excessive bile secretion.

hyperglycemia (hi"per-gli-se'me-ah): excessive concentration of glucose in the blood.

hyperinsulinism (hi"per-in'su-lin'izm): excessive pancreatic secretion of insulin (also called ***insulin shock***).

hypersplenism (hi"per-splen'izm): abnormally increased hemolytic function of the spleen.

hypervitaminosis: condition caused by excessive ingestion of vitamins, especially A and B.

hypochlorhydria: deficiency of hydrochloric acid in the stomach.

hypocholesteremia (hi"po-ko-les'ter-e'me-ah): abnormal decrease of cholesterol in the blood.

hypochylia: deficiency of chyle.

hypoglycemia (hi"po-gli-se'me-ah): low blood glucose level.

hypovitaminosis: disease caused by deficiency of one or more of the essential vitamins.

ileus (il'e-us): mechanical obstruction of the intestines, with colic, vomiting, fever, and dehydration.

incontinence of feces: inability to restrain fecal evacuation.

intussusception (in″tus-sus-sep′shun): prolapse of a portion of the intestine into the lumen of an immediately adjacent portion.

jaundice (jawn′dis): yellowish tinge of skin, sclerae, and other tissues, with deposits of bile pigments in the excretions.

leukoplakia (lu″ko-pla′ke-ah): development of white plaques (patches) on the mucous membranes.

malocclusion: failure of proper closure of jaws because of malposition of teeth.

marasmus (mah-raz′mus): a type of protein and calorie malnutrition chiefly occurring in infants and children.

mucocele (mu′ko-sel): cyst or polyp containing mucus.

nausea: sick sensation, often resulting in vomiting.

obstipation: extreme constipation due to intestinal obstruction.

oligopepsia: lack of digestive tone.

oligotrophy: insufficient nutrition.

pellagra (pel-lag′rah): niacin-deficiency condition characterized by inflamed mucous membranes, dermatitis, and diarrhea.

phytobezoar (fi″to-be′zor): gastric mass composed of vegetable matter.

polydipsia: extreme thirst.

polyphagia: ravenous eating.

proctalgia: pain in or near rectum and anus.

proctocele: hernia of the rectum (also called ***rectocele***).

proctoptosis (prok″top-to′sis): rectal prolapse.

pruritus ani: chronic, intense itching of the anal region.

pylorospasm: spasm of the pylorus of the stomach.

rickets: vitamin D deficiency disorder, usually in infants and children, chiefly affecting calcification of bones, with resulting bending and deformation of the bones.

scurvy: disease due to vitamin C (*ascorbic acid*) deficiency, resulting in anemia, mucocutaneous bleeding, and hardening of the leg muscle.

splanchnoptosis (splank″no-to′sis): prolapse of the viscera (also called ***visceroptosis***).

sprue (sproo): chronic condition of malabsorption characterized by intolerance to certain foods, resulting in anorexia, anemia, diarrhea, and weight loss.

stenosis: narrowing of an opening or passage.

tenesmus (te-nez′mus): painful, ineffective straining at stool.

ulcer: lesion on the surface of a mucous membrane or skin, caused by disintegration of inflamed necrotic tissue.

volvulus: intestinal obstruction caused by twisting of the bowel.

vomiting: forcible expulsion of gastric contents through the mouth.

*Oncology**

Some tumors of the gastrointestinal tract are listed below. Various types of tumors occur in other parts of the body, as well as in the gastrointestinal tract. Particular to the large intestine is a method of describing the stages of colorectal tumors called Dukes' classification (developed by and named for a British cancer specialist): Dukes'-A tumor is superficial, confined to mucosa and submucosa, with a high survival rate; Dukes'-B tumor has invaded the fat or muscle tissue, but does not involve the lymphatic system, and has a survival rate of about 55 percent; Dukes'-C tumors involve greater penetration of the muscles, and involve the lymph nodes; Dukes'-D tumors have metastasized to other organ tissues. C and D have only a slight chance of survival.

ameloblastoma (ah-mel″o-blas-to′mah): normally benign tumor of the jaw.

cementoma (se″men-to′mah): mass composed of cementum lying at the apex of a tooth, probably the result of trauma.

cholangiohepatoma (ko-lan″je-o-hep″ah-to′mah): tumor composed of liver cord cells and bile ducts in mixed masses.

cholangioma (ko-lan″je-o′mah): bile duct tumor.

dentigerous cyst (den-tij′er-us): cyst containing a tooth or teeth.

epulis: any tumor of the gingivae such as an abscess or gumboil.

hepatoma* (hep″ah-to′mah): malignant tumor of the liver (also called ***hepatocarcinoma***).

odontogenic fibrosarcoma*: malignant tumor of the jaw that develops from the formative components of a tooth.

odontoma (o-don-to′mah): tumor of dental tissue.

polyp: small, tumorlike growth on a mucous membrane surface, especially the throat or the intestines.

polyposis* (pol″e-po′sis): potentially malignant condition of multiple polyps in mucous membrane lining the intestine, particularly the colon.

signet ring cell carcinoma*: malignancy most frequently found in the stomach and large intestine.

Surgical Procedures

Due to the large number of surgical procedures applicable to the gastrointestinal system, they have been organized into groups involving puncture (***-centesis***), suture (***-rrhaphy***), incision (***-otomy***), excision (***-ectomy***), repair (***-plasty***), fixation (***-pexy***), and opening and anastomasis (***-stomy***).

*Indicates a malignant condition.

Puncture for Drainage or Aspiration

abdominocentesis (ab-dom″i-no-sen-te′sis): paracentesis of the abdominal cavity (also called *celiocentesis*).

colocentesis (ko″lo-sen-te′sis): paracentesis of the colon.

paracentesis: surgical puncture of a cavity for fluid aspiration.

peritoneocentesis (per″i-to″ne-o-sen-te′sis): paracentesis of the peritoneal cavity.

Suture and Repair of Wounds, Lesions, Injuries, Ruptures, and Displacements

cecorrhaphy (se-kor′ah-fe): suture or repair of the cecum.

celiorrhaphy (se″le-or′ah-fe): suture or repair of the abdominal wall (also called *laparorrhaphy*).

cheilorrhaphy (ki-lor′ah-fe): suture or repair of the lip.

cholecystorrhaphy (ko″le-sis-tor′ah-fe): suture or repair of the gallbladder.

choledochorrhaphy (ko″led-o-kor′ah-fe): suture or repair of the common bile duct.

colorrhaphy (ko-lor′ah-fe): suture or repair of the colon.

duodenorrhaphy (du″o-de-nor′ah-fe): suture or repair of the duodenum.

enterorrhaphy (en″ter-or′ah-fe): suture or repair of the intestine.

gastrorrhaphy (gas-tror′ah-fe): suture or repair of the stomach.

glossorrhaphy (glo-sor′ah-fe): suture or repair of the tongue.

hepatorrhaphy (hep″ah-tor′ah-fe): suture or repair of the liver.

herniorrhaphy (her″ne-or′ah-fe): suture or repair of a hernia.

ileorrhaphy (il″e-or′ah-fe): suture or repair of the ileum.

jejunorrhaphy (je″joo-nor′ah-fe): suture or repair of the jejunum.

omentorrhaphy (o″men-tor′ah-fe): suture or repair of the omentum.

proctorrhaphy (prok-tor′ah-fe): suture or repair of the rectum.

Incision to Explore, Drain, or Remove a Foreign Body

celioenterotomy (se″le-o-en-tero-to′o-me): incision into intestine through abdominal wall (*celio* refers to abdomen).

celiogastrotomy (se″le-o-gas-trot′o-me): incision into the stomach through the abdominal wall.

celiotomy: incision into the abdominal cavity.

cheilotomy: incision into the lip.

cholangiotomy: incision into the bile duct.

cholecystotomy: incision into the gallbladder (also called *cholecystomy*).

choledocholithotomy (ko-led″o-ko-li-thot′o-me): incision into the common bile duct for removal of a stone.

choledochotomy (ko″led-o-kot′o-me): incision into common bile duct.

cholelithotomy: incision into the gallbladder for removal of stones.

colotomy: incision into the colon.

duodenotomy: incision into the duodenum.

enterocholecystotomy (en″ter-o-ko″le-sis-tot′o-me): incision into the intestine and gallbladder.

enterotomy: incision into the intestine.

esophagotomy: incision into the esophagus.

gastrotomy: incision into the stomach.

hepatotomy: incision into the liver.

ileotomy: incision into the ileum.

jejunotomy: incision into the jejunum.

laparotomy: incision into abdominal wall for exploratory purposes.

pancreatomy: incision into the pancreas (also called *pancreatotomy*).

pharyngotomy: incision into the pharynx.

proctotomy: incision into the rectum (usually for rectal stricture).

pylorotomy: incision into the pylorus.

sialoadenotomy (si″ah-lo-ad″e-not′o-me): incision and drainage of a salivary gland.

sialolithotomy: removal of a stone from a salivary gland.

sigmoidotomy: incision into the sigmoid.

sphincterotomy (sfingk″ter-ot′o-me): incision into sphincter muscle.

Excision to Remove All or Part of an Organ

alveolectomy: partial excision of an alveolar process of a tooth.

appendectomy: excision of the vermiform appendix.

cecectomy (see-kek″toe-me): excision of the cecum.

cholangiocholecystocholedochectomy (ko-lan″ge-o-ko″le-sis″to-ko″le-do-kek′to-me): excision of the gallbladder, hepatic duct, and common bile duct.

cholecystectomy: excision of the gallbladder.

choledochectomy (kol″e-do-kek′to-me): excision of a portion of the common bile duct.

colectomy: partial excision of the colon.

duodenectomy (du″o-de-nek′to-me): partial or total excision of the duodenum.

esophagectomy: partial excision of the esophagus.

gastrectomy: total or partial excision of the stomach.

gastropylorectomy (gas″tro-pi″lo-rek′to-me): excision of the pyloric portion of stomach.

glossectomy: surgical removal of part or all of the tongue.

hemorrhoidectomy: excision of hemorrhoids.

hepatectomy: excision of a portion or all of the liver.

ileectomy: excision of the ileum.

jejunectomy: excision of the jejunum.

omentectomy: excision of a portion or all of the omentum.

omphalectomy (om″fah-lek′to-me): excision of the umbilicus (navel), or an attached tumor.

pancreatectomy: surgical removal of all or part of the pancreas.

parotidectomy (pah-rot″i-dek′to-me): excision of the parotid gland.

pharyngectomy (far″in-jek′to-me): partial or total excision of the pharynx.

proctectomy: excision of the rectum.

proctosigmoidectomy (prok″to-sig″moidek′to-me): excision of rectum and sigmoid flexure.

sialoadenectomy (si″ah-lo-ad″e-nek′to-me): excision of a salivary gland.

sigmoidectomy (sig″moid-ek′to-me): excision of the sigmoid flexure.

Plastic Surgery for Repair

anoplasty (a′no-plas″te): repair of the anus.

cheiloplasty (ki′lo-plas″te): repair of the lip.

choledochoplasty (koled′o-ko-plas″te): common bile duct repair.

esophagoplasty (e-sof′ah-go-plas″te): repair of the esophagus.

gastroplasty: repair of the stomach.

glossoplasty: repair of the tongue.

hernioplasty: repair of a hernia.

palatoplasty: repair of palate, including cleft palate.

pharyngoplasty: (fah-ring′go-plas″te): repair of the pharynx.

proctoplasty: repair of rectum or anus.

pyloroplasty (pi-lo′ro-plas″te): repair to remove a pyloric obstruction and expedite emptying of the stomach.

sialodochoplasty (si″ah-lo-do′ko-plas″te): plastic repair of the salivary ducts.

sphincteroplasty (sfingk′ter-o-plas″te): repair of a sphincter.

stomatoplasty (sto′mah-to-plas″te): repair of mouth.

Fixation to Suspend or Fasten

cecopexy: fixation of the cecum.

cholecystopexy: fixation of the gallbladder.

colopexy: fixation of the colon.

enteropexy: fixation of the intestine to the abdominal wall.

gastropexy: fixation of the stomach.

hepatopexy: fixation of the liver.

mesenteriopexy: fixation or attachment of a torn mesentery (also called **mesopexy**).

omentopexy: fixation of omentum to the abdominal wall or an organ.

proctococcypexy (prok″to-kok′si-pek″se): fastening of the rectum to tissues in front of the coccyx.

proctopexy: fixation of a prolapsed rectum to adjacent tissues.

sigmoidopexy: attachment of the sigmoid colon to another structure.

Ostomies and Anastomoses

Ostomies are surgically created openings, usually in the intestines after partial resection to remove diseased or damaged parts, through which body waste is expelled. Anastomoses are surgically created openings, to produce communication between normally separated organs or spaces.

apicostomy (a″pe-kos′to-me): surgical creation of an opening through bone and gum to root portion of the tooth.

cecocolostomy (se″ko-ko-los′to-me): anastomosis between the cecum and colon (also called **colocecostomy**).

cecoileostomy (se″ko-il″e-os′to-me): anastomosis between the cecum and ileum (also called **ileocecostomy**).

cecostomy: creation of an artificial opening into the cecum.

cholangioenterostomy (ko-lan″je-o-en″ter-os′to-me): anastomosis between intestine and bile duct.

cholangiogastrostomy (ko-lan″je-o-gas-tros′to-me): anastomosis between bile duct and stomach.

cholangiojejunostomy (ko-lan″je-o-je-joo-nos′to-me): anastomosis between a bile duct and the jejunum.

cholangiostomy: creation of an opening into a bile duct.

cholecystenterostomy (ko″le-sis-ten″teros′to-me): anastomosis between the gallbladder and intestine (also called **enterocholecystostomy**).

cholecystocolostomy (ko″le-sis″to-ko-los′to-me): anastomosis between the gallbladder and colon (also called **cystocolostomy**).

cholecystogastrostomy (ko″le-sis″to-gas-tros′to-me): anastomosis between the gallbladder and stomach.

cholecystoduodenostomy (ko″le-sis″to-du″o-de-nos′to-me): anastomosis between the gallbladder and duodenum.

cholecystoileostomy (ko″le-sis″to-il′e-os′to-me): anastomosis between the gallbladder and ileum.

cholecystojejunostomy (ko″le-sis″to-je-joo-nos′to-me): anastomosis between the gallbladder and jejunum.

choledochocholedochostomy (ko-led′o-ko-ko-led′o-kos′to-me): anastomosis between two portions of the common bile duct.

choledochoduodenostomy (ko-led″o-ko-du″o-de-nos′to-me): anastomosis between the common bile duct and duodenum.

choledochoenterostomy (ko-led″o-ko-en″ter-os′to-me): anastomosis between the common bile duct and intestine.

choledochogastrostomy (ko-led″o-ko-gas-tros′to-me): anastomosis between the common bile duct and stomach.

choledochoileostomy (ko-led″o-ko-il-e-os′to-me): anastomosis between the common bile duct and ileum.

choledochojejunostomy (ko-led″o-ko-je-joo-nos′to-me): anastomosis between the common bile duct and jejunum.

choledochostomy (ko-led-o-kos′to-me): formation of an opening into the common bile duct for drainage.

colocolostomy (ko″lo-ko-los′to-me): anastomosis between two portions of the colon.

coloproctostomy (ko″lo-prok-tos′to-me): anastomosis between the colon and rectum (also called *colorectostomy*).

colosigmoidostomy (ko″lo-sig″moi-dos′to-me): anastomosis between the sigmoid and any other part of the colon.

colostomy: formation of an artificial opening into the colon from the surface of the body.

duodenoenterostomy (du″o-de″no-en″ter-os′to-me): anastomosis between the duodenum and another part of the intestine.

duodenoileostomy (do″o-de″no-il″e-os′to-me): anastomosis between the duodenum and ileum.

duodenojejunostomy (du″o-de″no-je-joo-nos′to-me): anastomosis between the duodenum and jejunum.

duodenostomy (du″od-e-nos′to-me): creation of an opening into the duodenum.

enteroanastomosis (en″ter-o-ah-nas″to-mo′sis): anastomosis between two sections of the intestine (also called *enteroenterostomy*).

enterocolostomy: anastomosis between the small intestine and colon.

enterostomy (en″ter-os′to-me): creation of an opening into the intestine through the abdominal wall.

esophagoduodenostomy (e-sof″ah-go-du″o-de-nos′to-me): anastomosis between the esophagus and duodenum.

esophagoenterostomy (e-sof′ah-go-en″ter-os′to-me): anastomosis between the esophagus and intestine.

esophagogastrostomy (e-sof′ah-go-gas-tros′to-me): anastomosis between the esophagus and stomach.

esophagojejunostomy (e-sof′ah-go-je-joo-nos′to-me): anastomosis between the esophagus and jejunum.

esophagostomy: creation of an artificial opening into the esophagus.

gastroanastomosis (gas″tro-ah-nas″to-mo′sis): anastomosis between pyloric and cardiac ends of stomach (also called *gastrogastrostomy*).

gastrocolostomy (gas″tro-ko-los′to-me): anastomosis between the stomach and colon.

gastroduodenostomy (gas″tro-du″o-de-nos′to-me): anastomosis between the stomach and duodenum.

gastroenterocolostomy (gas″tro-en″ter-o-ko-los′to-me): anastomosis between the stomach and intestines.

gastroenterostomy (gas″tro-en-ter-os′to-me): anastomosis between the stomach and colon.

gastroileostomy (gas″tro-il-e-os′to-me): anastomosis between the stomach and ileum.

gastrojejunostomy (gas″tro-je-joo-nos′to-me): anastomosis between the stomach and jejunum.

gastrostomy (gas-tros′to-me): creation of an opening into the stomach.

hepaticoduodenostomy (he-pat″i-ko-du″o-de-nos′to-me): anastomosis between hepatic ducts and duodenum (also called *hepatoduodenostomy*).

hepaticoenterostomy (he-pat″i-ko-en″ter-os′to-me): anastomosis between the hepatic ducts and intestine (also called *hepaticocholangioenterostomy*).

hepaticogastrostomy (he-pat″i-ko-gas-tros′to-me): anastomosis between the hepatic duct and stomach.

hepaticojejunostomy (he-pat″i-ko-je″joo-nos′to-me): anastomosis between the hepatic duct and jejunum.

hepaticostomy: creation of an opening into the hepatic duct.

hepatocholangiostomy (he-pat″o″ah-to-ko-lan′je-os′to-me): creation of an opening into the hepatic duct for drainage.

ileocolostomy (il″e-o-ko-los′to-me): anastomosis between the ileum and colon.

ileoileostomy (il″e-o-il″e-os′to-me): anastomosis between two different parts of the ileum.

ileoproctostomy (il″e-o-prok-tos′to-me): anastomosis between the ileum and rectum.

ileosigmoidostomy (il″e-o-sig″moid-os′to-me): anastomosis between the ileum and sigmoid colon.

ileostomy: creation of an opening into the ileum through the abdominal wall.

jejunocolostomy (je-joo″no-ko″los-′to-me): anastomosis between the jejunum and colon (also called *jejunoileostomy*).

jejunojejunostomy (je-noo″no-jee″joo-nos′to-me): anastomosis between two parts of the jejunum.

jejunostomy: creation of an opening through the abdominal wall into the jejunum.

pancreaticoduodenostomy (pan″kre-at″i-ko-du″o-de-nos′to-me): anastomosis of the pancreatic duct and the duodenum.

pancreaticoenterostomy (pan″kre-at″i-ko-en″ter-os′ to-me): anastomosis of the pancreatic duct and the intestine.

pancreaticogastrostomy (pan″kre-at″i-ko-gas-tros′to-me): anastomosis of the pancreatic duct and the stomach.

pancreaticojejunostomy (pan″kre-at″i-ko-je″joo-nos′ to-me): anastomosis of the pancreatic duct and the jejunum.

proctostomy (prok-tos′to-me): creation of an opening into the rectum from the surface of the body (also called **rectostomy**).

pylorostomy (pi″lo-ros′to-me): creation of an opening through the abdominal wall near the pyloric end of the stomach.

sigmoidoproctostomy (sig-moi″do-prok-tos′to-me): anastomosis between the sigmoid flexure and the rectum (also called **sigmoidorectostomy**).

sigmoidosigmoidostomy (sig-moi″do-sig-moi-dos′to-me): anastomosis between two portions of the sigmoid.

sigmoidostomy: creation of an artificial opening into the sigmoid flexure from the body surface.

Other Surgical Procedures

cholecystolithotripsy (kol″le-sis″to-lith′o-trip″se): crushing of stones in the gallbladder (also called **cholelithotripsy** or **cholelithotrity**).

choledocholithotripsy (ko-led″o-ko-lith′o-trip″se): crushing of a stone within the common bile duct.

exteriorize: transpose an internal organ to the outside of the body.

proctotoreusis (prok″to-to-roo′sis): creating an artificial anus.

ptyalectasis (ti″ah-lek′tah-sis): dilation of a salivary duct.

pylorodiosis (pi-lo″ro-di-o′sis): dilating a stricture of pylorus with the finger, which is either inserted through a gastrotomy incision (*Loreta's method*), or the anterior stomach wall (*Hahn's method*).

Laboratory Tests and Procedures

biopsy: insertion of needle to obtain sample of tissue in organs such as the liver, to detect abnormalities and diseases.

Blood Tests:

amylase: pancreatic enzyme elevated in disease of pancreas or salivary glands.

Australian antigen: detects serum hepatitis B, and differentiates between it and serum hepatitis A.

bilirubin: a pigment of bile measurably present in liver and gallbladder diseases.

carcinoembryonic antigen: to detect the presence of cancer in the colon and pancreas.

C-peptide test: to determine the ability of diabetics to make their own insulin.

insulin test: to determine amount of insulin secreted by the pancreas after fasting and again after receiving glucose.

Liver Function Tests:
to determine damage or disease, normal enzymes or injected chemicals are measured for elevation or retention in the blood serum:

aminotransferases: aspartate aminotransferase (AST) (formerly called *serum glutamic-oxaloacetic transaminase [SGOT]*) and **alanine aminotransferase (ALT)** (formerly called *serum glutamic-pyruvic transaminase [SGPT]*) levels are measured for elevation to detect liver disease.

argininosuccinic lyase: normally present enzyme.

bromsulphalein: injected and found retained in blood over a specified time period.

cephalin-cholesterol flocculation: reaction of blood serum mixed with cephalin and cholesterol.

complement C3: elevated levels in cancer, decreased levels in liver disease.

guanase: enzyme level elevated in hepatitis and other types of liver disease.

lactic dehydrogenase isoenzymes: pattern of distribution is diagnostic for liver disease.

ornithine carbamoyl transferase: level of this enzyme elevated in liver disease.

plasma volume: elevated in liver and spleen disease.

protein: elevated in liver disease.

total alkaline phosphatase: increased levels indicate liver disease.

total cholesterol: elevated or decreased in particular liver diseases.

transferrin: iron-binding protein that decreases in liver disease.

Endoscope Examinations:
tube-like device with light and refracting mirrors that is used to examine internal body areas for abnormalities and to remove tissue samples and small growths.

colonoscopy: examination of the colon.

esophagoscopy: examination of the esophagus.

gastroscopy: examination of stomach and upper GI tract.

proctoscopy: examination of anus and rectum.

proctosigmoidoscopy: examination of rectum and sigmoid colon.

sigmoidoscopy: examination of sigmoid colon.

Gastric Fluid Analysis:
series of tests on fluid aspirated from the stomach, to detect various diseases.

Radiologic Studies:

barium enema: studies using contrast media to visualize the colon and rectum.

celiac angiography: studies of the blood vessels of the liver, spleen, stomach and pancreas, using contrast medium.

cholangiography: studies of the gallbladder and its ducts.

cholecystography (oral): studies of the gallbladder after ingestion of a fatty meal, using contrast media to outline structures.

computerized tomography (CT): imaging device using X-rays at multiple angles through specific sections of the body, analyzed by computer to provide a total picture of the part being examined (also called ***computerized axial tomography [CAT]***).

gastrointestinal series: X-ray studies of esophagus, stomach, and small intestine, after swallowing a contrast medium such as barium. The large intestine is visualized by use of barium enema.

magnetic resonance imaging (MRI): noninvasive method of scanning the body by use of an electromagnetic field and radio waves, which provides visual images on a computer screen and magnetic tape recordings (also called ***nuclear magnetic resonance [NMR]***). Used to examine soft tissues such as visceral contents.

nuclear magnetic resonance (NMR): see magnetic resonance imaging.

percutaneous transhepatic cholangiography: X-ray study of bile duct by use of dye injected to detect obstruction.

sialography: X-ray studies of salivary glands using contrast medium.

splenoportography: X-ray studies of spleen, liver, and blood vessels using a contrast medium.

X-ray scans: X-ray studies of liver, spleen and pancreas, to detect tumors or other abnormalities by use of radioactive substances injected intravenously.

Stool Tests:

combined fatty acids test: to determine ability to digest fat.

guaiac test: for detection of blood in intestinal tract.

mucus test: elevation in stool indicates bowel abnormality.

parasites test: microscopic examination of fecal matter to detect parasitic infection.

pus: presence indicates intestinal tract infection.

stool culture: fecal matter incubated in growth media to detect presence of microorganisms.

total nitrogen: content measured to detect pancreatic insufficiency or poor protein digestion.

trypsin activity: elevation indicates fibrocystic disease of pancreas.

urobilinogen: metabolic product that decreases in liver and gallbladder diseases.

Urine Tests:

amylase: elevated in pancreatitis.

copper: element found in elevated amounts in liver disease.

coproporphyrin: elevated in liver and metabolic disease.

diacetic acid: produced in metabolic diseases such as diabetes.

oral glucose tolerance test: measurable level of sugar present indicates metabolic disorder.

qualitative glucose: present in metabolic diseases such as diabetes.

5-Hydroxyindoleacetic acid: elevation indicates tumor in appendix or lower intestinal tract.

inulin clearance: rate of excretion of inulin indicates presence of liver disease.

CHAPTER 12

The Genitourinary System

Liquid Waste Processing and Human Reproduction

CHAPTER OVERVIEW

The genitourinary system includes the urinary and reproductive systems of both sexes. In this chapter, the structures and functions of the various parts of both systems are presented and discussed.

THE URINARY SYSTEM

The organs that produce and excrete the waste substance urine from the body are the two **kidneys**, which filter the blood and remove waste products of metabolism in the form of urine; two **ureters**, which carry the urine from the kidneys; a **bladder**, which receives and stores the urine; and a **urethra**, which excretes the urine from the body. These organs are common to both sexes, with essentially the same structure.

The Kidneys

The **kidneys** (Fig. 12-1) are two bean-shaped organs (**nephro-** and **reno-** refer to kidney) located on both sides of the vertebral column, behind the parietal peritoneum, and just above the waist. An average kidney weighs 4 to 6 ounces (152 to 240 g), is about 4 inches (11 cm) long, 2 to 3 inches (5 to 7.5 cm) wide, and 1 inch (2.5 cm) thick. The left kidney is usually a little larger and is suspended a little higher than the right one. Renal fasciae

(fibrous tissue) connecting to other structures, in conjunction with heavy encapsulating pads of fat surrounding the kidneys, hold them in place. Each kidney has a concave depression, the **hilus**, on its medial margin, for the entry of blood vessels, nerves, and its ureter.

Kidney Composition and Structure

The kidneys are dark reddish-brown and are solid organs except for the **renal sinus**, which is the space into which the hilus opens. Sectioning of the kidney shows it to be composed of an external **cortex** and an internal **medulla** (Fig. 12-3).

The renal sinus contains the **renal pelvis**, blood vessels, nerves, and fat. The renal pelvis, a funnel-shaped reservoir that occupies most of the renal sinus, is made up of the major and minor **calyces** (singular—**calyx**), irregular saclike structures that collect urine from all portions of the kidney. The broad portion of the renal pelvis lies within the renal sinus, and its apical portion passes out through the hilus to unite with the **ureter**, the outlet tube of the kidney extending to the bladder (Fig. 12-1).

Twelve to eighteen small cone-shaped structures called **medullary pyramids**, which make up the medulla, stud the walls of the renal sinus, with their **bases** facing the cortex and their narrow ends, the **papillae**, extending into the renal pelvis calyces, where the urine collects through ducts in the papillae. The cortex extends between the pyramids, forming the renal columns (see Fig. 12-3).

The Functional Unit of the Kidney

The **nephron** is the functional unit of the kidney, consisting of the **renal corpuscle** and the **renal tubule**. There are about 1 million nephrons in the human kidney. The renal corpuscle consists of a double-walled, cup-shaped structure called the **glomerular** or **Bowman's capsule**, which contains a twisted cluster of cap-

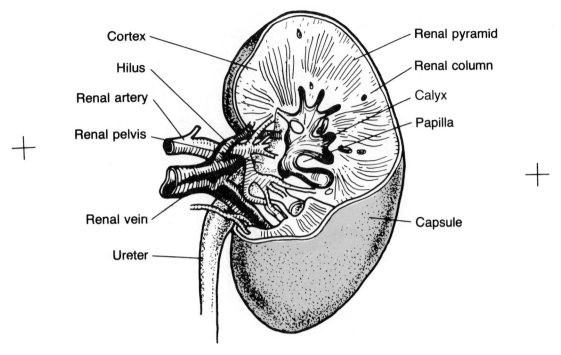

Figure 12-1.   Structure of the kidney.

illary channels called the **glomerulus** forming a rounded body.

The renal tubule is divided into the **proximal convoluted tubule**, the **descending limb** of the **loop of Henle**, the **ascending limb** of the **loop of Henle**, the **distal convoluted tubule**, and the **collecting tubule** (Figs. 12-2 and 12-3).

The renal corpuscles and the attached proximal convoluted tubules into which they drain lie in the cortical portion of the kidney, with the tubules making up the largest part of the renal cortex. The loop of Henle follows the proximal convoluted tubule and is divided into a descending and an ascending limb, lying for the most part within the renal medulla. The distal convoluted tubule resembles the proximal convoluted tubule in structure, except that it is much shorter when uncoiled, and drains into the collecting tubules, which convey the urine to the renal pelvis by way of the papillary ducts of the pyramids.

Functions of the Kidneys

The main function of the kidneys is to filter waste materials from the blood and excrete them in the urine. The waste products include nitrogenous wastes from the breakdown of proteins, toxic substances, mineral salts, excess glucose, and water (both ingested water and that produced during metabolism). In the blood-filtering pro-

cess, water and solutes from blood in the glomeruli pass through the capillaries and the glomerular walls into the tubules. The tubules have the ability to select substances needed by the body and return them to the blood.

The speed at which the blood filters through the kidneys is affected by the blood pressure. If the systemic blood pressure drops, as in shock, it may cause filtration of blood to slow to a point where the kidneys stop functioning. Similarly, if the systemic pressure is too high, kidney damage may result causing a loss of substances that normally would have been reabsorbed for use by the body.

The kidneys affect the rate of secretion of some hormones, synthesize other hormones, and maintain the pH of the blood so that it does not become too acid or too alkaline.

The Ureters

The **ureters**, one from each kidney, are about 15 to 18 inches (38 to 46 cm) long and are less than $\frac{1}{2}$ inch (1.25 cm) in diameter, extending from the renal pelvis of the kidney down to the urinary bladder. The ureter on the left is slightly longer because of the higher position of the left kidney. The walls of the ureters are made up of an outer fibrous tissue layer, two center layers of smooth muscle, and a mucous membrane lining.

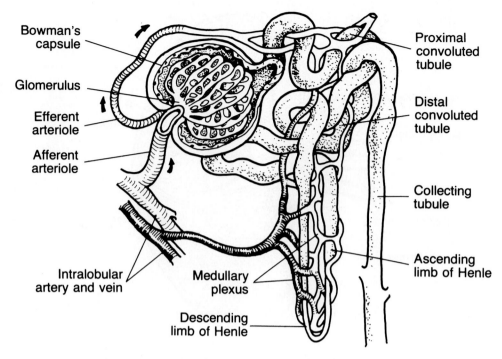

Figure 12-2.   The nephron, the functional unit of the kidney.

Urine enters the bladder through the ureters every 10 to 30 seconds, in spurts rather than in a continuous flow. The spurts are produced by the action of successive peristaltic waves, beginning in the renal pelvis and passing down throughout the extent of the ureters. Situated at the bladder entrance is a ureteral orifice, which opens for 2 to 3 seconds and then closes until a succeeding peristaltic wave opens it again, serving to prevent urine from flowing back to the ureters during bladder contraction.

The Urinary Bladder

The **urinary bladder** is an extremely elastic, musculomembranous sac, lying in the pelvis, formed of three layers of smooth muscle tissue lined with mucous membrane containing **rugae** (wrinkles or ridges). It contains two openings to receive urine from the two ureters, and another opening into the urethra, through which urine is excreted. The bladder has two functions, to serve as a storage place for urine, and to excrete urine through the urethra.

The average bladder will hold more than 250 ml of urine, but that amount will usually create a desire to empty the bladder. The contraction of the bladder and the relaxation of the internal sphincter muscle are involuntary actions, but the external sphincter muscle is controlled by voluntary action. The act of preventing or concluding voiding (urinating) is learned and voluntary in a mature, healthy human.

The Urethra

The **urethra** is a membranous, tubular canal that carries the urine from the bladder to the exterior of the body.

The male urethra is approximately 8 inches (20 cm) long and is narrower than in the female. It extends from the neck of the bladder, through the prostate gland, between the fascia connecting the pubic bones, and through the **penis** (external male reproductive organ). The male urethra is divided into three sections, **prostatic**, **membranous**, and **cavernous**. The exterior opening of the urethra in the male is also called the **urinary meatus**. In males, the urethra has a dual function, carrying both urine and the reproductive organ secretions (Fig. 12-4).

In the female, the urethra is approximately 1 to 1½ inches (2.5 to 4 cm) in length, extending from the neck of the bladder to the exterior surface of the body. The exterior opening of the urethra, called the **urinary meatus**, is located between the vagina and clitoris. In the female, the only function of the urethra is urination (Fig. 12-6).

Characteristics of Normal Urine

Normal urine is usually clear, pale amber in color, with a characteristic odor. It is approximately 95% water, containing many dissolved substances, such as nitrogenous wastes, electrolytes, toxins, pigments, hormones,

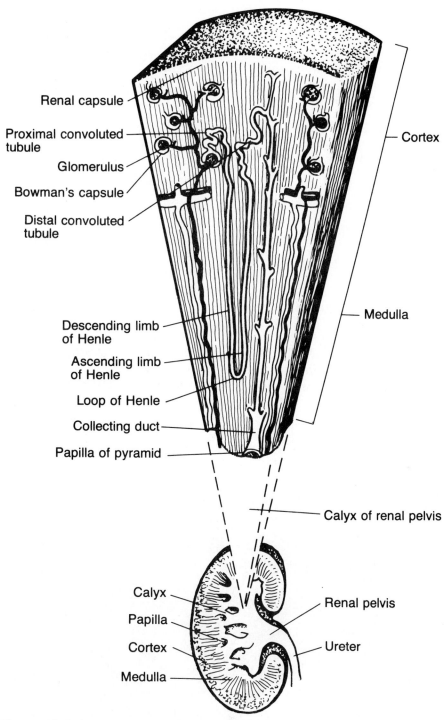

Figure 12-3. Magnification showing renal corpuscles, proximal and distal convoluted tubules, and loops of Henle and collecting tubules.

and at times abnormal substances such as glucose, albumin, or blood.

The average urinary output in a 24-hour period ranges from 1000 to 2000 ml. The normal specific gravity of urine varies from 1.015 to 1.025, with an acid reaction.

Review A

Complete the following:

1. The organs of the urinary system are the _____, _____, _____, and

   _____.

2. The concave depression on the medial margin of the kidney is called the _____.

3. The _____ is the functional unit of the kidney.

4. The main function of the kidneys is to _____ waste from the blood.

5. The wrinkles on the mucous membrane lining the bladder are called _____.

THE MALE REPRODUCTIVE ORGANS

The basic male reproductive organs (*gonads*) are the *testes*. The accessory organs are ducts, glands, and supporting structures. The ducts are the *epididymides*, *vas deferens*, *ejaculatory ducts*, and the urethra. The glands are the *seminal vesicles*, *prostate*, and *bulbourethral* (*Cowper's*) glands, with the *penis*, *scro-*

tum, and *spermatic cords* functioning as supporting structures (Fig. 12-4).

The Testes

The *testes*, or *testicles*, are a pair of egg-shaped glands normally located in a saclike structure called the *scrotum*. Each testicle is enclosed in a fibrous white

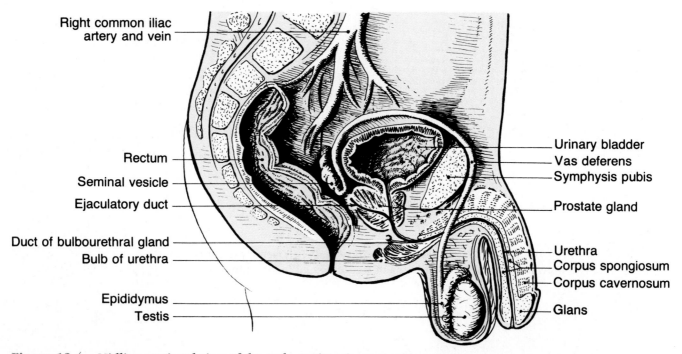

Right common iliac artery and vein

Rectum

Seminal vesicle

Ejaculatory duct

Duct of bulbourethral gland

Bulb of urethra

Epididymus

Testis

Urinary bladder

Vas deferens

Symphysis pubis

Prostate gland

Urethra

Corpus spongiosum

Corpus cavernosum

Glans

Figure 12-4.   Midline sectional view of the male genitourinary system.

capsule that continues into the gland to divide it into numerous conical *lobules*, or compartments, each of which contains one or more coiled *seminiferous tubules* and *interstitial cells* (*Leydig cells*). The seminiferous tubules join into a cluster from which several ducts emerge and enter the head of the *epididymis*.

The testes have two functions, producing *spermatozoa* (sperm cells, or male reproductive cells—singular is *spermatozoon*) and secreting hormones. The sperm cells are produced by the seminiferous tubules. The chief hormone *testosterone* is an *androgen* (male sex hormone) that is secreted by the Leydig cells, which are specialized interstitial cells. Testosterone has several functions. It induces and maintains male secondary sex characteristics, such as hair growth and pitch of voice, as well as having an influence on growth of muscles and bones, accounting in part for the observed sex differences. Testosterone has an influence on general, as well as fluid and electrolyte metabolism, has an excitory effect on kidney tubule reabsorption, and suppresses anterior pituitary secretion of gonadotropins.

The Epididymis

The *epididymides* (singular—*epididymis*), a pair of tightly coiled, tubelike structures, each about 20 feet (6 meters), lie along the posterior borders of each testis. The functions of each epididymis are to serve as a passageway for sperm from the testis to the body surface, store sperm before ejaculation, and secrete a part of the *semen* (seminal fluid).

The Vas Deferens (Ductus Deferens)

The *vas deferens* are a pair of tubes, each about 1/8 inch (0.3 cm) in diameter, a continuation of the epididymis. The vas extends from the epididymis up through the inguinal canal, where it is encased by the *spermatic cord*, into the abdominal cavity and down the posterior of the bladder where it connects with the seminal vesicle duct and forms the *ejaculatory duct*. The function of the vas deferens is to act as a duct for the testis and connect the epididymis with the ejaculatory duct.

The Ejaculatory Ducts

The *ejaculatory ducts* are two short tubes formed by the joining of the vas deferens with the ducts of the seminal vesicles. They pass through the prostate gland and extend to the urethra.

The Seminal Vesicles

The *seminal vesicles* are two twisted pouches lying along the lower posterior surface of the bladder, in front of the rectum. They secrete the mucid, liquid part of the semen, and prostaglandins.

The Prostate Gland

The *prostate gland* is composed of smooth muscle and glandular tissue, is doughnut-shaped, about the size of a large walnut, and surrounds the urethra. The prostate secretes a viscous, alkaline substance that makes up most of the seminal fluid (semen). The alkalinity protects the sperm from acid present in the urethra of the male and the vagina of the female and increases its motility.

The Bulbourethral Glands

The *bulbourethral* (*Cowper's*) glands are two rounded, pea-sized bodies below the prostate gland, on either side of the membranous part of the urethra, and connected to it by a duct about 1 inch (2.5 cm) in length. These glands secrete an alkaline substance that has a protective action similar to that of the prostate secretion.

The Scrotum

The *scrotum* is a saclike, skin-covered structure that hangs from the perineal area. It is separated into two sacs internally, each containing one testis, one epididymis, and the inferior part of a spermatic cord.

The Penis

The *penis* is made up of three rounded masses of cavernous (erectile) tissue, encased in individual fibrous coats, and held together by an outer skin covering. The *glans penis* (*balanus*), a slight bulge at the distal end of the penis, is covered with a retractable, loose, double fold of skin, the *prepuce* (*foreskin*).

The penis contains the urethra, which carries both reproductive tract secretions and urine, and is the organ by means of which sperm are introduced into the vagina.

The Spermatic Cords

The *spermatic cords* are formed of white fibrous tissue, encasing the vas deferens, blood and lymph vessels, and nerves. They are located in the *inguinal* (groin) *canals*, between the scrotum and abdominal cavity.

Review B

Complete the following:

1. The basic male reproductive organs are the _____.

2. The two functions of the male reproductive organs are _____ and _____.

3. The coiled, tubelike passages for sperm, from the testes to the body surface, are the _____.

4. The doughnut-shaped, walnut-sized gland in the male reproductive system is the _____.

5. The vas deferens are encased by the _____.

THE FEMALE REPRODUCTIVE ORGANS

The basic female reproductive organs (gonads) are a pair of **ovaries**. The accessory organs consist of an internal group that include a pair of **fallopian** (**uterine**) **tubes** or **oviducts**, a **uterus**, and a **vagina**, and an external group consisting of the **vulva** (external **genitalia**) and a pair of **mammary glands** (breasts) (Figs.12-5 through 12-7).

The Ovaries

The adult **ovaries** are two almond-shaped and sized glands located on each side of the uterus, behind and below the **fallopian tubes**. Each ovary is connected to the uterus by a ligament. The end of each uterine tube is suspended over the corresponding ovary so that the **fimbriated** (fingerlike) end of the tube does not come in contact with the ovary, making it a gland with an unattached duct (Fig. 12-5).

Structure of the Ovaries

A single layer of epithelial cells forms the ovarian surface. The interior consists primarily of a network of connective tissue, in which are embedded countless numbers of microscopic formations, called **follicles**, containing **ova** (eggs, or female sex cells) in different stages of development.

Functions of the Ovaries

The functions of the ovaries are ovulation and hormonal secretion. The ova develop in the ovaries, and when an **ovum** (singular of ova) matures, it is expelled by the ovary to be caught up by the fimbriated end of the fallopian tube over that ovary.

Estrogen and **progesterone** are the ovarian hormones. Estrogen is also produced in the adrenal cortex (male and female), the testes (male), and the fetal-placental unit (during pregnancy), and has a variety of functions in both sexes.

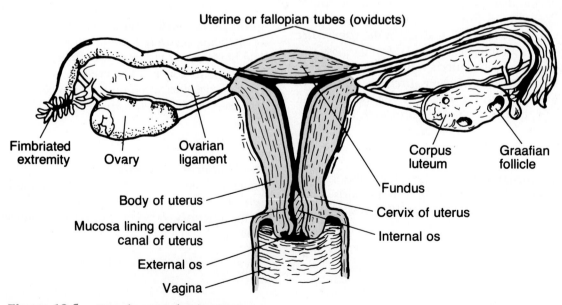

Figure 12-5.   **Female reproductive tract.**

Ovarian estrogen has several functions. It induces the development of the female secondary sex characteristics and the cyclic (menstrual) changes in the uterus in preparation for the implantation and developmental support of a fertilized ovum. Progesterone, which is produced in the adrenal cortex as well as in the *corpus luteum* of the ovary and the placenta, also prepares the uterus to receive and nurture the fertilized ovum, in addition to having an effect on the female secondary sex characteristics.

The Fallopian (Uterine) Tubes

Structure of the Fallopian Tubes

There are two fallopian tubes, each about 4 inches (10 cm) in length, consisting of an inner, ciliated mucous membrane layer, a middle, smooth layer, and an outer layer of serous tissue. The proximal ends of the fallopian tubes are attached to the uterus, and the distal ends, the *infundibula* (singular—*infundibulum*), are funnel-shaped, with fringed, fingerlike processes called *fimbriae*. The fimbriated ends are suspended over, but not attached to, or touching, the ovaries (Fig. 12-5).

Function of the Fallopian Tubes

The fallopian tubes act as ducts to the uterus for the ova produced by the ovaries. Normally, *fertilization* (ovum and sperm cell union) takes place in a fallopian tube.

The Uterus

The *uterus* is a thick-walled, hollow, pear-shaped organ (*metro-* and *hystero-* refer to the uterus), lying in the pelvic cavity between the bladder and rectum. The upper portion of the uterus, the *body*, has a rounded swelling, just above and between the entry points of the fallopian tubes, called the *fundus*. The lower, narrower portion of the uterus is the *cervix* (neck). The opening from the cervix of the uterus into the cervical canal is called the *internal os* (mouth or opening) and the opening from the cervical canal into the vagina is called the *external os* (Figs. 12-5 and 12-6).

Structure of the Uterus

The uterine walls are formed of three layers. The internal lining is a specialized epithelial mucous membrane called the *endometrium*. The middle layer, the *myometrium*, is formed of layers of smooth muscle, extending diagonally, crosswise, and lengthwise. The external layer, the *perimetrium*, is an extension of the parietal peritoneum serous membrane, which covers only the upper two thirds of the body of the uterus.

Functions of the Uterus

The uterus has several functions. *Menstruation* provides a way to clear the uterus and build a fresh environment for a fertilized ovum. During pregnancy the uterus maintains and supports the developing fetus. In labor the uterus completes childbirth by contracting and evacuating its contents.

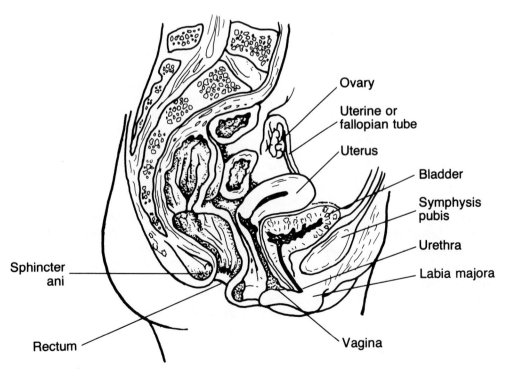

Figure 12-6.   **Side view of the female reproductive tract.**

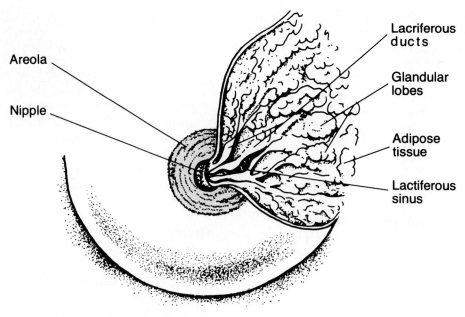

Figure 12-7. The lactating breast.

The Vagina

The **vagina** is located in front of the rectum and behind the urethra and bladder, extending from the cervix of the uterus to the external genitalia (Fig. 12-6).

Structure of the Vagina

The vagina is an extremely elastic tube of smooth muscle, lined with a mucous membrane forming rugae, and is approximately 4 inches (10 cm) long at the back of the tube and 3 inches (8 cm) long at the front, because of the protrusion of the cervix into the upper portion of the anterior wall. In the virginal condition the external vaginal orifice may be partly occluded (blocked) by a fold of mucous membrane, the **hymen**.

Functions of the Vagina

The functions of the vagina in reproduction are to receive the fluid of the male sex organ, and to provide passage out of the body for the menstrual flow, secretions of the uterus, and the neonate at birth.

The Vulva

The vulva, or external genitalia, includes the **mons pubis**, **labia majora**, **labia minora**, **clitoris**, **vaginal orifice**, and **Bartholin's** (or **greater vestibular**) **glands** (Fig. 12-6).

The **mons pubis** is a pad of fat located in front of the **symphysis pubis**, which is covered by skin until after puberty, when hair grows in the area.

The **labia majora** (large lips) are two folds of fat-filled skin, covered with hair after puberty, and extending backward from the mons pubis. Within these two folds of skin are two smaller folds of thin-skinned mucous membrane called the **labia minora** (small lips), which unite anteriorly to enclose the clitoris, and contain numerous sebaceous glands in their lateral and medial surfaces. The area between the labia minora is known as the **vestibule**.

The **clitoris** is an organ formed of erectile tissue, located beneath the point of union of the labia minora, similar in structure to the glans penis of the male, and also covered with a prepuce (foreskin).

The **vaginal orifice** is located posterior to the urinary meatus. (Although the urinary meatus is located between the clitoris and the vaginal orifice, it is not a genital organ in the female).

Bartholin's (**greater vestibular**) **glands** are two pea-size mucus glands, on each side of the vaginal orifice, that secrete a lubricant.

The muscular, skin-covered area between the vaginal orifice and anus is called the **perineum**.

The Mammary Glands (Breasts)

The **mammary glands** (breasts) are the milk-producing glandular structures located over the pectoral muscles of the thorax, whose development is controlled by estrogen and progesterone, two hormones secreted by the ovaries.

Structure of the Mammary Glands

Each breast is composed of connective and adipose tissue in lobes and lobules with milk-secreting cells around a duct. The individual ducts join with others to form larger ducts, which circle the nipple, ending in minute openings on the nipple surface. The halo of pigment surrounding the nipple is called the **areola** (Fig. 12-7).

Function of the Mammary Glands

The only function of the mammaries is to produce milk for the feeding of the neonate. Milk production is stimulated by the lactogenic hormone prolactin produced by the anterior lobe of the pituitary gland.

Review C

Complete the following:

1. The basic female reproductive organs are the _____.

2. Microscopic _____ contain ova in different stages of development.

3. The rounded swelling at the top of the body of the uterus is called the _____.

4. The smooth muscled, elastic tube extending from the uterine cervix to the external genitalia is the

_____.

5. The halo of pigment around the nipple is called the _____.

THE MENSTRUAL CYCLE

In the human female, secondary sex characteristics begin to develop and the ability to sexually reproduce is achieved at puberty.

The onset of **menstruation** (also called **menarche**) occurs at puberty and normally continues for approximately 40 years, with variations due to heredity, diet, and other factors. Cessation of menstruation is known as **menopause** (also called **climacteric**).

The female reproductive system undergoes cyclical changes about every 28 days in order to prepare the uterus to receive a fertilized ovum. At the beginning of each monthly menstrual cycle (**men-** means month), ova within the **graafian follicles** in the ovaries begin to develop. The follicles secrete estrogen and progesterone. One graafian follicle ruptures (**ovulation**) and its ovum is expelled from the ovary to the uterine tube. The ruptured follicle grows larger, filling with a yellow lipoid material, and becomes the **corpus luteum** (yellow body). The corpus luteum also secretes estrogen and progesterone. If fertilization occurs, the corpus luteum will continue to secrete these hormones. If fertilization does not take place, these secretions will slowly diminish and the reduced levels of the hormones will lead to a new menstrual cycle. This cycle can be divided into four stages.

Stages of Menstruation

The stages of menstruation are the **menses** (menstrual period), the **postmenstrual** (preovulatory, proliferative, or follicular) stage, **ovulation**, and the **premenstrual** (postovulatory) stage, with individual variations as to time span (Fig. 12-8).

Menses

The menstrual period occurs on days 1 through 5, during which the disintegrated endometrial lining of the uterus, blood, and other secretions are evacuated through the vagina.

Postmenstrual Stage

The endometrial lining of the uterus, which was sloughed off during the menses, builds up under the influence of the ovarian hormone estrogen, and the ova within the graafian follicles also grow at this time. This stage usually lasts from days 6 through 13.

Ovulation

Ovulation normally takes place midway between menstrual periods, on days 14 and 15, although the precise day is uncertain and is dependent on the postmenstrual phase. In the ovary the mature graafian follicle ruptures and the ovum is released and expelled into the fallopian tube.

Premenstrual Stage

During this stage, from days 15 through 28, the corpus luteum secretes progesterone and estrogen, which help to prepare the uterus to receive a fertilized ovum. If pregnancy does not occur, a new cycle will begin.

PREGNANCY

At conception the ovum is normally penetrated by one sperm cell while it is in the fallopian tube. After fertilization, the fertilized ovum begins to form a rounded mass of cells and slowly moves from the tube into the uterus,

Stages of Menstruation

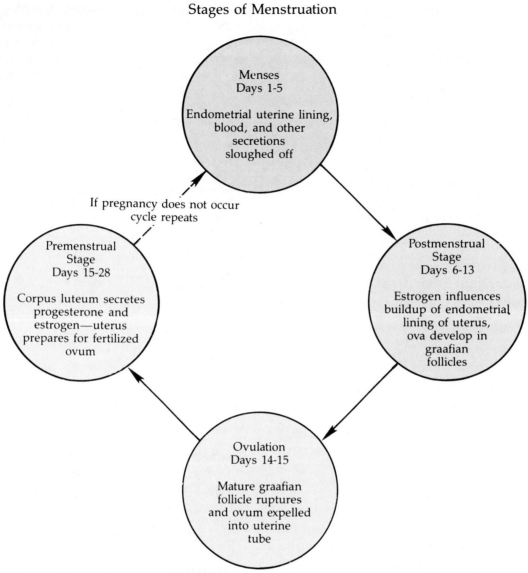

Figure 12-8.   Stages of menstruation.

where it attaches itself to the endometrial lining and begins to develop. The ***embryonic*** stage lasts from the second through the eighth week of pregnancy, and the developing organism is called an ***embryo***. The inner cells of the rounded cell mass form the embryo and its ***amnion***, which is the thin, clear sac filled with ***amniotic fluid*** in which the embryo floats. The outer cells of the rounded cell mass (***chorion***) help to form the ***placenta***, along with the endometrium of the uterus.

The placenta is the only connection between the mother and the developing ***fetus***. The ***fetal stage*** lasts from the end of the eighth week until birth. Although the maternal and fetal circulations are independent of each other, the placenta carries nutrients, oxygen, and antibodies from the maternal blood to that of the fetus, and carries fetal metabolic waste back to the maternal blood for disposal. The placenta secretes estrogen, progesterone, and ***human chorionic gonadotropin*** (***HCG***), which stimulates ovarian secretion of estrogen and progesterone.

Review D

Complete the following:

1. The onset of menstruation is called _____.

2. The cessation of menstruation is called _____.

3. The menstrual stages are _____

_____

_____.

4. The _____ stage lasts from the second through the eighth week of pregnancy.

5. The only connection between the mother and the fetus is the _____.

Answers to Review Questions: The Genitourinary System

Review A
1. kidneys (two), ureters (two), bladder, urethra
2. hilus
3. nephron
4. filter
5. rugae

Review B
1. testes
2. produce spermatozoa, secrete hormones
3. epididymides
4. prostate
5. spermatic cords

Review C
1. ovaries
2. follicles
3. fundus
4. vagina
5. areola

Review D
1. menarche
2. climacteric
3. menses or menstrual period, postmenstrual or preovulatory or follicular or proliferative, ovulation, premenstrual or postovulatory
4. embryonic
5. placenta

CHAPTER 12 EXERCISES

THE GENITOURINARY SYSTEM: LIQUID WASTE PROCESSING AND HUMAN REPRODUCTION

Exercise 1: Complete the following:

1. The urinary organs are _____, _____, _____, and _____.

2. Sectioning of the kidney shows it to have an external _____.

3. Sectioning of the kidney shows it to have an internal _____.

4. Within the renal sinus are irregular saclike structures that collect the urine from all portions of the kidney, called _____.

5. The functional unit of the kidney is the _____.

6. The twisted cluster of capillary channels called the _____ is contained in _____ capsule.

7. The tubes extending down from the kidneys to the bladder for the passage of urine are called the

   _____.

8. The musculomembranous sac lying in the pelvis, which serves as a reservoir for urine, is called the

   _____.

9. In addition to the excretion of urine, the kidneys play a role in maintaining the _____ of the blood.

10. A _____ prevents urine from flowing back to the ureters during bladder contraction.

Exercise 2: Using the terms below, identify the parts in Fig. 12-9 by placing the part name in the corresponding blank.

Cortex   Renal vein
Renal pyramid   Ureter
Hilus   Capsule
Renal column   Papilla
Renal artery   Calyx (calix)
Renal pelvis

1. _____   7. _____

2. _____   8. _____

3. _____   9. _____

4. _____   10. _____

5. _____   11. _____

6. _____

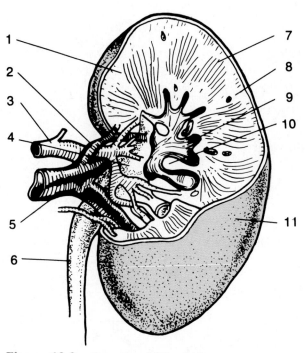

Figure 12-9.   **Structure of the kidney.**

Exercise 3: Complete the following:

  1. The accessory organs of the male reproductive system are _____
  _____ .

  2. The supporting structures of the male reproductive system are _____
  _____ .

  3. The male reproductive cell is called _____ .

  4. The chief male sex hormone is _____ .

  5. The accessory organs of the female reproductive system are _____
  _____ .

  6. The tube through which urine is voided, common to both male and female, is called the _____ .

  7. The functions of the ovaries are _____
  and _____ .

  8. The female cycle beginning with puberty is called _____ .

  9. The cessation of this cycle is called _____ .

  10. The female reproductive cells are called _____ .

Exercise 4: Using the following terms, identify each structure in Fig. 12-10 by writing its name in the corresponding blank.

Bulb of urethra
Corpus cavernosum
Corpus spongiosum
Duct of bulbourethral gland
Ejaculatory duct
Epididymis

Glans
Prostate gland
Rectum
Right common iliac artery and vein
Seminal vesicle

Symphysis pubis
Testis
Urethra
Urinary bladder
Vas deferens

  1. _____
  2. _____
  3. _____
  4. _____
  5. _____
  6. _____
  7. _____
  8. _____
  9. _____
  10. _____
  11. _____
  12. _____
  13. _____
  14. _____
  15. _____
  16. _____

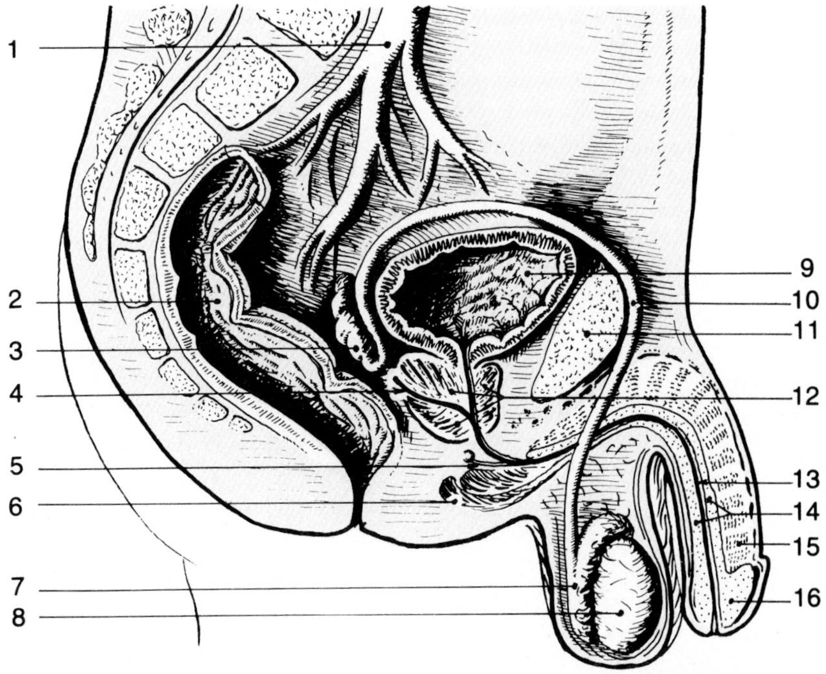

Figure 12-10.   Midline sectional view of the male genitourinary system.

Exercise 5: Using the terms below, identify each part in Fig. 12-11 by writing the appropriate name in the corresponding blank.

Corpus luteum

Fallopian, or uterine, tubes (oviducts)

Graafian follicle

Cervical canal of uterus

Ovary

Vagina

Ovarian ligament

External os

Body of uterus

Fimbriated extremity

1. _____

2. _____

3. _____

4. _____

5. _____

6. _____

7. _____

8. _____

9. _____

10. _____

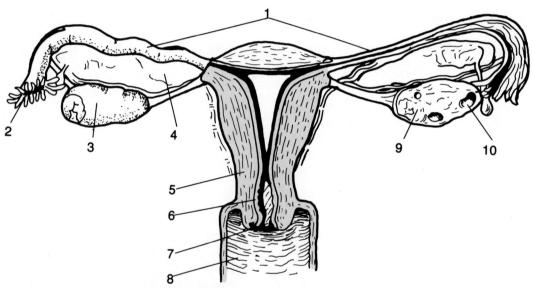

Figure 12-11.   Female reproductive tract.

Exercise 6: Using the terms below, identify each part in Fig. 12-12 by placing its name in the corresponding blank.

Vagina

Ovary

Fallopian, or uterine, tube (oviduct)

Uterus

Urethra

Labia majora

Rectum

Symphysis pubis

Bladder

Sphincter ani

1. _____

2. _____

3. _____

4. _____

5. _____

6. _____

7. _____

8. _____

9. _____

10. _____

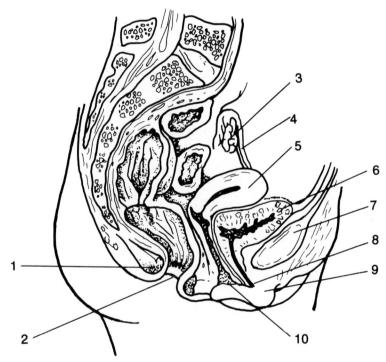

Figure 12-12.   Side view of the female reproductive tract.

Exercise 7: Matching:

____ **1.** pouches just above the prostate whose duct unites with the vas deferens to form the ejaculatory duct		**A.** scrotum
____ **2.** pair of tubes encased by spermatic cords		**B.** seminal vesicles
____ **3.** male gland producing spermatozoa		**C.** semen
____ **4.** specialized interstitial cells secreting the male sex hormone (testosterone), responsible for secondary sex characteristics		**D.** spermatozoa
____ **5.** reproductive cells of the male		**E.** Leydig cells
____ **6.** reproductive cells of the female		**F.** endometrium
____ **7.** pigmented portion of nipple		**G.** prostate
____ **8.** mucous membrane lining of the uterus		**H.** mons pubis
____ **9.** early or developing stage of any organism		**I.** fimbriae
____**10.** secretion discharged by male reproductive organ		**J.** endocervix
____**11.** developing human beginning with ninth week		**K.** cervix
____**12.** fingerlike processes at ends of fallopian (uterine) tubes		**L.** ova
____**13.** interior of cervix		**M.** testis
____**14.** foreskin of penis		**N.** embryo
____**15.** pad of fat in front of symphysis pubis		**O.** vulva
____**16.** external female genitalia		**P.** prepuce
____**17.** elastic muscular tube below cervix, extending to body exterior		**Q.** vagina
____**18.** saclike male structure		**R.** vas deferens
____**19.** walnut-size, doughnut-shaped male gland		**S.** areola
____**20.** neck of uterus		**T.** fetus

Exercise 8: Give the meaning of the components in the following words and then define the word as a whole. Suffixes meaning *pertaining to* or *state or condition*, shown following a slash mark (/), are not to be defined separately. Before reaching for your medical dictionary, check the glossary at the end of the chapter.

1. Pyuria:

py _____

ur/ia _____

_____

2. Ovotestis:

ovo _____

testis _____

_____

3. Metrosalpingitis:

metro _____

salping _____

itis _____

_____

4. Hematometra:

hemato _____

metra _____

_____

5. Oophorosalpingitis:

oophoro _____

salping _____

itis _____

_____

6. Metrocolpocele:

metro _____

colpo _____

cele _____

_____

7. Episiotomy:

episio _____

tomy _____

_____

8. Hysterolaparotomy:

hystero _____

laparo _____

tomy _____

_____

9. Oophorohysterectomy:

oophoro _____

hyster _____

ectomy _____

_____

10. Balanitis:

balan _____

itis _____

_____

11. Nephropyelitis:

nephro _____

pyel _____

itis _____

_____

12. Pyelitis:

pyel _____

itis _____

_____

Chapter 12 Crossword Puzzle

Across

3. the longer ureter
5. union of ovum and sperm
8. cluster of capillary channels
10. human chorionic gonadotropin
12. a tube that excretes urine
13. rupture of graafian follicle
14. fluid in which embryo floats
16. foreskin
17. finger-like processes
22. upper portion of uterus
23. where urine collects
25. stores urine
26. mammaries
27. halo of pigment around nipple
29. combining form meaning kidney

Down

1. menopause
2. concave depression on kidney
4. minute formations embedded in ovary surface
5. uterine tube(s)
6. wrinkles or ridges in bladder
7. male sex hormone
9. female reproductive organs
11. root meaning kidney
12. tubes carrying urine to storage
15. onset of menstruation
18. internal part of kidney
19. menstrual period
20. root for uterus
21. functional unit of kidney
24. female sex cells
28. openings from cervix to canal and canal to vagina

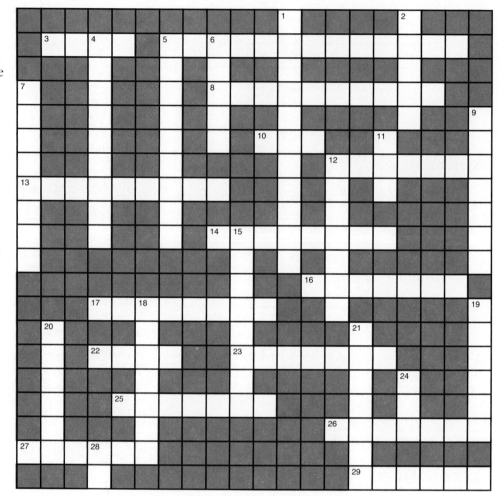

Chapter 12 Hidden Words Puzzle

```
R  K  M  U  T  S  K  R  U  S  B  S  C  K  U  Q  C  G  W  R  J  L  N
N  Y  Q  N  D  D  Y  L  E  P  F  C  I  U  S  P  V  X  S  T  H  A  M
R  F  P  T  E  A  C  M  B  N  Q  M  A  M  M  A  R  Y  S  D  R  I  H
D  R  N  K  U  P  Y  Y  L  X  A  B  S  P  J  U  M  E  A  T  U  S  R
E  K  T  V  U  I  H  O  C  P  E  L  V  I  S  O  U  F  P  B  C  B  E
F  Q  R  R  U  X  X  R  C  A  V  E  R  N  O  U  S  D  G  U  H  W  E
O  P  H  I  P  D  H  N  O  T  C  M  T  L  C  I  L  C  X  U  C  Q  X
H  C  R  Z  S  M  X  M  N  N  G  E  S  T  R  O  G  E  N  B  F  E  Y
D  U  C  O  H  T  H  K  V  B  M  M  R  P  P  L  R  P  I  K  N  I  U
F  I  I  U  S  N  T  Y  O  B  O  B  M  V  N  L  I  T  E  S  T  E  S
V  X  E  R  L  T  J  I  L  P  Y  R  A  M  I  D  S  X  E  T  O  Q  L
Y  Z  N  P  D  M  A  H  U  D  Q  A  B  P  I  X  S  Y  L  X  Y  L  E
Z  E  U  S  V  N  D  T  T  P  Q  N  T  S  B  U  G  U  O  L  B  M  R
C  O  R  P  U  S  C  L  E  N  D  O  M  E  T  R  I  U  M  V  A  K  S
S  L  C  Y  F  O  D  V  D  P  K  U  T  P  D  P  K  A  D  E  I  V  I
C  O  L  U  Y  C  N  W  C  B  I  S  F  J  B  F  R  E  B  W  R  J  E
T  P  D  U  J  O  G  R  J  B  D  D  S  U  M  K  R  W  M  Y  O  V  K
F  H  Q  C  B  G  L  Y  U  W  N  U  I  B  A  B  L  H  O  G  U  U  G
H  J  C  N  I  X  Q  I  U  D  E  L  I  D  A  F  J  K  P  G  Z  I  N
L  Q  T  F  Q  P  K  W  E  R  Y  L  G  Y  Y  X  H  K  U  Q  M  X  C
S  A  H  I  C  Q  M  Q  N  Q  S  A  S  O  U  M  V  Q  Y  O  Y  M  B
M  W  S  N  A  S  E  M  I  E  V  T  R  W  S  I  I  R  G  U  B  E  E
H  V  Y  H  N  V  J  G  K  W  H  N  T  K  D  D  P  S  F  U  V  Q  D
```

Can you find the 20 words hidden in this puzzle?

ENDOMETRIUM	CONVOLUTED	EPIDIDYMIS	MEMBRANOUS
CAVERNOUS	CORPUSCLE	ESTROGEN	PROSTATE
PYRAMIDS	CAPSULE	KIDNEYS	MAMMARY
NEPHRON	PREPUCE	CERVIX	CORTEX
MEATUS	PELVIS	TESTES	RENAL

CHAPTER 12 ANSWERS

Exercise 1
1. kidneys, ureters, bladder, urethra
2. cortex
3. medulla
4. major and minor calices
5. nephron
6. glomerulus, Bowman's
7. ureters
8. bladder
9. pH
10. ureteral orifice

Exercise 2
1. cortex
2. hilus
3. renal artery
4. renal pelvis
5. renal vein
6. ureter
7. renal pyramid
8. renal column
9. calyx (calix)
10. papilla
11. capsule

Exercise 3
1. ducts, glands, supporting structures
2. penis, scrotum, spermatic cords
3. spermatozoon or sperm cell
4. testosterone
5. fallopian (uterine) tubes, uterus, vagina, vulva, mammaries (breasts)
6. urethra
7. ovulation, hormonal secretion
8. menstruation (menses)
9. menopause (climacteric)
10. ova

Exercise 4
1. right common iliac artery and vein
2. rectum
3. seminal vesicle
4. ejaculatory duct
5. duct of bulbourethral gland
6. bulb of urethra
7. epididymis
8. testis
9. urinary bladder
10. vas deferens
11. symphysis pubis
12. prostate gland
13. urethra
14. corpus spongiosum
15. corpus cavernosum
16. glans

Exercise 5
1. fallopian, or uterine, tubes
2. fimbriated extremity
3. ovary
4. ovarian ligament
5. body of uterus
6. cervical canal of uterus
7. external os
8. vagina
9. corpus luteum
10. Graafian follicle

Exercise 6
1. sphincter ani
2. rectum
3. ovary
4. fallopian, or uterine, tube
5. uterus
6. bladder
7. symphysis pubis
8. urethra
9. labia majora
10. vagina

Exercise 7
1. B
2. R
3. M
4. E
5. D
6. L
7. S
8. F
9. N
10. C
11. T
12. I
13. J
14. P
15. H
16. O
17. Q
18. A
19. G
20. K

Exercise 8
1. pyuria: pus; urine—pus in the urine
2. ovotestis: ovary; testis—gonad containing both ovarian and testicular tissue
3. metrosalpingitis: uterus; fallopian, or uterine, tube; inflammation—inflammation of uterus and fallopian, or uterine, tube
4. hematometra: blood; uterus—accumulation of blood in the uterus
5. oophorosalpingitis: ovary; fallopian, or uterine, tube; inflammation—inflammation of ovary and fallopian, or uterine, tube
6. metrocolpocele: uterus; vagina; hernia—herniation of uterus into vagina
7. episiotomy: vulva; incision—surgical incision of vulval orifice for obstetric purposes
8. hysterolaparotomy: uterus; abdomen; incision—surgical incision of uterus through abdominal wall
9. oophorohysterectomy: ovary; uterus; removal—removal or excision of ovary or ovaries, and uterus
10. balanitis: glans penis; inflammation—inflammation of glans penis
11. nephropyelitis: kidney; kidney pelvis; inflammation—inflammation of kidney and its pelvis
12. pyelitis: kidney pelvis; inflammation—inflammation of kidney pelvis

Answers: Chapter 12 Crossword Puzzle

```
                                  1:C               2:H
        3:L  E  F  T     5:F  6:  F  E  R  T  I  L  I  Z  A  T  I  O  N
                4:O       A   U           I              L
     7:A         L        L  8:G  L  O  M  E  R  U  L  U  S        9:O
        N         L        L     A                    S              V
        D         I        O     E   10:H  C  G     11:R              A
        R         C        P         T        12:U   R  E  T  H  R  A
    13:O  V  U  L  A  T  I  O  N            E      R        N        R
        G         E        A        R      E                        I
        E         S        N     14:A 15:M  N  I  O  T  I  C        E
        N                        E      C              E           S
                                 N    16:P  R  E  P  U  C  E
             17:F  I  M  B  R  I  A  E        S              19:M
        20:H        18:E        R        21:N              E
        Y      22:B  O  D  Y     23:C  A  L  Y  C  E  S        N
        S         U           H           P     24:O        S
        T      25:B  L  A  D  D  E  R        H     V        E
        E         L              26:B  R  E  A  S  T  S
    27:A  R  E 28:O  L  A              O
        S         S           29:N  E  P  H  R  O
```

Answers: Chapter 12 Hidden Words Puzzle

```
.   .   .   .   .   .   R   .   .   .   .   .   .   .   .   .   .   .   .
.   .   N   .   .   .   E   .   .   C   .   .   .   P   .   .   .   .   .
.   .   .   E   .   .   .   N   .   M   A   M   M   A   R   Y   .   .   .   .
.   .   .   .   P   .   .   .   A   .   P   .   .   M   E   A   T   U   S   .
.   .   .   .   .   H   .   .   P   E   L   V   I   S   .   .   .   P   .   .
.   .   .   .   .   .   R   C   A   V   E   R   N   O   U   S   .   .   U   .
.   P   .   .   .   .   .   O   .   C   M   .   .   C   .   L   .   .   C   .
.   .   R   .   .   .   .   N   N   .   E   S   T   R   O   G   E   N   .   .   E
.   .   .   O   .   .   .   V   .   .   M   R   .   .   R   .   .   .   .   .
.   .   .   .   S   .   .   O   .   .   B   .   V   .   .   .   T   E   S   T   E   S
.   .   .   .   .   .   T   .   L   P   Y   R   A   M   I   D   S   .   E   .   .   .
.   .   .   .   .   .   A   .   U   .   A   .   .   X   .   .   .   .   X   .
.   .   .   .   .   .   T   T   .   N   .   .   .   .   .   .   .   .   .
C   O   R   P   U   S   C   L   E   N   D   O   M   E   T   R   I   U   M   .   .   .
.   .   .   .   .   .   .   D   P   K   U   .   .   .   .   .   .   .   .
.   .   .   .   .   .   .   I   S   .   .   .   .   .   .
.   .   .   .   .   .   .   D   D   .   .   .   .   .
.   .   .   .   .   .   .   N   .   I   .   .   .   .
.   .   .   .   .   .   .   E   .   .   D   .   .   .
.   .   .   .   .   .   .   Y   .   .   Y   .   .   .
.   .   .   .   .   .   .   S   .   .   .   M   .   .
.   .   .   .   .   .   .   .   .   .   .   I   .   .
.   .   .   .   .   .   .   .   .   .   S   .   .   .
```

Words:

- > ENDOMETRIUM
- > CAVERNOUS
- > PYRAMIDS
- \ NEPHRON
- > MEATUS
- ∨ CONVOLUTED
- > CORPUSCLE
- \ CAPSULE
- \ PREPUCE
- > PELVIS
- \ EPIDIDYMIS
- > ESTROGEN
- ∨ KIDNEYS
- \ CERVIX
- > TESTES
- ∨ MEMBRANOUS
- \ PROSTATE
- > MAMMARY
- \ CORTEX
- \ RENAL

CHAPTER 12 GLOSSARY

Urinary Tract Organs and Related Anatomic Terms

bladder: elastic musculomembranous sac for storing urine.

Bowman's capsule: the glomerular capsule of the kidney containing the cluster of capillary channels (*glomerulus*).

calyx or **calix** (ka′liks): urine-collecting, irregular saclike structure of the renal pelvis.

collecting tubules: terminal collection passages that carry urine to the renal pelvis.

distal convoluted tubules: portion of the convoluted tubules between Henle's loop and the collecting tubules.

glomerulus: coils of capillaries within Bowman's capsule (plural—***glomeruli***).

Henle's loop: U-shaped turn in a convoluted tubule of the kidney, located between the proximal and distal ends, with both ascending and descending limbs.

hilus: concave depression on medial margin of the kidney through which the ureters, blood vessels, and nerves enter.

kidneys: two glandular bodies that filter blood and secrete urine.

nephron (nef′ron): functional and structural unit of the kidney, including a renal corpuscle and a renal tubule.

renal corpuscle: glomerular or Bowman's capsule (also called ***Malpighian corpuscle***).

renal cortex (kor′teks): outer part of the kidney, extending between the renal pyramids to form the renal columns.

renal medulla: inner part of the kidney composed of conical structures, called renal pyramids.

renal papillae: the narrow, conical ends of renal pyramids.

renal pelvis: the reservoir that collects urine, made up of the major and minor calices.

renal pyramid: see ***renal medulla***.

renal sinus: kidney cavity containing renal pelvis, blood vessels, nerves and fat.

renal tubule: minute tubule of the kidney that secretes, collects and transports urine, and forms part of the functional unit, the nephron (also called ***uriniferous tubule***).

uresis: normal passage of urine.

ureter: tube that carries urine from the kidney to the bladder.

urethra: tube that carries urine from the bladder to the surface of the body.

Pathologic Conditions of the Urinary Tract

Inflammations and Infections

balanitis (bal″ah-ni′tis): inflammation of the glans penis.

cystitis: bladder inflammation.

glomerulonephritis (glo-mer″u-lo-ne-fri′tis): kidney disease with inflammation of the glomeruli, not caused by a kidney infection.

nephritis (ne-fri′tis): inflammation of the kidneys.

nephrotuberculosis: tuberculosis of the kidney.

perinephritis (per″i-ne-fri′tis): inflammation of tissues surrounding the kidney.

pyelitis (pi″e-li′tis): inflammation of the kidney pelvis.

pyelocystitis (pi″e-lo-sis-ti′tis): inflammation of the kidney pelvis and bladder.

pyelonephritis (pi″e-lo-ne-fri′tis): inflammation of the kidney caused by infection (also called ***nephropyelitis***).

pyonephritis (pi″o-ne-fri′tis): pus-producing inflammation of the kidney.

pyonephrosis (pi″o-ne-fro′sis): presence of pus in the kidney causing distention, usually because of obstruction.

ureteritis (u″re-ter-i′tis): inflammation of a ureter.

ureteropyelitis (u-re″ter-o-pi-e-li′tis): inflammation of a ureter and its kidney pelvis (also called ***ureteropyelonephritis***).

ureteropyosis (u-re″ter-o-pi-o′sis): presence of pus in the ureter.

urethritis (u″re-thri′tis): inflammation of the urethra.

urethrocystitis (u-re″thro-sis-ti′tis): inflammation of the urethra and bladder.

Hereditary, Congenital, and Developmental Disorders

epispadias (ep″i-spa′de-as): urethral opening on dorsum of penis (*spadias* refers to cleft).

fused kidney: one single kidney resulting from fusion during development.

horseshoe kidney: fusion of the adjacent developing poles of the kidney so that the concavity formed faces upward, resembling a horseshoe.

hypospadias (hi″po-spa′de-as): urethra opens on the under surface of the penis or on the perineum.

renal ectopia: displaced kidney.

supernumerary kidney: developmental anomaly, with more than the normal two kidneys.

Other Abnormalities

albuminuria: presence of albumin and other proteins in the urine.

anuria: lack of urine being excreted (also called *anuresis*).

arteriolar nephrosclerosis (nef″ro-skle-ro′sis): scarring of the kidney caused by hypertension (also called *nephroangiosclerosis*).

azotemia (az″o-te′me-ah): presence of urea or other nitrogenous elements in the blood.

blennorrhea (blen″o-re′ah): excess mucus discharge from the urethra or vagina (also called *blennorrhagia*).

cylindruria (sil″in-droo′re-ah): presence of cylindrical casts in the urine.

cystocele: hernia of the urinary bladder through the vaginal wall.

dysuria: painful or difficult urination.

glycosuria: presence of sugar in the urine (also called *glucosuria* or *glycuresis*).

hematuria: presence of blood in the urine.

hydronephrosis (hi″dro-ne-fro′sis): distention of the kidney caused by an obstruction of the ureter.

hypercalciuria (hi″per-kal′si-u′re-ah): excessive calcium in the urine.

incontinence (in-kon′ti-nens): inability to control urination.

nephrolith (nef′ro-lith): kidney stone.

nephrolithiasis (nef″ro-li-thi′ah-sis): condition characterized by the presence of kidney stones (*renal calculi*).

nephromalacia (nef″ro-mah-la′she-ah): softening of the kidney.

nephromegaly (nef″ro-meg′ah-le): enlargement of the kidney.

nephroptosis (nef″rop-to′sis): downward displacement of the kidney.

nephrorrhagia (nef″ro-ra′je-ah): hemorrhage into or from the kidney.

nephrosis (ne-fro′sis): any disease of the kidney.

oliguria: scanty urine output.

phosphaturia (fos″fat-u′re-ah): excess of phosphates excreted in the urine.

polycystic kidney disease (PKD): multiple cysts of the kidney.

polyuria: excessive urination.

pyelonephrosis (pi″e-lo-ne-fro′sis): any disease of the kidney pelvis.

pyuria: pus in the urine.

renal colic: pain due to passage of a calculus in the kidney or ureter.

renal infarction: ischemia of kidney due to thrombus or embolus.

retention: keeping within the body a substance that is usually excreted, such as urine.

uraturia: excess of urates in the urine.

uremia: disturbed kidney function in which products of protein metabolism are found in the blood and produce a toxic condition.

ureteralgia: pain in the ureter.

ureterectasis (u-re″ter-ek′tah-sis): dilation of the ureter.

ureterolith (u-re′ter-o-lith): stone in the ureter.

ureterolithiasis (u-re″ter-o-li-thi′ah-sis): formation of a stone in a ureter.

ureterolysis (u-re″ter-ol′i-sis): rupture or paralysis of a ureter.

ureterorrhagia (u-re″ter-o-ra′je-ah): hemorrhage of a ureter.

ureterostenosis (u-re″ter-o-ste-no′sis): ureteral stricture.

urethralgia: pain in the urethra (also called *urethrodynia*).

urethremphraxis (u″re-threm-frak′sis): obstruction of the urethra.

urethrorrhagia (u-re″thro-ra′je-ah): urethral bleeding (also called *urethremorrhagia*).

urethrorrhea (u-re″thro-re′ah): abnormal urethral discharge.

urethrostaxis (u-re″thro-stak′sis): urethral oozing of blood.

urinary calculus (kal′ku-lus): stone or concretion in the kidney, ureter, or bladder.

Oncology*

The following list pertains specifically to tumors of the urinary system. Other tumors, both benign and malignant, occur in other parts of the body as well as the urinary system. Some of these are epidermoid carcinoma, sarcoma, fibrosarcoma, liposarcoma, leiomyoma, leiomyosarcoma, myxoma, myxosarcoma, and papillary carcinoma.

adenomyosarcoma*: malignant tumor of the kidneys in young children (also called *Wilms' tumor*, *nephroblastoma*, and *embryoma of the kidney*).

renal cell carcinoma*: malignancy of the kidneys invading all essential parts and frequently metastasizing (also called *hypernephroid carcinoma*).

transitional cell carcinoma*: malignancy chiefly affecting the urinary bladder, ureters, and renal pelvis, arising from a transitional type of stratified epithelium.

Surgical and Other Procedures

cystectomy: total or partial resection of the bladder.

cystendesis: suturing of a wound of the urinary bladder.

*Indicates a malignant condition.

cystidolaparotomy (sis″ti-do-lap″ah-rot′o-me): incision of the bladder through the abdominal wall.

cystidotrachelotomy (sis″ti-do-tra-kel-ot′o-me): incision of the neck of the urinary bladder (also called **cystotrachelotomy** and **cystauchenotomy**).

cystolithectomy (sis″to-li-thek′to-me): removal of a stone by incising the urinary bladder (also called **cystolithotomy**).

cystopexy (sis′to-pek″se): surgical fixation of the urinary bladder to a supporting structure such as the abdominal wall.

cystoplasty: plastic repair of the bladder.

cystoproctostomy: surgical communication of the posterior bladder wall to the rectum (also called **cystorectostomy**).

cystorrhaphy (sis-tor-ah-fe): suturing of the urinary bladder.

cystostomy: creation of an opening into the bladder.

cystotomy: incision into the urinary bladder.

hemodialysis: in cases of kidney failure, cleansing of waste from blood, using a dialysis machine, which filters the blood through a semipermeable membrane.

lithotripsy: the use of shock waves to crush kidney stones, as a substitute for surgical removal.

nephrectomy (ne-frek′to-me): excision of a kidney.

nephrocapsectomy (nef″ro-kap-sek′to-me): excision of the renal capsule.

nephrocystanastomosis (nef″ro-sist″ah-nas″to-mo′sis): formation of a passage between the kidney and the urinary bladder due to ureteral obstruction.

nephrolithotomy (nef″ro-li-thot′o-me): removal of a kidney stone by incising the kidney.

nephropexy (nef′ro-pek″se): fixation of a floating kidney.

nephropyelolithotomy (nef″ro-pi″e-lo-li′thot′o-me): incising the substance of the kidney to remove a stone from its pelvis.

nephrorrhaphy (nef-ror′ah-fe): suturing the kidney.

nephrosplenopexy (nef″ro-sple′no-pek″se): fixation of the kidney and the spleen.

nephrostomy (ne-fros′to-me): creation of a permanent passage leading directly into the kidney pelvis.

nephrotomy (ne-frot′o-me): incision into the kidney.

nephrotresis (nef″ro-tre′sis): creating a passage into the kidney by stitching the parietal muscles to the edges of the kidney incision.

nephroureterectomy: excision of the kidney and all or part of the ureter.

nephroureterocystectomy (nef″ro-u-re″ter-o-sis-tek′to-me): excision of the kidney, ureter, and a section of the wall of the bladder.

pyelocystostomosis (pi″e-lo-sis″to-sto-mo′sis): creation of a passage between the renal pelvis and the bladder (also called **pyelocystanastomosis**).

pyelolithotomy (pi″e-lo-li′thot′o-me): excision of a stone from the kidney pelvis.

pyeloplasty (pi′e-lo-plas″te): repair of the pelvis of the kidney.

pyelostomy: creation of an opening into the pelvis of the kidney to temporarily divert urine away from the ureter.

pyelotomy: incision of the renal pelvis.

pyeloureterolysis (pi″e-lo-u-re″ter-ol′i-sis): removal of adhesions near the attachment of the ureter and the renal pelvis.

pyeloureteroplasty: plastic repair of the kidney pelvis and ureter.

ureterectomy: removal of all or part of a ureter.

ureterocolostomy (u-re″ter-o-ko-los′to-me): transplantation of the ureter into the colon.

ureterocystanastomosis (u-re″ter-o-sis″tah-nas″to-mo′sis): creation of a new attachment between a ureter and the bladder (also called **ureterocystoneostomy**, **ureteroneocystostomy**, **ureterocystostomy**, and **ureterovesicostomy**).

ureteroenteroanastomosis (u-re″ter-o-en″ter-o-ah-nas″to-mo′sis): formation of an attachment between the ureter and the intestine (also called **ureteroenterostomy**).

ureterolithotomy (u-re″ter-o-li-thot′o-me): surgical incision for the removal of a calculus from the ureter.

ureterolysis: freeing up of a ureter from adhesions or surrounding disease.

ureteroneopyelostomy (u-re″ter-o-ne″o-pi″e-los′to-me): excision of a urethral stricture and creation of an opening into the kidney pelvis for insertion of the newly formed end of the ureter (also called **ureteropelvioneostomy**).

ureteronephrectomy (u-re″ter-o-ne-frek′tome): excision of an entire kidney and its ureter.

ureteroplasty (u-re″ter-o-plast″te): plastic repair of a ureter to widen a stricture.

ureteroproctostomy (u-re″ter-o-prok-tos′to-me): creation of an attachment between the ureter and the lower part of the rectum (also called **ureterorectoneostomy** and **ureterorectostomy**).

ureteropyeloneostomy (u-re″ter-o-pi″elo-ne-os′to-me): creation of a new passage to the ureter from the kidney pelvis (also called **ureteropyelostomy**).

ureteropyelonephrostomy (u-re″ter-o-pi″e-lo-ne-fros′to-me): surgical creation of an attachment between the kidney pelvis and the ureter.

ureteropyeloplasty: repair of the ureter and renal pelvis.

ureterorrhaphy (u″re-ter-or′ah-fe): suturing a fistula of the ureter.

ureterosigmoidostomy: insertion and attachment of the ureter into the sigmoid flexure.

ureterostomy (u″re-ter-os′to-me): creation of a passage by which a ureter may discharge its contents.

ureterotomy: incision of a ureter.

ureterotrigonoenterostomy (u-re″ter-o-tri-go″no-en″ter-os′to-me): a ureter and a portion of its surrounding bladder wall, at its terminal point, is inserted and attached into the intestine.

ureterotrigonosigmoidostomy (u-re″tero-tri-go″no-sig″moid-os-′to-me): a ureter and a portion of its surrounding bladder wall, at its terminal point, is inserted and attached into the sigmoid flexure.

ureteroureterostomy (u-re″ter-o-u-re″ter-os′to-me): surgical end-to-end attachment of two parts of a transected ureter.

urethrectomy: excision of all or part of the urethra.

urethrocystopexy (u-re″thro-sis′to-pek″se): fixation of the junction between the urethra and bladder and the bladder area above, to the back of the pubic bones, to relieve stress incontinence.

urethroplasty: plastic repair of the urethra for a wound or defect.

urethrorrhaphy (u″re-thror′ah-fe): suturing of the urethra to close a urethral fistula.

urethrostomy: creation of an opening passage into the urethra to relieve a stricture.

urethrotomy: cutting of the urethra to relieve a stricture.

Laboratory Tests and Procedures for the Urinary System

Addis count: urine test to determine presence of kidney disease.

antideoxyribonuclease B: blood test to determine the presence of a specific kidney disease, poststreptococcal glomerulonephritis.

catheterized urine specimen: obtaining a urine specimen under sterile conditions, to check for microorganisms in the urinary system.

computerized tomography (CT): imaging device using X-rays at multiple angles through specific sections of the body, analyzed by computer to provide a total picture of the part being examined (also called **computerized axial tomography [CAT]**).

concentration test: to determine the kidney's ability to concentrate and dilute urine.

creatinine test: urine test for creatinine, a metabolic product elevated in kidney function disturbance.

creatinine clearance, endogenous: measure of the rate at which the kidneys remove creatinine from the blood, to evaluate kidney function.

cystogram: X-ray study of the bladder.

cystoscope: fiberoptic endoscope to examine the interior of the bladder.

Diodrast clearance: used to evaluate kidney function: a blood test to determine the rate at which an injected substance is removed from the blood by the kidneys; and a urine test to determine the rate of excretion of the injected substance by the kidneys.

glucose: urine test using paper strips impregnated with enzymes to determine the presence of glucose in the urine (for example, Clinistix, Diastix, or Tes-Tape).

hemoglobin: urine test to determine the presence of hemoglobin in the urine, indicating an abnormal condition or disease of the genitourinary tract.

intravenous pyelogram (IVP): X-ray record of the kidneys and urinary tract after intravenous injection of a dye substance.

magnetic resonance imaging (MRI): noninvasive method of scanning the body by use of an electromagnetic field and radio waves, which provides visual images on a computer screen and magnetic tape recordings (also called **nuclear magnetic resonance [NMR]**).

nuclear magnetic resonance (NMR): see **magnetic resonance imaging**.

renal angiography and arteriography: x-ray studies of the blood vessels surrounding the kidneys, the renal artery, and related blood vessels, after the injection of a contrast medium.

renal scan: x-ray scan using intravenous injection of a radioactive substance to determine the size, shape, and exact location of the kidneys, and to diagnose abnormalities.

retrograde pyelogram: x-ray record of the kidneys and urinary tract, using injection of a contrast medium directly into the bladder.

total volume: measurement of urine excreted in a 24-hour period, to evaluate kidney function.

Male Reproductive Organs and Related Anatomic Terms

bulbourethral glands: glands located on either side of the urethra whose alkaline secretion has a protective function for sperm (also called **Cowper's glands**).

corpora cavernosa penis (kor′po-rah kav″er-no′sah): columns of erectile tissue of the penis, forming the sides and posterior portion that attaches to the pubic bone.

corpus spongiosum penis (kor′pus spun″je-o′sum): column of erectile tissue surrounding the urethra.

ejaculatory ducts: two short tubes formed by the joining of the vas deferens and the ducts of the seminal vesicles, which pass through the prostate and extend to the urethra.

epididymis (ep″i-did′i-mis): pair of tightly coiled tubelike structures that secrete a part of the semen, serve as storage areas for sperm before ejaculation, and provide passageways for sperm from the testes to the body surface (plural—**epididymides**).

glans penis: slight bulge at the distal end of the penis.

Leydig's cells (li′digz): specialized interstitial cells that secrete the male sex hormone testosterone.

penis: the male sex organ, containing the urethra, which carries both reproductive tract secretions and urine to the body surface.

prepuce (pre′puse): retractible, double fold of skin, covering the glans penis (also called *foreskin*).

prostate: doughnut-shaped, walnut-sized gland surrounding the urethra, secreting a thick alkaline substance that makes up most of the seminal fluid.

scrotum (skro′tum): saclike, skin-covered structure, hanging from the perineal area, containing the testes, epididymides, and part of the spermatic cords.

semen: thick, whitish secretion discharged by the male reproductive organs, containing the spermatozoa.

seminal vesicles: two twisted pouches lying along the lower posterior surface of the bladder, in front of the rectum, which secrete the liquid part of semen, and prostaglandins.

seminiferous tubules (se″mi-nif′er-us): coiled tubules within the testes that produce sperm cells.

Sertoli's cells (ser″to′lez): cells in the testis that support and nourish the sperm germ cells.

spermatic cords: white, fibrous tissue encasing the vas deferens, blood and lymph vessels, and nerves.

spermatid (sper′mah-tid): germ cell developing into a spermatozoon (also called *spermatoblast*).

spermatozoa (sper″mah-to-zo′ah): male reproductive (sperm) cells (singular—*spermatozoon*).

testis (tes′tis): egg-shaped male gland (also called *testicle*), that produces spermatozoa and secretes hormones (*orchis* refers to testis).

vas deferens: excretory duct of the testis that joins the epididymis with the ejaculatory duct (also called *ductus deferens*).

Female Reproductive Organs and Related Anatomic Terms

areola (ah-re′o-lah): pigmented halo around the breast nipple.

Bartholin's glands (bar′to-linz): two pea-sized glands, one on each side of the vaginal orifice, which secrete a lubricant (also called *greater vestibular glands*).

cervix (ser′viks): neck of the uterus.

climacteric: menopause.

clitoris (kli′to-ris): small mound of erectile tissue located beneath the point of union of the labia minora, similar to the penis, and also covered with a prepuce.

corpus (kor′pus): body (plural—*corpora*).

corpus cavernosum clitoridis (ka-ver-no′sum kli-tor′id-is): one of the two columns of erectile tissue that form the clitoris.

corpus luteum (lu′te-um): yellow body formed by the graafian follicle that has discharged its ovum (*luteum* means yellow).

ectopic pregnancy (ek-top′ik): fertilized ovum implanted outside uterus, most commonly in a uterine tube (*ectopic* means out of normal position).

endocervix: mucous membrane lining the cervical canal and/or the opening of the cervix into the uterus.

endometrium (en-do-me′tre-um): mucous membrane lining the uterus.

estrus: cyclical period relating to sexual activity.

fallopian tubes: pair of tubes extending from the uterus to the ovary on each side, which pick up and convey expelled ova to the uterus (also called *uterine tubes* and *oviducts*).

fimbriae (fim′bre-aye): finger-like processes at the ends of the fallopian (uterine) tubes over the ovaries.

graafian follicles (graf′e-an): mature ovarian follicles.

hymen: fold of mucous membrane partially blocking vaginal orifice.

labia majora (la′be-ah ma-jo′rah): two folds of skin that extend backward from the mons pubis.

labia minora: two smaller folds of thin-skinned mucus membrane within the labia majora.

mammary glands: breasts (also called *mammae*).

menopause (men′o-pawz): cessation of menstruation (also called *climacteric*).

menstruation (men″stroo-a′shun): flow of blood, tissue, and other secretions, evacuated through vagina, occurring monthly, after puberty, when an ovum has not been fertilized (*mensis* means month).

mons pubis (monz pu′bus): pad of fat located in front of the symphysis pubis.

myometrium (mi-o-me′tre-um): middle, muscular coat of the uterus.

os: mouth; the *internal os* is the opening from the cervix into the cervical canal, and the *external os* is the opening from the cervical canal into the vagina.

ovary: female gland that produces ova or eggs.

ovum: female reproductive cell (plural—*ova*).

pudendum (pu-den′dum): human external genitalia, especially referring to females.

Skene's gland (skenz): two ducts just within the meatus of the urethra that drain a particular group of glands into the vestibule (also called *paraurethral glands*).

uterus: thick-walled, hollow, pear-shaped organ in the pelvic cavity of the female, that houses and nourishes the embryo and fetus.

Pregnancy and Related Anatomic Terms

amnion (am'ne-on): membrane containing the fetus floating in amniotic fluid.

chorion (ko're-on): outermost layer of the fertilized ovum that helps form the placenta.

cyesis (si-e'sis): pregnancy (**cyema** means embryo).

decidua (de-sid'u-ah): mucosa of the uterus thrown off after birth.

ectoderm: outer of three germ layers of the embryo.

embryo: developing stage of an organism, from the second through the eighth week in humans.

endoderm: innermost of three germ layers of the embryo (also called **entoderm**).

fetus: developing offspring, from the end of the eighth week until birth in humans.

gravid (grav'id): pregnant.

gravida (grav'i-dah): pregnant female, referred to as gravida I in the first pregnancy, gravida II in the second pregnancy, and so forth.

lactiferous ducts (lak-tif'er-us): ducts that carry the milk secretions of the breast to and through the nipples (also called **galactophorous ducts**).

mesoderm: middle of three germ layers of the embryo, lying between the ectoderm and the endoderm.

neonate: newborn.

omphalus (om'fah-lus): see **umbilicus**.

para: female who has produced living young (para I, para II, and para III designate one, two, and three pregnancies, respectively, and so forth.)

parturition (par"tu-rish'un): process of giving birth.

placenta (plah-sen'tah): vascular fetal organ within the uterus that connects the fetus to the mother by way of the umbilical cord, for the exchange of nutrients, oxygen, antibodies, and waste products.

presentation: the presenting part of the fetus, at birth.

primigravida: female in her first pregnancy (also called **gravida I**).

primipara: female who has had one pregnancy that resulted in viable young or who is giving birth for the first time (also called **para I**).

umbilical cord: communicating channel between the placenta and fetus.

umbilicus (um-bil'i-kus): scar that marks the site of the connection of the umbilical cord in the fetus (also called **navel** and **omphalus**).

zygote (zi-got): fertilized ovum.

Pathologic Conditions of the Male and Female Reproductive Systems

Inflammation and Infections

bartholinitis: inflammation of Bartholin's gland.

cellulitis: inflammation of the cellular or connective tissues of the pelvic area.

cervicitis: inflammation of the mucous membrane tissues of the uterine cervix, with frequent involvement of deeper tissues.

chronic cystic mastitis: inflammation of the breast with fluid-filled cyst formation (also called **fibrocystic disease of the breast**).

decidual endometritis (de-sid'u-al en"do-me-tri'tis): inflammation of the decidual endometrial membranes of the uterus during pregnancy.

endometritis (en'do-me-tri'tis): inflammation of the endometrium.

epididymitis: inflammation of the epididymis.

mammillitis (mam"i-li'tis): inflammation of the nipple.

mastadenitis (mas"tad-e-ni'tis): inflammation of the breast (also called **mastitis**).

metritis (me-tri'tis): inflammation of the uterus.

metroperitonitis (me"tro-per'i-ti-ni'tis): inflammation of the peritoneum around the uterus.

metrophlebitis (me"tro-fle-bi'tis): inflammation of the uterine veins.

metrosalpingitis (me"tro-sal"pin-ji'tis): inflammation of the uterus and fallopian tubes.

myometritis (mi"o-me-tri'tis): inflammation of the uterine wall muscles.

oophoritis (o"of-o-ri'tis): ovarian inflammation.

oophorosalpingitis (o-of'o-ro-sal"pin-ji'tis): inflammation of an ovary and fallopian tube.

orchitis: inflammation of the testicles.

perioophoritis: inflammation of the covering of the ovary.

priapism: persistent erection of penis, related to excessive amounts of androgens or to disease.

priapitis: inflammation of penis.

prostatitis: inflammation of the prostate gland.

pyocolpos (pi"o-kol'pos): accumulation of pus in the vagina.

pyometra (pi"o-me'trah): collection of pus in the uterine cavity.

pyosalpinx (pi"o-sal'pinks): accumulation of pus in a fallopian tube.

salpingitis (sal"pin-ji'tis): fallopian tube inflammation.

seminal vesiculitis: seminal vesicle inflammation.

vaginitis: inflammation of the vagina.

vulvitis: inflammation of the vulva.

Sexually Transmitted Diseases (STD)

This category covers diseases transmitted by sexual contact, formerly referred to as venereal diseases

acquired immune deficiency syndrome (AIDS): see Chapter 16.

bacterial vaginitis: vaginal infection caused by *Hemophilus vaginalis* or *Gardnerella vaginalis*, characterized by discharge, itching and pain on urination.

chlamydia: highly contagious, common infection, caused by *Chlamydia trachomatis* bacterium. A major cause of infection of the cervix and fallopian tubes, which, if untreated, may result in pelvic inflammatory disease (PID). Also may be transmitted to newborns in the birth canal, resulting in eye and ear, and possibly fatal lung, infections.

condyloma acuminatum (kon″di-lo′mah ah-ku″mi-nah′tum): infectious wart or papilloma caused by the *human papilloma virus (HPV)*, a common STD source (see ***carcinoma of cervix***), usually found on the external genitalia, cervix, vagina, or anus (also called ***venereal wart*** and ***genital wart***).

genital candidiasis: fungal infection caused by *Candida albicans*, usually affecting moist cutaneous area, especially the vagina (also called ***monilia*** and ***candidosis***).

gonorrhea (gon″o-re′ah): second most common STD, a contagious infection of genital mucous membranes by *Neisseria gonococcus*, usually contracted through sexual intercourse, but can be acquired by contact with exudates. It is a major cause of pelvic inflammatory disease.

herpes genitalis: infection caused by the *herpesvirus* marked by clusters of herpes simplex vesicles on the genitalia, with no known cure (also called ***genital herpes***). Treatment is palliative.

lymphogranuloma venereum (lim″fo-gran″u-lo′mah ve-ne′re-um): infection usually due to *Chlamydia trachomatis* bacteria (now considered the most common source of STD), characterized by genital ulcerative lesions and hypertrophy of inguinal lymph nodes (also called ***lymphopathia venereum*** and ***lymphogranuloma inguinale***).

pelvic inflammatory disease (PID): a bacterial infection usually due to *gonorrhea* or *Chlamydia trachomatis*, with inflammation of fallopian tubes, ovaries, or other structures found in the pelvic cavity; a common cause of sterility.

syphilis: acute, contagious infection caused by the spirochete *Treponema pallidum*, with a first symptom of chancre sore, progressing through primary, secondary, and tertiary stages. The latter involves many organ systems, such as the integumentary, skeletal, cardiovascular and central nervous systems.

trichomoniasis (trik″o-mo-ni′ah-sis): protozoan infection, usually producing a leukorrhea of the vagina and vulva.

Hereditary, Congenital, and Developmental Disorders

anorchism (an-or′kizm): absence of one or both testes.

atresia of vagina (ah-tre′za-ah): absence of vaginal opening.

bifid clitoris: clitoris divided into two parts.

cryptorchism (krip-tor′kizm): testes do not descend into the scrotum (also called ***cryptorchidism***).

ectopia of testis: one or both testes misplaced in other location.

hermaphroditism (her-maf″ro-di′tizm): individual having both ovarian and testicular tissue.

hypoplasia of cervix: under-development of the cervix.

ovotestis: gonad that contains both ovarian and testicular tissue (see ***hermaphroditism***).

polymastia: more than two breasts.

polyorchism: more than two testes.

polythelia: more than the normal number of nipples, on the breast or elsewhere on the body.

pseudohermaphroditism: presence of gonads of one sex, with physical characteristics of both sexes.

rudimentary uterus: under-developed or imperfectly developed uterus.

supernumerary: more than the normal number, referring, for example, to nipples, ovaries, or fallopian tubes.

synorchism (sin′or-kizm): the testes are fused together in the abdomen rather than the scrotum (also called ***synorchidism***).

Other Abnormalities

abruptio placentae: placenta that separates prematurely.

adenomyosis of the uterus (ad″e-no-mi-o′sis): benign invasion of the endometrium into the muscle wall of the uterus.

amenorrhea (ah-men″o-re′ah): absence of the menses.

aspermatogenesis (ah-sper″mah-to-jen′e-sis): failure to develop spermatozoa.

aspermia (ah-sper′me-ah): failure to form or emit semen.

benign prostatic hyperplasia: enlargement of the prostate gland due to proliferation of cells.

corpus hemorrhagicum: blood clot in a corpus luteum, or blood in an ovarian follicle.

displacement of uterus: retroflexion, retroversion, or anteflexion of the uterus.

dysmenorrhea (dis″men-o-re′ah): painful menstruation.

dyspareunia (dis″pah-roo′ne-ah): painful coitus (sexual intercourse or copulation) in women.

gynecomastia (jin″e-ko-mas′te-ah): unusual enlargement of male breast.

hematocele (hem′ah-to-sel): effusion of blood into a body cavity or canal such as the scrotum, testis, pelvis, or pudendum.

hematocolpos (hem″ah-to-kol′pos): menstrual blood collected in the vagina because of obstruction.

hematometra (hem″ah-to-me′trah): blood collected in the uterine cavity.

hematosalpinx (hem″ah-to-sal-pinks): blood collected in a fallopian tube.

hydatidiform mole (hi″dah-tid′i-form): abnormal pregnancy, with a mass of cystic tissue in the uterus resembling a bunch of grapes.

hydrocele: collection of fluid in a testis.

hydrorrhea gravidarum (hi″dro-re′ah gra″vi-dah′rum): discharge of thin, watery fluid from the pregnant uterus.

hyperplasia of the endometrium: over-development of the lining of the uterus.

hysterolith (his′ter-o-lith): stone, or calculus, in the uterus.

hysterorrhexis (his″ter-o-rek′sis): rupture of the uterus (also called **metrorrhexis**).

impotence: lack of copulative power in the male.

kraurosis vulvae (kraw-ro′sis): shriveling of the skin of the vagina and vulva.

lactation: secretion of milk.

leukorrhea (lu″ko-re′ah): whitish discharge from the vagina.

lithopedion (lith′o-pe′de-on): calcified dead fetus out of the uterus.

mammalgia (mam-mal′je-ah): pain in the breast (also called **mastalgia** and **mastodynia**).

mastoptosis (mas″to-to′sis): pendulous breast.

mastorrhagia (mas″to-ra′je-ah): hemorrhage from the breast.

menometrorrhagia (men″o-met″ro-ra′je-ah): excessive uterine bleeding during and between menstrual periods.

menorrhagia (men″o-ra′je-ah): profuse menstruation.

menoschesis (men″o-ske′sis, men-os′ke-sis): suppression of the menses.

menostasis (men-os′tah-sis): amenorrhea or absense of menses.

metratrophia (me″trah-tro′fe-ah): atrophy of the uterus.

metrorrhagia (me″tro-ra′je-ah): abnormal uterine bleeding, especially between menstrual periods.

metrostenosis (me″tro-ste-no′sis): narrowing of the uterine cavity.

nabothian cyst (nah-bo′the-an): cystlike formation in a nabothian gland (one of many small mucus-secreting glands) of the uterine cervix.

oligohydramnios (ol′i-go-hi-dram′ne-os): presence of less than normal amount of amniotic fluid.

oligomenorrhea (ol′i-go-men″o-re′ah): scanty menstruation.

oligospermia (ol″i-go-sper′me-ah): diminished amount of spermatozoa in the semen.

parovarian cyst: cyst located beside the ovary.

phimosis (fi-mo′sis): constriction of the skin of the prepuce over the glans penis.

placenta accreta: abnormal form of placenta adherence to the uterine wall.

placenta bipartita: bilobate placenta.

placenta circumvallata: cup-shaped placenta.

placenta previa: placenta that develops in the lower segment of the uterus.

placenta tripartita: trilobate placenta.

premenstrual syndrome (PMS): cyclical disorder involving physical and emotional symptoms preceding menstrual period, with fatigue, edema, tension, irritability, and depression.

prolapse of uterus: protrusion of the uterus through the vaginal orifice.

prostatic hypertrophy: enlargement of the prostate due to increase in cell size.

pruritus vulvae (proo-ri′tus): intense itching of the vulva.

puerperal eclampsia: convulsions occurring in female following delivery, associated with high blood pressure, edema, and protein in the urine.

salpingocele (sal-ping′go-sel): hernia of the fallopian tube.

salpingo-oophorocele (sal-ping″go-oof′or-o-sel): hernia of both an ovary and a fallopian tube.

spermatocele (sper′mah-to-sel): epididymal cyst with sperm cells.

spermaturia (sper″mah-tu′re-ah): discharge of semen in urine (also called **seminuria**).

spontaneous abortion: premature discharge of an embryo or nonviable fetus from the uterus.

Stein-Leventhal syndrome: female disorder characterized by facial hair, overweight, and infrequent or absent menstrual periods, caused by adrenal gland malfunction or excessive androgen secretion of the ovaries.

sterility: inability to reproduce.

vaginismus (vaj″i-niz′mus): painful spasm of the vagina.

varicocele (var′i-ko-sel): varicose condition of the veins of the spermatic plexus that causes a swelling to form in the scrotum.

velamentous placenta: placenta in which the umbilical cord is attached to the adjoining membranes.

Oncology*

The following list pertains only to tumors of the reproductive systems, although other benign and malignant tumors, which occur in other parts of the body, also occur in the reproductive system. Some of these are fibrosarcomas, fibromas, adenocarcinomas, sarcomas, lipomas, medullary carcinomas, and lymphangiomas.

*Indicates a malignant condition.

arrhenoblastoma (ah-re"no-blas-to'mah): ovarian neoplasm sometimes causing secondary male sex characteristics.

Brenner tumor: ovarian tumor consisting of groups of epithelial cells lying in fibrous connective tissue.

carcinoma of cervix*: malignant, epithelial tissue neoplasm, believed to be caused by the *papilloma virus* (STD-producing virus), also suspect in cancers of the vagina, vulva, and penis.

choriocarcinoma*: highly malignant tumor that invades the myometrium and blood vessels (also called ***chorioepithelioma***).

cystadenoma (sis"tad-e-no'mah): benign ovarian cystic tumor, with serous or pseudomucinous fluid.

dysgerminoma* (dis"jer-mi-no'mah): rare, malignant, ovarian neoplasm derived from undifferentiated gonadal germ cells.

fibroadenoma: benign tumor, of several different types, involving the mammary gland.

granulosa cell tumor*: ovarian tumor, benign or malignant, that begins in the graafian follicle, and may produce estrogen, creating endometrial hyperplasia.

neomammary carcinoma*: malignant tumor of breast (also called ***medullary carcinoma***).

Paget's disease of the nipple*: malignant tumor of the nipple, usually associated with deeper carcinomas.

prostatic carcinoma*: malignant tumor of the prostate gland, with growth stimulated by male hormones, especially testosterone.

sclerosing adenosis: benign nodular lesion of the breast, which may resemble carcinoma microscopically.

seminoma*: malignant testicular tumor, similar to dysgerminoma.

teratoma* (ter"ah-to-mah): benign neoplasm of ovary, and malignant neoplasm of testis.

thecoma* (the-ko'mah): malignant ovarian tumor composed of theca cells.

Surgical Procedures

abortion: termination of pregnancy.

amniotomy (am"no-ot'o-me): surgical rupture of fetal membranes to induce labor.

basiotripsy (ba'se-o-trip"se): surgical crushing of the head of a dead fetus to facilitate removal (also called ***cranioclasis***).

cervicectomy: excision of uterine cervix (also called ***trachelectomy***).

cesarean section: surgical incision through abdominal and uterine walls for delivery of neonate.

circumcision: excision of all or part of the prepuce of the glans penis.

clitoridectomy (kli"to-rid-ek'to-me): excision of the clitoris.

colpectomy: excision of the vagina.

colpocleisis (kol"po-kli'sis): closing of the vaginal canal (***cleisis*** refers to closure).

colpohysterectomy (kol-po-his"ter-ek'to-me): removal of the uterus via the vagina.

colpohysteropexy (kol"po-his'ter-o-pek"se): fixation of the uterus via surgery through the vagina.

colpohysterotomy: incision of the uterus via the vagina.

colpomyomectomy (kol"po-mi"o-mek'to-me): removal of a myoma through the vagina.

colpoperineoplasty (kol"po-per"i-ne-o-plast"te): surgical repair of the vagina and perineum.

colpoperineorrhaphy (kol"po-per"i-ne'or'ah-fe): suture to repair a torn vagina and perineum.

colpopexy (kl'po-pek"se): suturing of a relaxed vagina to the abdominal wall for support.

colpoplasty: plastic repair of the vagina.

colpopoiesis (kol"po-poi-e'sis): creation of a vagina by plastic surgery.

colporrhaphy (kil-por'ah-fe): suturing repair of the vagina.

colpotomy: surgical incision of the vaginal wall.

dilatation and curettage (D&C) (ku-reh-tahzh'): cervical dilation and scraping of inside of uterus for diagnostic purposes, removal of endometrial tissue, or removal of uterine contents.

embryotomy (em"bre-ot'o-me): removal of a dead embryo or fetus from uterus by means of dissection.

epididymectomy (ep"i-did"i-mek'to-me): excision of the epididymis.

epididymotomy (ep"i-did"i-mot'o-me): incision into the epididymis, usually for drainage purposes.

epididymovasotomy (ep-i-did'i-mo-vaz-o'to-me): anastomosis of the epididymis to the vas deferens.

episioplasty (e-piz'e-o-plas"te): repair of the vulva.

episiorrhaphy (e-piz"e-or'ah-fe): repair of torn vulva or an episiotomy.

episiotomy: incision of the vulva to prevent tearing on delivery of neonate.

hymenectomy (hi"men-ek'to-me): excision of the hymen.

hymenotomy (hi"men-ot'o-me): incision of the hymen.

hysterectomy: removal of the uterus.

hysterolaparotomy (his"ter-o-lap"ah-rot'o-me): incision of the abdomen to remove or incise the uterus.

hysteromyotomy (his"ter-o-mi-ot'o-me): incision into the uterine muscle wall.

hysteropexy: fixation of the uterus to correct misplacement or abnormal mobility.

hysterorrhaphy (his-ter-or'ah-fe): suturing of a torn uterus.

hysterosalpingostomy (his"ter-o-sal"ping-gos'to-me): surgical clearing of the lumen of a fallopian tube.

lumpectomy: excision of a tumor leaving surrounding tissue and lymph nodes intact.

mammilliplasty (mah-mil′i-plas″te): plastic repair of the nipple (also called *theleplasty*).

mastectomy: excision of the breast (also called *mammectomy*).

mastopexy (mas′to-pek-se): surgical reconstruction of a pendulous breast (also called *mastoplasty*).

mastotomy: incision of the breast (also called *mammotomy*).

oophorectomy (o″of-o-rek′to-me): excision of one or both ovaries (also called *ovariectomy*).

oophorocystectomy: excision of an ovarian cyst.

oophorohysterectomy (o-of′o-ro-his″ter-ek′to-me): removal of the uterus and ovaries.

oophoropexy (o-of′o-ro-pek″se): fixation of an ovary.

oophoroplasty (o-of′o-ro-plas″te): plastic repair of an ovary.

oophorosalpingectomy (o-of′o-ro-sal″pin-jek′to-me): removal of an ovary and a tube (also called *salpingooophorectomy* and *salpingoovariectomy*).

oophorotomy: incision of an ovary.

orchidorrhaphy: surgical fixation of an undescended testicle into the scrotum (also called *orchiopexy*).

orchiectomy (or″ke-ek′to-me): excision of one or both testes.

orchioplasty (or′ke-o-plas″te): plastic repair of a testicle.

ovariocentesis (o-va″re-o-sen-te′sis): puncture of an ovarian cyst or an ovary.

ovariostomy (o″va-re-os′to-me): creation of an opening in an ovarian cyst for purposes of drainage (also called *oophorostomy*).

ovariotomy: incision of an ovary, usually for biopsy purposes.

panhysterectomy (pan″hist-er-ek′to-me): complete removal of the uterus and cervix.

perineal prostatectomy: removal of the prostate gland through the perineum.

prostatectomy (pros″tah-tek′to-me): removal of all or part of the prostate gland.

prostatomy: incision into the prostate gland (also called *prostatotomy*).

prostatovesiculectomy (pros″tah-to-ve-sik″u-ke″to-me): excision of the prostate gland and seminal vesicles.

radical mastectomy: excision of the breast, pectoral muscle, axillary lymph nodes, skin, and other tissues.

retropubic prostatectomy: excision of the prostate gland through the lower abdomen.

salpingectomy (sal″pin-jek′to-me): removal of a fallopian tube.

salpingopexy: surgical fixation of a fallopian tube.

salpingorrhaphy (sal″ping-gor′ah-fe): suturing of a fallopian tube.

salpingostomatomy (sal-ping″go-sto-mat′o-me): procedure to create an opening in a fallopian tube when the fimbriated end is closed (also called *salpingostomy*).

salpingotomy: incision into a fallopian tube.

scrotoplasty (skro′to-plas″te): repair of the scrotum.

tracheloplasty (tra′ke-lo-plas″te): plastic repair of the cervix.

trachelorrhaphy (tra″ke-lor′ah-fe): suturing of a torn cervix.

trachelotomy: incision into the cervix.

transurethral resection of prostate (TURP): resection of the prostate gland through the urethra.

vasectomy: excision of all or part of the vas deferens.

vasotomy: incision into the vas deferens.

vesiculectomy (ve-sik″u-lek′to-me): excision of all or a portion of a seminal vesicle.

vesiculotomy (ve-sik″u-loto′-me): incision into the seminal vesicles to open them.

vulvectomy (vul-vek′to-me): excision of the vulva.

Laboratory Tests and Procedures of the Reproductive Systems

alpha-fetoprotein (AFP): blood test between the fourteenth and eighteenth weeks of pregnancy to screen for neural tube defects in the fetus.

amniocentesis (am″ne-o-sen″te′sis): aspiration of fluid from the amniotic sac for sampling of fetal cells after 5 months to diagnose genetic defects and diseases and to determine sex of fetus.

chorionic villus sampling (CVS): biopsy technique, between the eighth and twelfth weeks of pregnancy, using a catheter to suction up a minute amount of the chorionic villi, which has the same cells as the fetus, in order to detect fetal defects (also called *chorionic villus biopsy [CVB]*).

darkfield examination: microscopic test of the fluid from the chancre lesion in the suspected primary stage of syphilis.

hysterostoscopy: examination of the uterus using a fiberoptic endoscope.

karyotyping: analysis of chromosomes of fetal cells or somatic cells of children and young adults to detect genetic diseases and abnormalities.

Papanicolaou smear: microscopic examination of cell samples from the cervix and vagina, to detect cancer and infections (also called *Pap smear*).

percutaneous umbilical blood sampling (PUBS): blood sample from fetal umbilical cord to detect genetic abnormalities, blood disorders, and infections.

Pregnancy Tests

agglutination inhibition test (AIT): urine test as early as 10 days after conception, based on the the presence of the human chorionic gonadotropin (HCG), the hormone secreted by the female pituitary gland to stimulate ovaries, which indicates pregnancy.

radioimmunoassay (RIA): sensitive, reliable blood test, to detect the beta unit of HCG, which can diagnose pregnancy before the first menstrual period is missed.

radioreceptor assay (RRA): sensitive, reliable blood test to detect human chorionic gonadotropin (HCG) by means of a gamma counter to reveal radioactivity, taking about an hour to complete and being almost 100% reliable in detecting pregnancy as early as 1 week after conception.

prostatic acid phosphatase (PAP): blood test to detect a substance normally present, that increases when prostate cancer has spread.

prostate specific antigen (PSA): blood test to detect the presence of a specific antigen that increases in cases of prostate cancer and other prostate diseases.

Radiographic Studies

amniography (am″ne-og′rah-fe): an X-ray of the gravid uterus after injection of contrast media into the amniotic sac to visualize the contents.

computerized tomography (CT): imaging device using x-rays at multiple angles through specific sections of the body, analyzed by computer to provide a total picture of the part being examined (also called ***computerized axial tomography [CAT]***).

hysterogram: X-ray of the uterus using contrast medium injected into the uterine cavity.

hysterosalpingography: X-ray of uterus and fallopian tubes, using contrast medium.

magnetic resonance imaging (MRI): noninvasive method of scanning the body by use of an electromagnetic field and radio waves, which provides visual images on a computer screen and magnetic tape recordings (also called ***nuclear magnetic resonance [NMR]***).

mammography: x-ray of breast tissue to detect tumors.

seminal fluid tests: series of tests of seminal fluid to determine the percentage and motility of spermatozoa, the makeup of the fluid, the amount produced in ejaculation, and so forth.

transrectal ultrasonography: a procedure using ultrasound waves, made by an instrument inserted into the rectum, to visualize the prostate and nearby structures.

ultrasonography: use of ultrasound to visualize deep body structures, to monitor the fetus and placenta.

venereal disease research laboratory test (VDRL): test for syphilis.

Section Four

The Adaptive and Defense Mechanisms of the Body

This is the fourth of the five sections of **LEARNING MEDICAL TERMINOLOGY.** This section contains four chapters that describe those systems that aid the body in coordinating with and adapting to the external and internal environments, and one chapter devoted to a glossary of multiple-system diseases.

Chapter 13, the **Endocrine System,** details the activity of the glands of internal secretion, and their regulation of body functions through chemical means.

Chapter 14, the **Nervous System,** describes the separate divisions of this system and their functions in coordinating the complexities of human life.

Chapter 15 describes the **Special Senses,** through which the body receives stimulation from the world around it.

Chapter 16 presents the **Lymphatic and Immune Systems** which work together to protect and defend the integrity of the body.

Chapter 17 consists of a glossary containing a relatively comprehensive listing of pathologic conditions that affect more than one system of the body.

As in the previous section, there are drawings within the chapters illustrating the principal parts of the anatomy in that particular chapter. In addition, there are colored plates at the front of the text that provide more vivid detail.

CHAPTER 13

The Endocrine System

The Chemical Stimulators

It's a Fact:
The finding that urine from a diabetic person contains sugar identical to grape sugar pointed the way to the recognition of diabetes mellitus as a sugar metabolic disorder.

CHAPTER OVERVIEW

This chapter describes the ductless glands (pituitary, hypothalamus, thyroid, parathyroids, adrenals, pineal, pancreas, ovaries, testes, and thymus), which constitute the endocrine system. The structure and function of the glands and their secretions are detailed narratively and in chart form.

THE ENDOCRINES

The complex activities of the body are controlled by the endocrine and central nervous systems. The central nervous system acts directly and instantaneously, while the action of the endocrine system is more subtle, discharging its secretions slowly into the circulatory system, and controlling organs from a distance.

The endocrine system (Fig. 13-1) is made up of ductless glands of internal secretion, so-called because they have no ducts to carry away their secretions and depend on the capillaries and, to a certain extent, the lymph vessels, for this function. The secretions of these glands are called **hormones** (which means to rouse or set in motion). Although most hormones are excitatory in function, some are inhibitory.

The secretion of hormones is controlled by a feedback mechanism. The presence and amount of a hormone, and any substances released by tissue excited by that hormone, regulate further secretion of that hormone by its gland. This ensures that the right amount of the hormone, no more and no less, will maintain the proper balance of bodily functioning.

The Pituitary Gland

The **pituitary gland**, or **hypophysis**, despite all its important functions, is no larger than a pea. It is about 1/2 inch (1.3 cm) in diameter and weighs about 0.02 oz (0.5 gm). It has been called the "orchestra leader" and "master gland" because it exerts control over all other glands.

Structure of the Pituitary Gland

The pituitary gland lies protected within the sphenoid bone in a saddle-shaped depression called the **sella turcica**. It is further protected by an extension of the **dura mater** (membrane covering the brain) called the **pituitary diaphragm**. A stemlike portion of the pituitary gland, the **pituitary stalk**, extends through the diaphragm and provides a connection (the **infundibulum**) to the **hypothalamus** portion of the brain, located on the underside.

The pituitary gland is actually made up of two separate glands with different embryonic origins and functions: the **anterior lobe**, or **anterior pituitary gland** (**adenohypophysis**), develops as an upgrowth from the embryonic pharynx, while the **posterior lobe**, or **posterior pituitary gland** (**neurohypophysis**), develops as a downward extension of the brain (Fig. 13-2).

Functions of the Anterior Lobe

The master role is played by the anterior lobe, with its numerous anterior pituitary hormones influencing the actions of other endocrines. This internal regulation is further coordinated by the action of the hypothalamus on the anterior lobe, controlling the release of six major types of anterior pituitary hormones. The combining forms *-tropic* and *-tropin* mean influence or stimulation (see Table 13-1 on pp. 266-267).

Growth hormone (**GH**), also called **somatotropin**, promotes bodily growth of both bony and soft tissues.

Thyroid-stimulating hormone (**TSH**), a **thyrotropic hormone**, influences the thyroid gland and causes secretion of the thyroid hormone.

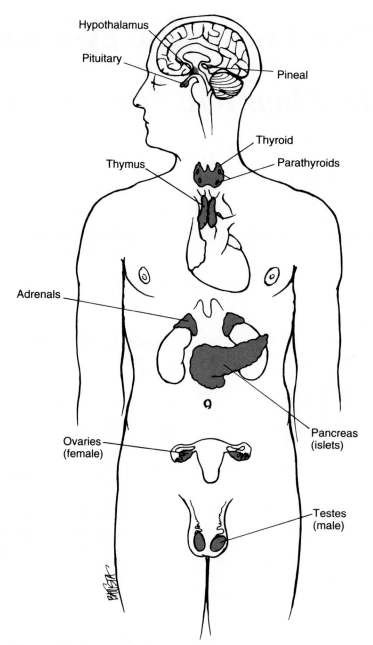

Figure 13-1.   Location of the endocrine glands.

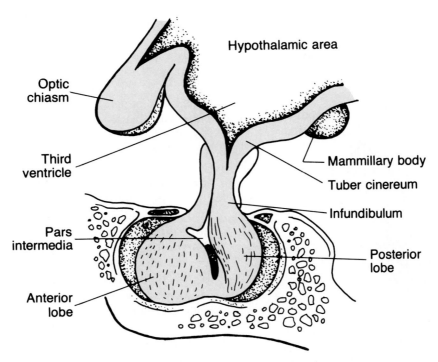

Figure 13-2.   Pituitary gland and brain structures in proximity.

Two **gonadotropic hormones** influence the ovaries and testes and are necessary for the proper development and function of the reproductive system:

Follicle-stimulating hormone (FSH) stimulates the growth of graafian follicles and the secretion of estrogen in the female, and the development of the seminiferous tubules and sperm cells in the male.

Luteinizing hormone (LH) stimulates, in the female, ovarian follicle and ovum maturation, formation of the corpus luteum, secretion of estrogen, and ovulation. In the male this hormone stimulates the interstitial cells of the testes to produce and secrete testosterone.

Prolactin, or **lactogenic hormone**, is responsible for breast development during pregnancy and, as its name implies, for production of milk.

Adrenocorticotropic hormone (ACTH) or **adrenocorticotropin**, influences growth of the adrenal glands and also stimulates the adrenal cortex to synthesize and release corticosteroids. ACTH also appears to have a relationship to pigmentation of the skin.

Melanocyte-stimulating hormone (MSH), the last of the anterior pituitary hormones, stimulates formation of melanin pigment in the skin.

Functions of the Posterior Lobe

The posterior lobe of the pituitary gland secretes two hormones, which are actually made in the hypothalamus and passed through the infundibulum into the posterior lobe, where they are stored and secreted into the circulation.

Antidiuretic hormone (ADH), or **vasopressin**, limits the development of large volumes of urine by stimulating water reabsorption by the distal and collecting tubules of the kidneys.

Oxytocin stimulates both the ejection of breast milk into the mammary ducts and contraction of the uterus after pregnancy.

The Hypothalamus

The **hypothalamus** is a part of the brain, made of neural tissue, but also has endocrine functions (Chapter 14).

As previously noted, both **antidiuretic hormone** and **oxytocin** are produced by the hypothalamus and stored and released from the posterior pituitary. In addition, the hypothalamus produces hormones that cause stimulation or inhibition of the release of anterior pituitary hormones.

The Thyroid

The **thyroid gland** is composed of two pear-shaped lobes separated by a middle strip of tissue, the **isthmus**, which crosses in front of the second and third tracheal cartilages (Fig. 13-3). The thyroid perches like a butterfly with wings extended on the front part of the neck below the larynx. The lobes are molded to the trachea and esophagus down as far as the sixth tracheal cartilage, and they extend upward to the sides of the cricoid and thyroid cartilages. The thyroid may be felt slightly and may even be visible as a swelling in some diseases of the gland.

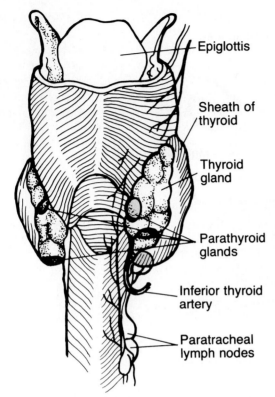

Figure 13-3. **Posterior view of thyroid and parathyroid glands.**

The thyroid weighs about one ounce (28 to 30 gm) in the normal adult, and has a rich vascular supply from the inferior and superior thyroid arteries, with a wide capillary network for diffusion of blood to the veins, and a rich lymphatic system that drains the lymph spaces around the follicles. Although lymph vessels drain some of the hormones, the major portion is carried away by the capillaries. The hormone secreted by the thyroid is under the control of the anterior pituitary lobe.

Functions of the Thyroid

The main function of the thyroid is the secretion of two iodine-laden hormones, **thyroxine** and **triiodothyronine**, which together are referred to as **thyroid hormone**. This hormone is high in iodine and vital for growth and metabolism, and, through variations in the activity of the gland, it alters the metabolic rate in accordance with changing physiologic demands. Growth and differentiation of tissue during development is also regulated by the thyroid hormone.

Iodine is the essential element of the thyroid hormone. Most disorders of the thyroid are caused by either over- or under-production of the thyroid hormone and its iodine-containing substance. The iodine in the thyroid hormone is combined with a protein in the blood, which is then referred to as **protein-bound iodine** (**PBI**). However, when the hormone enters the tissue, the separate components become unbound from the protein.

A secondary function of the thyroid gland is the secretion of **calcitonin**, which produces a decrease in the concentration of calcium in the blood, helping to maintain the balance of calcium necessary for a variety of bodily processes. This balance is achieved in conjunction with the functioning of the parathyroid glands.

Structure of the Thyroid

The thyroid is a soft, highly vascular mass, brownish-red in color, consisting of tiny sacs, or follicles, that are filled with a gelatinous yellow fluid called **colloid**. The colloid contains the hormone secreted by the thyroid. It is stored in the colloid and passed into the capillaries to be sent to the tissues as required.

Review A

Complete the following:

1. Endocrine gland secretions are called _____.

2. The endocrine glands are the: _____

    _____

    _____ .

3. The two parts of the pituitary gland are the _____ and _____ lobes.

4. The thyroid gland is made up of _____ lobes and a strip called the_____.

5. The essential element of the thyroid hormone is _____.

The Parathyroid Glands

The **parathyroid glands** (**para** means alongside of or next to) are small, reddish-brown, oval glands, about 1/4 inch (6 mm) at their widest dimensions. There are usually two on each side, lying behind the thyroid gland and embedded in its posterior surface (Fig. 13-3). The

blood supply of the parathyroid glands is from the inferior thyroid artery, and their functional activity is controlled by a hormone of the anterior lobe of the pituitary gland.

Parathyroid hormone (**PTH**), secreted by the glands, regulates the calcium and phosphorus content of the blood and bones. The regulation of calcium content is very important in certain tissue activities, such as blood formation and coagulation, milk production in pregnant females, and maintenance of normal neuromuscular excitability.

Parathyroid hormone promotes calcium absorption in the blood, increasing its calcium concentration. This mechanism is antagonistic (opposite) to that of the hormone calcitonin from the thyroid gland. These two hormones together maintain calcium balance.

The Adrenal Glands

The *adrenal* (*suprarenal*) *glands* resemble small caps perched on the top of each kidney. They are flattened, yellowish bodies about 2 inches (52 mm) high, 1 inch (25 mm) wide, and 1/2 inch (13 mm) thick, slightly smaller in the female than in the male, and may vary in weight.

Structure of the Adrenal Glands

The adrenal glands are composed of two distinct parts, the *cortex* (outer part), and the *medulla* (inner part), with each having different glandular functions. The cortex is indispensable to life, but the medulla is not. The cortex, which is about 1/4 inch thick (6 mm), makes up the bulk of the gland and is divided into three zones, *zona glomerulosa* (outer), *zona fasiculata* (middle), and *zona reticularis* (inner).

Functions of the Adrenal Glands

All of the known adrenal hormones of the cortex are called *corticoids*, any of which can be manufactured synthetically. They are classified as:

Mineralocorticoids (*MC*), secreted by the outer zone are concerned with the regulation of sodium and potassium and their excretion. The principal one is *aldosterone*, which is responsible for electrolyte and water balance, by acting on the blood sodium and potassium concentration.

Glucocorticoids (*GC*), secreted mainly by the middle zone, including *cortisol* (*hydrocortisone*), and *corticosterone*. The glucocorticoids affect literally all cells in the body, but their general effect is in the metabolism of carbohydrates, fats, and proteins, resistance to stress, antibody formation, lymphatic functioning, and recovery from injury and inflammation.

Sex hormones, secreted by the inner zone, which include, in both sexes, small amounts of the male hormone *androgen*, which stimulates the sex drive in the female, but, because of its relative insignificance in the male, compared to testosterone, has little influence.

The presence of adrenocorticotropin (ACTH), a pituitary hormone in the blood supply, is necessary for the anatomic integrity and functioning of the adrenal cortex in secreting androgens and cortisol.

The adrenal medulla secretes *epinephrine* (*adrenaline*) and *norepinephrine* (*noradrenalin*). Epinephrine, particularly, aids the body in meeting stressful situations, such as defense flight, attack, or pursuit. By stimulating or boosting the sympathetic nervous system, epinephrine aids in coping with stress. The effects of these secretions include increases in heartbeat, blood pressure, blood glucose level, and rate of blood clotting.

The Pineal Gland

The *pineal gland*, or *body* (*epiphysis cerebri*), which derives its name from its resemblance to a pine cone, is a small, firm, oval body about 1/4 inch (6 mm) long, located near the base of the brain. Although exact functions have not been established, it secretes *melatonin*, a skin-lightening agent, which is believed to inhibit ovarian function and secretion of the pituitary luteinizing hormone, and may be related to the circadian (24-hour cycle) rhythms of the body.

The Pancreas

The *pancreas*, as part of the gastrointestinal system, is described in Chapter 11.

As an endocrine gland, microscopic, specialized cells of the pancreas, called the *islands* (or *islets*) *of Langerhans*, secrete *insulin*, *glucagon*, and *pancreatic polypeptide* (*PP*) into the circulation.

Insulin is necessary for the use and storage of carbohydrates, and acts to decrease blood glucose levels, while glucagon acts to increase them. The level of glucose in the blood is also dependent on the action of many of the other endocrine secretions, such as the pituitary growth hormone, epinephrine, ACTH, and the glucocorticoids, all of which act to increase it, and the thyroid hormone, which acts to decrease it. Pancreatic polypeptide plays a role in the production of glucagon and gastric juices, and has been identified as having additional functions in digestion and metabolism.

The Gonads

The male and female *gonads*, as parts of the genitourinary system, are described in Chapter 12. As endocrine glands, the female ovaries produce the hormones *estrogen* and *progesterone*, and the male testes produce the hormone *testosterone*. All of these hormones are important to the functioning of the reproductive system. These glands become active at puberty under the influence of the anterior pituitary lobe, producing both sexual behavior and secondary sex characteristics of pubic and axillary hair in both sexes, sperm development, deep voice and facial hair in the male, and breast development and the menstrual cycle in the female. Table 13-1 and the glossary at the end of the chapter contain descriptions of the gonadal hormones.

Table 13-1   THE ENDOCRINE GLANDS AND THEIR HORMONES

Gland	Hormone	Function
Pituitary		
Anterior lobe	growth hormone (GH) (somatotropin)	promotes body and soft tissue growth
	thyroid stimulating hormone (TSH) (thyrotropic hormone)	stimulates thyroid gland production of thyroid horomone
	follicle-stimulating hormone (FSH)	stimulates graafian follicle growth
		stimulates secretion of estrogen in ovaries
		stimulates development of seminiferous tubules in testes
		stimulates development and production of sperm cells
	luteinizing hormone (LH)	stimulates ovarian follicle and ovum maturation
		stimulates formation of corpus luteum
		stimulates secretion of estrogen
		stimulates ovulation
		stimulates interstitial cells of testes to produce and secrete testosterone
	prolactin (lactogenic hormone)	stimulates breast development and milk production
	adrenocorticotropic hormone (adrenocorticotropin) or ACTH	influences growth of the adrenal glands
		stimulates adrenal cortex to synthesize and release corticosteroids
		affects skin pigmentation
	melanocyte-stimulating hormone (MSH)	stimulates formation of melanin pigment in the skin
Posterior lobe	antidiuretic hormone (ADH) (vasopressin)	stimulates water reabsorption by kidney tubules
	oxytocin	stimulates ejection of breast milk and uterine contractions after pregnancy
Hypothalamus	antidiuretic hormone (ADH)	passes hormone on to posterior pituitary
	oxytocin	passes hormone on to posterior pituitary
	releasing and inhibiting hormones	stimulate or inhibit production and release of anterior pituitary hormones
Thyroid	thyroid hormone (thyroxine, triiodothyronine)	regulates growth, development, and metabolism
	calcitonin	promotes calcium absorption in bones and reduces concentration in blood
Parathyroid	parathyroid hormone (PTH)	regulates phosphorus content of blood and bones
		promotes calcium concentration in blood and reduces concentration in bones

Table 13-1 THE ENDOCRINE GLANDS AND THEIR HORMONES—CONT'D.

Gland	Hormone	Function
Adrenal		
Cortex	mineralocorticoids (e.g. aldosterone)	regulate sodium and potassium
	glucocorticoids (cortisol, and corticosterone)	metabolism of carbohydrates, fats, and proteins
		resistance to stress, antibody formation, lymphatic functioning, recovery from injury and inflammation
	sex hormones (androgen)	stimulate female sex drive
Medulla	epinephrine (adrenaline), norepinephrine (noradrenalin)	stimulate sympathetic nervous system responses to stress
Pineal	melatonin	promotes lightening of skin
		inhibits ovarian function and secretion of the anterior pituitary luteinizing hormone
Pancreas: Islands of Langerhans	insulin	regulates use and storage of carbohydrates
		reduces glucose in blood
	glucagon	increases glucose in blood
	pancreatic polypeptide (PP)	stimulates production of glucagon and gastric juices
		functions in digestion and metabolism
Gonads		
Ovaries	estrogen and progesterone	produces secondary sex characteristics and sexual behavior
		produces menstrual cycle
Testes	testosterone	produces secondary sex characteristics and sexual behavior
		promotes sperm development
Thymus	thymosin	functions in the immune system

The Thymus

The **thymus**, located in the mediastinum, produces the hormone **thymosin**, which plays an important part in the body's immune system (Chapter 16).

Review B

Complete the following:

1. The parathyroid hormone regulates the _____ and _____ content of blood and bones.

2. The two little caplike glands on top of the kidneys are the _____ glands.

3. The pineal gland secretion is _____.

4. The islands of Langerhans in the pancreas secrete _____, and

_____.

5. The gonads become active at puberty under the influence of the _____ pituitary lobe.

Answers to Review Questions: The Endocrine System

Review A
1. hormones
2. pituitary, hypothalamus, thyroid, parathyroids, adrenals, pineal gland (or body), pancreas, ovaries, testes, and thymus
3. anterior, posterior
4. two, isthmus
5. iodine

Review B
1. calcium, phosphorus
2. adrenal
3. melatonin
4. insulin, glucagon, and pancreatic polypeptide (or PP)
5. anterior

CHAPTER 13 EXERCISES

THE ENDOCRINE SYSTEM: THE CHEMICAL STIMULATORS

Exercise 1: Complete the following:

1. The thyroid gland is located in_____

_____.

2. The normal location of the parathyroid glands is_____

_____.

3. The part of the brain that has an endocrine function is the _____.

4. The function of the hormone secreted by the parathyroids is to_____

_____.

5. The pituitary gland is located _____.

6. The connection between the hypothalamus and the pituitary gland is called the _____.

7. The pituitary is called the "master gland" because it _____

_____.

8. The _____ lobe of the pituitary gland secretes an antidiuretic hormone that stimulates water reabsorption by tubules of the kidneys.

9. The two distinct parts of the adrenals whose functions differ are the _____ and the

_____.

10. The _____ of the adrenal gland is indispensable to life.

11. The _____ of the adrenal gland secretes glucocorticoids, mineralocorticoids, and sex hormones.

12. The _____ of the adrenal gland secretes epinephrine and norepinephrine.

13. The endocrine system is made up of _____ glands of internal secretion.

14. The secretions of the endocrine glands are called _____.

15. The secretion of the thymus is called _____.

Exercise 2: Matching:

A. growth hormone
B. mineralocorticoids
C. melatonin
D. oxytocin
E. prolactin
F. thyrotropic hormone
G. somatotropin
H. releasing and inhibiting hormones
I. luteinizing hormone
J. estrogen and progesterone
K. pancreatic polypeptide
L. glucagon
M. posterior lobe

N. anterior lobe
O. follicle-stimulating hormone (FSH)
P. calcitonin
Q. testosterone
R. glucocorticoids
S. antidiuretic hormone
T. adrenocorticotropic hormone
U. thymosin
V. parathyroid hormone
W. epinephrine
X. insulin
Y. melanocyte-stimulating hormone (MSH)

____ **1.** pigmentation hormone of the anterior lobe of the pituitary gland

____ **2.** a skin-lightening hormone of the pineal gland

____ **3.** hormones of the adrenal cortex that regulate sodium and potassium levels

____ **4.** hormones of the hypothalamus that act on the anterior pituitary

____ **5.** thyroid-stimulating hormone (TSH) of the anterior lobe of the pituitary gland that stimulates it to secrete thyroxine and triiodothyrine

____ **6.** thyroid hormone that helps to regulate calcium levels in the blood

____ **7.** growth hormone secreted by the anterior lobe of the pituitary gland

____ **8.** hormone secreted by the posterior lobe of the pituitary gland that stimulates uterine contractions

____ **9.** hormone responsible for development of the breast in pregnancy

____ **10.** hormone from the anterior lobe of the pituitary gland that stimulates formation of the corpus luteum and secretion of testosterone by interstitial cells of the testis

____ **11.** hormone, secreted by the islands of Langerhans, which increases blood glucose

____ **12.** functions in production of glucagon and gastric juices

____ **13.** pituitary lobe that is an upgrowth of the embryonic pharynx

____ **14.** pituitary lobe that is a downward extension of the brain

____ **15.** ovarian hormones that promote menses after puberty

____ **16.** anterior pituitary hormone that stimulates the growth of graafian follicles and secretion of estrogen in the female, and the development of sperm cells in the male

____ **17.** hormone that plays an important part in the immune system

____ **18.** hormone secreted by the adrenal medulla that helps the body to meet stresses by stimulating the symphathetic nervous system

____ **19.** adrenal cortex hormones concerned with fat, protein, and carbohydrate metabolism

____ **20.** male hormone producing secondary sex characteristics

____ **21.** hormone regulating calcium and phosphorus in blood and bone

____ **22.** meaning of ACTH

____ **23.** meaning of ADH

____ **24.** hormone that reduces glucose in the blood

____ **25.** meaning of GH

Exercise 3: Using the list of terms below, identify each part in Fig. 13-4 by writing the name in the corresponding blank.

Adrenal gland   Pituitary gland (hypophysis)   Pancreas
Ovary (female)   Parathyroid glands   Thymus
Pineal gland or body   Testis (male)   Hypothalamus
Thyroid gland

1. _____

2. _____

3. _____

4. _____

5. _____

6. _____

7. _____

8. _____

9. _____

10. _____

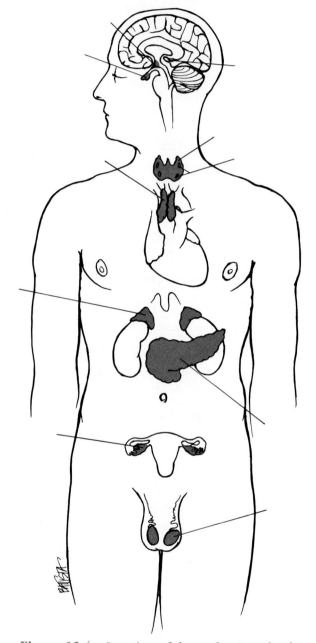

Figure 13-4.   Location of the endocrine glands.

Exercise 4: Give the meaning of the components in the following words and then define the word as a whole. Suffixes meaning *pertaining to* or *state or condition* shown following a slash mark (/), are not to be defined separately. Before reaching for your medical dictionary, check the glossary at the end of the chapter.

1. Adrenalitis:

adrenal _____

itis _____

_____

2. Acromegaly:

acro _____

megaly _____

_____

3. Adiposogenital dystrophy:

adiposo _____

genital _____

dys _____

trophy _____

_____

4. Hypothyroidism:

hypo _____

thyroid/ism _____

_____

5. Hypoadrenocorticism:

hypo _____

adreno _____

cortic/ism _____

_____

6. Hypogonadism:

hypo _____

gonad/ism _____

_____

7. Hyperthyroidism:

hyper _____

thyroid/ism _____

_____

8. Adrenal hyperplasia:

adrenal _____

hyper _____

plas/ia _____

_____

9. Thyrotoxicosis:

thyro _____

toxic/osis _____

_____

10. Eosinophilic adenoma:

eosinophil/ic _____

aden _____

oma _____

_____

11. Hemithyroidectomy:

hemi _____

thyroid _____

ectomy _____

_____

12. Isthmectomy:

isthm _____

ectomy _____

_____

Chapter 13 Crossword Puzzle

Across

1. hormone of milk production
3. element in thyroid hormone combined with protein in blood
6. inner part of adrenals
9. hormone that stimulates ovaries and testes
10. pituitary gland
12. endocrine secretions
13. female sex hormone
15. ductless gland
19. male sex hormone
20. a pituitary lobe
21. increases blood glucose
24. reduces blood glucose
25. gland resembling pine cone

Down

2. thyroid hormone promoting calcium absorption in bones
4. separating strip of thyroid
5. a pituitary lobe
7. hormone stimulating ejection of breast milk
8. butterfly-shaped gland in neck
11. abbr. for hormone also known as somatotropin
13. master gland
14. hormone promoting body and soft tissue growth
16. female sex hormone
17. skin-lightening agent
18. gland resembling small cap on kidney
22. outer part of adrenals
23. hormone stimulating skin pigment

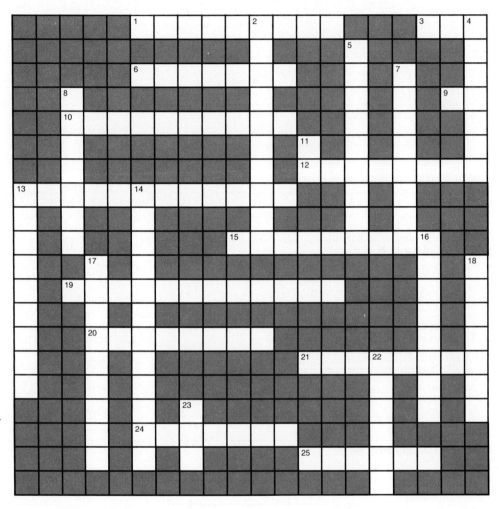

Chapter 13 Hidden Words Puzzle

```
T F J P V Z W K Q E Z K W D I C D S P H T N L F V U L
G O N A D S D N P Q B O J B X Y N Q V C O N U Y A C I
L R E N H B S G O W H N C J W Q C S Y H W J I R K R R
N O G C K Y G T H Y R O I D F S S H J M B P Q D Y O S
D I B R T Q P C C O W V E G K T P A U Q A D A V D Q Y
P E P E S T R O G E N A Y D L P N U M U Q X C A X N E
I M J A G T T L P H N R C O U G E P Y E L B K G L I O
T A N S M N G L O H N I K C W I C B I I D B K H D S L
Z K V N O O B O D O Y E R R I Q M F H N W K V T S H H
K V W S K H R I H M A S T E R P J W T T U W T S K F S
H N M H W E P D E R V Q I V L A F S O W I G M V S P C
B H U C W U K B S I B X D S D R Q H Q T K F O J S Y D
G N N Y V S R T O E U I K O J A I N V E R M U C Z S B
Q N S L N A Z Z T H R F J M S T A C Q R O K Y B U X B
B E Z K R Q S R H E P N U A E H U J M O B P H X W H V
Q P R F J P T O S H P M O T C Y Y L B N N T Y H W Y W
N N G O G J T H P D H E A O R R I P S S Q Q Y W T L B
N M P W E I H Q Y R R O I T E O S J O H R H W R S S F
I I Q S F P I D Q R E R K R T I T G L T C Z H I S G F
P V F P Y G L R M Q O S V O I D H Q N V H K R O K S T
I Q A G E L L M D Q V X S P O S M J S O K A W C B H N
L F I V D N O A B H F O I I N F U N D I B U L U M F M
W R M X S X X O N A J L Y N N Q S Q H U N D A A O P B
D X R P H Y J M A D U C T L E S S D A H O S O T M C L
V X Y C E J O U B R F Y F E U G G T F T T B I Y R U W
W B L D G G H L Q E E M G O N Y E R X D F L Y X A Q S
V C H Q T B Q D X N F Q B Q P X Y U S X G L O L Z Q X
T W Q D W L H Q E A J Q J U J X S E C P N V H R N G F
P Q J N X I U A L L B Y W U C R J X T X B X R T H J F
```

Can you find the 20 words hidden in this puzzle?

HYPOTHALAMUS	INFUNDIBULUM	PARATHYROIDS	SOMATOTROPIN
VASOPRESSIN	HYPOPHYSIS	SECRETION	THYROXINE
DUCTLESS	ESTROGEN	PANCREAS	ADRENAL
COLLOID	ISTHMUS	OVARIES	THYROID
GONADS	MASTER	GLAND	LOBE

CHAPTER 13 ANSWERS

Exercise 1
1. front part of neck below the larynx
2. behind the thyroid and embedded in its posterior surface
3. hypothalamus
4. regulation of calcium and phosphorus content of the blood and bones
5. within depression of sphenoid bone
6. infundibulum
7. exerts control over all the endocrine glands
8. posterior
9. cortex, medulla
10. cortex
11. cortex
12. medulla
13. ductless
14. hormones
15. thymosin

Exercise 2

1. Y	6. P	11. L	16. O	21. V
2. C	7. G	12. K	17. U	22. T
3. B	8. D	13. N	18. W	23. S
4. H	9. E	14. M	19. R	24. X
5. F	10. I	15. J	20. Q	25. A

Exercise 3

1. hypothalamus
2. pineal body
3. pituitary gland (hypophysis)
4. parathyroid glands
5. thyroid gland
6. thymus
7. adrenal gland
8. pancreas
9. testis (male)
10. ovary (female)

Exercise 4
1. adrenalitis: adrenals; inflammation—inflammation of the adrenals
2. acromegaly: extreme or extremities; enlarged or huge—enlarged bones of hands, feet, and facial bones (jaws)
3. adiposogenital dystrophy: fat; genitalia; disordered, difficult, bad; nourishment—adiposity of feminine type; hypoplasia of genitals, with retarded sexual development
4. hypothyroidism: under, decreased; thyroid—decreased function of the thyroid gland
5. hypoadrenocorticism: under, decreased; adrenal; cortex—underfunctioning of adrenal cortex
6. hypogonadism: under; gonads (testes or ovaries)—decreased functions of gonads
7. hyperthyroidism: over, increased; thyroid—overproduction of thyroid hormone
8. adrenal hyperplasia: adrenals; over, increased; growth or development—overdevelopment of adrenals, or enlarged adrenals
9. thyrotoxicosis: thyroid; toxic; condition—toxic thyroid condition; thyroid crisis
10. eosinophilic adenoma: eosinophil cells; gland; tumor—glandular tumor composed mainly of eosinophilic cells
11. hemithyroidectomy: partial or half; thyroid—surgical excision of part of the thyroid gland
12. isthmectomy: isthmus; excision—surgical excision of the isthmus

Answers: Chapter 13 Crossword Puzzle

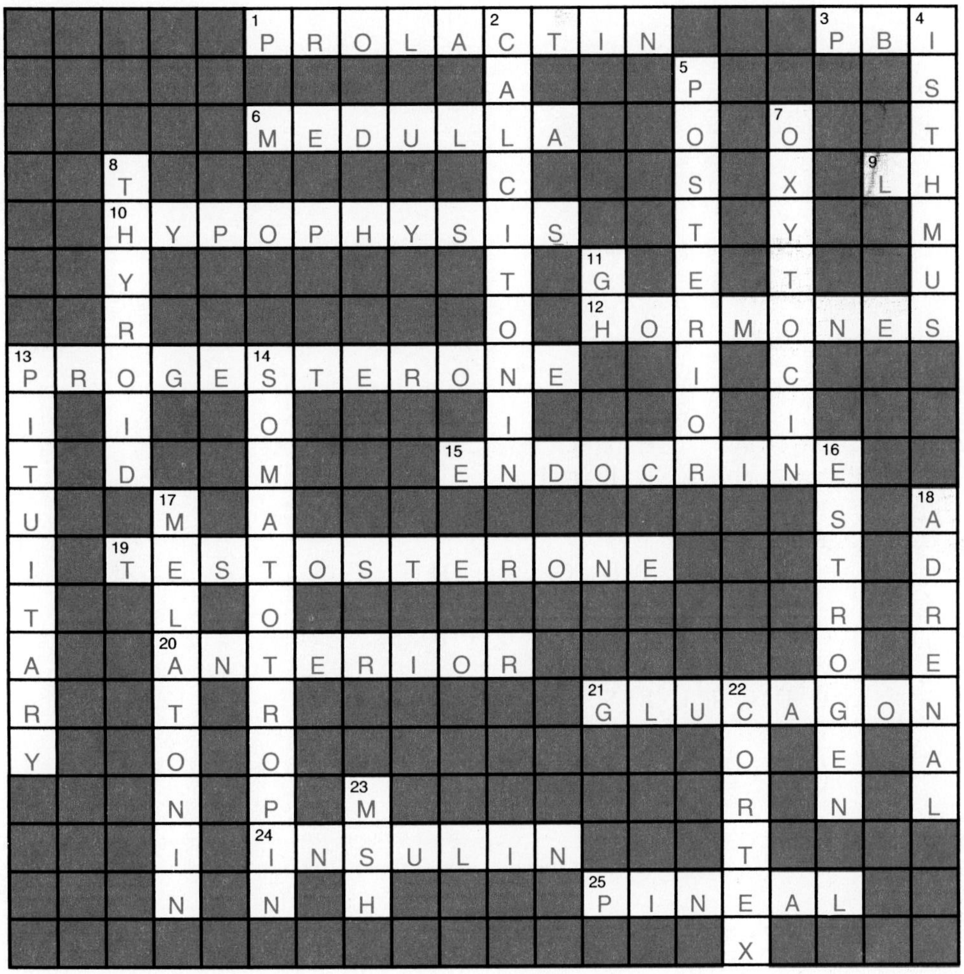
1 PROLACTIN
2 CALCITONIN
3 PBI
4 ISTHMUS
5 POSTERIOR
6 MEDULLA
7 OXYTOCIN
8 THYROID
9 LH
10 HYPOPHYSIS
11 GH
12 HORMONES
13 PROGESTERONE
PITUITARY
14 SOMATOTROPIN
15 ENDOCRINE
16 ESTROGEN
17 MELATONIN
18 ADRENAL
19 TESTOSTERONE
20 ANTERIOR
21 GLUCAGON
22 CORTEX
23 MSH
24 INSULIN
25 PINEAL

Answers: Chapter 13 Hidden Words Puzzle

```
.   .   .   P   .   .   .   .   .   .   .   .   .   .   .   .   .   .   .   .
G   O   N   A   D   S   .   .   .   .   .   .   .   .   .   .   .   .   .   .
L   .   .   N   H   .   .   .   .   .   .   .   .   .   .   .   .   .   .   .
.   O   .   C   .   Y   .   T   H   Y   R   O   I   D   .   .   .   .   .   .
.   .   B   R   .   P   C   .   .   V   .   .   .   .   .   .   .   .   .   .
.   .   .   E   S   T   R   O   G   E   N   A   .   .   .   .   .   .   .   .
.   .   .   A   .   .   L   P   .   .   R   .   .   .   .   .   .   .   .   .
.   .   .   S   .   .   L   .   H   .   I   .   .   .   .   .   .   .   .   .
.   .   .   .   .   .   O   .   .   Y   E   .   .   .   .   .   .   .   .   .
.   .   .   .   .   .   I   .   M   A   S   T   E   R   P   .   .   .   .   .
.   .   .   .   .   .   D   .   .   .   I   .   .   A   .   .   .   .   .   .
.   .   .   .   .   .   .   .   .   .   S   .   R   .   .   .   .   .   .   .
.   .   .   .   V   .   .   .   .   .   O   .   A   .   .   .   .   .   .   .
.   .   .   .   .   A   .   .   .   .   M   S   T   .   .   .   .   .   .   .
.   .   .   .   .   .   S   .   .   .   A   E   H   .   .   .   .   .   .   .
.   .   .   .   .   .   T   O   .   .   .   T   C   Y   Y   .   .   .   .   .
.   .   .   .   .   .   .   H   P   .   .   O   R   R   I   P   .   .   .   .
.   .   .   .   .   .   .   Y   R   .   .   T   E   O   S   .   O   .   .   .
.   .   .   .   .   .   .   R   E   .   R   T   I   T   .   .   T   .   .   .
.   .   .   .   .   .   G   .   .   .   O   S   .   O   I   D   H   .   .   .   .   .   H
.   .   .   .   .   .   L   .   .   .   X   S   P   O   S   M   .   .   .   A   .   .   .
.   .   .   .   .   .   A   .   .   .   I   I   N   F   U   N   D   I   B   U   L   U   M   .   .
.   .   .   .   .   .   N   A   .   .   N   N   .   S   .   .   .   .   A   .   .   .
.   .   .   .   .   .   D   U   C   T   L   E   S   S   .   .   .   .   .   .   M   .   .
.   .   .   .   .   .   R   .   .   .   .   .   .   .   .   .   .   .   .   U   .
.   .   .   .   .   .   E   .   .   .   .   .   .   .   .   .   .   .   .   .   S
.   .   .   .   .   .   N   .   .   .   .   .   .   .   .   .   .   .   .   .
.   .   .   .   .   .   N   .   .   .   .   .   .   .   .   .   .   .   .   .
.   .   .   .   .   .   L   .   .   .   .   .   .   .   .   .   .   .   .   .
```

Words:

\ HYPOTHALAMUS	> INFUNDIBULUM	∨ PARATHYROIDS	∨ SOMATOTROPIN
\ VASOPRESSIN	\ HYPOPHYSIS	∨ SECRETION	\ THYROXINE
> DUCTLESS	> ESTROGEN	∨ PANCREAS	∨ ADRENAL
∨ COLLOID	∨ ISTHMUS	∨ OVARIES	> THYROID
> GONADS	> MASTER	\ GLAND	\ LOBE

CHAPTER 13 GLOSSARY

Endocrine System Glands, Hormones, and Related Anatomic Terms

acidophil (ah-sid′o-fil): acid-staining cell of the anterior lobe of the pituitary gland, which secretes growth and lactogenic hormones.

adenohypophysis (ad″e-no-hi-pof′i-sis): anterior lobe of the pituitary gland (*hypophysis*), as distinguished from the posterior lobe (*neurohypophysis*).

adrenal glands: glands located at the top of each kidney (also called ***suprarenal glands***).

adrenaline (ad-ren′ah-lin): adrenal medulla hormone, which stimulates smooth muscle, cardiac muscle, and glands, to assist the body in meeting stress (also called ***epinephrine***).

adrenalopathy (ad-re″nal-op′ah-the): any adrenal gland pathology (also called ***adrenopathy***).

adrenocorticotropin (ACTH) (ad-re″no-kor″tik-o-trop′in): hormone of the anterior pituitary gland that promotes growth and development of the adrenal cortex and stimulates the cortex to secrete glucocorticoids (also called ***adreno-corticotrophin***).

aldosterone: hormone of the adrenal cortex responsible for electrolyte and water balance.

androsterone (an-dros′ter-on): an androgen, or male sex hormone, secreted by the adrenal gland.

antidiuretic hormone (ADH): hormone secreted by the posterior pituitary, which stimulates water reabsorption by the distal and collecting kidney tubules (also called ***vasopressin***).

basophils: basic-staining cells of the anterior lobe of the pituitary which secrete thyrotropin, a thyroid-stimulating hormone (TSH), adrenocorticotropin (ACTH), follicle-stimulating hormone (FSH), luteinizing hormone (LH), and melanocyte-stimulating hormone (MSH).

calcitonin: hormone secreted by the thyroid that promotes calcium absorption in the bones and reduced concentration of calcium in the blood.

chorionic gonadotropin: hormone secreted by the cells of the placental chorion.

chromophobe (kro′mo-fob): nonstaining cell of the anterior pituitary lobe.

colloid (kol′oid): gelatinous substance in the follicles of the thyroid glands that contains the hormone secreted by the thyroid.

cortex (kor′teks): outer portion of the adrenal gland that secretes mineralocorticoids, glucocorticoids, androgens, and some estrogen.

corticosterone (kor″ti-kos′ter-on): adrenocortical glucocorticoid hormone.

cortisol (kor′ti-sol): adrenocortical glucocorticoid hormone (also called ***hydrocortisone***).

estrogenic hormones: ovarian hormones that influence the development of secondary sex characteristics, sexual behavior, and the menstrual cycle.

euthyroid (u-thi′roid): normally functioning thyroid gland.

follicle-stimulating hormone (FSH): anterior pituitary hormone that stimulates the growth of graafian follicles, and the secretion of estrogen in the female, and the development of the seminiferous tubules and sperm cells in the male.

glucocorticoid: group of adrenocortical steroids that are concerned with protein, fat, and carbohydrate metabolism, and aid the body in resisting stress.

gonadotropic hormones: pituitary hormones that influence the gonads.

growth hormone (GH): hormone secreted by the anterior pituitary gland that promotes bodily growth (also called ***somatotropin*** and ***somatotrophin***).

hormone: chemical substance secreted by an endocrine gland.

hypophysis cerebri (hi-pof′i-sis): another name for pituitary gland.

infundibulum (in″fun-dib′u-lum): funnel-shaped passage with neural tracts from the hypothalamus of the brain to the pituitary gland.

iodine (i-o′din): essential element of the thyroid hormone.

islands of Langerhans (lahng′er-hanz): specialized pancreatic cells secreting insulin, glucagon, and pancreatic polypeptide (PP) into the circulation.

lactogenic hormone: pituitary hormone responsible for breast development and milk production in pregnancy (also called ***prolactin***).

luteinizing hormone (LH): anterior pituitary hormone that stimulates the formation of the corpus luteum, secretion of estrogen and progesterone in the female, and the development and secretion of testosterone in the interstitial cells of the testes.

medulla: inner portion of the adrenal glands producing epinephrine and norepinephrine.

mineralocorticoid: adrenocortical steroid that affects sodium and potassium balance.

neurohypophysis: posterior lobe of pituitary gland.

norepinephrine: hormone secreted by the adrenal medulla (also called ***noradrenalin***).

oxytocin (ok″se-to′sin): hormone of the posterior lobe of the pituitary gland that stimulates uterine contractions.

parathyroids: glands, normally two on each side, behind or embedded in the thyroid gland.

parathyroid hormone: parathyroid gland secretion that regulates calcium and phosphorus content of blood and bones.

pineal body: small gland located near the base of the brain.

pituicyte (pi-tu'i-sit): fusiform cell of the posterior lobe of the pituitary gland.

pituitary gland (pi-tu'i-tar"e): master gland, attached to the base of the brain, that exercises control over the other endocrine glands.

progesterone: hormone produced by the corpus luteum, whose function is to prepare the uterus to receive the fertilized ovum by causing growth and development of the uterine endometrial lining (also called *corpus luteum hormone*).

prolactin: see *lactogenic hormone*.

suprarenals: adrenal glands.

testosterone: hormone of the testis that induces and maintains secondary sex characteristics.

thyroid (thi'roid): large gland situated on the front part of the neck just below the larynx.

thyroid-stimulating hormone (TSH): hormone of the anterior pituitary gland that promotes growth and development of the thyroid gland and stimulates it to secrete thyroxine and triiodothyronine, which make up thyroid hormone (also called *thyrotropin* and *thyrotrophin*).

thyroxine (thi-rok'sin): one of two iodine-laden hormones making up the thyroid hormone whose main function is to regulate the metabolic rate and processes of growth and tissue differentiation (also called *thyroxin*).

triiodothyronine (tri"i-o"do-thi'ro-nen): second of two hormones that make up the thyroid hormone, containing less iodine than thyroxine, but having the same functions.

vasopressin: see *antidiuretic hormone*.

Pathologic Conditions

Inflammations and Infections

adrenalitis: inflammation of the adrenal glands.

thyroiditis: inflammation of the thyroid gland.

Hereditary, Congenital, and Developmental conditions

acromegaly (ak"ro-meg'ah-le): disease caused by pituitary hypersecretion of the growth hormone after completion of bone development, characterized by enlargement of the bones of the hands, feet, and face.

adiposogenital dystrophy (ad"i-pi"so-jen'i-tal): developmental disorder of adolescent males caused by anterior pituitary tumor or malfunction of the hypothalamus, with symptoms of under-development of genitals, female secondary sex characteristics, and adiposity of a feminine type (also called *Froblich's syndrome*).

congenital adrenal hyperplasia: congenital condition of hypersecretion of adrenocortical androgens in both sexes, causing virilization of females and under-development of gonads in males.

congenital goiter: goiter present at birth.

cretinism (kre'tin-izm): infantile hypothyroidism with symptoms including permanently stunted growth and mental development due to thyroid hormone deficiency, which may be related to maternal iodine deficiency (also called *infantile hypothyroidism*).

dwarfism: developmental disorder caused by anterior pituitary growth hormone hypofunction (also called *Lorain-Levi syndrome*).

giantism: developmental disorder caused by excessive secretion of growth hormone before completion of bone development, with over-growth of the long bones producing excessively large stature.

Hashimoto's disease (hash"i-mo'toz): chronic lymphomatous thyroiditis of auto-immune origins, with marked hereditary pattern, predominantly affecting females, with hypothyroidism and degeneration of the secreting cells of the thyroid gland (also called *chronic lymphomatous thyroiditis* and *struma lymphomatosa*).

hypogonadism: developmental disorder caused by inadequate secretion of pituitary gonadotropins, resulting in sexual immaturity and decreased functional activity of the gonads in males and females.

hypoparathyroidism: insufficiency of the parathyroid glands, which may be familial or due to excision, disease, or injury of the thyroid or parathyroid glands, resulting in hypocalcemia, with increased bone density due to decreased bone resorption.

Other Abnormalities

Addison's disease: life-threatening condition of adrenal insufficiency that may be caused by immune system processes, tumor, infection or adrenal gland hemorrhage, characterized by darkening of the skin, severe weakness, progressive anemia, low blood pressure, anorexia, and digestive disturbance.

adrenocortical hyperfunction: over-functioning of the adrenal cortex.

adrenocortical hypofunction: under-functioning of the adrenal cortex.

adrenogenital syndrome: developmental disorders due to hyperplasia, or tumor, of the adrenal glands, with masculinizing symptoms such as hirsutism, deepening of voice, and absence of menses in females, and feminizing of males with gynecomastia and lack of sperm.

aldosteronism (al"do-ster'on-izm"): disorder caused by adrenocortical hyperfunction, with muscular weakness, tetany, and excessive thirst and urination (primary type also called *Conn's syndrome*).

anorexia (an"o-rek'se-ah): lack or loss of appetite, a symptom in some endocrine disorders.

cachexia (kah-kek'se-ah): general ill health and malnutrition, which may be symptomatic of some endocrine disorders.

Cushing's syndrome: pituitary basophilism, with excessive secretion of adrenocortical hormone, characterized by obesity, moon-face, oligomenorrhea in women, and lowered testosterone levels in men (also called ***hypercortisolism***).

diabetes insipidus (di"ah-be'tez in"sip'i-dus): metabolic disorder characterized by polyuria and excessive thirst due to insufficient production of antidiuretic hormone (ADH).

diabetes mellitus: metabolic disease caused by a deficiency of production of the insulin hormone by the islands of Langerhans, with symptoms of sugar in the urine, loss of electrolytes and water, and degeneration of blood vessels. This disease appears in two forms: an insulin-dependent condition (formerly called juvenile-onset type) treated by insulin injections, and a non-insulin-dependent condition (formerly called adult-onset type) treated by diet control.

exophthalmos (ek"sof-thal'mos): protruding eyes, a symptom of one type of goiter.

fibrous thyroiditis: enlarged thyroid with progressive fibrosis of the normal tissue, with the gland adhering to adjacent structures (also called ***ligneous thyroiditis*** and ***Riedel's struma***).

goiter (goi'ter): enlargement of the thyroid, having a characteristic swelling at the front of the neck (also called ***struma***).

Graves' disease: hyperplasia of the thyroid gland (also called ***Basedow's disease***).

hirsutism (her'sut-izm): abnormal hairiness, which may occur in some endocrine disorders.

hyperparathyroidism: hyperfunction of the parathyroid gland of a primary type due to neoplasms or unknown causes, and a secondary type due to a metabolic disorder, producing calcium imbalance in the bodily systems, with osteoporosis and deposition of calcium in tissues.

hyperthyroidism: over-production of the thyroid hormone.

hypophyseal cachexia (kah-kek'se-ah): hypofunction of the anterior pituitary gland due to trauma, lesions, or tumors, resulting in generalized ill health with weakness, and overall insufficiency of adrenal, thyroid, and gonadal functions (also known as ***Simmonds' disease*** and ***pituitary cachexia***).

hypothyroidism: under-function of the thyroid gland.

myxedema: form of adult hypothyroidism, with metabolic slowdown resulting from deficient thyroid hormone secretion, having symptoms ranging from milder forms with skin dryness, intolerance for cold, and some intellectual slippage, to severe forms with obesity, slowness of motor function, and severe intellectual dullness.

parathyroid tetany: muscular cramps and spasms, resulting from hypocalcemia due to excision of, or injury to, the parathyroids.

polydipsia: excessive thirst, a symptom of diabetes.

polyuria: excessive urination, a symptom of diabetes.

seasonal affective disorder (SAD): dysfunction linked to pineal gland production of melatonin, which is produced in darkness (night), and inhibited in daylight, becoming a problem for people residing in areas of extended darkness, such as in polar regions, producing symptoms of depression, known as "winter blues".

Sheehan's syndrome: hypopituitarism due to a post-partum circulatory collapse, sometimes related to uterine hemmorhage, resulting in pituitary necrosis.

tetany: muscle spasm and cramp, a symptom of hypoparathyroidism.

thyroid crisis: exacerbation of pre-existing hyperthyroidism as a result of trauma, surgery, or severe adrenocortical insufficiency (also called ***thyrotoxic crisis*** or ***thyroid storm***).

thyrolytic: pertaining to substances destructive to thyroid tissue.

thyropathy: any disease or disorder of the thyroid gland.

thyroprivia (thi"ro-priv'e-ah): condition caused by lack of thyroid hormone.

virilism (vir'i-lizm): masculinization of a female, at birth or later in life, because of adrenocortical or gonadal dysfunction, or hormonal treatment.

*Oncology**

adrenal cortical carcinomas*: large, malignant, metastisizing tumors of the adrenal cortex, which produce virilism or Cushing's syndrome.

basophilic adenoma: pituitary gland tumor whose cells stain with basic dyes.

chromophobic adenoma (kro'mo-fob-ik): benign tumor of pituitary gland whose cells resist staining with dyes.

craniopharyngioma of pituitary gland (kra"neo-o-fah-rin"je-o'mah): tumor arising from the epithelium of the pituitary stalk.

eosinophilic adenoma of pituitary gland: tumor of the eosinophilic cells of the anterior hypophysis, associated with acromegaly and giantism.

feminizing adenocarcinoma of adrenal gland*: malignant tumor that produces female secondary sex characteristics in the male.

feminizing adenoma of adrenal gland: benign tumor causing development of female secondary sex characteristics in the male.

*Indicates a malignant condition.

glioma of pineal gland: benign tumor of neuroglial tissue in the pineal gland.

Hurthle cell adenoma of thyroid gland (her'tel): adenoma containing Hurthle (large eosinophilic) cells.

Hurthle cell carcinoma of thyroid gland*: malignant tumor of the thyroid.

pheochromocytoma (fe'o-kro-mo-si-to'mah): tumor of the adrenal medulla, usually benign.

pinealoma: rare tumor of the pineal gland, sometimes associated with hydrocephalus or precocious puberty.

virilizing adenocarcinoma of adrenal gland*: malignant tumor of the adrenal gland, with development of male secondary sex characteristics in the female.

virilizing adenoma of adrenal gland: tumor of the adrenal glands, with development of male secondary sex characteristics in the female.

Surgical Procedures

adrenalectomy (ad-re"nal-ek'to-me): excision of the adrenal glands.

hemithyroidectomy: partial excision of the thyroid gland.

hypophysectomy (hi"po-fiz-ek'to-me): excision of the hypophysis, or anterior pituitary gland.

isthmectomy: excision of the thyroid isthmus.

lobectomy: excision of a lobe of the thyroid gland.

parathyroidectomy: excision of a parathyroid gland.

pinealectomy (pin"e-al-ek'to-me): excision of the pineal body.

thyroidectomy: excision of the thyroid gland.

thyroidotomy: incision of the thyroid gland for exploration or drainage of an abscess or cyst.

Laboratory Tests and Procedures

aldosterone assay: twenty-four-hour urine or blood collection test to determine the presence of the hormone aldosterone, which is normally present and necessary for electrolyte balance.

catecholamine test: urine test to measure amounts of adrenaline (epinephrine) and noradrenaline (norepinephrine), which are elevated in tumors of the adrenal gland (see also *vanillylmandelic acid*).

computerized tomography (CT): imaging device using X-rays at multiple angles through specific sections of the body, analyzed by computer to provide a total picture of the part being examined (also called *computerized axial tomography [CAT]*).

cortisol tests: tests of blood plasma and urine to measure levels of cortisol, to detect disorders of the adrenal glands.

estrogen receptor test: to determine whether hormonal treatment will be useful in cancer treatment, by measuring the response of the cancer to estrogen.

Goetsch's skin reaction: test for hyperthyroidism involving localized reaction to epinephrine injection.

17-hydrocorticosteroid test (17-OCHS): twenty-four-hour urine collection to determine the functioning of the adrenal glands as diagnostic of hyper- or hypoadrenalism.

17-ketosteroids tests (17-KS): twenty-four-hour urine test to measure the levels of a group of adrenal cortex hormones involved in Addison's disease, Cushing's syndrome, stress, precocious puberty disorders, feminization in males, and virilization in females.

luteinizing hormone assay: blood or urine test to determine the amount of pituitary hormones FSH and LH present, to detect gonadal failure or insufficiency, precocious puberty, testicular feminization, anorchia, and menopause.

magnetic resonance imaging (MRI): noninvasive method of scanning the body by means of an electromagnetic field and radio waves, which provides visual images on a computer screen and magnetic tape recordings (also called *nuclear magnetic resonance [NMR]*).

protein-bound iodine (PBI) test: test of thyroid function in which blood protein-bound iodine is measured to estimate the amount of available thyroid hormone in peripheral blood.

radioactive iodine uptake (RAIU) or **thyroid ^{131}I uptake test:** thyroid function is evaluated by introducing radioactive iodine orally or intravenously during a selected time period, and measuring its absorption by the thyroid with a gamma ray detector.

Thyroid hormone tests: Blood tests to determine thyroid hormone levels and diagnose disorders of the thyroid.

> **triiodothyronine (T_3) thyroxine (T_4) thyroxine-binding globulin (TBG)**

thyroid scan: intravenous injection of radioactive substance for organ imaging to detect abnormalities in the size, shape, location, and function of the thyroid gland.

thyroid stimulation test: anterior pituitary thyroid-stimulating hormone (TSH) is injected to determine if thyroid problems are due to pituitary or thyroid dysfunction.

thyroid ultrasonography: noninvasive procedure to detect cysts and tumors of the thyroid by directing ultrasonic pulses at the gland that are reflected back for display on an oscilloscope.

vanillylmandelic acid (VMA) assay: twenty-four-hour urine test to detect VMA (a metabolite of catecholamines), to evaluate adrenal function.

CHAPTER 14

The Nervous System

The Central Processing Unit

CHAPTER OVERVIEW

This chapter explores the structure and functions of both divisions of the nervous system, central and peripheral, including the brain, spinal cord, nerves, and fluids.

CHARACTERISTICS OF THE NERVOUS SYSTEM

The nervous system has been compared to a computer system, with the brain acting as the central processing unit, relaying messages by way of the spinal cord, through nerve fibers that radiate to every structure in the body, to provide connections for input and output data. Sensory nerves bring impulses, or information, from the various systems of the body, whereas motor nerves carry impulses from the central coordinating point to muscles or glands that need to respond for appropriate adjustment of the body.

The nervous system is divided into the ***central nervous system*** (***CNS***), which includes the ***brain*** and ***spinal cord***, and the ***peripheral nervous system*** (***PNS***), composed of the ***craniospinal nerves*** and the ***autonomic nervous system*** (***ANS***), which controls and coordinates the functioning of the vital organs. Nervous tissue is composed of many types of cells and fibers, working together in one central mass, with many peripheral strands.

Nerve Structure and Function

Nervous system cells are called ***neurons***. All neurons are similar in that they have one ***axon***, one or more

dendrites, and a grayish ***cell body*** in between, containing a nucleus responsible for maintaining the life of the whole cell. The dendrites are numerous short branches that conduct nerve impulses toward the cell body. The axons are longer branches that carry impulses away from the cell body, either to other neurons, through contact with their dendrites, to the cell body itself, or directly to other organs or tissues (see Fig. 5-5). It is estimated that each neuron interconnects with about 1000 other neurons.

Neurons are divided into ***sensory*** (or ***afferent***), ***motor*** (or ***efferent***), and ***connector*** (or ***interneuron***) neurons. In sensory neurons, the dendrites are connected to receptors (eyes, ears, and other sense organs), and the axons are connected to other neurons. The receptors change information from external sources, such as light waves or sound vibrations, into electrical impulses. In motor neurons, the dendrites are connected to other neurons, and the axons to effectors (muscles and glands). In connector neurons, the dendrites and axons are both connected to other neurons.

Normally, impulses pass in only one direction. Sensory neurons conduct impulses from the sense organs to the spinal cord and brain. Motor neurons conduct impulses from the brain and spinal cord to muscles and glands. Sensory or afferent impulses are transmitted to the brain through the ascending tracts of the spinal cord, whereas motor or efferent impulses are carried from the brain through the descending tracts of the spinal cord.

The impulses are essentially the same in all types of neurons, and may be compared to the wavelike action of peristalsis. The initiating stimulus of the impulse in one section of a nerve fiber causes a similar reaction in the next connecting section, and this chain reaction continues until the impulse reaches the end of the nerve fiber. Nerve impulses differ only in terms of the body part affected: an impulse caused by light rays entering the eye may result in vision; an impulse received in the ear may result in hearing; other impulses may result in muscle movement, and still others may result in glandular secretions.

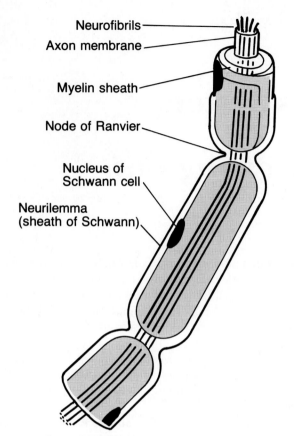

Neurofibrils

Axon membrane

Myelin sheath

Node of Ranvier

Nucleus of
Schwann cell

Neurilemma
(sheath of Schwann)

Figure 14-1.   Diagram of a nerve and its coverings.

The threadlike dendrites and axons are also called nerve *fibers*. Bundles of these fibers bound together are called *nerves*. Groups of neuron cell bodies within the brain and spinal cord are called *nuclei*, whereas those outside are called *ganglia* (singular—*ganglion*). A side branch of the axon is called a *collateral*, which ends in a fine, spreading branch called a *terminal twig*, deriving its name from its resemblance to a twig or branch of a tree.

The point at which an impulse is transmitted from the axon of one neuron to the dendrite of another is a microscopic space called a *synapse*. The electrical impulses carried by the neuron do not directly jump the synapse, but instead produce a *neurotransmitter* chemical, which activates other electrical impulses in the dendrites of the connecting neuron.

Nerve fibers are of different types. Some are myelinated, with a coat of white fatty material called a *myelin sheath* surrounding them, found mainly in the central nervous system. Nonmyelinated fibers have a tubelike membrane covering called the *neurilemma* or *Schwann's sheath*, and are found especially in the autonomic nervous system. A myelin sheath and a neurilemma are found in peripheral somatic fibers, and there are axon fibers that have no sheath, found in the central nervous system and within organs (Fig. 14-1).

The nerve cells and their gossamer filaments are held together and supported by a specialized type of tissue called *neuroglia*. Neuroglial cells have many processes, or branches, that form a dense network between neurons. They are divided into four main types—*astrocytes* (*astro*—star), *microglia*, *oligodendroglia*, and *Schwann cells*. Astrocytes cover the surfaces of the capillaries of the brain, and, together with the walls of the capillaries, form the blood-brain barrier, which regulates the passage of nutritive and chemical molecules to the brain neurons. Microglia are phagocytic cells that fight infection and help in healing. Oligodendroglia aid in holding nerve fibers together and in forming the myelin sheath within the central nervous system. Schwann cells, which are found only outside the central nervous system, form the neurilemma and a thin layer of myelin around nerve fibers.

The central nervous system contains both white and gray matter. The white color is created by the the myelinated fibers of the bundles of axons and dendrites, and the gray color is due to the masses of nerve cell bodies.

The cell body is vital to the neuron, and, if the cell body dies, the neuron dies and can never be replaced. Neurons are so specialized that they have lost their power to reproduce new cells. When an axon is severed, that part distal to the cell body dies, with both the fiber and its surrounding myelinated sheath degenerating. A new axon may gradually grow and restore the nerve, but such regeneration occurs only in the peripheral nervous system. Once a connection is broken within the central nervous system, it is broken forever, although other nerve structures may take over the functions of the injured nerves.

Review A

Complete the following:

1. The nervous system is divided into the _____ and _____ nervous systems.

2. All neurons have one _____ and one or more _____, with a grayish

_____ in between.

3. The three types of neurons are _____, _____, and _____.

4. Threadlike dendrites and axons are also called _____.

5. Groups of neuron cell bodies within the brain and spinal cord are called _____.

6. The microscopic space over which an impulse is transmitted is called a _____.

7. The sheath of Schwann is also called the _____.

8. The nerve cells and their filaments are held together and supported by a type of tissue called

_____.

9. Receptors change information from external sources such as light waves into electrical _____.

10. Groups of neuron cell bodies outside the brain and spinal cord are called _____.

CENTRAL NERVOUS SYSTEM

The central nervous system (CNS) includes the brain and the spinal cord. This system is also referred to as the cerebrospinal system. The brain lies in the cranial cavity, and the spinal cord, continuous with the lower end of the brain, passes through the *foramen magnum*, an opening in the occipital bone of the head, and continues down through the vertebral column. The brain and spinal cord are both protected from injury by the skeletal system, the brain by the bones of the skull, and the spinal cord by the vertebrae.

The Meninges

The *meninges* (plural of *meninx*—meaning membrane) are three membranes that envelop the central nervous system, separating the brain and spinal cord from the body cavities in which they lie, and aiding in their support and protection (Fig. 14-2). The meninges are composed predominantly of white fibrous connective tissue.

The *dura mater*—the outermost layer, is the hardest, toughest, and most fibrous of the three.

The *arachnoid* (*arachno* means spider)—the middle membrane is much less dense, and weblike in appearance.

The *pia mater*—the innermost, thin, compact membrane that is closely adapted to the surface of the brain and spinal cord, is very vascular and supplies the blood for the central nervous system tissues.

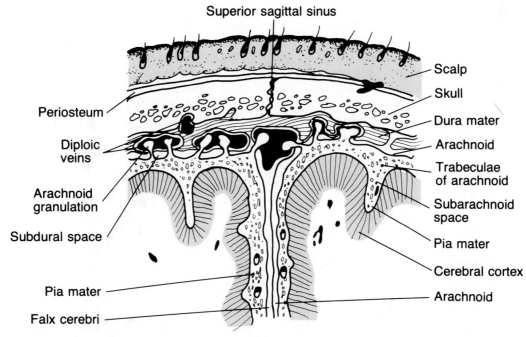

Figure 14-2.   Coronal section through skull.

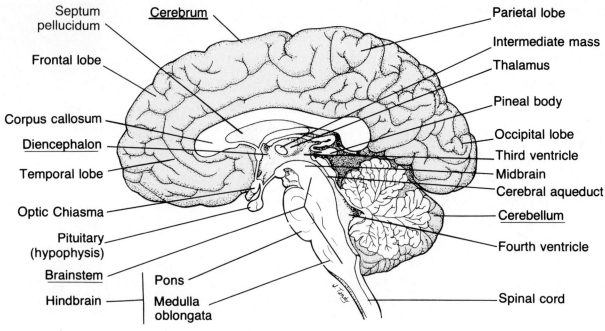

Figure 14-3. Structures of the brain, with major divisions underlined.

The Brain

The brain is the greatly enlarged part of the central nervous system, weighing about 40 to 60 oz (1.1 to 1.7 kg) in the average adult, and in proportion to the size of the body, it is much larger in the neonate than in the adult. The size of the cranium (skull) furnishes only a general index as to the size of the brain, for the shape and thickness of the skull and the subarachnoid space vary in individuals. It is estimated that the average brain contains about 100 to 200 billion neurons at birth, and of these 50 to 100 thousand neurons die each day.

The divisions of the brain are the ***brainstem***, the ***diencephalon***, the ***cerebellum***, and the ***cerebrum*** (Fig. 14-3).

The Brainstem

The brainstem is divided into the ***medulla oblongata***, the ***pons***, and the ***midbrain***, with the pons and medulla together commonly referred to as the ***hindbrain*** (Fig. 14-3).

The Medulla Oblongata.   The medulla oblongata, the lowest and most posterior part of the brain, about 1 inch (2.5 cm) in length, is an extension of the spinal cord at the point where the central canal of the spinal cord enlarges to form the fourth ventricle, extending to the

The pia mater and arachnoid are often viewed as one membrane, the ***pia-arachnoid*** (also called the ***leptomeninges***). The space between the pia mater and the arachnoid is known as the ***subarachnoid space***, and that between the arachnoid and the dura mater as the ***subdural space***.

pons. The fourth ventricle, a large kite-shaped cavity that secretes some of the cerebrospinal fluid, contains openings that connect the cavity with the subarachnoid space and with the lateral ventricles in the cerebral hemispheres.

The medulla oblongata is composed of white matter, and a reticular formation, or network, composed of gray and white matter. This network has a ***reticular activating system***, connecting with all of the sensory systems and the cortex, controlling and regulating the degree of cortical arousal and alertness. The reticular formation also contains groups of nuclei, some of which are highly specialized structures, called nerve centers, that regulate heart action, respiration, and blood pressure.

Nerve fibers (the white matter) in the medulla oblongata establish communication between the cerebrum and the spinal cord. As these nerve fibers pass through the medulla, about 75% cross from one side to the other. This is the basis for the right side of the brain controlling the left side of the body, and the left side of the brain controlling the right side of the body.

The Pons.   The pons, about 1½ inches (3.8 cm.) long and made up of reticular formation and white matter, is the portion of the brain that serves as a bridge (pons means bridge) connecting the medulla oblongata, cerebellum, and cerebrum. A portion of the reticular formation, which figures significantly in respiration, extends into the pons. The pons is also associated with the fifth, sixth, seventh, and eighth cranial nerves. These nerves provide sensory input from face and head, muscles and other internal tissues, sense of taste, hearing and balance. They also provide motor control of facial muscles, including the muscles of mastication, and salivary secretion.

The Midbrain. The midbrain, or ***mesencephalon***, is the uppermost part of the brainstem, above the pons, and, like the hindbrain, is also composed of reticular formation and white matter. It contains auditory, visual, and muscle control centers, and is also involved in body posture and equilibrium.

The third and fourth cranial nerves originate in the midbrain, which also contains a small central canal called the ***cerebral aquaduct*** (***aqueduct of Sylvius***), that connects the third ventricle of the brain, located in the diencephalon, with the fourth ventricle, located between the cerebellum and the hindbrain.

Review B

Complete the following:

1. Another name for the central nervous system is the _____ system.

2. The three meningeal membranes are the _____,

   _____, and _____.

3. The four divisions of the brain are the _____,

   _____, _____, and

   _____.

4. The brainstem consists of the _____,

   _____, and _____.

5. The hindbrain is made up of the _____ and the

   _____.

The Cerebellum

The cerebellum is the second largest division of the brain, situated just above the medulla, and beneath the rear portion of the cerebrum, resembling a partially opened shell in appearance, and comprising about 10% of the weight of the entire brain. It consists of a central portion called the ***vermis***, and two larger sections, one on each side, called the right and left ***cerebellar hemispheres*** (Fig. 14-3).

The chief functions of the cerebellum are to balance, harmonize and coordinate muscular activity initiated by the cerebrum. The cerebellum, through its vestibular portion, is connected with the semicircular canals of the ear, which, together with the movements of the eyes, react to gravity and sudden changes or movement of the head. These are further integrated and correlated, by the cerebellum, with nerve impulses from the muscles, tendons, and joints. Through these functions, the cerebellum fine-tunes motor activity and muscle tone, which is essential for precise and complicated voluntary movement, and the maintenance of posture. It also enables the various muscle groups to act harmoniously or as a cooperative whole at a given moment. Many motor activities, originally initiated by the cerebrum and coordinated by the cerebellum, such as walking, running, and other skilled movements, eventually become automatic and are not consciously initiated or coordinated.

The Diencephalon

The diencephalon is the part of the brain between the midbrain and the cerebrum, containing the ***thalamus***, the ***epithalamus***, and the ***hypothalamus*** (***thalamus*** means chamber). The diencephalon also contains the third ventricle, a narrow chamber between the right and left halves of the thalamus (Fig. 14-3).

The thalamus is a large, gray, oval mass, that acts as a center to receive sensory impulses and transmit them on to the cerebral cortex. The thalamus has been referred to as the great integrating center of the brain, because it plays a role in integrating visual, auditory, tactile, temperature, pain, and taste sensations with pleasant and unpleasant emotions, and with memory storage.

The ***epithalamus*** contains the pineal body (Chapter 13) and olfactory centers.

The ***hypothalamus*** is located beneath the thalamus. It connects the endocrine and nervous systems, which coordinate the maintenance functions of the body (Chapter 13). The hypothalamus also regulates the autonomic nervous system, and contains centers for control of body temperature, carbohydrate and fat metabolism, appetite and emotions. It is a key center for the interaction of emotional and bodily functioning, and plays a crucial role in psychosomatic illness. The hypothalamus contains the posterior lobe of the pituitary gland, the infundibulum (previously discussed in the Endocrine System), and the *optic chiasma*. The optic chiasma, which is also a part of the cerebral hemispheres, is formed chiefly of nerve fibers, and beyond the chiasma these fibers continue as the optic tract.

The Cerebrum

The cerebrum, the largest part of the brain, is divided into two hemispheres called the ***cerebral hemispheres***, which occupy most of the brain cavity (Fig. 14-3).

Structure.   The outer surface, or ***cortex***, is made up of gray matter, beneath which is white matter that forms the central portion of the brain. As the brain develops, the cerebral hemispheres increase greatly in size in relation to the rest of the brain. As the gray matter of the cortex increases in amount, the surface of each cerebral hemisphere is thrown into folds called ***gyri*** (singular—***gyrus***), or ***convolutions***, which are separated from each other by furrows called ***sulci*** (singular—***sulcus***), with the deeper furrows called ***fissures***.

Each cerebral hemisphere contains a ***lateral ventricle***, which projects an anterior horn into the frontal lobe, a posterior horn into the occipital lobe, and an inferior horn into the temporal lobe. These horns are also called ***cornua*** (***cornu*** means horn). The lateral ventricles, in conjunction with the third and fourth ventricles, produce the cerebrospinal fluid.

Connecting the structures of one cerebral hemisphere with the other are three groups of ***commissural tracts*** (connections between corresponding anatomic parts):

> ***corpus callosum***—the largest, consisting of dense masses of white matter that transversely unite the two hemispheres.
>
> ***anterior commissure***—contains fibers that connect different parts of the temporal lobes with one another.
>
> ***posterior commissure***—formed by a thin sheet of fibers that cross transversely under the posterior part of the corpus callosum, and connect to the olfactory centers.

The Functional Areas of the Cerebral Cortex

The cerebral cortex is divided into lobes: ***frontal***, ***temporal***, ***parietal***, and ***occipital***, corresponding

with the bones in the region in which they are located (Fig. 14-3). Some anatomists consider a fifth area, the ***insula*** or ***island of Reil***, hidden below the frontal lobe, to be an additional lobe.

Frontal Lobe.   The frontal lobe, the most anterior of all the lobes, is the center for voluntary movement, and is often referred to as the motor area, containing areas for the control of gross, fine, and complicated muscle movements. One of these areas, the ***premotor***, is viewed as the highest level of motor control because it is concerned with learned motor activity of a highly complicated nature, such as playing a musical instrument, dancing, and athletic skills. The most anterior portion of the frontal lobe, the ***prefrontal*** area, is also the seat of the highest of human functions, including intelligence, creativity, memory, and association of ideas.

Parietal Lobe.   The parietal lobe collects, recognizes, and organizes sensations of pain, temperature, touch, position and movement. From these sensations we perceive the size, shape, and weight of external objects and of our own physical being.

Temporal Lobe.   The temporal lobe contains the centers for awareness and correlation of auditory stimuli, and functions in storage of auditory and visual memory as well as language development. One area, ***Broca's speech area***, is especially concerned with speech.

Occipital Lobe.   The occipital lobe forms the posterior extremity of each cerebral hemisphere, involves visual perception, visual memory and associations, and plays a role in eye movements.

Hemispheric Differences in Function

As previously noted, the left hemisphere of the cerebrum controls the right side of the body, and the right hemisphere controls the left side of the body, because the descending nerve fibers cross over in the medulla and spinal cord, with fibers from the left crossing to the right, and fibers from the right crossing to the left.

General differences in hemispheric function appear to exist, with the left, which is usually dominant, being involved in language, logic, analytic thinking, and ordering of events and symbols, whereas the right hemisphere has been linked to imagination, creativity in art and music, and to spatial and depth perception.

Review C

Complete the following:

1. The cerebellum is divided into right and left _____.

2. The diencephalon contains the _____, _____, _____, and

_____.

3. The outer surface of gray matter in the cerebrum is called the _____.

4. The four lobes of the cerebrum are the _____, _____, _____, and

_____.

5. The left cerebral hemisphere controls the _____ side of the body, and the right cerebral

hemisphere controls the _____ side of the body.

Limbic System

The limbic system appears to be a center for emotional experience, emotional behavior, and memory, and has been referred to as "the emotional brain." Emotions that have been identified with the limbic system include sadness, pleasure, fear, anger, and sexual arousal, which are subject to moderation by the cerebral cortex.

The limbic system involves areas of the diencephalon and the cerebrum, including the *cingulate gyrus*, *isthmus*, *hippocampal gyrus*, *uncus*, *hippocampus*, *septum*, *amygdala*, and the *hypothalamus*. The hippocampus has been called the "gatekeeper for memory," and has been related to learning and memory problems in diseases like Alzheimer's.

Cerebrospinal Fluid

Cerebrospinal fluid is a thin, transparent, watery fluid found within the ventricles of the brain, the central canal of the spinal cord, and the subarachnoid space. It is produced by a network of capillaries that filter plasmalike fluids from blood into the ventricles, with the lateral ventricles producing the major part.

Cerebrospinal fluid drains from the lateral ventricles into the third ventricle, through the cerebral aqueduct (aqueduct of Sylvius) into the fourth ventricle, from which it passes into the subarachnoid space. The cerebrospinal fluid surrounds the brain, providing support for its weight and serving as a protective cushion. The spinal cord is also surrounded and cushioned by the fluid. In addition to the protection provided by the cerebrospinal fluid, it also supplies some nutrients.

SPINAL CORD

The spinal cord is an essential extension of the central processing unit, the brain. Sensations received by the sensory nerves are relayed to the spinal cord, where they are transferred either to the brain or to motor nerves. If the sensation is transferred to a motor nerve, it travels out to a muscle or gland and produces an action.

The spinal cord resembles a flattened cylinder and is about the thickness of a pencil. It extends from the medulla oblongata to the level of the first lumbar vertebra.

Structure

The spinal cord, constituting about 2% of all the central nervous system, is enclosed in the vertebral column, which protects it from injury. Like the brain, it has three membranous coverings, the pia mater, arachnoid, and dura mater, which have been described in the section on the meninges, and, like the brain, it is bathed in cerebrospinal fluid. The spinal cord is made up of an inner core of gray matter and an outer core of white matter, which, in cross section, resembles a butterfly, with its wings divided into two dorsal and two ventral parts called *horns*.

Both ascending and descending tracts are contained in the spinal cord. These tracts are white fibers made up of axons and dendrites. The ascending tracts conduct the afferent (sensory) nerve impulses to the brain, and the descending tracts conduct the efferent (motor) nerve impulses from the brain. Centers for connections between the afferent and the efferent nerve impulses are provided by the gray matter (Fig. 14-7).

It is through the spinal cord, and the attachment of 31 pairs of spinal nerves along its sides, that the brain maintains intimate association with all the organs of the body (Figs. 14-4 and 14-5). Each of the 31 pairs of spinal nerves is attached to the spinal cord by one posterior afferent root and one anterior efferent root, at approximately equal distances throughout the entire length of the cord.

The spinal cord is divided into sections, with 8 pairs of cervical nerves, 12 pairs of thoracic nerves, 5 pairs of lumbar nerves, 5 pairs of sacral nerves, and 1 pair of coccygeal nerves. The functions of these nerves are discussed in the section on the peripheral nervous system.

Injury of the spinal cord in any segment can imperil any or all of its functions. When the spinal cord is injured, the part above the injury functions normally, but there is paralyis of the part below the injury, and the brain receives no impulses from that area.

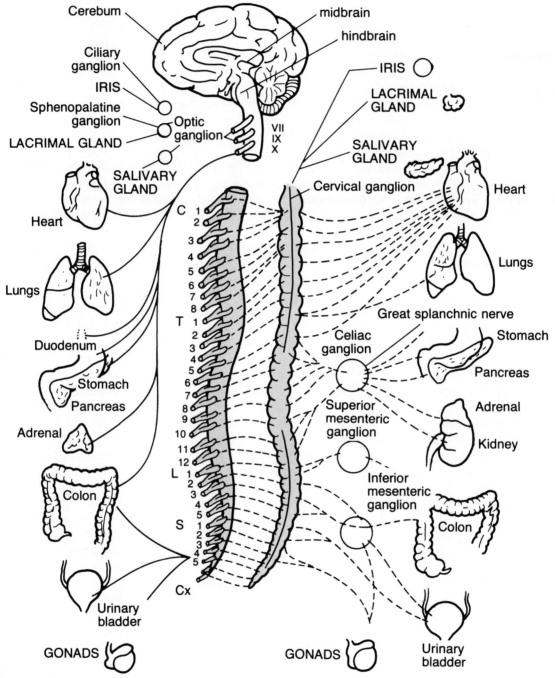

Figure 14-4. Sympathetic and parasympathetic nervous systems. The sympathetic system is represented by broken lines and the parasympathetic by solid lines.

Review D

Complete the following:

1. The limbic system is referred to as the _____ brain.

2. The cerebrospinal fluid is found within the _____, the _____, and the

_____.

3. The spinal cord has _____ membranous coverings.

4. The spinal cord has both _____ and _____ tracts.

5. There are _____ pairs of spinal nerves along the spinal cord.

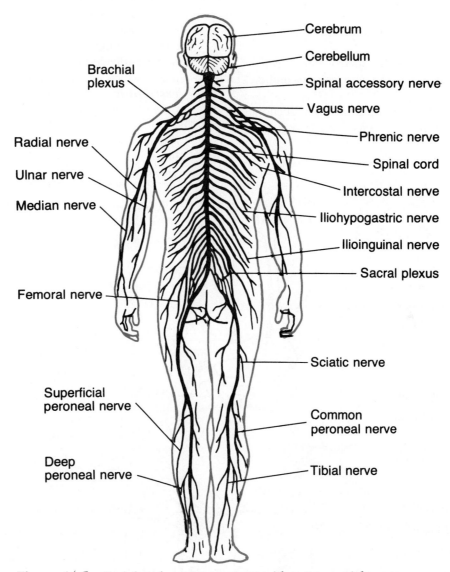

Figure 14-5. Peripheral nervous system, with some cranial nerves.

THE PERIPHERAL NERVOUS SYSTEM

The peripheral nervous system (PNS) includes all of the nerves and ganglia located outside of the brain and spinal cord, including the autonomic nervous system (Figs. 14-4 and 14-5). Due to the closeness of the connections, the peripheral nervous system overlaps the central nervous system, the spinal cord, and their functions.

Cranial Nerves

The first segment of the peripheral nervous system is the 12 pairs of cranial nerves arising from the brain, especially the brain stem (Fig. 14-6).

The first cranial nerve, the **olfactory**, is for the sense of smell.

The second cranial nerve, the **optic**, extends from the retina of the eye to the optic chiasma and is for vision.

The third cranial nerve, the **oculomotor**, functions in movement of the eye, focus, pupil changes, and eye muscle sense.

The fourth cranial nerve, the **trochlear**, functions in movement of the eye.

The fifth cranial nerve, the **trigeminal**, is the largest of the cranial nerves, with both sensory and motor functions, and is divided into three parts, the **ophthalmic**, the **maxillary**, and the **mandibular**. The trigeminal receives sensations from the head and face, and innervates the chewing muscles.

The sixth cranial nerve, the **abducens**, innervates the muscles of the eye.

The seventh cranial nerve, the **facial**, is both a sensory and a motor nerve, controlling muscles of the face, ears, and scalp, and functioning in facial expression, salivary gland secretion, and in taste sensation.

The eighth cranial nerve, the **acoustic** or **auditory** nerve, is divided into two parts, the **cochlear** nerve, which functions in hearing, and the **vestibular** nerve, which functions in maintaining balance and equilibrium.

The ninth cranial nerve, the **glossopharyngeal**, is both a motor and a sensory nerve, which functions in taste sensations, swallowing, and salivary secretion.

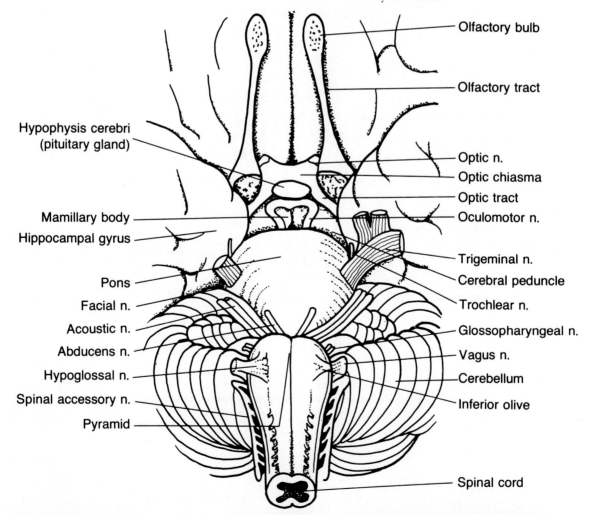

Figure 14-6.   Attachment of the cranial nerves to the underside (ventral surface) of the brain.

The tenth cranial nerve, the *vagus*, is the longest of the cranial nerves, and is both a motor and a sensory nerve. It is extensive in distribution, with many branches to the pharynx, larynx, trachea, esophagus, and the thoracic and abdomino-pelvic viscera, receiving sensations from, and activating, these organs.

The eleventh cranial nerve, the *spinal accessory*, is a motor nerve divided into two parts, *cranial* and *spinal*, and functions in swallowing, head and shoulder movements, visceral movements, and voice production.

The twelfth cranial nerve, the *hypoglossal*, is a motor nerve that controls the muscles of the tongue, and functions in speech and swallowing.

Spinal Nerves

As noted previously, 12 pairs of cranial nerves arise from the brain, and 31 pairs of spinal nerves stem from the spinal cord. Both voluntary and involuntary impulses are carried by these nerves. In general, the cranial nerves are voluntary, except for those serving the heart, the smooth muscles of the lungs, the salivary glands, and the stomach and eye muscles. The spinal nerves send fibers to all the muscles of the trunk and extremities, with involuntary fibers going to smooth muscles and glands of the gastrointestinal tract, genitourinary tract, and cardiovascular system.

The spinal nerves are attached to the spinal cord by anterior (efferent) and posterior (afferent) roots. After leaving the spinal cord, the nerves are named after their corresponding vertebra. The first pair of cervical nerves emerge between the first cervical vertebra and the occipital bone, thus providing for 8 pairs of cervical nerves, although there are only seven cervical vertebrae. The next 12 pairs are the thoracic spinal nerves, followed by

5 pairs of lumbar, 5 pairs of sacral, and 1 pair of coccygeal spinal nerves. The lower spinal nerves supply the lower extremities and extend below the level of the spinal cord in parallel strands, resembling a horse's tail, the *cauda equina* (*cauda* means tail, and *equina* means horse). Through openings in the sacrum they extend down the thigh.

Spinal nerves are composed of sensory and motor fibers of both the autonomic and the voluntary nervous systems. In some areas of the body they merge to form an interlacing network called a *plexus*. These plexuses are the *cervical plexus* in the neck, the *brachial plexus* in the shoulder, and the *lumbosacral plexus* in the lumbar, sacral, and coccygeal areas of the back. The names and areas served by a number of the peripheral nerves, many of which are named for bones, organs, or body regions, are shown in Figs. 14-4 and 14-5.

The cervical plexus is formed by the first four cervical nerves and supplies the skin and muscles of the shoulders, neck, and head, with phrenic branches going to the diaphragm.

The lower cervical and first thoracic nerves supply the upper limbs through the brachial plexus, which lies in the shoulder area, serving the skin and the arm and hand muscles.

The lumbosacral plexus supplies the skin and muscles of the back, abdomen, buttocks, lower limbs, perineum, and external genitalia. The sciatic nerve is a part of the lumbosacral plexus, and is the largest nerve in the body.

Nerve Pathways

Somatic (*soma* means body) motor pathways involve the conduction of impulses from the central nervous system to skeletal muscles. These pathways are classified into *pyramidal* (*corticospinal*) and *extrapyramidal* tracts. The pyramidal tracts conduct impulses that

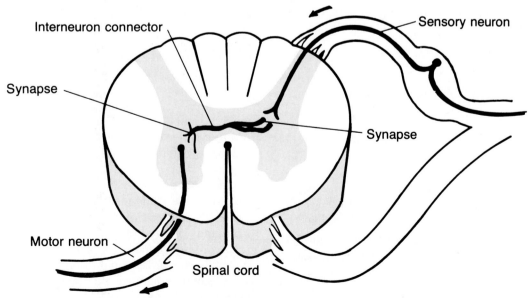

Figure 14-7.   **Reflex arc in the spinal cord.**

facilitate conscious, voluntary actions of the muscles. Impulses from the extrapyramidal tracts produce larger, more automatic movements by contracting groups of muscles in sequence, such as those involved in walking, running, and swimming.

Reflex Action

The arrangement of sensory, connector, and motor nerves is referred to as a *reflex arc*, and the action produced is a *reflex action*. An example of a reflex action is that which occurs when a hand touches a hot stove, and the instantaneous pain sensation causes quick withdrawal of the hand. The sensation, in this instance, is relayed to the spinal cord level, because there is not enough time to think of removing the hand, which would be a brain function. When consciousness is involved in an action, it is under the control of the brain. A reflex action occurs below the brain level, within the spinal cord, and is not conscious or voluntary (Fig. 14-7).

We have many reflex actions that are automatic, such as walking, dancing, skating, typing, or even driving an automobile, which are learned by experience or education. When a child is learning to walk, every step taken requires concentration, but in time, experience establishes reflexes, which allow the child the freedom of walking without concentrating. Some reflexes, such as sucking, chewing, swallowing, urination, and defecation, appear to be inherited, because they are present at birth.

Among the most common reflexes are:

> *knee jerk reflex*—the leg extends in response to tapping of the patellar ligament.
> *Babinski reflex*—dorsiflexion of the big toe in response to stroking the sole of the foot.
> *biceps reflex*—contraction of the biceps muscles in response to tapping of the tendon.
> *Achilles tendon reflex*—the foot extends in response to tapping the Achilles tendon.
> *pupillary reflex*—the pupil of the eye contracts in response to exposure of the retina to a bright light.

THE AUTONOMIC NERVOUS SYSTEM

Although a part of the peripheral nervous system, the autonomic system is an integral part of the entire nervous system. It functions automatically, and is divided into the **sympathetic** and **parasympathetic** systems, which act upon the involuntary, smooth and cardiac muscles, and glands (Fig. 14-4). It also serves the vital systems that function automatically, such as the digestive, circulatory, respiratory, urinary, and endocrine systems.

Structure

Sympathetic System

The sympathetic trunk lies close to the vertebrae and is composed of a series of ganglia (nerve cell clusters) on each side, forming a nodular cord resembling a string of beads (Fig. 14-4). These ganglia extend from the base of the skull to the front of the coccyx and are the basis of the sympathetic (or ***thoracolumbar***) system. These ganglia are connected with the thoracic and lumbar spinal cord and with the muscles, organs, and glands they affect through spinal nerves.

Parasympathetic System

The parasympathetic (or ***craniosacral***) system centers are located in the brainstem and the sacral regions (Fig. 14-4). The centers in the brainstem send out impulses through the oculomotor, facial, glossopharyngeal, and vagus cranial nerves, and the second, third, and fourth sacral nerves make up the sacral group.

Functions of the Autonomic System

The sympathetic and parasympathetic divisions oppose each other in function, and maintain balance in the body mechanisms they serve. They are under the control of the hypothalamus, cerebral cortex, and medulla oblongata in the brain, which coordinates their actions, and keeps the body in **homeostasis** (normal stability of the internal environment). In general, the parasympathetic system maintains the routine functioning of the body, whereas the sympathetic system is called on to respond under additional stress or emergency conditions.

Some examples of opposition of the sympathetic and parasympathetic systems are the sympathetic system dilating the pupils and the parasympathetic system contracting them; the sympathetic decreasing ciliary muscle tone so that eyes are accommodated to distant objects and the parasympathetic contracting these muscles to accommodate the eyes to near objects. The sympathetic dilates the bronchial tubes, and the parasympathetic contracts them. The action of the heart is quickened or strengthened by the symphathetic system, whereas the parasympathetic system slows its action. The blood vessels of the skin and viscera are contracted by the sympathetic system so that more blood goes to the muscles where it is needed for "fight or flight" under stress, and the parasympathetic system dilates the blood vessels when the need has passed. The gastrointestinal tract and bladder are relaxed by the sympathetic system and contracted by the parasympathetic. The sympathetic system causes contractions of the sphincters to prevent leakage from anus or urethra, and the parasympathetic system relaxes these sphincters so that waste matter can be expelled. In similar fashion they regulate the body temperature, salivary digestive secretions, and the endocrine glands.

Review E

Complete the following:

1. The peripheral nervous system includes the _____ system, the _____ nerves, and the _____ nerves.

2. There are _____ pairs of cranial nerves.

3. The spinal nerves are named for the corresponding _____.

4. Somatic motor pathways are classified into _____ and _____ tracts.

5. An unconscious, involuntary action occurring below the brain level is a _____ action.

6. The autonomic nervous system has two divisions: _____ and _____.

7. The two (above named divisions) work in _____ to each other.

8. The first cranial nerve, for the sense of smell, is the _____ nerve.

9. The second cranial nerve, the _____, is the nerve of vision.

10. In the _____ reflex, the leg extends in response to tapping of the patellar ligament.

Answers to Review Questions: The Nervous System

Review A
1. central, peripheral
2. axon, dendrites, cell body
3. sensory, motor, connector
4. (nerve) fibers
5. nuclei
6. synapse
7. neurilemma
8. neuroglia
9. impulses
10. ganglia

Review B
1. cerebrospinal
2. dura mater, arachnoid, pia mater
3. brainstem, diencephalon, cerebellum, cerebrum
4. medulla oblongata, pons, midbrain
5. medulla oblongata and pons

Review C
1. hemispheres
2. thalamus, epithalamus, hypothalamus, third ventricle
3. the cortex
4. frontal, temporal, parietal, occipital
5. right, left

Review D
1. emotional
2. ventricles of the brain, central canal of the spinal cord, subarachnoid spaces
3. three
4. ascending, descending
5. 31

Review E
1. autonomic, cranial, spinal
2. 12
3. vertebrae
4. pyramidal, extrapyramidal
5. reflex
6. sympathetic, parasympathetic
7. opposition
8. olfactory
9. optic
10. knee jerk

CHAPTER 14 EXERCISES

THE NERVOUS SYSTEM: THE CENTRAL PROCESSING UNIT

Exercise 1: Complete the following:

1. The brain and spinal cord are located in the _____ system.

2. The craniospinal nerves are located in the _____ system.

3. The sympathetic and parasympathic systems are located in the _____ system.

4. The groups of neuron cell bodies outside the central nervous system are called _____.

5. The membranes that envelop the central nervous system are called _____.

6. The three membranes that envelop the nervous system are the _____, the _____, and the _____.

7. The portion of the brain that is referred to as a bridge is the _____.

8. The part of the brain in which the thalamus, epithalamus, and hypothalamus are located is the _____.

9. The thin, transparent, watery fluid found in the ventricles of the brain, central canal of the spinal cord, and the subarachnoid space is called _____.

10. The passage for the spinal cord through the occipital bone of the cranium is called the _____.

Exercise 2: Using the list of terms below, identify each part in Fig. 14-8 by writing the name in the corresponding blank.

Cerebrum	Midbrain	Diencephalon
Frontal lobe	Occipital lobe	Medulla oblongata
Corpus callosum	Pons	Third ventricle
Pineal body	Parietal lobe	Optic chiasma
Septum pellucidum	Temporal lobe	Cerebellum
Pituitary (hypophysis)	Cerebral aqueduct	Spinal cord
Fourth ventricle	Intermediate mass	Thalamus
Brainstem		

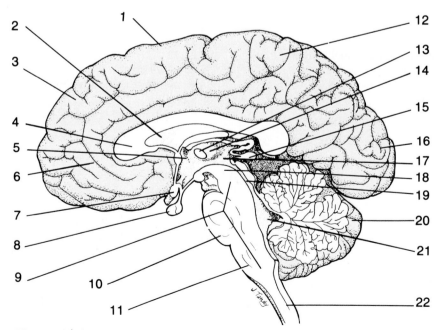

Figure 14-8.   Structures of the brain.

1. _____
2. _____
3. _____
4. _____
5. _____
6. _____
7. _____
8. _____
9. _____
10. _____
11. _____

12. _____
13. _____
14. _____
15. _____
16. _____
17. _____
18. _____
19. _____
20. _____
21. _____
22. _____

Exercise 3: Matching:

____ **1.** long nerve cell processes that carry impulses from the cell body

____ **2.** numerous short nerve cell processes that conduct nerve impulses toward the cell body

____ **3.** neurons concerned with muscle or gland action

____ **4.** peripheral neurons that conduct afferent impulses from the sense organs to the spinal cord

____ **5.** region of connection between processes of two adjacent neurons for transmission of impulses

____ **6.** peripheral nerve endings

____ **7.** space between the pia mater and the arachnoid

____ **8.** space between the dura mater and arachnoid

____ **9.** central body of the cerebellum, shaped like a worm

____ **10.** a furrow, or groove, separating folds of the brain

____ **11.** second cranial nerve, which innervates the retina of the eye

____ **12.** third cranial nerve, which innervates the eye muscles and the sphincter of the pupil and ciliary processes

____ **13.** interlacing network of spinal nerves

____ **14.** nerve that originates in the spinal cord and innervates the diaphragm

____ **15.** a so-called wandering nerve, both motor and sensory, with an extensive distribution, with some gastric, pyloric, hepatic, and celiac branches

A. subarachnoid
B. vagus
C. sulcus
D. synapse
E. oculomotor
F. dendrites
G. terminal twigs
H. axon
I. subdural
J. plexus
K. sensory neurons
L. optic
M. vermis
N. motor neurons
O. phrenic

Exercise 4: Give the meaning of the components in the following words and then define the word as a whole. Suffixes meaning "pertaining to" or "state or condition" shown following a slash mark (/), are not to be defined separately. Before reaching for your medical dictionary, check the glossary at the end of the chapter.

1. Encephalomyelitis:

   encephalo_____

   myel_____

   itis_____

   _____

2. Arachnoiditis:

   arachnoid_____

   itis_____

   _____

3. Meningoencephalitis:

   meningo_____

   encephal_____

   itis_____

   _____

4. Pachymeningitis:

   pachy _____

   mening _____

   itis _____

   _____

5. Polioencephalomeningomyelitis:

   polio_____

   encephalo_____

   meningo_____

   myel_____

   itis_____

   _____

6. Rachiomyelitis:

   rachio_____

   myel_____

   itis_____

   _____

7. Anencephalia:

   an_____

   encephal/ia_____

   _____

8. Cephalocele:

   cephalo_____

   cele_____

   _____

9. Encephalomyelocele:

   encephalo_____

   myelo_____

   cele_____

   _____

10. Heterotopia spinalis:

    hetero_____

    top/ia_____

    spinal/is_____

    _____

Chapter 14 Crossword Puzzle

Across

1. web-like membrane
4. deeper furrows
5. neuron cell body groups in CNS
10. fluid of central nervous system
12. kite-shaped ventricle
13. a division of the brain
16. craniospinal and autonomic nerves
18. bridge
19. hold and support nerve cells
21. aqueduct (of Sylvius)
22. peripheral nervous system abbr.
23. posterior lobe of cerebral cortex
25. nerve cell clusters outside CNS

Down

2. interneuron neuron
3. a lobe of the cerebral cortex
6. means horn
7. cerebral hemisphere convolutions
8. Schwann's sheath
9. a division of the brain
11. afferent neurons
14. a division of the brain
15. the mesencephalon
17. pons and medulla together
18. a lobe of the cerebral cortex
20. anterior lobe of cerebral cortex
24. central nervous system abbr.

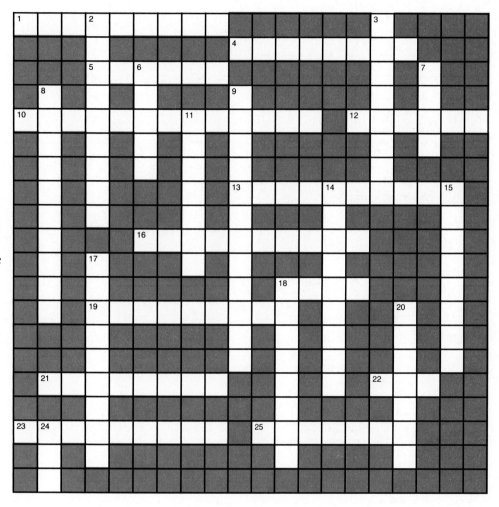

Chapter 14 Hidden Words Puzzle

```
A  G  Y  Z  E  Z  Y  F  B  G  Y  M  S  O  T  U  V  K  D  N  M
I  X  W  R  E  C  E  P  T  O  R  R  T  F  M  P  J  Y  T  F  L
E  Y  O  J  V  L  O  Z  Y  W  J  J  Y  E  N  N  W  N  J  U  U
L  C  E  N  T  R  A  L  P  D  I  Y  V  C  C  J  H  I  C  M  U
L  T  I  V  L  K  U  O  L  I  X  G  Y  C  Y  V  C  I  U  S  K
S  Y  H  N  Q  S  Y  M  P  A  T  H  E  T  I  C  O  M  W  S  H
D  Y  A  F  M  R  U  U  P  D  T  J  H  Z  X  M  R  Y  O  B  D
H  T  N  V  Q  Z  R  B  E  X  D  E  N  D  R  I  T  E  X  U  P
J  H  Y  A  T  G  B  T  A  F  F  E  R  E  N  T  L  L  J  H  G
K  J  U  O  P  K  W  C  U  R  F  F  W  A  E  E  T  I  J  R  X
Q  L  K  H  L  S  P  S  T  J  A  E  D  V  L  H  X  N  U  Y  P
B  O  U  C  B  U  E  Q  O  S  H  C  R  M  U  S  Q  K  D  S  V
F  M  M  E  M  B  R  A  N  E  P  S  H  E  Q  V  X  M  P  G  H
E  Q  M  F  S  D  M  I  O  Y  T  I  T  N  N  O  L  I  B  S  F
O  A  X  K  O  U  U  Y  M  K  J  W  U  I  O  T  P  W  I  S  G
U  K  K  T  T  R  U  H  I  P  B  N  J  N  M  I  M  A  Y  B  Q
E  X  H  D  R  A  A  V  C  I  U  N  D  G  B  U  D  H  G  L  W
W  Q  Y  I  U  L  D  M  V  Y  I  L  O  E  S  W  L  X  B  R  C
K  V  F  B  Y  O  S  R  E  C  S  E  S  S  C  N  E  U  R  O  N
X  F  W  G  M  O  W  J  Y  N  W  C  U  E  C  L  W  D  S  A  I
```

Can you find the 20 words hidden in this puzzle?

SUBARACHNOID	SYMPATHETIC	COLLATERAL	AUTONOMIC
AFFERENT	DENDRITE	EFFERENT	MEMBRANE
MENINGES	RECEPTOR	STIMULUS	SUBDURAL
CENTRAL	FORAMEN	IMPULSE	SYNAPSE
MYELIN	NEURON	AXON	TWIG

CHAPTER 14 ANSWERS

Exercise 1
1. central nervous system
2. peripheral nervous system
3. autonomic nervous system
4. ganglia
5. meninges
6. dura mater (or pachymeninx), arachnoid, pia mater
7. pons
8. diencephalon
9. cerebrospinal fluid
10. foramen magnum

Exercise 2
1. cerebrum
2. septum pellucidum
3. frontal lobe
4. corpus callosum
5. diencephalon
6. temporal lobe
7. optic chiasma
8. pituitary (hypophysis)
9. brainstem
10. pons
11. medulla oblongata
12. parietal lobe
13. intermediate mass
14. thalamus
15. pineal body
16. occipital lobe
17. third ventricle
18. midbrain
19. cerebral aqueduct
20. cerebellum
21. fourth ventricle
22. spinal cord

Exercise 3
1. H
2. F
3. N
4. K
5. D
6. G
7. A
8. I
9. M
10. C
11. L
12. E
13. J
14. O
15. B

Exercise 4
1. encephalomyelitis: brain; spinal cord; inflammation—inflammation of the brain and spinal cord
2. arachnoiditis: arachnoid membrane; inflammation—inflammation of the arachnoid membrane
3. meningoencephalitis: meninges; brain; inflammation—inflammation of the brain and meninges
4. pachymeningitis: dura mater, or pachymeninges; inflammation—inflammation of the pachymeninges
5. polioencephalomeningomyelitis: gray matter of the brain; brain; meninges; spinal cord; inflammation—inflammation of the gray matter of the brain, spinal cord, and meninges
6. rachiomyelitis: spinal cord; inflammation—inflammation of spinal cord
7. anencephalia: no; brain—absence of cerebral hemispheres and cranial vault
8. cephalocele: brain; hernia—herniation of a part of cranial contents
9. encephalomyelocele: brain; spinal canal; hernia—herniation of brain substance and spinal cord at foramen magnum
10. heterotopia spinalis: other; place; spinal—displaced spinal cord, or spinal cord displaced to other than normal position

Answers: Chapter 14 Crossword Puzzle

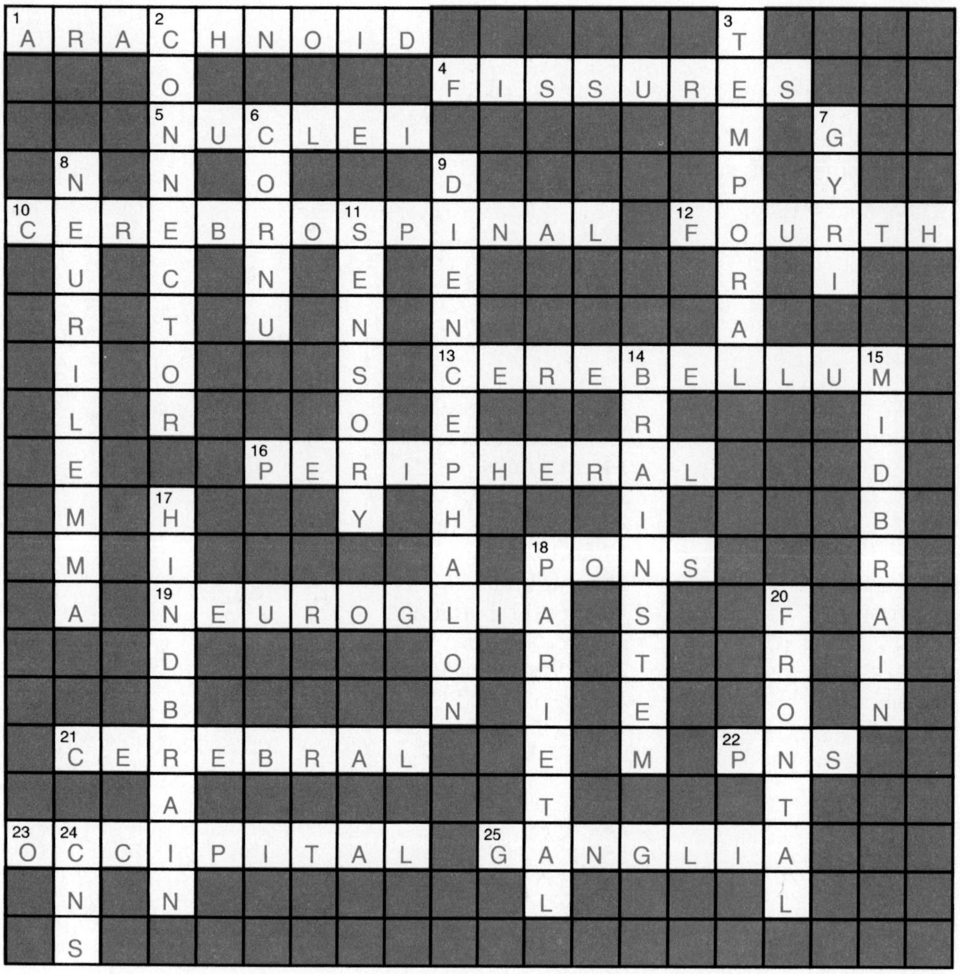

Answers: Chapter 14 Hidden Words Puzzle

```
A   .   .   .   .   .   .   .   .   .   .   .   .   .   .   .   .   .   .
.   X   .   R   E   C   E   P   T   O   R   .   .   .   .   .   .   .   .
.   .   O   .   .   .   O   .   .   W   .   .   .   .   .   .   .   .   .
.   C   E   N   T   R   A   L   .   .   I   .   .   .   .   .   .   .   .
.   .   .   .   .   .   .   L   .   .   G   .   .   .   .   .   .   .   .
S   .   .   .   S   Y   M   P   A   T   H   E   T   I   C   .   M   .   .
.   Y   .   .   .   U   .   .   .   T   .   .   .   .   .   Y   .   .   .
.   .   N   .   .   .   .   B   E   .   D   E   N   D   R   I   T   E   .
.   .   .   A   .   .   .   .   A   F   F   E   R   E   N   T   .   L   .
.   .   .   .   P   .   .   .   U   R   F   .   .   A   .   .   .   I   .
.   .   .   .   .   S   .   .   T   .   A   E   .   .   L   .   .   N   .
.   .   .   .   .   U   E   .   O   .   .   C   R   M   .   .   .   .   .
.   .   M   E   M   B   R   A   N   E   .   S   H   E   .   .   .   .   .
.   .   .   F   .   D   .   I   O   .   .   .   T   N   N   .   .   .   .
.   .   .   .   O   U   .   .   M   .   .   .   .   I   O   T   .   .   .
.   .   .   .   R   .   .   I   P   .   .   .   N   M   I   .   .   .   .
.   .   .   .   A   A   .   C   .   U   .   .   G   .   U   D   .   .   .
.   .   .   .   L   .   M   .   .   .   L   .   E   .   .   L   .   .   .
.   .   .   .   .   E   .   .   .   .   S   S   .   N   E   U   R   O   N
.   .   .   .   .   .   N   .   .   .   E   .   .   .   S   .   .   .   .
```

Words:

\ SUBARACHNOID	> SYMPATHETIC	\ COLLATERAL	V AUTONOMIC
> AFFERENT	> DENDRITE	\ EFFERENT	> MEMBRANE
V MENINGES	> RECEPTOR	\ STIMULUS	V SUBDURAL
> CENTRAL	\ FORAMEN	\ IMPULSE	\ SYNAPSE
V MYELIN	> NEURON	\ AXON	\ TWIG

CHAPTER 14 GLOSSARY

Divisions of the Nervous System

autonomic: part of the peripheral nervous system that functions automatically and normally cannot be controlled voluntarily, that activates glands serving the vital systems, and involuntary (smooth) and cardiac muscles.

central: division of the nervous system that includes the brain and spinal cord (also called the *cerebrospinal system*).

parasympathetic: one of two divisions of the autonomic system, arising from the central nervous system by preganglionic neurons, with cell bodies located in the brain or in the second, third, and fourth sacral segments of the spinal cord (also called the *craniosacral system*).

peripheral: division of the nervous system that consists of nerves and ganglia peripheral to, or outside, the spinal cord and brain, including the cranial and spinal nerves and the autonomic nervous system.

sympathetic: one of two divisions of the autonomic system, arising from the central nervous system by preganglionic neurons, with cell bodies located in the thoracic and first three lumbar segments of the spinal cord, and with ganglia extending from the base of the skull to the coccyx (also called the *thoracolumbar system*).

Brain, Spinal Cord, and Related Anatomic Terms

anterior commissure: band of white fibers that connects the temporal lobes of the two cerebral hemispheres.

arachnoid (ah-rak'noid): middle meningeal membrane resembling a spider's web (*arachnoid* means spider).

ascending tracts: tracts located in the spinal cord, carrying afferent or sensory nerve fibers that conduct nerve impulses to the brain.

brain: central mass of nerve tissue within the cranium, including the cerebrum, cerebellum, diencephalon, midbrain, pons, medulla oblongata, and other structures.

cerebellum (ser"e-bel'um): second largest division of the brain, situated above the medulla oblongata and beneath the rear portion of the cerebrum, commonly referred to as the little, or small, brain.

cerebral aqueduct (ak'we-dukt): canal for the passage of cerebrospinal fluid between the third and fourth ventricles (also called the *aqueduct of Sylvius*).

cerebral cortex: outer portion of the cerebrum containing the gray matter or cell bodies of the neurons.

cerebrospinal fluid (ser"e-bro-spi'nal): thin, transparent, watery fluid found around the spinal cord and in the ventricles of the brain, central canal of the spinal cord, and subarachnoid space, providing support for the weight of the brain, and serving as a protective cushion and source of nutrients for the brain and spinal cord.

cerebrum (ser'e-brum): largest part of the brain, occupying most of the cranial cavity, and divided into two cerebral hemispheres.

commissure (kom'i-shur): band of white fibers that joins the two halves of the cerebral hemispheres.

convolution: fold in the surface of the cerebral hemisphere (also called *gyrus*).

cornu (kor'nu): hornlike projection, used to describe various projections in the nervous system (plural— *cornua).*

corpus callosum (kor'pus kah-lo'sum): largest commissure of the brain that connects one cerebral hemisphere with another.

descending tracts: tracts located in the spinal cord, carrying nerve fibers that conduct efferent, or motor, impulses from the brain.

diencephalon (di"en-sef'ah-lon): part of the brain between the midbrain and the cerebrum (*dia* means through, across, or between; *cephalon* refers to brain).

dura mater (du'rah ma'ter): outermost membrane of the brain and spinal cord.

endorphins: natural, opiate-like substances, produced in both the brain and pituitary gland, that have narcotic action upon receptor sites in the brain, and are believed to play a role in pain experience, emotions, and problems of substance addiction.

ependyma (e-pen'di-mah): membrane lining the ventricles of the brain and the central canal of the spinal cord, producing cerebrospinal fluid.

epithalamus (ep"i-thal'ah-mus): portion of the diencephalon that includes the pineal body and olfactory (smell) centers.

fissure: deep groove, or furrow, of the brain on the cortical surface of the cerebrum.

foramen magnum: passage for the spinal cord through the occipital bone of the cranium.

fourth ventricle: kite-shaped cavity in the hindbrain that produces some of the cerebrospinal fluid.

hemisphere (hem'i-sfer): either lateral half of the cerebrum or cerebellum.

hippocampus: part of the limbic system often called the "gatekeeper for memory", in which damage or defect has been linked to learning and memory problems such as those in Alzheimer's disease.

hypothalamus (hi"po-thal'ah-mus): portion of the diencephalon located below and between the lobes of the thalamus, containing the optic chiasma, the posterior lobe of the pituitary gland, and the infundibulum.

lateral ventricle: space in each hemisphere that projects an anterior cornu (horn) into the frontal lobe, a posterior cornu into the occipital lobe, and an inferior cornu into the temporal lobe, and produces most of the cerebrospinal fluid.

leptomeninges (lep″to-me-nin′jez): pia mater and arachnoid membranes of the brain together (singular—*leptomeninx*).

limbic system: structures of the cerebrum that lie on the medial surface close to the corpus callosum, and together are described as the "emotional brain" because of their importance in experiencing a wide range of emotions from pleasure and sexual feelings to anger, fear, and sorrow. The hippocampal portion has been related to memory problems.

lobes of cerebrum: the cerebral cortex is divided into four lobes named for the cranial bones above them: occipital, frontal, temporal, and parietal.

medulla oblongata (me-dul′ah ob″long-ga′tah): posterior part of the brain, continuous with the spinal cord.

meninges (me-nin′jez): three membranes enveloping the central nervous system, the dura mater, pia mater, and arachnoid (singular—*meninx*).

midbrain: upper part of the brain stem, above the pons

nucleus: mass or cluster of gray matter in the brain or spinal cord (see **ganglion** under Nerve Structures).

optic chiasma (op′tic ki′azm-ah): crossing of the optic nerves on the ventral surface of the brain (*chiasm* means crossing).

pachymeninx (pak″e-me′ninks): dura mater (plural— *pachymeninges*).

pia-arachnoid (pi″ah-ah-rak′noid): both the pia mater and arachnoid membranes when considered as one membrane (*pia* means tender).

pia mater: innermost, thin, compact membrane closely adapted to the surface of the spinal cord and brain.

pons: portion of the brain that serves as a bridge to connect the cerebellum, cerebrum, and medulla oblongata (*pons* means bridge).

posterior commissure: thin sheet of fibers that cross transversely under the posterior part of the corpus callosum, connecting the olfactory centers in the cerebral hemispheres.

spinal cord: lowest part of the central nervous system, extending from the medulla oblongata to the coccyx, and containing the ascending and descending nerve tracts.

subarachnoid: space between the pia mater and arachnoid.

subarachnoid cisterns: subarachnoid reservoirs containing cerebrospinal fluid (*cisterna* means closed place).

subdural space: space between the dura mater and the arachnoid.

subthalamus: portion of the diencephalon that lies between the thalamus and the midbrain.

sulcus (sul′kus): a furrow (groove), separating the gyri from each other (plural—*sulci*).

thalamus (thal′ah-mus): middle portion of the diencephalon that forms part of the lateral wall of the third ventricle and lies between the epithalamus and the hypothalamus (plural—*thalami*).

third ventricle: cavity, located below and between the cerebral central hemispheres, producing cerebrospinal fluid.

vermis: central body of the cerebellum, shaped something like a worm (*vermis* means worm).

Nerve Structures and Related Anatomic Terms

afferent neurons: neurons that conduct impulses from the sense organs to the spinal cord and brain.

astrocyte (as′tro-site): star-shaped cell of the neuroglia (*astro* means star).

axon: long nerve cell process carrying impulses from the cell body.

collaterals: side branches of the axon.

connectors: neurons in which the dendrites and axons are connected to other neurons.

dendrites: numerous short nerve cell processes that conduct nerve impulses toward the cell body.

efferent neurons: motor neurons that convey impulses from the brain and spinal cord to the muscles and glands.

ganglion (gang′gle-on): mass of nerve cells, located outside the brain and spinal cord, that serves as a center for nerve impulses (plural—*ganglia*).

microglia (mi-krog′le-ah): phagocytic cells of the nervous system.

motor neurons: see **efferent neurons**.

myelinated nerves (mi′-eli-nat″ed): nerves covered with a sheath of white fatty material called myelin (also called *medullated nerves*).

myelin sheath: white, fatty coat surrounding nerve fibers, found mainly in the central nervous system.

nerve trunk: white, glistening, cordlike bundle formed by nerve fibers running together.

neurilemma (nu″ri-lem′mah): tubelike membrane covering nerve fibers, which may or may not be myelinated (also called *nucleated membrane* and *sheath of Schwann*; also spelled *neurolemma*).

neuroglia (nu-rog′le-ah): specialized type of nervous tissue that holds nerve cells and their gossamer filaments together.

neuron: single nerve cell, the structural unit of the nervous system, with a cell body, axon, and dendrites.

neurotransmitters: chemical substances that act at the synapse to stimulate or inhibit the transmission of impulses, of numerous types including acetylcholine, norepinephrine (adrenaline), dopamine, and serotonin.

oligodendroglia (ol"i-go-den-drog′le-ah): cells that aid in holding nerve fibers together and forming the myelin sheath of nerves.

plexus (plek′sus): interlacing network of spinal nerves, in several areas of the body.

Ranvier's node (rahn-ve-ay′s): interruption or constriction in the myelin sheath, at regular intervals.

receptors: organs of sensation.

reflex action: arrangement of sensory, connector, and motor nerves forming the reflex arc, acting together to produce a reflex action.

sensory neurons: peripheral nerves that conduct afferent impulses from the sense organs to the spinal cord.

synapse (sin′aps): microscopic space between an axon of one neuron and the dendrites of another, across which an impulse is transmitted (**synapse** means connection).

terminal twigs: peripheral nerve endings, identified according to their action, as vascular, articular, muscular, and cutaneous.

Cranial Nerves

The following list includes the 12 cranial nerves and some of their branches.

abducens (ab-du′senz): sixth cranial nerve; motor nerve that supplies the lateral rectus muscle of the eye.

acoustic: eighth cranial nerve, having two sensory divisions, the *cochlear*, which supplies the cochlea of the ear, and the *vestibular*, which supplies the vestibule and semicircular canals of the ear (also called ***auditory nerve***).

alveolar: two branches of the maxillary division of the trigeminal nerve, *superior* and *inferior*, which receive sensations from the head and innervate the chewing muscles.

auricular, posterior: sensory and motor branch of the facial nerve that supplies the ear muscles and the occipitofrontal muscle.

auriculotemporal: sensory branch of the mandibular division of the trigeminal nerve, which supplies the skin of the scalp and temple, the superior part of the ear, the external accoustic meatus, and the tympanic membrane.

buccinator: sensory branch of the mandibular division of the trigeminal nerve, which supplies the skin of the cheek and gums, and mucous membranes of the cheek (also called **buccal**).

cranial nerves: twelve pairs of cranial nerves, originating in the brain, with their branches and ganglia.

facial: seventh cranial nerve, a sensory and motor nerve, which originates in the pons and supplies facial muscles and some taste buds.

glossopharyngeal: ninth cranial nerve, both sensory and motor, which originates in the medulla oblongata and supplies the tongue, pharynx, and eardrum.

hypoglossal: twelfth cranial nerve, a motor nerve that originates in the medulla oblongata and innervates the muscles of the tongue.

infraorbital: sensory branch of the maxillary division of the trigeminal nerve, supplying part of the nose, lip, the skin and conjunctiva of the lower eyelid, and some of the upper teeth and gums.

intermediate nerve: sensory root of the facial nerve, supplying salivary glands, palate, tonsils, and tongue.

lacrimal: sensory branch of the ophthalmic division of the trigeminal nerve, supplying the lacrimal gland, conjunctiva, and upper eyelid.

laryngeal: branches of the vagus nerve, both sensory and motor, that supplies the laryngeal, pharyngeal, and tracheal structures.

lingual: sensory branch of the mandibular division of the trigeminal nerve, that supplies parts of the tongue and mouth.

mandibular: sensory and motor division of the trigeminal nerve, with a posterior and anterior division, that gives rise to the lingual, inferior alveolar, and auriculotemporal nerves.

maxillary: sensory division of the trigeminal nerve that supplies the mucous membranes of maxillary sinus and nasal cavity, skin of face and scalp, and some teeth, through its branches, the zygomatic, alveolar, and infraorbital nerves.

oculomotor: third cranial nerve, both sensory and motor, which supplies eye muscles, pupillary sphincter, and ciliary processes.

olfactory: first cranial nerve, a sensory nerve that supplies the sense of smell.

ophthalmic: sensory division of the trigeminal nerve that supplies the skin of the forehead, upper eyelid, external nose, frontal sinus, and the eye, through its branches, the lacrimal, nasal, and frontal nerves.

optic: second cranial nerve, a sensory nerve supplying the retina of the eye.

palatine: two sensory branches of the maxillary division of the trigeminal nerve that supply the soft and hard palates, uvula, and tonsils.

spinal accessory: eleventh cranial nerve, a motor nerve, supplies the sternocleidomastoid and trapezius muscles, cervical lymph glands, pharynx, larynx, and thoracic viscera.

trigeminal: fifth cranial nerve, both sensory and motor, with three divisions: ophthalmic, maxillary, and mandibular.

trochlear: fourth cranial nerve, a motor nerve that supplies the superior oblique muscles of the eye.

tympanic: sensory branch of the glossopharyngeal nerve, supplying the tympanic cavity membranes, mastoid air cells, and parotid gland.

vagus: tenth cranial nerve, with meningeal, auricular, pharyngeal, superior laryngeal, superior and inferior cardiac, recurrent laryngeal, bronchial, esophageal, gastric, pyloric, hepatic, and celiac branches that serve the structures for which they are named.

zygomatic: sensory branch of the maxillary division of the trigeminal nerve, supplying the skin over the cheekbone and temple.

Spinal Nerves

The following list includes only a portion of the many spinal nerves. Spinal nerve origins are identified using letters to show their anatomical locations, and numbers to indicate positions in the spinal column. C refers to cervical, T to thoracic, L to lumbar, and S to sacral. The number following the letter indicates the corresponding vertebra (e.g., C1 indicates the first cervical vertebra).

cauda equina: nerves that supply the lower extremities, extending below the level of the spinal cord, deriving their name from the arrangement of their strands, which resembles a horse's tail.

dorsal scapular: motor nerve that originates in the spinal cord (C5 to C7) and supplies muscles of the upper back.

femoral: sensory and motor nerve that originates in the spinal cord (L2 to L4) and supplies the muscles of the hip, thigh, and leg.

genitofemoral: sensory and motor nerve that originates in the spinal cord (L1 to L2) and serves the genitalia and lumboinguinal regions.

gluteal: sensory and motor nerve, with inferior and superior branches, originating in the spinal cord (L4 to S2), supplying the gluteal muscles and hip joint.

hypogastric: branches of the superior hypogastric plexus that supply the pelvic and ureter areas.

iliohypogastric: sensory and motor nerve that originates in the spinal cord (L1) and supplies the abdominal muscles and the skin above the pubis and lateral gluteal region.

ilioinguinal: sensory nerve that originates in the spinal cord (L1) and supplies the skin of the upper thigh, scrotum and labia majora.

intercostobrachial: sensory nerve that originates in the spinal cord (T2 to T3) and supplies the skin of the axilla and medial side of the arm.

interosseus: group of sensory and motor nerves supplying muscles and membranes of the upper and lower extremities.

long thoracic: motor nerve that originates in the spinal cord (C5 to C7) and supplies muscles that move the scapula.

median: sensory nerve that originates in the spinal cord (C6 to T1) and supplies the muscles of the forearm and muscles and skin of the hand.

musculocutaneous: sensory and motor nerve that originates in the spinal cord (C5 to C7) and supplies the brachial and biceps muscles and skin of the radial side of the forearm.

obturator: sensory and motor nerve that originates in the spinal cord (L2 to L4) and supplies muscles of the thigh, and skin of the hip, thigh, and knee joint.

peroneal: sensory and motor, deep and superficial nerves that originate in the sciatic nerve and supply the muscles of the lower leg and skin of the foot and toes.

phrenic: sensory and motor nerve that originates in the spinal cord (C4 to C5) and supplies the diaphragm, lungs, pericardium and peritoneum.

pudendal: sensory and motor nerve that originates in the spinal cord (S2 to S4) and supplies skin, erectile tissue, and muscles of the perineal area.

radial: sensory and motor nerve that originates in the spinal cord (C5 to T1, and C6 to C8) and supplies the skin and muscles of the arm and hand.

saphenous: sensory branch of the femoral nerve that supplies the skin of the leg and foot.

sciatic: sensory and motor nerve, the largest in the body, originates from the sacral plexus (L4 to S3), and supplies the lower limbs.

tibial: sensory and motor division of the sciatic nerve that supplies the hamstring muscles and the muscles and skin of the back of the leg and the sole of the foot

ulnar: sensory and motor nerve that originates in the spinal .cord (C7 to T1) and supplies muscles of the forearm and hand, and skin of the hand.

Pathologic Conditions of the Nervous System

Inflammations and infections

arachnoiditis (ah-rak″noid-i′tis): inflammation of the arachnoid membrane (also called ***arachnitis***).

cerebrospinal syphilis: syphilitic infection of the brain and spinal cord, or syphilis of the central nervous system (also called ***Erb's paralysis***).

choriomeningitis (ko″re-o-men″in-ji′tis): inflammation of the cerebral meninges (meningitis), with infiltration by lymphocytes of the choroid plexuses of the ventricles.

encephalitis (en″sef-ah-li′tis): inflammation of the brain, with a variety of types. One recent virulent type is *Eastern equine encephalitis*, a rare but usually fatal virus, transmitted by the Asian tiger mosquito.

encephalomyelitis (en-sef″ah-lo-mi″e-li′tis): inflammation of the brain and spinal cord, with a variety of types.

ependymitis (ep″en-di-mi′tis): inflammation of the ependymal lining of the ventricles of the brain and the central canal of the spinal cord.

ganglionitis (gang″gle-on-i′tis): inflammation of a nerve ganglion.

Guillain-Barre syndrome (ge-yan′bar-ray): a post-infectious neurologic condition with symptoms of fever, pain, tenderness, weakness or paralysis of muscles, with suspected viral or immune response causes (also called ***Landry's paralysis, polyradiculitis, Landry-Guillain-Barre-Strohl syndrome, polyneuropathy, radiculoganglionitis, radiculoneuritis, infectious polyneuritis*** and ***acute idiopathic polyneuritis***).

herpes zoster (her′pez zos′ter): infection caused by a herpes virus (*varicella-zoster* or *VZV*) that follows nerve pathways, characterized by small blisters or vesicles on the skin (also called ***shingles***).

leptomeningitis (lep″to-men″in-ji′tis): inflammation of the leptomeninges (pia-arachnoid membrane) of the brain and spinal cord.

meningitis (men″in-ji′tis): inflammation of the meninges of the brain or spinal cord, caused by viral or bacterial infection. (In children, the most common bacterial cause is Haemophilus influenza Type B).

meningoencephalitis (me-ning″go-en-sef″ah-li′tis): inflammation of the brain and meninges (also called ***cerebromeningitis*** and ***encephalomeningitis***).

meningoencephalomyelitis (me-ning″go-en-sef″ah-lo-mi″e-li′tis): inflammation that involves the brain, meninges, and spinal cord.

meningomyelitis (me-ning″go-mi″e-li′tis): inflammation of the spinal cord and its membranes.

meningomyeloradiculitis (me-ning″go-mi″e-lo-rah-dik″u-li′tis): inflammation of the meninges, spinal cord, and spinal cord roots (***radiculo*** refers to root).

meningoradiculitis (me-ning″go-rah-dik″u-li′tis): inflammation of the meninges and the nerve roots.

myelitis (mi″e-li′tis): inflammation of the spinal cord (***myel*** refers to both spinal cord and bone marrow and the context in which it is used will determine which tissue is involved).

myeloradiculitis (mi″e-lo-rah-dik″u-li′tis): inflammation of the spinal cord and nerve roots.

myelosyphilis: syphilis of the spinal cord.

neuritis: inflammation of a nerve or nerves, caused by infection, toxicity, or trauma.

neuroamebiasis (nu″ro-am″e-bi′ah-sis): neuritis that results from infection by amebae.

neurochorioretinitis (nu″ro-ko″re-o-ret″i-ni′tis): inflammation of the optic nerve, retina, and choroid of the eye.

neuromyelitis (nu″ro-mi″e-li′tis): spinal cord inflammation with neuritis (also called ***myeloneuritis***).

neuromyositis (nu″ro-mi″o-si′tis): neuritis with inflammation of corresponding muscles.

pachyleptomeningitis (pak″e-lep″to-men″in-ji′tis): inflammation of all three membranes of the brain or spinal cord.

pachymeningitis (pak″e-men″in-ji′tis): inflammation of the dura mater (also called ***perimeningitis***).

polioencephalitis (po″le-o-en-sef″ah-li′tis): inflammation of the gray matter of the brain, caused by polio virus (***polio*** refers to gray or the gray matter of the nervous system).

polioencephalomeningomyelitis (po″le-o-en-sef″ah-lo-me-nin″go-mi″e-li′tis): inflammation of gray matter of the brain and spinal cord and their covering membranes.

poliomyelitis (po″le-o-mi″e-li′tis): acute viral infection and inflammation of the gray matter of the spinal cord caused by one of three polio viruses, resulting in asymptomatic, paralytic, or mild types; relatively uncommon since the development of preventive viral vaccines, of which the Salk and Sabin vaccines are best known.

poliomyeloencephalitis (pol″e-o-mi″el-o-en-sef′a-li′tis): inflammation of the gray matter of the brain and spinal cord due to the polio virus (also called ***poliomyelencephalitis***).

polyneuritis: inflammation of a large number of spinal nerves at the same time.

polyneuroradiculitis (pol″e-nu″ro-rah-dik″uli′tis): inflammation of the spinal ganglia, nerve roots, and peripheral nerves.

polyradiculitis (pol″e-rah-dik″u-li′tis): inflammation of nerve roots.

rabies (ra′bez): a once-fatal viral disease infecting the central nervous system and salivary glands, transmitted by the bite of an infected animal or an existing wound coming in contact with infected saliva (also called ***hydrophobia*** because of the painful glottal and throat spasms produced by drinking water).

rachiomyelitis (ra″ke-o-mi″e-li′tis): inflammation of the spinal cord.

radiculitis (rah-dik″u-li′tis): inflammation of a spinal nerve root.

radiculomeningomyelitis (rah-dik″u-lo-me-ning″go-mi″e-li′tis): inflammation of the nerve roots, the spinal cord, and its covering (also called ***rhizomeningomyelitis***).

Reye's syndrome (riz): encephalopathy associated with fatty degeneration of the liver occurring in children as a rare sequela to influenza and other viral infections, with late stages showing intracranial pressure and cerebral edema (Chapter 17).

tetanus (tet′ah-nus): acute, bacterial infectious disease caused by *Clostridium tetani* whose source is in soil, street dust, or animal and human feces, transmitted by spores at the site of an injury, burn, or wound, primarily affecting the nervous system and involving the peripheral nerves and anterior horn cells (*Lockjaw* is a popular synonym and symptom, along with generalized muscle spasms and seizures).

Hereditary, congenital, and developmental disorders

adrenoleukodystrophy (ALD): rare, fatal disease caused by a sex-linked X chromosome defect, affecting males, resulting in myelin sheath deterioration, and degeneration of brain tissue, with symptoms of muscular spasticity, optic neuritis, deafness, and mental and emotional deterioration (also called *Siemerling-Creutzfeldt disease*).

amyelencephalia (a-mi″el-en-seh-fa′le-ah): absence of both brain and spinal cord.

amyelia (a″mi-e′le-ah): absence of the spinal cord.

anencephaly (an″en-se-fa′le): congenital defective development of cranial bones, with failure of brain and spinal cord to develop (also called *anencephalia*).

Arnold-Chiari syndrome (ke-ar′e): malformation, with downward displacement of the cerebellum into the fourth ventricle and underdevelopment of hindbrain, and internal hydrocephalus, usually associated with an opening in the spinal column (also called *cerebellomedullary malformation syndrome*).

ataxia telangiectasia (AT) (tel-an′gie-ek-tas″eah): hereditary, progressive disorder of immunoglobulin metabolism that appears when a child begins walking, with symptoms of lack of coordination, dilation of the ends of blood vessels in ears, eyes, and face, and susceptibility to respiratory infection, which usually causes death in early adulthood (also called *Louis-Bar's syndrome*).

atelencephalia (a-tell′en-se-fa′le-ah): incomplete or imperfect development of the brain (*atel* means incomplete).

atelomyelia (at″e-lo-mi-e′le-ah): incomplete development of the spinal cord.

atelorachidia (at″e-lo-rah-kid′e-ah): incomplete development of the spinal column.

cephalocele (se-fal′o-sel): protrusion of a part of the cranial contents through a defect in the skull (also called *encephalocele* and *craniocele*).

cerebral sphingolipidosis (sfing′go-lip′i-do′sis): group of inherited diseases characterized by excessive muscle tone, underdevelopment, spastic paralysis, blindness, convulsions, and mental deterioration, associated with abnormal retention of lipids in the brain (includes *Tay-Sachs disease*, an infantile form formerly called amaurotic family idiocy; *Jansky-Bielschowsky disease*, an early

juvenile type; *Spielmeyer-Vogt disease*, a late juvenile form; and *Kufs' disease*, an adult form).

Charcot-Marie-Tooth disease (shar′ko): inherited neuromuscular disease, characterized by atrophy of peroneal muscles of the fibula, producing footdrop, clubfoot, and ataxia.

craniomeningocele (kra″ne-o-me-nin′go-sel): herniation of the cerebral membranes through a defect in the skull.

craniorachischisis (kra″ne-o-rah-kis′ki-sis): congenital incomplete closure of the skull and spinal column.

diastematomyelia (di″ah-stem″ah-to-mi-e′le-ah): separation of the lateral halves of the spinal cord by a septum of bone or cartilage (also called *diastomyelia; diastasis* means separation).

encephalomyelocele (en-sef″ah-lo-mi-el′o-sel): herniation of the spinal cord, meninges and medulla due to abnormality of the foramen magnum.

epilepsy (ep′i-lep″se): hereditary or idiopathic nervous system disorder, with or without convulsions, that may also develop following infection or trauma. Characterized by a temporary disturbance of brain impulses, with several types: *grand mal*, loss of consciousness with convulsions; *petit mal*, temporary loss of awareness and suspension of activity; *psychomotor*, brief clouding of consciousness accompanied by meaningless repetition of movement, such as handclapping; and *focal*, in which the seizures are one-sided or affect limited body areas (*epilepsy* means a condition of seizure).

Friedreich's ataxia (fred′riks): progressive heredofamilial spinocerebellar degeneration with an early onset characterized by kyphoscoliosis, cardiac abnormalities, nystagmus, and ataxia.

heterotopia (het″er-o-to′pe-ah): displacement of gray matter into the white matter of the brain and spinal cord.

Huntington's chorea: rare, progressive, hereditary disease of the brain, usually beginning after age 30, associated with degenerative changes of the basal ganglia and cerebral cortex, producing symptoms of personality change, such as irritability, poor judgment, indifference, and memory loss, progressing to total incapacitation and eventual death within 10 to 20 years. There is a 50:50 chance of inheriting the disease if either parent has the defective gene (also called *chronic chorea* and *degenerative chorea*).

hydrencephalocele (hi″dren-sef′ah-lo-sel): hernial protrusion of the brain substance through a cranial defect, with an accumulation of cerebrospinal fluid in the sac (also called *hydrocephalocele*).

hydrencephalomeningocele (hi″dren-sef′ah-lo-me-nin′go-sel): hernial protrusion of the meninges through a cranial defect, with accumulations of cerebrospinal fluid and brain substance in the sac.

hydrocephalus (hi-dro-sef'ah-lus): abnormal accumulation of fluid in the cerebral ventricles, with thinning of the cortex and enlargement of the head due to separation of the cranial bones.

hydromeningocele (hi″dro-me-nin′go-sel): protrusion of the meninges through a defect in the skull or spine, with an accumulation of cerebrospinal fluid in the sac.

hydromyelia (hi″dro-mi-e′le-ah): accumulation of fluid in the spinal cord, resulting in an enlarged central canal.

hydromyelocele: protrusion, through a spina bifida, of membranes and tissue of the spinal cord, forming a sac containing cerebrospinal fluid (also called **_hydromyelomeningocele_**).

Krabbe's disease (krab'ez): rare, infantile, familial cerebral sclerosis, with death usually occurring in 1 to 2 years (also called **_globoid cell leukodystrophy_**).

Lesch-Nyhan cerebral palsy: an X-linked, inherited disorder of males, associated with an enzyme formation defect, and characterized by spastic cerebral palsy and mental retardation.

macrocephaly (mak″ro-se-fa′le): excessively large size of head (also called **_macrocephalia_** and **_megacephaly_**).

Marie's sclerosis: hereditary form of sclerosis of the cerebellum.

meningocele (me-ning′go-sel): herniation of the meninges through a cranial or spinal column defect.

meningoencephalocele (me-ning″go-en-sef′ah-lo-sel): herniation of the meninges and brain substance through a defect in the skull.

meningomyelocele (me-ning″go-mi-el′o-sel): herniation of a part of the spinal cord and meninges through a defect in the spinal column.

Menkes' syndrome: rare, congenital, genetically determined, fatal nerve disorder involving inability to metabolize copper, affecting only males, producing a characteristic kinky hair, failure to thrive, seizures, and brain deterioration (also called **_kinky hair disease_**).

microcephalus (mi″kro-sef′ah-lus): person with an excessively small head.

microcephaly: condition of excessive smallness of the head (also called **_microcephalia_**).

microgyrus (mi″kro-ji′rus): abnormally small, narrow convolution of the brain.

micromyelia (mi″kro-mi-e′le-ah): abnormally short or small spinal cord.

Moebius syndrome (me″be-us): rare, congenital, developmental, facial palsy, often accompanied by oculomotor disorders (inability to control facial and eye muscles).

myelocele (mi′e-lo-sel): herniation of the substance of the spinal cord through a defect in the vertebral column (also called **_myelocystocele_**,

myelocystomeningocele, and **_myelomeningocele_**).

myelodysplasia (mi″e-lo-dis-pla′ze-ah): defective development of the spinal cord.

myeloradiculodysplasia (mi″e-lo-rah-dik″u-lo-dis-pla′ze-ah): developmental abnormality of the spinal cord and spinal nerve roots.

myeloschisis (mi″e-los′ki-sis): developmental anomaly in which there is a cleft spinal cord.

neurofibromatosis: hereditary disorder that affects not only the nervous system but other systems as well (Chapter 17).

porencephaly (po″ren-se-fa′le): abnormal presence of cavities in the brain substance usually opening into the lateral ventricles (also called **_porencephalia_** and **_spelencephaly_**; **_spel_** means cavity).

spina bifida (spi′nah bif′i-dah): developmental anomaly characterized by a defective formation of the bony spinal canal through which spinal membranes and/or cord may protrude.

spina bifida occulta (ok-kul′tah): spina bifida without associated protrusion of the spinal cord or meninges.

syringobulbia (si-ring″go-bul′be-ah): presence of a cavity filled with fluid in the brainstem.

syringoencephalomyelia (si-ring″go-en-sef″ah-lo-mi-e′le-ah): presence of a tubular cavity in the substance of the brain and spinal cord.

syringomyelia (si-ring″go-mi-e′le-ah): cavities, lined with dense tissue, within the spinal cord, producing deterioration of sensation, paralysis, and scoliosis of the spine.

syringomyelocele (si-ring″go-mi′e-lo-sel): protrusion of the spinal cord through the bony defect in spina bifida, in which the cavity of the herniated sac is connected with the central canal of the spinal cord (also called **_syringocele_**).

Tay-Sachs disease: a form of inherited cerebral sphingolipidosis (occurring largely in families of Eastern European Jewish background), with destruction of ganglion cells, myelin degeneration, and glial proliferation that results in blindness, dementia, and psychomotor retardation, with death within four years of age.

tuberous sclerosis: congenital familial disease, producing tumors on the surfaces of the lateral ventricles, and sclerotic patches on the surface of the brain, resulting in marked mental deterioration and epilepsy (also called **_Bourneville's disease_**).

Circulatory disturbances

cerebral hemorrhage: bleeding into the structure of the cerebrum, usually caused by rupture of an artery or a congenital aneurysm, that may be followed by destruction of brain tissue, with ensuing paralyses, sensory losses, and cognitive confusion and losses.

cerebrovascular accident (CVA): commonly called *stroke*, includes rupture (hemorrhagic stroke) or obstruction (ischemic stroke) of an artery of the brain, producing severe headache, nausea, vomiting, confusion, and, depending upon area affected, possible neck rigidity, fever, and photophobia, accompanied by localized and widespread neurologic deterioration, with possible coma, paralysis, and aphasia; may be fatal, with survival often leaving some residual damage and reduced functioning (see also **transient ischemic attack**).

encephalomalacia: softening of brain tissue caused by reduced blood supply.

epidural hematoma: collection of blood outside the dura mater.

intracranial hemorrhage: cranial blood vessel leakage leading to escape of blood within the cranium and development of hematomas.

subarachnoid hemorrhage: escape of blood into the subarachnoid space, usually caused by rupture of an aneurysm.

subdural hemorrhage: escape of blood between dura mater and arachnoid membranes (also called *subdural hematoma* and *hemorrhagic pachymeningitis*).

transient ischemic attack (TIA): condition that may precede an ischemic stroke, producing symptoms of double vision, or loss of vision, numbness in upper extremities, dizziness and falling, usually lasting about 24 hours.

Other organic abnormalities

Alzheimer's disease (altz'hi-merz): one of a group of brain degenerative disorders classified as *primary degenerative dementias, Alzheimer's type (SDAT)* is a progressive brain atrophy disease characterized by neuronal degeneration, neurofibrillary tangles, and senile plaques in the brain, usually occurring in persons over age 65, with rare cases under age 50 classified as *presenile dementia*, with prognosis of death within 10 years. Possible factors implicated in the disease include impairment of the proteins that make up the structure of cells, viral infection, and low neurotransmitter activity.

amyotrophic lateral sclerosis (ALS): chronic progressive disease of the nervous system, occurring in later life, in which there is atrophy of muscles and hardening of the lateral columns of the spinal cord, characterized by disturbance in motility, weakness and wasting of afflicted muscles, and irregular twitching (also called *Lou Gehrig's disease* and *Charcot's disease*).

aphasia: loss of oral or written language due to brain damage, of various types, mainly receptive and expressive.

ataxia: muscular incoordination.

athetosis (ath'e-to-sis): recurring series of purposeless motions of the extremities, due to brain lesion or drug toxicity (*athetos* means not fixed).

aura: experience that precedes and marks the onset of a paroxysmal attack such as an epileptic seizure, that may take the form of visual, auditory, olfactory, or tactile sensations.

Bell's palsy: palsy characterized by peripheral facial weakness with retraction of the angle of the mouth and impaired closure of the eye on the affected side.

bradylalia: abnormally slow speech, due to a brain lesion (*lalia* means talking).

Brown-Sequard syndrome: paralysis of motion on one side of the body and of sensation on the other due to a lesion on one side of the spinal cord.

cephalalgia: headache (also called *cephalodynia* and *cerebralgia*).

cerebral ataxia: lack of muscular coordination caused by disease of the cerebrum (*ataxia* means lack of order).

cerebral palsy: group of conditions with a variety of symptoms due to brain damage, affecting muscular control and coordination, described by symptoms as *spastic, athetoid, rigid, ataxic,* and *tremor*.

chorea (ko-re'ah): a convulsive nervous disease with involuntary jerky movements (*chorea* means to dance).

coma: stuporous condition of depressed responsiveness, with absence of response to strong stimuli.

decerebration: loss of higher mental functions because of brain damage.

delirium: mental disturbance marked by hallucinations, excitement, physical restlessness, and incoherence, that may occur as a result of fever, disease (especially alcoholic psychosis), or injury (*delirium* means off the track).

dementia: mental deterioration of the brain because of organic disease.

diplegia: paralysis of like parts on both sides of the body.

dysbasia: difficulty in walking, because of central nervous system lesion (*basia* means step).

dyskinesia: impaired voluntary movement resulting in fragmentary, incomplete, or involuntary movements, because of brain damage or disorder.

dysphasia: speech impairment caused by central nervous system lesion.

dyspraxia: partial loss of ability to perform coordinated motions.

Erb-Duchenne paralysis: paralysis of the upper arm, with the absence of involvement of the small hand muscles (also called *Erb's paralysis*).

hemiplegia: paralysis of one side of the body, of several types.

Horner's syndrome: paralysis of the cervical sympathetic fibers, causing inward sinking of the eyeball, ptosis of the upper eyelid, constriction of the pupil, and narrowing of the opening between the eyelids.

hyperpathia: exaggerated response to stimuli, marked by severe pain or discomfort in response to light stimulation of the skin, caused by damage to the thalamus.

Jacksonian seizure: focal seizure or convulsion, beginning with distal twitching of a group of muscles such as the fingers, and progressing proximally in "march-like" fashion, reflecting cortical activity in a particular form of epilepsy.

monoplegia: paralysis of one part.

multi-infarct dementia: one of the dementias of aging caused by a series of small strokes that cause brain cell damage, giving rise to mental function decline (previously called *senile dementia*).

multiple sclerosis (MS): an immune system disorder, the most common demyelinating disorder of the brain and spinal cord (CNS), appearing in early adulthood, with intermittent progressions and remissions, characterized by sporadic sclerotic patches on the myelin sheath, which form scars so that nerve impulses are interrupted, lost, or misrouted, resulting in a variety of symptoms including paralysis, nystagmus, lack of coordination, ataxia, tremor, paresthesia, visual and speech disturbances (also known as *insular*, *disseminated*, or *focal sclerosis*).

myeloplegia: spinal paralysis.

narcolepsy: uncontrollable urge to sleep or sudden attacks of sleep (*narco* refers to sleep).

neuralgia: pain in a nerve or nerves (also called *neurodynia*).

opisthotonos (o″pis-thot′o-nos): tetanic spasm with head and heels bent backward and body bowed forward (*opistho* means backward).

palsy (pawl′ze): paralysis (see **entries under individual types**).

panplegia: total or complete paralysis (also called *pamplegia*).

paralysis: loss or impairment of motor function in a part as the result of disease or a lesion of the neural or muscular mechanism.

paraparesis: partial paralysis.

paraphasia: partial aphasia in which wrong words with senseless meaning are used (also called *paraphrasia*).

paraplegia (par″ah-ple′je-ah): paralysis of the lower torso and extremities.

paresis: a form of paralysis.

Parkinson's disease: disease primarily of late life, usually caused by changes in the basal ganglia, producing a masklike expression, rigidity, tremor of the resting muscles, and a drooping posture (also called *paralysis agitans* and *parkinsonism*).

Pick's disease: one of the primary degenerative dementia disorders. Classified as a presenile dementia, with insidious onset occurring around ages 45 to 50, involving vascular and degenerative changes in the brain, with symptoms including thinking and memory difficulties, fatigue, and personality changes, and, as the disease progresses, increasing disorientation, apathy, and impairment of thought and judgment are noted, with death within 8 years.

pragmatagnosia: inability to recognize formerly known objects.

progressive bulbar paralysis: progressive paralysis of the muscles, as well as atrophy of the lips, tongue, mouth, and throat (also called *Duchenne's paralysis*).

retrograde amnesia: loss of memory for events preceding the event causing brain damage.

senility: deterioration, both physical and mental, related to aging.

shaken infant syndrome (SIS): brain damage in infants and young children, caused by severe shaking, exuberant play, or physical abuse, that produces intracranial hemorrhage and pressure on brain tissue.

syncope (sin′ko-pe): transient loss of consciousness resulting from a decrease in cerebral blood flow, usually accompanied by a fall in blood pressure, and commonly referred to as fainting.

tabes dorsalis: degeneration of the dorsal columns of the spinal cord and sensory nerve trunks as a result of tertiary syphilis.

torpor: no response to normal stimuli.

Tourette's disease or syndrome: onset in childhood, characterized by facial and vocal tics, progressing to generalized lack of coordination and coprolalia (uncontrollable urge to say obscenities), believed to be caused by a defect in the basal ganglia of the brain, with resulting excess of the neurotransmitter dopamine, treatable with dopamine-blocking tranquilizers (named for French physician, Gilles de la Tourette).

Wernicke's disease (ver′ni-kez): encephalopathy attributed to thiamine deficiency associated wtih chronic alcoholism, often found in individuals with a variety of debilitating diseases caused by diets consisting primarily of carbohydrates, and characterized by ataxia, mental dullness, impaired retentive memory, diplopia, nystagmus, with symptoms of alcohol withdrawal.

Oncology*

astroblastoma (as″tro-blas-to′mah): tumor composed of immature astrocytes (preastrocyte cells).

astrocytoma (as″tro-si-to′mah): tumor made up of adult astrocytes (star-shaped cells).

ependymoblastoma (ep-en″di-mo-blas-to′mah): tumor derived from embyronic ependymal cells.

ependymoma (ep-en″di-mo′mah): tumor derived from adult ependymal cells.

gangliocytoma (gang″gle-o-si-to′mah): tumor derived from mature ganglion cells (also called *ganglioneuroma*).

glioblastoma multiforme* (gli″o-blas-to′mah): malignant cystic tumor of the cerebrum or spinal cord (also called *glioma multiforme*).

glioma (gli-o′mah): any tumor composed of any of the various cells forming the interstitial tissue of the brain, spinal cord, pineal body, posterior pituitary and the retina.

glioneuroma (gli″o-nu-ro′mah): tumor composed of gliomatous and neural elements.

medulloblastoma* (me-dul″o-blas-to′mah): malignant tumor of the cerebellum.

meningematoma (me-nin″jem-ah-to′mah): hematoma of the dura mater of the meninges (also called *meninghematoma*).

meningioma (me-nin″je-o′mah): benign, encapsulated tumor originating in the arachnoid.

meningofibroblastoma (me-ning′go-fi″bro-blas-to′mah): type of meningioma.

neurilemoma (nu″ri-le-mo′mah): tumor of the peripheral nerve sheath of Schwann (also called *neurolemmoma*, *neurinoma*, and *Schwannoma*).

neuroblastoma* (nu″ro-blas-to′mah): malignant tumor of the nervous system composed mainly of neuroblasts.

neurocytoma (nu″ro-si-to′mah): brain tumor composed of undifferentiated ganglionic nerve cells (also called *medulloepithelioma*).

neuroepithelioma (nu″ro-ep″i-the″le-o′mah): rare type of glioma usually occurring in the retina.

neurofibroma (nu″ro-fi-bro′mah): tumor of peripheral nerve cells resulting from abnormal proliferation of Schwann cells.

neurogliocytoma (nu-rog″le-o-si-to′mah): tumor made up of neuroglial cells.

neuroglioma (nu″ro-gli-o′mah): tumor made up of neuroglial tissue.

oligodendroblastoma (ol″i-go-den″dro-blas-to′mah): tumor composed of young oligodendroglial cells.

oligodendroglioma (ol″i-go-den″dro-gli-o′mah): tumor composed of oligodendroglia.

paraganglioma (par″ah-gang″gle-o′mah): tumor that contains chromaffin cells and occurs in the sympathetic nervous system (also called *chromaffinoma*).

spongioblastoma (spon″je-o-blas-to′mah): tumor composed of spongioblasts (also called *spongiocytoma*).

sympathicoblastoma* (sim-path″i-ko-blas-to′mah): malignant tumor that contains embryonic sympathetic nerve cells (also called *sympathoblastoma* and *sympathogonioma*).

Surgical Procedures

chordotomy (ko-dot′o-me): any operation on the spinal cord.

craniectomy (kra″ne-ek′to-me): excision of a part of the skull.

cranioplasty (kra′ne-o-plas″te): repair of defects of the skull.

craniotomy (kra″ne-ot′o-me): surgical opening of skull to remove a tumor, or relieve intracranial pressure.

duraplasty: plastic repair of the dura mater.

gangliectomy (gang″gle-ek′to-me): excision of a ganglion (also called *ganglionectomy*).

hemicraniectomy (hem″e-kra″ne-ek′to-me): procedure for exposing part of the brain in preparation for surgery (also called *hemicraniotomy*).

hemidecortication (hem″e-de-kor″ti-ka′shun): removal of half of the cerebral cortex.

hemispherectomy (hem″i-sfer-ek′to-me): removal of a cerebral hemisphere.

leukotomy (lu-kot′o-me): cutting of the white matter in the frontal lobe of the brain (also spelled *leucotomy*).

lobectomy (lo-bek′to-me): excision of a lobe of the brain.

lobotomy (lo-bot′o-me): incision into the frontal lobe of the brain through drilled holes in the skull.

meningeorrhaphy (me-nin″je-or′ah-fe): suture of the meninges, especially those of the spinal cord.

neurectomy (nu-rek′to-me): excision of a part of a nerve.

neuroanastomosis (nu″ro-ah-nas″to-mo′sis): anastomosis, or connection, between nerves.

neurolysis (nu-rol′i-sis): surgical freeing of perineural adhesions.

neuroplasty: plastic repair of a nerve.

neurorrhaphy: suturing of a nerve.

neurotomy: dissection of a nerve.

neurotripsy (nu″ro-trip′se): surgical crushing of a nerve.

phrenemphraxis (fren″em-frak′sis): surgical crushing of the phrenic nerve (also called *phreniclasia* and *phrenicotripsy*).

*Indicates a malignant condition.

phrenicectomy (fren"i-sek'to-me): excision or resection of part of the phrenic nerve (also called **phreniconeurectomy** and **phrenectomy**).

phrenicotomy: surgical division of the phrenic nerve.

rachicentesis (ra"ke-sen-te'sis): lumbar puncture (also called **rachiocentesis**).

radicotomy (rad"i-kot'o-me): sectioning of nerve roots of the spine to relieve pain or spastic paralysis (also called **radiculectomy** and **rhizotomy**).

sympathectomy: resection of a sympathetic nerve or ganglion (also called **sympathetectomy** and **sympathicectomy**).

sympathicotripsy (sim-path"i-ko-trip'se): surgical crushing of a sympathetic ganglion.

tractotomy (trak-tot'o-me): surgical interruption of a nerve tract.

vagotomy: sectioning of a vagus nerve.

ventriculocisternostomy (ven-trik"u-lo-sis"ter-nos'to-me): surgical creation of an opening or shunt between the ventricles and the cisterna magna (enlarged subarachnoid space) to relieve cerebrospinal fluid pressure (also called **ventriculostomy**).

volumetric interstitial brachytherapy (VIB): the use of radiation implants through catheters inserted into small holes drilled in the skull and left in place for 3-4 days, delivering radiation directly to a tumor and preserving surrounding tissue, after which catheters are removed, producing comparatively long remission.

Laboratory Tests and Procedures

amyloid beta-protein precurser (APP) test: antibody assay test of cerebrospinal fluid to measure the level of a substance that produces the protein plaques in the brains of Alzheimer's victims.

brain electrical activity map (BEAM): computer-generated map of the brain emitting electrical activity evoked by flashes of light, with the patterns of wavelike electrical activity revealing the presence of tumors or other lesions.

brain scan: a scanner is used, in conjunction with intravenous injection of radioactive substance, which circulates to the brain, concentrating in areas of abnormality, to diagnose lesions, tumors and areas of necrosis.

cerebral angiography: using a contrast medium injected into the carotid, brachial, subclavian or femoral arteries, a series of x-rays is taken to visualize the blood vessels of the brain.

cerebrospinal fluid scan: injection of radioactive material into the spinal canal in conjunction with a brain scan to detect abnormalities of the skull or spinal fluid leaks.

cerebrospinal fluid tests: series of tests to detect the presence of blood, infection, and other abnormalities, including a cell count to detect infection in the brain or spinal canal, abnormal levels of calcium present in tuberculous meningitis, and culture to detect disease-causing microorganisms.

coccidioidomycosis antibodies: blood test to identify a fungal infection that affects the central nervous system and other body parts.

computerized tomography (CT): use of a thin beam of x-rays to derive cross-sectional images (tomograms) of the head that are put together and analyzed to form a picture on a computer screen that shows tumors, tissue atrophy, and other anatomic abnormalities; a more effective tool for diagnosis than ordinary x-ray and pneumoencephalography (also called **computerized axial tomography [CAT]**).

diffusion-weighted magnetic resonance imaging: imaging method to detect the flow of fluid through the brain after trauma; for early detection of ischemic and infarct problems.

echoencephalogram: scan of the brain using ultrasound to detect abnormalities.

echo-planar imaging (EPI): a type of fMRI that reduces imaging time from minutes to fractions of a second, using changes in blood oxygenation to highlight active areas of the brain.

electroencephalograph (EEG): a machine used to reveal patterns of electrical activity of the brain in the form of brain waves; aids in diagnosing epilepsy, tumors, and other abnormalities reflected in electrical activity, and with advanced computer technology used with the EEG in what is called the "evoked potential" or neurometrics technique, shows promise in diagnosing even more difficult conditions including senility, learning disorders, stroke, and traumatic injury disorders.

magnetic resonance imaging (MRI): noninvasive method of scanning the body by use of an electromagnetic field and radio waves that provides visual images on a computer screen and magnetic tape recordings; used to examine soft tissue, and especially useful for diagnosis of multiple sclerosis and tumors (also called **nuclear magnetic resonance [NMR]**).

magnetoencephalography (MEG): measure of the magnetic fields produced by electrical activity of the brain. Used to detect neural activity too rapid for MRI or PET methods.

multiplane imager: brain scanning device using injected radioactive isotopes in the bloodflow of the brain, to study brain function.

myelography: x-ray of the spinal cord and subarachnoid space, using a contrast medium, to identify spinal lesions caused by disease or trauma.

perfusion magnetic resonance imaging: rapid method of MRI scanning, using a contrast agent in the blood to detect brain damage at the capillary level. (Together with diffusion-weighted MRI, provides a complete picture of an acute ischemic attack.)

pneumoencephalography: injection of gas such as air or oxygen into cerebral ventricles and subarachnoid spaces to allow x-ray visualization (pneumoencephalogram) of the cranium and contents for diagnosis of tumors, atrophy of tissue, and similar abnormalities.

positron emission transaxial tomography (PET): a further refinement of CT scan technology, PET uses a thin beam of x-ray scans to take computer-assisted, cross-sectional images of the brain after injection of a radioactive substance, to visualize the metabolism of this substance, and, consequently, the biochemical activity within the cells of the brain.

serum ammonia: blood test to detect elevated levels of ammonia; helps in diagnosing Reye's syndrome.

single photon emission computed tomography (SPECT): imaging method to reveal abnormal metabolic action of the brain, for diagnosis of cancer, stroke, Alzheimer's disease, some mental illnesses, localization of seizures in epilepsy, and for monitoring the treatment of tumors. A solution of radioactive sugar is injected into the patient, and as the sugar is metabolized by the brain, the imaging device rotates around the head, scanning, analyzing, and recording by computer.

stereotaxic neuroradiography: x-ray procedure frequently used during neurosurgery to guide a needle into a specific area of the brain.

vitamin B tests: group of tests done for vitamin B_2 on blood and urine and vitamin B_6 on urine to detect a vitamin deficiency that relates to nervous system problems.

Psychiatric Disorders

The following disorders, which are largely nonorganic or functional in origin, are named and described according to the most recent manual of mental disorders (DSM IV) of the American Psychiatric Association.* This list is only a sampling, and is not intended to describe all disorders listed in the manual.

affective disorders: a group of disorders ranging from mild to psychotic, including melancholia, despondency, hopelessness, sadness, and loss of interest in outside activities, classified as follows: *bipolar disorder*, involving both depression and elation (mania); *major depressive disorder*, a severe depressive condition; *cyclothymic disorder*, a persistent pattern of mood swings

without severe disruption of functioning; and *dysthymic disorder*, neurotic depression with mild rather than severe disruption of functioning.

alcoholic psychoses: disorders listed under substance abuse disorders, including: *pathologic intoxication*, a confused, disoriented state, with subsequent amnesia, following consumption of even moderate quantities of alcohol; *delirium tremens*, an acute mental disturbance characterized by delirium with trembling and great excitement, anxiety, disorientation, mental distress, hallucinations, restlessness, and convulsions, seen in alcoholic psychosis or following withdrawal of heavy alcohol or narcotic ingestion; *acute alcoholic hallucinosis*, a severe psychotic reaction with terrifying auditory hallucinations as the major symptom; and *Korsakoff's psychosis*, a psychosis characterized by memory defect, disorientation, delirium, hallucinations, and falsification of memory, symptoms that are believed to be caused by nutritional inadequacies, especially vitamin B deficiency, in chronic alcoholism.

anorexia nervosa: an *eating disorder* with high death potential from starvation, in which severe weight reduction is produced by voluntarily refusing food or vomiting ingested food, with onset in adolescent or young adult years, primarily seen in females (20:1 ratio) who have histories of unusual eating habits and tendencies to conscientiousness in school work and social behavior (both psychosocial and neurologic factors are believed to be involved in various stages of progression of the disorder).

anxiety disorders: category of disorders, including *phobic disorders*, *anxiety states*, *panic disorder*, *generalized anxiety disorder*, *post-traumatic stress disorder*, and *obsessive-compulsive disorder*, all of which involve anxiety (generalized apprehension) and defensive mechanisms that block anxiety to varying degrees, but, unlike psychoses, include continued contact with reality.

attention deficit hyperactivity disorder: a disorder of children and adolescents with symptoms of school underachievement, short attention span, restlessness, disorganization, and excessive physical activity.

bulimia (bu-lim′e-ah): abnormal appetite or hunger (*limia* refers to hunger), in which large amounts of food are consumed, and also referring to one variety of *eating disorder* in which food is vomited after eating large quantities, thus producing severe weight loss to the point of starvation and death (also called *phagomania* and *sitomania*).

conversion disorder: term for a disorder classified under *somatoform disorders* in which there is sensory or motor impairment in the absence of organic cause.

*American Psychiatric Association: Diagnostic and statistical manual of mental disorders, ed 4, Washington, D.C., 1994, American Psychiatric Association

depression: see **affective disorders**.

dissociative disorder: mental disorder in which a person escapes stress through altering the personality, including amnesia, fugue, multiple personality, and depersonalization, in which the person escapes stress by avoiding or escaping from (dissociating) the true self by varying degrees of memory or identity changes.

Down's syndrome: a form of mental retardation with multiple system involvement (Chapter 17).

factitious disorders: disorders that are characterized by physical or psychological symptoms that are produced voluntarily by the individual to gain attention (the chronic form is also called *Munchausen syndrome*). This category includes *factitious disorder by proxy*, in which the individual (usually a parent) induces symptoms in another (usually their child) to gain attention for themselves, without regard for the hazards to the other (also called *Munchausen by proxy disorder*).

fragile X syndrome: a form of X-linked moderate to severe mental retardation (Chapter 17).

Hurler's syndrome: a form of mental retardation with multiple system involvement (Chapter 17).

mania: abnormal mental state characterized by extreme excitement.

manic-depressive: obsolete term for the affective disorder called *bipolar affective disorder*.

mental retardation: condition of significantly below-average intellectual functioning, classified by level of function as mild, moderate and severe.

paranoia (par″ah-noi′ah): chronic form of psychosis characterized by delusions of persecution or grandeur.

paraphilias (para-fil′ee-yuhs): group of sexual disorders involving abnormal objects and types of sexual gratification.

personality disorders: group of disorders in which interpersonal problems are blamed on others, leading to lifetime histories of repetitive, irresponsible, manipulative and disturbed relationships, classified according to the most prominent characteristic pattern: *paranoid, schizoid, schizotypal, histrionic, narcissistic, antisocial, borderline, avoidant, dependent, compulsive, depressive, negativistic, self-defeating,* and *passive-aggressive*.

phobia (fo′be-ah): morbid fear, currently classified under *anxiety disorders*, referring to the generalized, unreasonable fear or anxiety that underlies the disorders, commonly referred to by their roots. (A simplified, limited list follows, with reference to medical dictionaries for additional listings).

    acrophobia: heights.

    agoraphobia (ag″o-rah-fo′be-ah): open spaces, crowded or public places.

    algophobia (al″go-fo′be-ah): pain.

    aquaphobia: water.

    astraphobia: lightning, thunder, and storms.

    claustrophobia (klaws″tro-fo′be-ah): closed spaces.

    cynophobia or kynophobia: dogs.

    entomophobia: insects.

    erotophobia: sexual love.

    gynephobia: women.

    microbiophobia: germs.

    mysophobia (mi″so-fo′be-ah): contamination or dirt.

    musophobia: mice.

    necrophobia: corpses.

    noctiphobia or nyctophobia: night or darkness.

    ophidiophobia (o-fid″e-o-fo′be-ah): snakes.

    thanatophobia (than″ah-to-fo′be-ah): death.

    xenophobia: strangers.

    zoophobia: animals or some particular animal.

post-traumatic stress disorder: classified as an *anxiety disorder*, the symptoms follow a traumatic event and involve reexperiencing the event, and/or symptoms of depression, autonomic arousal, dissociative states, and a variety of emotional problems (commonly seen in war veterans, rape and crime victims).

psychotic disorder: mental disorders in which there is a loss of contact with reality as well as personality disintegration, with major types including *affective, schizophrenic, organic,* and *schizoaffective*.

psychosomatic: pertaining to mind-body relationship, as in psychosomatic reactions, classified as a *somatization disorder*, in which the person is severely limited in effectively coping with stress and attaining goals, and defensive and self-defeating strategies are repeatedly used without success, leading to frustration and constant emotional arousal of the autonomic nervous system, which produces internal bodily changes, leading to breakdown of some organ systems.

schizophrenia (skiz″o-fre′ne-ah): this term, which literally means "split personality," covers a group of psychotic conditions in which there is a profound tendency to withdraw from reality, disorientation, and thought disorder, with subtypes including: *undifferentiated*, mixed-symptom type with delusions, hallucinations, thought disorder, and bizarre behavior; *paranoid*, illogical, changeable delusions and hallucinations with confused ideas of reference (object of others' interest) and grandiosity, that lead to unpredictable and sometimes dangerous behavior; *catatonic*, state of either excited or stuporous motor activity, sometimes changing abruptly to the opposite, with potential for dangerous behavior; *hebephrenic* or *disorganized*, a more severe form than the others, with greater personality breakdown, usually occurring at an earlier age, with silliness, peculiar mannerisms, bizarre behavior, and changeable and often fantastic hallucinations and delusions; and **residual**, involving individuals who have recovered from one of the other subtypes but who still manifest some mild schizophrenic thinking and behavior.

sociopathic personality: a person with an **antisocial personality disorder** whose characteristic behavior is antisocial, unconventional, or even criminal (also called **psychopathic personality**).

somatization disorder: see **psychosomatic**.

substance abuse disorders: this classification covers substance dependence and maladaptive behavior associated with the regular use of alcohol and/or drugs (barbiturates, sedatives, opioids, cocaine, amphetamines, hallucinogens, marijuana, tobacco, etc.), including interference with social or occupational functioning.

trance and possession disorder: trances and demonic possessions not recognized by one's culture or religion.

Other Psychiatric Descriptive and Diagnostic Terms

agraphia (ah-graf′e-ah): inability to express thoughts in writing; may be functional or the result of brain pathology.

alexia: inability to read, sometimes associated with cerebral dysfunction (**lexia** refers to word).

amentia (ah-men′she-ah): mental deficiency.

amnesia (am-ne′se-ah): loss of memory.

analgesia (an″al-je′ze-ah): insensibility to pain.

anepia (an-e′pe-ah): inability to talk (**epia** refers to speech).

anergic (an-er′jik): characterized by abnormal inactivity, with lack of energy (**ergic** means work).

anesthesia: loss of sensation.

anomia (ah-no′me-ah): loss of ability to recognize or name objects (**nomia** refers to name).

anosognosia (an-i″so-no′se-ah): loss of ability to recognize that one has a disease or bodily defect (**noso** means disease; **gnosia** means knowledge).

apathy: absence of emotion, or indifference to the environment or other people, with attention directed inward rather than outward.

aphonia: loss of voice.

apraxia (ah-prak′se-ah): loss of ability to perform intricate skilled acts that had been previously mastered.

asthenia (as-the′ne-ah): weakness or lack of strength and energy.

autism (aw′tizm): condition of being dominated by subjective, introspective thinking, and a symptom of schizophrenia, that may affect some children who show schizophrenic-like conditions in a disorder referred to as **infantile autism** or **Kanner's syndrome**.

autoeroticism (aw″to-e-rot′i-sizm): sexual gratification of self by various means without participation of another (**auto** means self).

automatism (aw-tom′ah-tizm): performance of undirected actions without evident conscious volition.

bestiality (bes-te-al′i-te): sexual relations between humans and animals, classified as a **paraphilia**.

bradykinesia (brad″e-ki-ne′se-ah): slow movement (**kinesis** means movement).

bradyphrenia: slowness of thinking (**phrenia** refers to mind).

bradypragia (brad″e-pra′je-ah): slowness of action.

bradypsychia (brad″e-si′ke-ah): slowness in mental reactions.

catalepsy (kat′ah-lep″se): waxy rigidity of the muscles, with limbs tending to remain in any position in which placed, observed in catatonic schizophrenia as well as other conditions.

cataphasia (kat″ah-fa′ze-ah): speech disorder involving constant repetition of the same word or phrase.

catatonia (kat″ah-to′ne-ah): form of schizophrenia (see **schizophrenia**).

cathexis (kah-thek′sis): concentration of mental or emotional energy that may be abnormal in intensity, on a person or object.

confabulation (kon-fab″u-la′shun): act of making up answers and concocting experiences without regard to truth.

coprolalia (kop″ro-la′le-ah): use of vulgar or obscene language (**copro** refers to dung or feces).

cyclothymia (si″klo-thim′e-ah): cyclic alternation of moods between elation and depression (see **affective disorders**).

deja entendu (da″zhah on-ton-doo′): impression, in a new situation, that one has heard the same thing previously.

deja vu (voo′): impression, in a new situation, that one has seen the same thing previously.

delusion: false belief or idea, a major symptom of psychosis.

dereism: irrational thinking or fantasy that is not in accord with logic, experience, and reality.

dipsomania (dip′so-ma′ne-ah): uncontrollable desire for alcohol.

disorientation: loss of proper bearings for time, place, and/or identity during mental confusion.

drug dependency: drug addiction or habituation.

dysarthria (dis-ar′thre-ah): imperfect articulation in speech, such as stuttering or stammering.

dysgraphia (dis-gra′fe-ah): inability to write properly.

dyslexia: impaired reading ability.

dyslogia (dis-lo′je-ah): impaired logical thinking.

dysphonia: difficulty in speaking, or any impairment of voice.

dysphoria (dis-fo′re-ah): sadness and depression.

dysthymia (dis-thim′e-ah): disorder of mood (***thymia*** refers to mind or emotion).

echolalia (ek″o-la′le-ah): meaningless repetition of words.

echopathy (ekop′ah-the): senseless repetition of words or actions.

egocentric: self-centered.

empathy: process of imaginative projection of one's own consciousness into other persons to understand their feelings and emotions.

erotic: relating to or producing sexual excitement or love.

erotomania (e-rot″to-ma′ne-ah): exaggerated sexual interest or behavior.

euphoria (u-fo′re-ah): exaggerated sense of well-being, the opposite of dysphoria.

euthymia (u-thi′me-ah): pleasant feeling, and state of well-being.

exhibitionism: exposing the genitals to public view or to members of the opposite sex, popularly referred to as "flashing" in lay terminology, classified as a ***paraphilia***.

extrovert: one whose interests are centered in external objects and actions.

fetishism: practice of attaching unusual or magical qualities to an object, or the investment of sexual feeling in an inanimate object, classified as a ***paraphilia***.

flagellantism: getting pleasure from whipping someone or being whipped, psychoanalytically viewed as sexual pleasure, related to sadism and masochism, classified as a ***paraphilia***.

folie a deux (foal-ee ah duh): disorder in which two closely associated people share the same deluded or distorted ideas (popularly called a "gruesome twosome").

fugue (fug): dissociated state in which a person seems rational and conscious and may perform purposeful acts, but later is unable to recall the occasion or events.

gay: popular term for homosexual; used more commonly for males.

glossolalia: speaking in an unknown or imaginary language.

hallucination (hah-lu″si-na′shun): sense perception not based upon objective reality.

haplology: omissions of syllables in speaking, found in manic speech.

hedonia (he-do′ne-ah): excessive interest in pleasure.

heterolalia : use of inappropriate or meaningless words in place of those intended (also called ***heterophasia***).

homosexuality (ho″mo-seks″u-al′i-te): sexual attraction to persons of the same sex (commonly called ***gay*** for males and ***lesbian*** for females), no longer considered a disorder unless it is

ego-dystonic (unacceptable to the person's deeper self).

hyperkinesis (hi″per′ki-ne′sis): increased motor function or activity, also used to refer to ***hyperkinetic disorder***, classified as an ***attention deficit disorder*** in children, characterized by hyperactivity, difficulty in sustaining attention, and reduced ability to perform tasks that require fine coordination.

hyperpragia (hi″per′a′je-ah): pronounced increase in mental activity (also called ***hyperphrenia***).

hypnosis (hip-no′sis): induced state of altered awareness or trance.

hypoalgesia: decreased sensitivity to pain (also called ***hypalgesia***).

hypochondria: term used to describe excessive somatic complaints without evident organic cause.

hypoesthesia (hi″po-es-the′ze-ah): decreased sensibility to pain.

hypokinesia: decrease of motor function.

hypomania: excitement, with increased activity and speech, but not as extreme as in mania.

hypophrasia: slow speech associated with psychosis.

id: Freudian term for the self-preservative and sexual instincts.

incest: sexual relations between close relatives (between parent and child, brother and sister, uncle and niece, etc.).

inertia (in-er′she-ah): inactivity.

insomnia (in-som′ni-a): sleeplessness.

introverted: thoughts and activities centered on self instead of toward others, with the person becoming isolated, introspective, and relatively uncommunicative, the opposite of extroverted.

inversion: turning inward.

kleptomania: impulse to steal (***klepto*** means steal).

lesbian: female homosexual.

lethargy: lack of energy.

libido (li-be′do): Freudian collective term for energy, motive, force, or striving, especially with reference to sexual drive.

logographia (log″o-graf′e-ah): inability to express ideas in writing.

malingering: simulating or feigning illness for purposes other than getting attention.

masochism (mas′o-kism): deriving gratification or pleasure by the recipient of cruel treatment or pain, classified as a ***paraphilia***.

misogyny (mis-oj′i-ne): aversion to women (***gyn*** refers to women).

misopedia (mis″o-pe′de-ah): hatred of children (***pedia*** refers to children).

mogilalia (moj-e-la′le-ah): stuttering, also called ***molilalia*** (***mogi*** means with difficulty).

narcissism (nar′si-sizm): excessive self-interest or self-love, and inability to love another.

necromania (nek″ro-ma′ne-ah): morbid preoccupation with death or the dead (***necro*** means death).

necrophilia (nek″ro-fil′e-ah): morbid attraction to a corpse or sexual intercourse with a dead person, classified as a ***paraphilia***.

necrosadism (nek″ro-sa′dizm): gratification of sexual needs through mutilation of a corpse, classified as a ***paraphilia***.

negativism (ne′ah-tiv-izm): abnormal opposition to suggestions or advice.

neurosis: obsolete term used to describe a less serious psychiatric problem than psychosis, and now referred to as a ***disorder***.

nosophilia: abnormal desire to be ill (***noso*** refers to disease).

nymphomania (nim″fo-ma′ne-ah): abnormally intense sexual desire in a female.

oligophrenia: mental deficiency.

onychophagy (on″i-kof′ah-je): habitual biting of nails.

palilalia (pal″i-la′le-ah): pathologic repetition of words (***pali*** means again).

paragraphia (par″ah-gra′fe-ah): disorder in which one word is written in place of another.

paralalia: speech disturbance.

paralgesia (par″al-je′se-ah): abnormally painful sensation.

paralogia (par″ah-lo′je-ah): impaired reasoning.

paraphilia (par″ah-fil′e-ah): aberrant sexual activity; sexual deviations.

pavor diurnus: attack similar to nightmare, but occurring during the daytime (***pavor*** means terror; ***diurnus*** means day).

pavor nocturnus: nightmare, night terror (***nocturnus*** means night).

phantom limb phenomenon: vivid feeling of still having an amputated limb, usually associated with subjective feelings of pain, perceived as originating in the lost limb.

pica (pi′ka): craving for ingestion of unnatural substances such as ashes, lead, hair, or dirt, usually seen in severely disturbed persons, although it may occur in pregnant women and in malnourished children.

poriomania (po″re-o-ma′ne-ah): tendency to wander from home.

pornographomania: morbid desire to collect pornographic or erotic literature, art, etc., as opposed to casual collection by relatively normal persons.

premenstrual syndrome (PMS): emotional counterpart of physiologic endocrine distress that precedes the onset of the menstrual period in females of reproductive age, with symptoms of fatigue, irritability, tension, anxiety, and depression.

pseudocyesis (su″do-si-e′sis): false pregnancy, classified as a ***somatoform disorder*** (***cyesis*** means pregnancy).

pseudographia (su″do-graf′e-ah): writing of meaningless symbols.

pseudologia (su″do-lo′je-ah): pathologic oral or written lying.

pseudomania: pretended mental disorder.

psychalia (si″ka′le-ah): hearing of voices or seeing images in mental disorders.

psyche (si′ke): term meaning soul or mind, including both conscious and unconscious processes.

psychogenic: originating from psychologic mechanisms and not from organic disease or disorder; for example, phobias are considered to be psychogenic in origin, but senile psychosis is regarded as organic.

psycholepsy (si-ko-lep′se): condition characterized by sudden changes in mood, tending toward depression.

psychosis: term for severe mental disorder with loss of reality contact, unlike neurotic disorder in which reality contact is retained.

pyromania: excessive preoccupation with fires and gaining pleasure from setting fires.

rationalization: one of many unconscious defense mechanisms, by which a plausible explanation is concocted to justify one's beliefs, behavior, needs, feelings, or motives, with the real motivation remaining hidden.

sadism (sad′izm): gratification through cruelty inflicted on others, classified as a ***paraphilia***.

sadomasochism (sad″o-maz′o-kizm): characterized by both sadism and masochism, classified as a paraphilia.

sodomy (sod′o-me): unusual sexual practices, classified under ***paraphilias***, including fellatio and anal intercourse between humans, and coitus between humans and animals (bestiality).

somnambulism: sleepwalking.

sophomania (sof″o-ma′ne-ah): exaggerated belief in one's own brilliance.

stress: term referring to physical or psychosocial adjustment demands placed on people, who differ in capacity to adapt, producing reactions that may be oriented either toward coping or toward protecting oneself from harm and damage. The body's reaction to sustained stress is described in Selye's concept of ***general adaptation syndrome (GAS)*** *, occurring in three major stages: ***alarm*** and ***mobilization***, in which the autonomic nervous system figures significantly; ***resistance***, in which psychosomatic symptoms appear and coping becomes more rigid and less effective; and ***exhaustion***, in which physical and emotional decompensation and breakdown occur and result in physical and mental abnormalities.

theomania: obsession with religion or with God or belief that one is God (***theo*** means God).

*Selye H: The stress of life, New York, 1956, McGraw-Hill Book Co

transvestism: sexual deviation, most common in males, classified as a ***paraphilia***, in which the individual gets sexual gratification from wearing clothes of the opposite sex, and may extend to wanting to be accepted as a member of the sex they are emulating, in which case they may even have sex change surgery to anatomically resemble the preferred sex identity, thereby becoming ***transsexual***.

trichophagia (tri-kof′ah-je-ah): practice of eating hair.

trichotillomania: uncontrollable urge to pull out one's own hair.

voyeurism (voi′yer-izm): sexual deviation in which sexual excitation or gratification is derived from looking at sexual organs or watching sexual activity by others, classified under ***paraphilias*** (also called ***scopophilia***).

zoosadism: deriving pleasure from cruelty to animals, classified as a ***paraphilia***.

Tests for Psychiatric and Neurologic Conditions

The following is a listing of a few of the many psychologic and psychiatric tests used to evaluate mental functioning and brain disorders.

Beck depression inventory: self-report measure of feelings, attitudes and behaviors that are diagnostic of depression.

brief psychiatric rating scale (BPRS): method of analyzing the clinical symptoms of patients with a standardized method of rating over 18 separate scales that cover a wide range of psychiatric conditions.

Minnesota multiphasic personality inventory (MMPI and MMPI-2): extensive self-report by patient using true-false inventory, that assesses psychiatric pathology.

Millon clinical multiaxial inventory (MCMI and MCMI-II): extensive self-report by patient using true-false inventory, that assesses personality traits, symptoms, and disorders.

neuropsychological tests: tests that assist in the diagnosis of brain damage or disorder and assess the extent of change from normal functioning. Some of the widely used tests for these purposes include:

  Bender visual motor gestalt test: drawing a set of geometric figures to assess perceptual impairment.

  Benton test of visual retention-revised: drawing, by memory, a set of complex geometric figures.

  Halstead-Reitan neuropsychological battery: a comprehensive battery of 11 basic tests of perception, cognition, and motor functioning, plus the use of the WAIS-R and MMPI, for diagnosing and assisting in localization of brain damage.

  Neurosurgery Center comprehensive examination of aphasia: battery of 24 tests evaluating visual, auditory, and tactile, sensory and motor aphasia problems.

  sorting tests: tests of abstract categorical function, using objects, colors, and shapes.

Rorschach test: a set of 10 standardized ink blots used to analyze thought processes, motives, characteristic defenses and effectiveness of coping, based on the "projective hypothesis" that, in trying to identify vague and unstructured materials, people will "project" their own feelings, motives and problems into the materials.

thematic apperception test (TAT): ambiguous and unstructured set of pictures about which patients make up stories by projecting their own conflicts into the pictures, revealing needs and motives, perception of reality, and characteristic coping or defensive strategies.

Wechsler Adult Intelligence Scale-Revised (WAIS-R): this measure of intelligence, which has a variety of different types of verbal and performance tests, is used to analyze cognitive competence, bizarre ideas, anxiety problems, and other structural components of psychiatric functioning.

Treatment Methods for Psychiatric Conditions

electroconvulsive therapy (ECT): form of shock therapy used in mental disorders (depression) in which electric currents are conveyed to the brain by electrodes applied to the scalp; results in loss of consciousness and muscle tonic and clonic contractions, followed by amnesia and confusion for varying periods after waking.

insulin coma therapy: rarely-used method of treating schizophrenics, involving administration of increasing amounts of insulin until the patient experiences hypoglycemic coma, which is terminated by providing glucose.

pharmacologic methods of treatment: drugs are extensively used in treatment of psychiatric conditions, and the following represent some of the chemical types and/or generic (non-trade name) drugs that have been used over a long period of time. New drugs are constantly being developed for use in this area, and some of the currently listed drugs may become obsolete.

  antianxiety drugs: group of minor tranquilizers that include the ***propanediols*** and ***benzodiazepines***.

  antidepressant drugs: two major groups are used to treat severe depressive symptoms, especially of the unipolar type: ***tricyclics*** and ***monoamine oxidase (MAO) inhibitors***.

antimanic drugs: primary drug used for manic states and bipolar affective disorders is *lithium carbonate*.

antipsychotic drugs: three major groups of antipsychotic drugs, or major tranquilizers, that are used to treat extreme agitation, delusions, hallucinations, and violent behavior, include the *phenothiazines*, *butyrophenomes*, and *thioxanthenes*.

neutoransmitter reuptake inhibitors: these drugs act by preventing absorption of the neurotransmitters serotinin and norepinephrine and are used primarily to reduce depression and produce feelings of well-being (one popular drug is *Prozac*).

stimulant drugs: these drugs, used primarily for hyperactivity in children, include *amphetamines* and *methylphenidates*.

prefrontal lobotomy: surgical procedure in which the frontal lobes are separated from the deeper centers in the diencephalon, producing significant personality changes, primarily used as a method for psychoses that do not respond to other methods, severe and debilitating obsessive-compulsive disorders, and for severe pain in terminal illness.

psychotherapies: this group of therapies involve the application of psychologic theory and knowledge to treatment of psychiatric disorders, with the following the best known of a large group.

behavior modification: the use of scientific principles of *contingency management* (rewarding desired behavior) to modify the symptoms and effect some personality change in a wide range of psychiatric disorders, including psychoses and personality disorders.

behavior therapy: this approach uses conditioning principles in the application of methods like *systematic desensitization*, *aversion therapy*, and *flooding* in the treatment of paraphilias, panic disorders, and phobias in particular.

client-centered therapy: this approach uses the overall relationship between the patient and therapist, and the therapist's positive attitudes, to open the patient to a theorized "growth potential" that encourages increased openness for the development of behavior change and insight.

cognitive therapy: this assists the patient to examine and analyze beliefs and attitudes that have produced and maintained their emotional disorders, and has been found especially effective with depression.

psychoanalytic therapy: this approach uses principles and methods of various psychoanalytic schools to produce insight in the patient about the origins of the pathology and the defensive tactics that the patient uses to maintain it.

CHAPTER 15

The Special Senses

The Sources of Information

> **It's a Fact:**
> Vision is so sensitive that, on a clear moonless night, a person on a mountain can detect the striking of a match 50 miles away.

CHAPTER OVERVIEW

In this chapter we discuss the five special senses: vision, hearing, smell, taste, and touch, and their unique structures and sensation mechanisms.

THE SENSE OF VISION

The organ of vision is the *eye*, with its various accessory organs, such as the *extrinsic muscles*, the *eyelids*, and the *tear apparatus*. Strictly speaking, the eye includes only the *bulb* of the eye (the *eyeball*) and the *optic nerve*, which connects it with the brain. This system constitutes the essential part of the organ of vision. (The term *optic* refers to the eye, as do the combining forms *oculo* and *ophthalmo*.)

The eye is the most important sense organ in the body. It is from the eye that we receive most of our information, not only in what we can see around us or in the near distance, but also in what we learn through the printed word.

The eyeball occupies the front half of the orbital cavity, where it is embedded (cushioned) in fat and connective tissue. The eyeballs lie on either side of the root of the nose, and are almost sphere-shaped. Attached to the eyeball and contained in its orbital cavity are the *optic nerve*, *ocular muscles*, and certain other nerves and vessels. A soft mucous membrane, called the *conjunctiva*, covers the anterior (or exposed) third of the eyeball, and lines the eyelids. The eyes are protected by the eyelids (referred to as *palpebrae*; combining form is *blepharo*), which are fringed with eyelashes (referred to as *cilia*), and, above the eyes another row of hairs,

usually arched in appearance, forms the eyebrows (referred to as *supercilia*). The eyes are moistened and kept clean by the tears from the *lacrimal glands*, and the eyelids blink frequently to spread the secretions of the lacrimal glands over the external surface of the eye, keeping it moist.

Movement of the eyeball is by six slender *extrinsic muscles*, attached to each eye, that act together. The movement of opening the eyes, however, is confined to the upper lid. The eyes are free to move in any direction, upward, downward, and sideways, or the gaze may be fixed and straight ahead.

The eyeball is like a hollow sphere whose wall is made up of three concentric coats and whose cavity is filled with transparent *refracting media* (tissues and fluid that transmit light). The outer fibrous coat, the *sclera*, has a white, opaque, posterior portion and a transparent anterior portion called the *cornea*. The intermediate coat, the *choroid*, is vascular and pigmented, and divided into a posterior portion and a smaller anterior portion, which has three structures, the *ciliary body*, the *suspensory ligament*, and the *iris*. The *retina* (internal coat), is the light-sensitive layer that is made up of differentiated nervous receptors continuous with the optic nerve. Three transparent refractive media fill the optic cavity; the *vitreous body* (semi-gelatinous substance contained in a thin, clear membrane) between the retina and the lens, and two *aqueous humor* (watery fluid) chambers anterior to the lens (Fig. 15-1).

The eye is like a camera, with an opening in front, the *pupil*, that lets light in, a *crystalline lens* behind the pupil focusing the rays of light to form an image on the retina, which contains the vision sense organs, the *rods* and *cones*. The optic nerve carries the impulses from the rods and cones to the visual area.

Structures of the Eye

Sclera

The *sclera* is the white, opaque portion of the eye, "the white of the eye," and constitutes the posterior five-sixths of the eyeball. It is composed of white fibrous

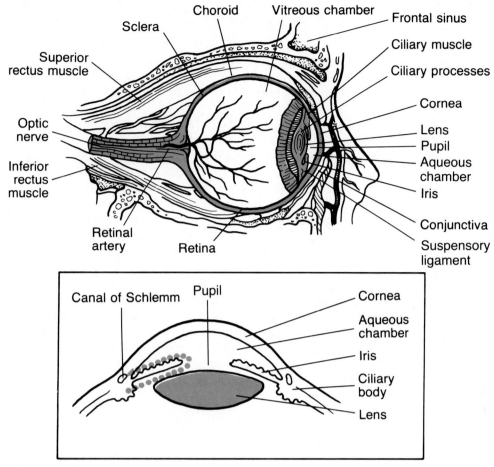

Figure 15-1.   Structures of the eye.

tissue and fine elastic fibers, with the front portion covered by a membrane called the ***conjunctiva***, through which small, superficial blood vessels can be seen. In children, the sclera is often very thin and allows the underlying choroidal pigment to show through, giving the sclera a bluish cast, and, in the aged, one often sees a yellowish cast. The conjunctival surfaces are lubricated and washed by the tears secreted by the lacrimal glands.

Cornea

The ***cornea*** is the anterior, transparent portion of the fibrous coat of the eyeball through which light enters the eye. It is nearly circular in shape, and its marked curvature makes it bulge with a dome-like protrusion that varies among individuals and diminishes somewhat with age. It is devoid of blood and lymph vessels, except at the extreme periphery, and this lack of vascularity makes the cornea subject to infection after injury.

Choroid

The ***choroid*** is located between the sclera and retina, and its posterior part is a thin membrane with a rich vascular layer. The cells of the choroid are filled with melanin, a black or dark brown pigment, which gives it a

dark brown appearance. Extra light is absorbed by the pigment which helps to prevent blurring of an image by internally reflected light. The chief function of the choroid is to maintain the nutrition of the retina through its capillary plexus and numerous small arteries and veins.

Ciliary Body

The ***ciliary body***, an extension of the choroid, is a thickened portion of the vascular layer which extends from the visual layer to the iris. The ciliary body is a wedge-shaped, flattened ring, with muscles connected to the ***suspensory ligament*** that attaches the lens to it, and ***processes*** (ridges) that secrete the ***aqueous humor*** (fluid). The ciliary processes consist of a rich vascular plexus embedded in pigmented ***stroma*** (connective tissue). Focusing on far or near objects (called ***accommodation***), is accomplished through changing the shape of the lens by action of the ciliary muscles.

Suspensory Ligament

The ***suspensory ligament*** is the second structure of the anterior extension of the choroid, continuous with the capsule that encloses the lens, and attaching it to the ciliary muscles.

Iris

The **iris**, the most anterior portion of the vascular layer, continuous with the ciliary body, is doughnut-shaped and its central opening, the **pupil**, appears to be black in color. The iris is composed of rings of muscle fibers, some of which are arranged circularly, contracting to reduce the size of the pupil, with others arranged radially, contracting to increase the size of the pupil, regulating the amount of light admitted to the lens. The iris is suspended in the aqueous space between the cornea and lens, dividing it into anterior and posterior chambers. The larger anterior chamber is between the iris and the cornea, and the posterior chamber is between the lens and the iris. These chambers are filled with the lymph-like aqueous humor, which aids in maintaining the shape of the eyeball, and empties into the **canal of Schlemm**, an oval channel circling the anterior chamber. The aqueous humor, which is secreted by the ciliary processes, flows through the pupil into the anterior chamber, and the pressure maintained by the balance between secretion and removal of fluid is known as the **intraocular pressure**.

The reflection of light scattered by pigment substances in the iris results in different colors, with dark eyes having abundant pigment, and blue eyes having less pigment. Some neonates have blue eyes because the pigment does not develop in the stroma (connective tissue fibers forming the major part of the iris) until after birth; however, others have brown eyes at birth because the stromal pigment is already developed.

Lens

The transparent crystalline **lens** is directly behind the iris of the eye, enclosed in an elastic capsule supported by the suspensory ligament, and focuses the light rays on the retina. The shape of the lens is altered by the action of the ciliary muscles, which affects the **refraction** (bending) of light rays.

Retina

The innermost of the three coats of the eyeball, the **retina**, is a soft, delicate membrane that is in contact with, and nourished by, the vascular coat. The retina is the nervous tissue layer with special neuroepithelial cells, the **rods** and **cones**, named for their shape, that serve as the photosensitive receptors of light stimuli. The cones are much less numerous than the rods, and are adapted to bright light and color perception as well as for fine details of an object. The rods are much more sensitive for low light vision, but are color blind. Near the center of the back of the retina is a small yellow area called the **macula lutea**, with a central depression, the **fovea centralis**, which is the region of clearest vision, in which the cones are most concentrated, and no rods are found. The retina also contains numerous sensory and connector neurons and their processes. At a point in the back of the retina, nearer the nose, there is an **optic disk**, where the nerve fibers from the entire eye converge to form the **optic nerve**, producing a blind spot because there are no rods or cones present. At the point where the optic nerve pierces the sclera, it is accompanied by the optic central artery and vein, which come from the choroid.

Lacrimal Glands

The **lacrimal glands**, about the size of an almond kernel, lie under the bones forming the upper, outer orbit, secreting **tears** which are carried to the conjunctiva by lacrimal ducts. There are several small accessory lacrimal glands lying in folds under the eyelids, which under ordinary circumstances secrete sufficient tears to lubricate and clean the eyes, with the main glands called into play only during crying or in response to irritation of the conjunctiva.

The blinking of the eyes spreads the tears over the conjunctival surfaces and directs the fluid into a lacrimal lake at the nasal corner, the **inner canthus**. The tears are drained from the lake by two small lacrimal ducts that lead into the nose. The opening of the tear ducts into the nose accounts for the "running" of the nose during crying.

The Mechanism of Vision

Vision occurs when light rays enter the pupil and are focused upon the retina by the lens, cornea, and aqueous and vitreous humors. This process of focusing is accomplished by all four components, any of which may develop defects. Light rays from objects 20 feet or more away are relatively parallel and are readily focused on the retina by the normal eye. Closer light rays must be bent more sharply to focus them on the retina. This process, called **accommodation**, involves an increase in convex curvature of the lens, which is elastic, by ciliary muscle contraction, along with some constriction of the pupil to restrict stray light that might blur the image.

Since both eyes must focus the light rays from an object on corresponding points on the retina to achieve single rather than double vision, the eyeballs are **converged** (moved together) by six extrinsic muscles that are attached to the outside of the eyeball and to the bones of the orbit. The slight difference in corresponding points of the retina on which the light rays from the same object are focused, caused by the few inches separating the eyes, as well as the individual's history of visual experiences with near and far objects, accounts for depth perception, or three-dimensionality.

Stimulations of the retinal receptors (rods and cones) are transmitted through the optic nerves to the **optic chiasma**, then to midbrain areas and the visual cortex areas of the occipital lobe. In the optic chiasma, the optic nerve fibers from the inner (or nasal) half of each retina cross over and join those from the outer (or temporal) half of the retina of the other eye before continuing on.

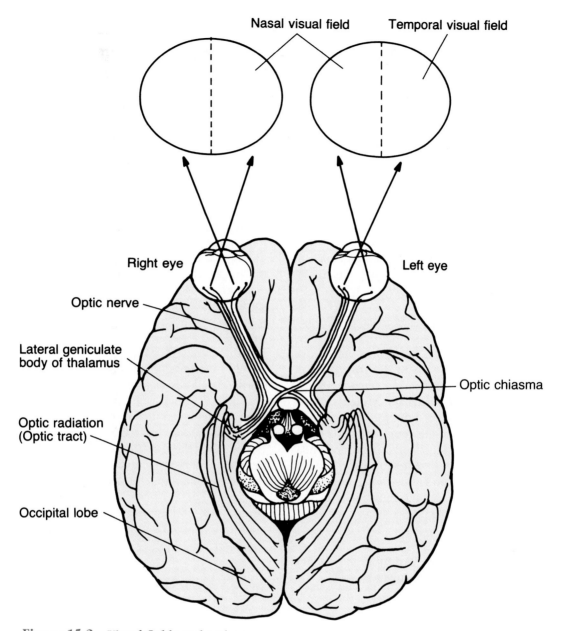

Figure 15-2. Visual fields and pathways.

For example, the fibers from the right half of the left eye link up with those from the right half of the right eye. This accounts for the finding that in conditions producing total loss of nerve transmission in the visual cortex of one hemisphere, there is partial loss of vision in both eyes rather than total loss in either (Fig. 15-2).

Review A

Complete the following:

1. The most important sense organ is the _____.

2. The mucous membrane covering the exposed third of the eyeball is the _____.

3. Tears are secreted by _____ glands.

4. There are _____ concentric coats making up the wall of the eyeball.

5. The receptors of light stimuli are the _____ and _____.

6. The "white of the eye" is called the _____.

7. Light enters the eye through the transparent part of the eyeball called the _____.

8. The pigment melanin fills the cells of the _____.

9. The process by which light rays are bent to focus them on the retina is called _____.

10. Stimulations of the retinal receptors are transmitted through the optic nerves to the _____.

THE SENSE OF HEARING

We usually think of the *ear* as the organ of hearing, which is divided into the *external ear*, *middle ear*, and *inner ear* (*oto* and *auris* refer to ear; *audi* refers to hearing). However, the ear also contains structures responsible for equilibrium.

Structures of the Ear

External Ear

The *external ear* is made up of the *auricle* (or *pinna*, meaning wing), the cartilaginous, cutaneous appendage, and the *external auditory meatus* (*meatus* means opening), which is a short, tortuous passage that leads to, and penetrates, the temporal bone. The external auditory canal is entirely lined by skin, and ends blindly at the *tympanic membrane* (eardrum). Sound waves reach the eardrum through this canal, are picked up by the inner bones of the ear, and transmitted by the auditory nerve to the brain (Fig. 15-3).

Middle Ear

This small, air-filled *tympanic cavity* in the skull is lined by a mucous membrane and situated between the inner ear and the tympanic membrane, communicating through the *eustachian tube* with the pharynx. This tube keeps the air pressure equal on both sides of the tympanic membrane, making the air pressure in the middle ear the same as that of the atmosphere. The pharyngeal orifice of the tube is normally closed, but opens during swallowing and yawning, or when a high pressure is created in the nasopharynx, as when blowing the nose or making a forced expiration with the nostrils and mouth closed. The tympanic membrane is very sensitive to any difference in pressure on its two surfaces, and during rapid changes in altitude, as in airplane ascents and descents, annoying aural effects may be produced, such as ringing sounds in the ears.

In the middle ear there are three tiny connected bones called the *auditory ossicles* (*ossicle* means little bone), deriving their names from their shape: the *malleus* (hammer), the *incus* (anvil), and the *stapes* (stirrup). These bones are connected by joints, and bridge the middle ear (tympanic cavity) to transmit sound waves, by the mechanical action of the ossicles, to the inner ear.

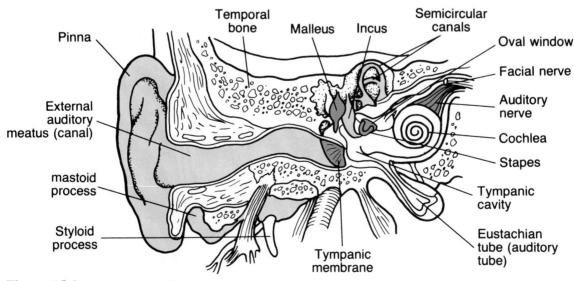

Figure 15-3.   Structures of the ear.

Inner Ear

The **inner ear** (**labyrinth**) begins at the **oval window**, against which the stapes presses, and continues in a labyrinthine **cochlea** (which means spiral or snail-shell shape), which contains three canals that are separated from each other by thin membranes and almost converge at the apex. Two of these canals are bony chambers filled with a **perilymph fluid**, one of which, the bony **vestibular canal**, is connected to the oval window that leads to the middle ear. Another, the **tympanic canal**, is also bony and is connected to the **round window** opening into the middle ear. The third canal, the **cochlear canal**, is a membranous chamber filled with **endolymph**, situated between the other two canals, containing the **organ of Corti**, a spiral-shaped organ located on the **basilar membrane** of the cochlear canal, made up of cells with projecting hairs that transmit auditory impulses to the cochlear nerve.

Mechanism of Hearing

Sound waves enter the external ear and strike the tympanic membrane, causing vibration, which sets into motion the three ossicles, the malleus, the incus, and the stapes, in that order. The stapes is the last to vibrate, and it strikes against the oval window of the vestibular canal, setting into motion the perilymph fluid in the vestibular and tympanic canals of the cochlea. The vibrating perilymph sets into motion the basilar membrane that separates these two canals, thereby disturbing the endolymph fluid in the membranous area of the cochlea. **Hair cells** of the organ of Corti, located in this area, are stimulated by the movement of the endolymph, and by bending against another membrane (the **tectorial**), the hair cells transmit the impulse to the brain by way of the auditory nerve. The final interpretation of sound is made by the brain.

Sense of Equilibrium

In addition to the structures just described, there are three **semicircular canals** in the labyrinth that lie in planes at right angles to each other, plus a **utricle**, and a **saccule** in each inner ear. These are the structures of equilibrium (see Fig. 15-3).

The saccule and utricle are small sacs that are lined with sensitive hairs and contain particles, called **otoliths** (**lith** refers to stone), that are made up of calcium carbonate. The otoliths press on the hair cells through the pull of gravity and stimulate the initiation of impulses from the hair cells to the brain through their basal sensory nerve fibers. The utricles and saccules, which together are called the **vestibule**, are responsible for the reactions that result from position change and change of **rectilinear** motion (movement in a straight line).

The semicircular canals, which are liquid-filled, respond to rotary, or turning, movement. They are positioned at right angles to each other, each corresponding to one of the three spatial planes. Turning the head in any direction stimulates at least one of the canals. Inside each canal are hair cell receptors that bend in response to rotary motion, stimulating nerve fibers that carry impulses to the vestibular branch of the auditory nerve, and then to the brain.

Review B

Complete the following:

1. The ear has two functions: _____ and _____.

2. The tympanic membrane is also known as the _____.

3. The _____ equalizes air pressure on both sides of the tympanic membrane.

4. The inner ear has a labyrinthine cochlea which contains _____ canals.

5. The three ossicles are the _____, _____, and _____.

6. The external auditory canal is entirely lined by _____.

7. The stapes presses against the _____.

8. Hair cells transmit sound stimulation to the brain by way of the _____ nerve.

9. The _____ membrane separates the vestibular and tympanic canals of the cochlea.

10. The structures of equilibrium are three _____ plus a _____ and a _____.

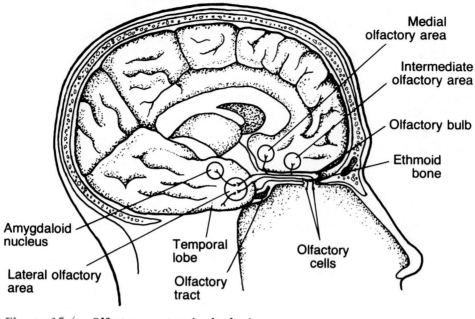

Figure 15-4. Olfactory centers in the brain.

THE SENSE OF SMELL

Smell is one of the most primitive senses. In many animals it is very acute and of paramount importance because it serves to warn the animal of approaching enemies, guides it in its quest for food, and even motivates the sex reflexes. In humans it also serves to warn of danger. Smoke is often smelled before the fire is located; escaping gas from a leaky burner or pipeline can be smelled before a person is overcome or carelessly lights the match that causes an explosion.

The peripheral organ for smell is the **nose** (**naso** and **rhino** refer to nose), with its external parts and nasal cavities. The organ of smell is the **olfactory epithelium** of the nose, and odor is perceived through stimulation of its cells. The olfactory (**olfact** refers to smell) receptors are confined to the nasal mucosa over a relatively small area in a narrow niche formed by the **superior nasal concha** (**concha** means shell-shaped), the upper part of the **septum** (wall between the two nasal cavities), and the **root** of the nose (Fig. 15-4).

The **root** of the nose is the upper, narrow end between the eyes, and the **bridge** of the nose is the part that extends from the root to the **tip** (**apex**). The **external nares** (**nostrils**) are the two oval openings separated from one another by the lower part of the **septum**, and the flexible lower portions on each side bordering the nostrils are the **alae** (**ala** is the singular form and means wing-like).

The nose is formed by the nasal bones and cartilage. The nasal bones are the **turbinates**, **superior** (upper), **medial** (middle), and **inferior** (lower) **conchae**. Nasal cartilages are connected to each other and to the bones by fibrous tissue. Just inside the nasal cavities is a lining of skin with a ring of coarse hairs, whose function is to trap dust and foreign particles during inspiration.

The mucous membrane lining the nose is continuous with particular connecting areas, and infections of this membrane are easily spread to them. These connecting areas include the nasopharynx, the eustachian tube (auditory canal), the middle ear cavity, the sphenoidal, ethmoidal, frontal, and maxillary sinuses, and the palatine bones and tear ducts.

The stimulation of the olfactory epithelium is initially transmitted to the **olfactory bulb**, and from there continues on to the olfactory centers in the brain. Six basic odors have been identified, interacting with each other to produce the variety we experience: flowery, fruity, spicy, resinous, burned, and putrid. The sense of smell is far more sensitive than the sense of taste, and complements it, as is evident when a respiratory infection blocks the sense of smell, causing food to lose its customary flavors.

THE SENSE OF TASTE

The organs of taste in humans are the **taste buds**, located mainly in the **papillae** (small projections) on the tongue, but a few may be found in the mucous membrane that covers the soft palate, the fauces (opening from the mouth to the pharynx), and the epiglottis.

The sense of taste is limited to four primary, or fundamental, tastes: sweet, sour (acid), salt, and bitter. The various other tastes that we experience are blends of these. For a substance to arouse a sensation of taste, it must be dissolved either in solution or by the saliva, which accounts for the location of the taste buds on a moist surface. Many substances that we think we taste are, in reality, only smelled, and their taste depends upon their odor. For this reason smell is sometimes described as "taste at a distance."

Review C

Complete the following:

1. The five special senses are _____, _____, _____, _____,

    and _____.

2. The _____ of the nose is the organ of smell.

3. Another term for nostrils is _____.

4. There are _____ basic odors.

5. Stimulation of the organ of smell is initially transmitted to the olfactory _____.

6. The organs of taste are located mainly on the _____.

7. The organs of taste are the _____.

8. There are _____ fundamental tastes.

9. Taste depends on _____.

10. To arouse a sensation of taste a substance must be _____.

TOUCH AND OTHER CUTANEOUS SENSES

The skin is a receptor for the sensations of touch as well as those of heat, cold, and pain (Chapter 8 and Table 15-1).

Touch (also called light pressure) is experienced as a function of stimulation of ***free sensory nerve endings*** (***dendrites***) everywhere in the skin, but especially around hair follicles. Tactile corpuscles in the epidermis called ***Merkel's disks*** relay light touch and superficial pressure, and other structures in the corium (layer below the epidermis) called ***Meissner's corpuscles*** are believed to mediate light pressure sensations. Heavier pressure stimulates the ***Pacinian corpuscles***, which are

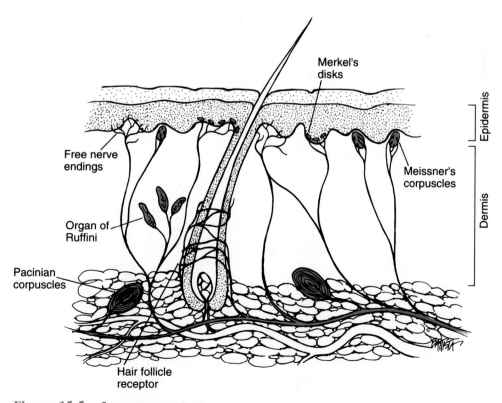

Figure 15-5.   Sensory receptors.

lamellated (layered) bodies of sensory nerve tissue located in the subcutaneous layer.

Thermal sensations of heat and cold are experienced in response to changes of even a few degrees from skin temperature, but the precise mechanisms are not known. Free nerve endings are believed to be the main receptors, along with **Ruffinian corpuscles**, which are sensory end structures located in the corium. Also considered as mediators of heat and cold are the **capillaries** of the skin (Fig. 15-5).

Pain sensations have not been linked to any specific

nerve structures, but are believed to be transmitted by free sensory nerve endings found just below the surface of the skin.

The skin areas of the body have varying sensitivities to sensation as a function of the distributions of receptors in the differing areas. The most sensitive areas generally are those most involved in obtaining information about oneself and the external world, such as the lips and fingers, whereas fewer receptors are found on the back of the hand or the dorsal surfaces.

Table 15-1   THE SPECIAL SENSES

Sense	Organ	Receptors	Stimulus
Sight (vision)	Retina of eye	Rods (120 million/eye)*, Cones (8 million/eye)*	Wavelengths of light
Hearing (audition)	Basilar membrane of cochlea (inner ear)	Hair cells of the organ of Corti	Sound vibrations
Balance (equilibrium)	Utricle, saccule, and semicircular canals of inner ear	Hair cells	Mechanical and fluid pressure
Smell (olfaction)	Mucous membranes of upper nasal cavity	Olfactory epithelium hair cells (60 million)	Chemical gas
Taste (gustation)	Surface of tongue	Taste buds on papillae (10,000)	Dissolved chemicals
Touch pressure	Layers of skin	Free nerve endings, Meissner's corpuscles, Pacinian corpuscles, Merkel's disks	Mechanical pressure
Pain		Free nerve endings	High intensity of stimuli
Warmth, cold		Free nerve endings, Ruffian corpuscles, skin capillaries	Thermal energy

*/means per (each)

Review D

Complete the following:

1. The skin is a receptor for _____, _____, _____, and _____.

2. Stimulation of free sensory nerve endings produces the sense of _____.

3. The most sensitive skin areas are the _____ and _____.

4. The least sensitive skin areas are the _____ surfaces.

5. The Pacinian corpuscles are stimulated by _____ pressure.

Answers to Review Questions: The Special Senses

Review A
1. eye
2. conjunctiva
3. lacrimal
4. three
5. rods and cones
6. sclera
7. cornea
8. choroid
9. accommodation
10. optic chiasma

Review B
1. hearing and equilibrium
2. eardrum
3. eustachian tube
4. three
5. malleus, incus, stapes
6. skin
7. oval window
8. auditory
9. basilar
10. semicircular canals, utricle, saccule

Review C
1. vision, hearing, smell, taste, touch
2. olfactory epithelium
3. external nares or nostrils
4. six
5. bulb
6. tongue
7. taste buds
8. four
9. odor
10. dissolved

Review D
1. touch, heat, cold, and pain
2. touch/pain
3. lips and fingers
4. dorsal
5. heavy/heavier

CHAPTER 15 EXERCISES

THE SPECIAL SENSES: THE SOURCES OF INFORMATION

Exercise 1: Complete the following:

1. The peripheral organ for smell is the _____.

2. The upper narrow end of the nose between the eyes is called the _____.

3. The structures that constitute the essential part of the eye are the _____ and the

   _____.

4. The movement of opening the eye is a function of the _____ eyelid.

5. The anterior, transparent portion of the fibrous coat of the eyeball, through which light enters the eye is the

   _____.

6. The part between the sclera and retina whose posterior part is a thin membrane with a rich vascular layer is the

   _____.

7. The innermost of the three coats of the eyeball, constituting the nervous layer on which light rays are focused is

   the _____.

8. The divisions of the ear are the _____, _____, and _____.

9. The malleus, incus, and stapes perform the important function of_____

   _____

10. The structures of equilibrium are the _____, _____, and

    _____.

Exercise 2: Using the list of terms below, identify each part in Fig. 15-6 by writing the name in the corresponding blank.

Vitreous chamber   **1.** _____

Conjunctiva   **2.** _____

Lens   **3.** _____

Retina   **4.** _____

Iris   **5.** _____

Sclera   **6.** _____

Aqueous chamber   **7.** _____

Optic nerve   **8.** _____

Cornea   **9.** _____

Ciliary processes   **10.** _____

Choroid   **11.** _____

Pupil   **12.** _____

Ciliary muscle   **13.** _____

Suspensory ligament   **14.** _____

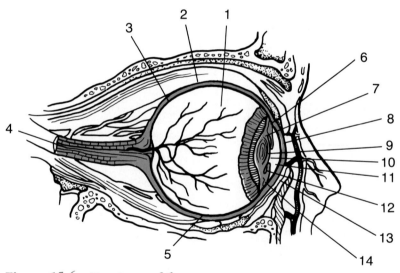

Figure 15-6.   **Structures of the eye.**

Exercise 3: Using the list of terms below, identify each part in Fig. 15-7 by writing the name in the corresponding blank.

Temporal bone   1. _____

Tympanic cavity   2. _____

Auditory nerve   3. _____

Pinna   4. _____

Cochlea   5. _____

Incus   6. _____

Mastoid process   7. _____

Eustachian tube   8. _____

Tympanic membrane   9. _____

External auditory meatus or canal   10. _____

Malleus   11. _____

Stapes   12. _____

Semicircular canals   13. _____

Styloid process   14. _____

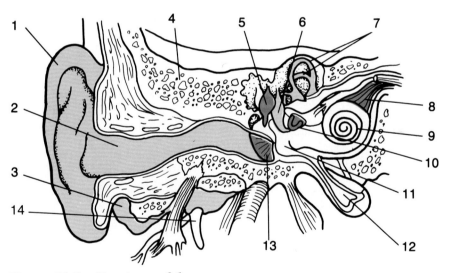

Figure 15-7.   **Structures of the ear.**

Exercise 4: Matching:

____ **1.** the depressed area in the center of the back of the retina, the area of clearest vision

A. eustachian tube

____ **2.** angles at the ends of the slits between the eyelids

B. canthi

____ **3.** specialized outer ends of the visual cells in the retina that are adapted to bright light, acute vision, and color perception

C. rods

____ **4.** special cylindrical neuroepithelial cells in the retina, highly sensititive to low light

D. semicircular canals

____ **5.** the partition separating the external nares

E. cones

____ **6.** special organ of hearing located on basilar membrane of the cochlea

F. tympanic membrane

____ **7.** the projecting posterior part of the ear that lies outside the head

G. septum

____ **8.** structures for equilibrium in the labyrinth

H. fovea

____ **9.** structure leading from the ear to the throat

I. pinna

____**10.** structure that separates the middle ear from the external ear

J. organ of Corti

Exercise 5: In the blank following each pair of words, indicate whether their meaning is the same or different.

1. inner ear
   labyrinth   _____

2. auricle
   external nares   _____

3. tympanic membrane
   eardrum   _____

4. eyelid
   palpebra   _____

5. earwax
   cerumen   _____

Exercise 6: Give the meaning of the components in the following words and then define the word as a whole. Suffixes meaning *pertaining to* or *state or condition* shown following a slash mark (/), are not to be defined separately. Before reaching for your medical dictionary, check the glossary at the end of the chapter.

1. Blepharitis:

blephar_____

itis_____

_____

2. Diplopia:

dipl_____

op/ia_____

_____

3. Nyctalopia:

nyct_____

al_____

op/ia_____

_____

4. Retinoblastoma:

retino_____

blast_____

oma_____

_____

5. Dacryoadenectomy:

dacryo_____

aden_____

ectomy_____

_____

6. Eustachitis:

eustach_____

itis_____

_____

7. Myringitis:

myring_____

itis_____

_____

8. Tympanomastoiditis:

tympano_____

mastoid_____

itis_____

_____

9. Xerophthalmus:

xer_____

ophthalm/us_____

_____

10. Otalgia:

ot_____

algia_____

_____

11. Dacryocystitis:

dacryo_____

cyst_____

itis_____

_____

12. Ageusia:

a_____

geus/ia_____

_____

13. Otorrhea:

oto_____

rrhea_____

_____

14. Optic neuritis:

op/tic_____

neur_____

itis_____

_____

15. Retinitis:

retin_____

itis_____

_____

Chapter 15 Crossword Puzzle

Across

1. colored portion of eye
6. membrane covering exposed eyeball
7. one of the special senses
9. free sensory nerve endings
12. stirrup (auditory ossicle)
14. utricles and saccules together
17. glands forming tears
18. organ of smell
20. tympanic membrane
22. visual sense receptors
24. sense of smell
27. anvil (auditory ossicle)
28. wall between nasal cavities
29. organ of vision
30. one of the special senses

Down

2. light-sensitive layer of eye
3. number of primary tastes
4. eyebrows
5. eyelashes
8. little bones
10. one of the special senses
11. one of the special senses
13. hammer (auditory ossicle)
15. inner ear
16. eyelids
19. combining form meaning ear
21. transparent portion of eyeball
23. white portion of eye
25. visual receptors for color
26. one of the special senses

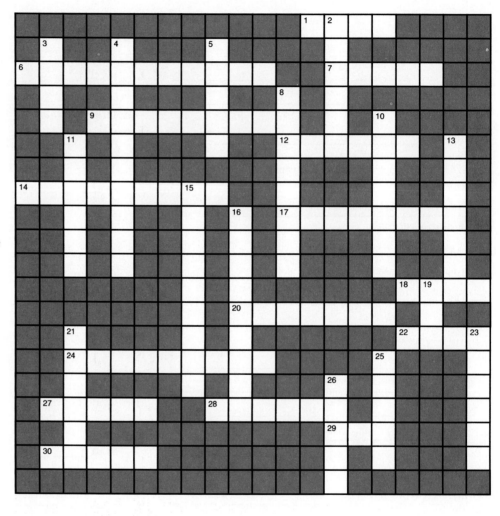

Chapter 15 Hidden Words Puzzle

```
H  V  L  T  V  T  H  V  T  N  M  U  H  E  J  C  C
E  H  S  A  W  Y  A  S  V  Y  N  S  I  F  Y  D  D
B  F  P  N  N  M  S  C  D  X  S  K  S  O  T  K  J
V  R  O  F  N  P  V  E  T  U  B  P  L  X  B  W  X
P  Q  K  Q  T  A  I  S  S  I  N  U  S  T  X  X  E
R  T  E  N  V  N  T  X  X  V  L  G  P  K  D  L  G
C  N  E  P  L  I  R  E  I  F  Z  E  D  A  P  M  P
B  Q  P  R  O  C  E  S  S  E  S  O  I  K  D  J  H
A  C  C  E  S  S  O  R  Y  L  K  R  U  C  P  X  E
N  G  X  X  R  U  U  B  X  Q  R  P  L  H  M  P  E
N  F  C  T  X  I  S  P  B  G  O  I  L  O  L  W  N
L  C  W  R  T  C  P  F  W  K  U  N  R  R  X  X  M
B  R  D  I  C  O  C  H  L  E  A  N  I  O  D  U  E
R  G  H  N  O  R  F  S  E  N  S  A  T  I  O  N  P
M  B  L  S  A  E  A  R  D  R  U  M  G  D  E  K  Q
A  E  Q  I  G  C  R  Y  S  T  A  L  L  I  N  E  O
P  I  O  C  V  E  A  U  R  I  C  L  E  R  N  U  W
X  I  F  B  M  P  Z  O  K  H  C  A  Y  I  T  N  Z
A  H  L  J  U  T  O  V  K  Y  O  I  P  S  D  E  I
N  R  I  P  V  O  R  L  V  N  M  Y  H  S  R  B  A
G  R  S  N  K  R  M  U  Y  J  M  Z  I  M  U  T  D
C  B  U  D  U  U  B  F  P  T  O  L  D  P  S  L  V
I  C  I  J  F  L  L  J  N  Y  D  W  K  H  D  I  E
S  S  V  H  R  N  P  R  R  N  A  R  E  S  K  W  J
D  T  W  C  W  W  M  P  U  C  T  K  A  O  C  Q  M
R  E  H  E  Y  T  L  E  Y  A  I  H  E  V  E  R  U
O  H  V  V  Y  L  G  E  R  V  O  X  B  Q  H  S  C
I  F  I  T  D  I  U  Y  T  E  N  G  Y  G  N  V  I
```

Can you find the 20 words hidden in this puzzle?

ACCOMMODATION	CRYSTALLINE	PERIPHERAL	ACCESSORY
EXTRINSIC	PROCESSES	SENSATION	RECEPTOR
TYMPANIC	VITREOUS	AURICLE	CAPSULE
CHOROID	COCHLEA	EARDRUM	TACTILE
NARES	PINNA	SINUS	IRIS

CHAPTER 15 ANSWERS

Exercise 1
1. nose
2. root
3. eyeball; optic nerve
4. upper
5. cornea
6. choroid
7. retina
8. external, middle, inner
9. transmission of sound waves to inner ear
10. semicircular canals, utricle, saccule

Exercise 2
1. vitreous chamber
2. choroid
3. sclera
4. optic nerve
5. retina
6. ciliary muscle
7. ciliary processes
8. cornea
9. lens
10. pupil
11. aqueous chamber
12. iris
13. conjunctiva
14. suspensory ligament

Exercise 3
1. pinna
2. external auditory meatus or canal
3. mastoid process
4. temporal bone
5. malleus
6. incus
7. semicircular canals
8. auditory nerve
9. cochlea
10. stapes
11. tympanic cavity
12. eustachian tube
13. tympanic membrane
14. styloid process

Exercise 4
1. H
2. B
3. E
4. C
5. G
6. J
7. I
8. D
9. A
10. F

Exercise 5
1. same
2. different
3. same
4. same
5. same

Exercise 6
1. blepharatis: eyelid; inflammation—inflammation of eyelid
2. diplopia: double; see—double vision
3. nyctalopia: night; blind; vision—night blindness
4. retinoblastoma: retina; germ cell; tumor—tumor arising from retinal blast (germ) cells
5. dacryoadenectomy: tear; gland; excision or removal—surgical excision of a tear gland
6. eustachitis: eustachian tube; inflammation—inflammation of eustachian tube
7. myringitis: eardrum; inflammation—inflammation of eardrum
8. tympanomastoiditis: tympanic membrane; mastoid; inflammation—inflammation of tympanic membrane and mastoid process
9. xerophthalmus: dry; eye—abnormally dry eyes
10. otalgia: ear; pain—earache
11. dacryocystitis: tear; sac; inflammation—inflammation of a tear, or lacrimal, sac
12. ageusia: not; taste—lack or impairment of sense of taste
13. otorrhea: ear; discharge—discharge from the ear
14. optic neuritis: optic, or eye; nerve; inflammation—inflammation of optic nerve
15. retinitis: retina; inflammation—inflammation of retina

Answers: Chapter 15 Crossword Puzzle

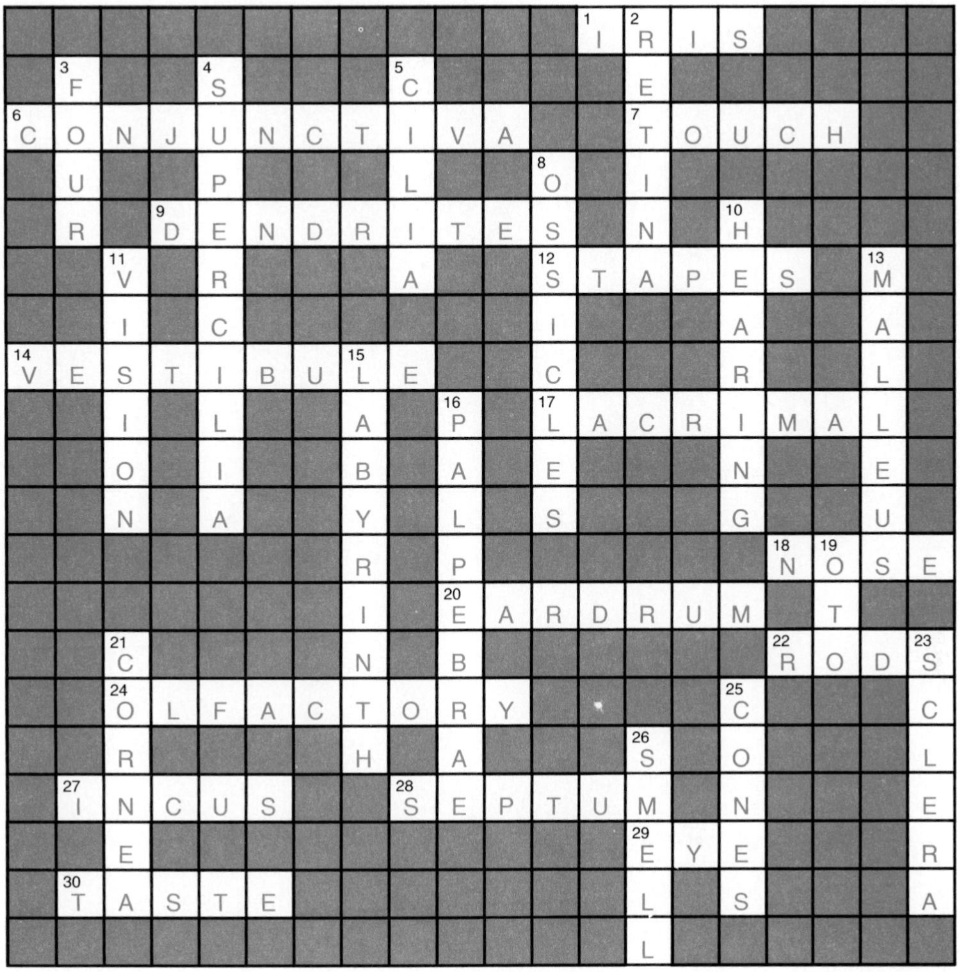

Answers: Chapter 15 Hidden Words Puzzle

```
                        T
                        Y    A
                        M         C
                        P    V         T
                        A    I         S    I    N    U    S
                        N    T                   L
                        I    R                        E
          P    R    O    C    E    S    S    E    S
A    C    C    E    S    S    O    R    Y                        C
                    X    R         U                   P         H
                    T         I    S                   I         O
                    R              P                   N         R
                    I    C    O    C    H    L    E    A    N         O
                    N         R         S    E    N    S    A    T    I    O    N
                    S         E    A    R    D    R    U    M         D
                    I         C    R    Y    S    T    A    L    L    I    N    E
                    C         E    A    U    R    I    C    L    E    R
                              P                        C    A         I
                              T                        O         P    S
                              O                        M         S
                              R                        M                   U
                                                       O                        L
                                                       D                             E
                                        N    A    R    E    S
                                                       T
                                                       I
                                                       O
                                                       N
```

Words:

∨	ACCOMMODATION	>	CRYSTALLINE	\	PERIPHERAL	>	ACCESSORY
∨	EXTRINSIC	>	PROCESSES	>	SENSATION	∨	RECEPTOR
>	TYMPANIC	∨	VITREOUS	>	AURICLE	\	CAPSULE
∨	CHOROID	>	COCHLEA	>	EARDRUM	\	TACTILE
>	NARES	∨	PINNA	>	SINUS	∨	IRIS

CHAPTER 15 GLOSSARY

SENSE OF VISION

Vision Related Anatomic and Other Terms

accommodation: process by which the lens and pupil adjust to focus light rays on the retina.

aqueous chamber: space within the eye that encloses the aqueous humor, divided by the iris into anterior and posterior chambers.

aqueous humor: watery fluid within the aqueous chamber between the cornea and vitreous humor.

blepharon: eyelid (also called *palpebra*).

canal of Schlemm: exit duct for aqueous humor, located in the anterior cavity, which keeps intraocular pressure constant under normal conditions.

canthus (kan'thus): angle at either end of the slit between the eyelids, the outer, temporal canthus, and the inner, nasal canthus (plural—*canthi*).

choroid (ko'roid): coat, located between the sclera and the retina, with cells filled with melanin, whose posterior part is a thin membrane with a rich vascular layer.

cilia: eyelashes.

ciliary body (sil'e-er"e): thickened extension of the choroid from the visual layer to the iris, consisting of the ciliary processes and muscles, assisting in accommodation, and secreting aqueous humor.

cones: specialized neuroepithelial cells of the retina which serve as the color and fine-detail receptors of vision.

conjunctiva (kon"junk-ti'vah): membrane that lines the eyelid and covers the eyeball.

cornea (kor'ne-ah): transparent structure that forms the anterior part of the external tunic of the eye.

emmetropia (em"e-tro'pe-ah): perfect vision (*emmetros* means in proper measure).

extrinsic muscles: six slender muscles attaching the outside of the eyeball to the bones of the orbit, acting together to move the eyeballs.

fovea (fo've-ah): depressed area in the center of the macula of the retina, with no rods and the greatest concentration of cones, producing the area of clearest vision.

intraocular pressure: pressure maintained by the balance between secretion and removal of aqueous humor in the anterior chamber.

iris: most anterior portion of the vascular layer of the eye, a doughnut-shaped, pigmented ring of muscles that regulates the size of the pupil.

lacrimal glands: organs of secretion of tears, which cleanse and lubricate the conjunctiva.

lens: transparent part of the eye, directly behind the iris, that focuses light rays on the retina (also called *crystalline lens*).

levator palpebrae muscles: muscles that raise upper lid.

macula: yellow spot near the center of the back of the retina with a central depression, the fovea (also called *macula lutea*).

optic: term referring to the eye.

optic chiasma: brain structure receiving transmissions of the optic nerves.

orb: eyeball.

orbit: bony socket that contains the eye.

palpebra: eyelid.

pupil: central hole or opening in the iris.

refracting media: transparent tissues and fluids in the eye through which light passes, and by which it is refracted (bent) and brought to focus.

retina: innermost, nervous tissue or sensory layer, of the three coats of the eyeball; contains the rods and cones.

rods: highly specialized, cylindric, neuroepithelial cells of the retina, that react to light but not color, and are most sensitive to low light intensity.

sclera (skle'rah): tough, white, supporting tunic of the eyeball.

supercilia: eyebrows.

suspensory ligament: ligament attaching the lens to the ciliary body.

uvea: term used to include the iris, ciliary body, and choroid.

vitelliform: resembling the yolk of an egg.

vitreous humor: semi-gelatinous transparent substance that fills the membrane-enclosed space between the lens and the retina.

Pathologic Conditions Relating to the Eye

Inflammations and Infections of the Eye

acute contagious conjunctivitis: purulent infection of the conjunctiva (also called *pinkeye*).

blepharitis: inflammation of the eyelid.

chorioretinitis (ko"re-o-ret"i-ni'tis): inflammation of the choroid and retina (also called *retinochoroiditis*).

choroiditis: inflammation of the choroid.

conjunctivitis: inflammation of the conjunctiva.

dacryoadenitis (dak"re-o-ad"e-ni'tis): inflammation of the lacrimal gland (also called *dacryadenitis*).

dacryocystitis: inflammation of the lacrimal sac.

episcleritis (ep"i-skle-ri'tis): inflammation of the tissue of the sclera.

hordeolum (hor-de'o-lum): inflammation of an eyelid sebaceous gland, commonly called a sty.

iridocyclitis (ir"i-do-si-kli'tis): inflammation of the iris and ciliary body.

iridocyclochoroiditis (ir"i-do-si"klo-ko"roid-i'tis): inflammation of the iris, the ciliary body, and the choroid coat.

iridokeratitis (ir"i-do-ker"ah-ti'tis): inflammation of the cornea and iris (also called *keratoiritis*).

iritis: inflammation of the iris.

keratitis: inflammation of the cornea.

keratoconjunctivitis (ker"ah-to-kon-junk"ti-vi'tis): inflammation of the cornea and conjunctiva.

keratoiridocyclitis (ker"ah-to-ir"i-do-sik-li'tis): inflammation of the cornea, iris, and ciliary body.

ophthalmitis: inflammation of the deeper structures of the eye (also called *ophthalmia*).

optic neuritis: inflammation of the optic nerve.

panophthalmitis: inflammation of all structures of the eye.

retinitis: inflammation of the retina.

scleritis: inflammation of the sclera.

sclerochoroiditis: inflammation of the sclera and choroid.

scleroconjunctivitis: inflammation of the sclera and conjunctiva.

sclerokeratitis: inflammation of the sclera and cornea.

trachoma: chronic, granulating, contagious infection of the conjunctiva, caused by the bacterium *Chlamydia*.

uveitis: inflammation of the uvea, which includes the iris, ciliary body, and choroid.

Hereditary, Congenital, and Developmental Disorders of the Eye

achromatopsia (ah-kro"mah-top'se-ah): total color-blindness (also called *achromatopia*).

albinism: absence of pigment in the eye.

aniridia (an"i-rid'e-ah): absence of the iris.

anophthalmos (an"of-thal'mos): absence of, or rudimentary development of, one or both eyes (also called *anophthalmia*).

congenital cataract: opacity of lens originating before birth.

corectopia (kor-ek-to'pe-ah): abnormal placement of the pupil (*core* refers to the pupil of the eye).

cyclopia (si-klo'pe-ah): developmental anomaly characterized by a single orbit.

deuteranomaly: partial color-blindness, involving subnormal perception of green due to a deficiency of green-sensitive cones.

deuteranopia: green color-blindness.

dichromatopsia (di"kro-mah-top'se-ah): partial color-blindness, with ability to distinguish only two of the primary colors (red, blue, yellow, green).

ectopia of lens: misplacement of the lens.

ectropion uveae: eversion or outward turning of the pupillary margin of the eye (also called *iridectropium*).

embryotoxon: congenital opacity at the margin of the cornea (*toxon* means a bow or anything arched).

megalocornea: developmental anomaly characterized by a large cornea.

megalophthalmos: abnormally large size of the eyes.

microcornea: abnormally small cornea.

microphakia: abnormally small lens.

microphthalmos: abnormally small eyes.

polycoria: existence of more than one pupil in an eye.

protanomaly (pro"tah-nom"ah-e): form of color-blindness, with an imperfect perception of red, due to deficiency of red-sensitive cones (also called *protanomalopsia*).

protanopia: red color-blindness, with absence of red-sensitive cones.

retinitis pigmentosa (pig"men-to'sah): group of retinal diseases that may be inherited, with retinal atrophy, weakening of the retinal vascular system, clumping of pigment, and narrowing of the visual field.

tritanomaly: partial color-blindness, with a deficiency of blue-sensitive pigment in the cones.

tritanopia (tri"tah-no'pe-ah): form of color-blindness, with an absence of blue-sensitive pigment in the cones, sometimes associated with drug effects, retinal detachment, or nervous system diseases (also called *tritanopsia*).

Other Abnormal Conditions of the Eye

adhesions of iris: fibrous bands or strictures in the iris or adhering the iris to other eye structures.

age-related macular degeneration (AMD): two types of degeneration of the retinal macula appearing in later life: the most common form, a dry type, causing visual dimming or distortion; and a much less common wet, or neovascular, type associated with abnormal growth of new blood vessels that leak into the macula, damaging the retina.

altered pupillary reflexes: hyper—(over), or hypo—(under) contraction of the pupil on exposure to light.

amblyopia (am"ble-o'pe-ah): dimness of vision (*ambly* means dimness).

ametropia (am"e-tro'pe-ah): defect in the refractive powers of the eye in which images are not brought into proper focus on the retina (*ametro* means disproportionate).

aniseikonia (an"i-si-ko'ne-ah): image seen by one eye differs in size and shape from that seen by the other eye (*anis* means unequal; *eikon* means image).

anisopia (an″i-so′pe-ah): inequality of vision in the two eyes.

anterior ischemic optic neuropathy (AION): sudden vision loss resulting from reduced blood supply to the optic nerve.

aphakia (ah-fa′keah): absence of lens, usually used to describe the absence of lens after cataract surgery but it may also be a congenital anomaly.

arcus senilis (ar-kus se-nil′is): white or gray ring around the cornea, caused by lipoid degeneration of the corneal tissue in the aged (**senilis** refers to old age).

astigmatism: defective curvature of the refractive surfaces of the eye, causing light rays to spread over a more or less diffuse area and not sharply focus on the retina (**stigma** means point).

blepharospasm: spasm of the eyelid or excessive winking of the eyes.

blindness: lack or loss of sight, with a variety of causes and a number of types.

  aknephascopia (ak″nef-ah-sko′pe-ah): reduced vision with poor lighting such as twilight (also called **twilight blindness—knepha** refers to twilight).

  cortical blindness: caused by lesion of cortical visual center.

  eclipse (solar) blindness: caused by viewing a partial eclipse of the sun, resulting in amblyopia due to retinal thermal lesion.

  hemeralopia: day blindness or defective vision in bright light.

  niphablepsia: dimness of vision, usually temporary, caused by glare of the sun upon the snow (also called **snow blindness—nipha** means snow).

  nyctalopia: night blindness.

cataract: opacity of the crystalline lens or its capsule, with a number of types and varying causes.

corneal opacity: opacity of the cornea.

corneal ulcer: lesion of the cornea.

diabetic retinopathy (ret″i-nop′ah-the): noninflammatory degeneration of the retina, characterized by retinal ischemia, hemorrhages, and exudation, which tends to develop in persons who have had diabetes for a long period of time.

diplopia: double vision (**diplo** means double).

enophthalmos (en-of-thal′mos): abnormal retraction of the eye into the orbit.

floaters: small bits formed of clumps of vitreous gel, that appear to float in the visual field.

glaucoma (glaw-ko′mah): disease characterized by excessive intraocular pressure, with hardness of the eye, atrophy of the retina, and possible progression to blindness.

hypermetropia: farsightedness, caused by insufficient refracting power to focus parallel rays on the retina (also called **hyperopia**).

hypertensive retinopathy: retinal degeneration caused by hypertension.

hypopyon (hi-po′pe-on): accumulation of pus in the anterior chamber of the eye.

lenticular opacity: opacity in the lens.

maculopathy (mak-u-lah′path-ee): degeneration of the retinal macula.

myopia: nearsightedness, caused by refraction error which focuses parallel rays in front of the retina.

nystagmus (nis-tag′mus): involuntary, rapid, horizontal, vertical, rotary, or mixed movements of the eyeball (**nys** means nod).

ophthalmoplegia: paralysis of eye muscles.

pannus: abnormal membrane-like corneal vascularization (**pannus** means cloth).

presbyopia: farsightedness resulting from normal aging changes in the lens (also called **hyperopia**).

ptosis: drooping or falling of the eyelid.

retinal detachment: separation of the retina from the choroid causing loss of vision; due to abscesses or hemorrhages in the vitreous body, trauma, complications of intraocular surgery, inflammation or tumors of the choroid, and passage of vitreous and/or aqueous humor through a hole in the retina.

Stargardt's disease: juvenile type of macular degeneration.

Stellwag's sign: infrequent or incomplete blinking of the eyelid, a sign of Graves' disease.

strabismus (strah-biz′mus): deviation of the eye, with various forms called **tropias** (meaning turning), including esotropia—turning inward (also called **convergent strabismus** or crossed eyes); **exotropia**—turning outward (also called **wall-eye**); **hypertropia**—upward deviation of one eye; **hypotropia**—downward deviation of one eye.

synechia (si-nek′e-ah): adhesion of one part of the eye to another, especially iris to cornea or lens (**synechia** means continuity).

Von Graefe's sign (gra′fez): lid lag, a sign of Graves' disease.

xerophthalmus (ze″rof-thal′mus): abnormally dry cornea and conjunctiva caused by vitamin A deficiency (also called **xerophthalmia**).

Oncology of the Eye*

Other tumors occur in the structure of the eye, as they do in other parts of the body, but only those peculiar to the eye are listed here.

angiomatosis retinae: condition of multiple and bilateral hemangiomas of the retina, which may be associated with hemangiomas of the cerebellum, fourth ventricle, and spinal cord.

*Indicates a malignant condition.

retinoblastoma* (ret″i-no-blas-to′mah): malignant tumor that arises from retinal germ cells, usually occurring in children under the age of three.

Surgical and Other Procedures of the Eye

blepharectomy (blef′ah-rek′to-me): excision or removal of all or part of an eyelid.

blepharoplasty (blef′ah-ro-plas″te): plastic repair of an eyelid.

blepharorrhaphy: suturing together of the eyelid margins (also called **tarsorrhaphy**).

blepharosphincterectomy (blef′ah-ro-sfingk″ter-ek′to-me): excision of some fibers of the eyelid muscle to relieve pressure on the cornea.

blepharotomy: incision of eyelid (also called **tarsotomy**).

canthectomy: surgical removal of a canthus.

canthoplasty (kan′tho-plas″te): plastic surgery of the palpebral fissure, especially the section of a canthus to lengthen the fissure, and surgical restoration of a defective canthus (also called **cantholysis**).

canthotomy: incision of a canthus.

capsulectomy: excision of the capsule of the crystalline lens.

capsulotomy: incision of the capusle of the crystalline lens.

cataract implant: procedure for the implantation of a permanent artificial lens after cataract removal.

conjunctivoplasty: plastic repair of the conjunctiva.

corectomedialysis (ko-rek″to-me″di-al′i-sis): formation of an artificial pupil by detachment of the iris from the ciliary body (also called **coretomedialysis** and **iridodialysis**).

coreoplasty: plastic repair of the pupil.

cyclodialysis (si″klo-di-al′i-sis): procedure for glaucoma, to form a communication between the anterior chamber of the eye and the suprachoroidal space.

cyclodiathermy (si″klo-di′ah-ther″me): treatment of a portion of the ciliary body by diathermy.

dacryoadenectomy (dak″re-o-ad″e-nek′to-me): excision of a tear gland.

dacryocystectomy: excision of a lacrimal (tear) sac.

dacryocystorhinostomy (dak″re-o-sis″to-ri-nos′to-me): anastamosis of the lacrimal sac to the nasal mucosa, through the lacrimal bone.

dacryocystosyringotomy (dak″re-o-sis″to-sir″in-got′o-me): incision of the lacrimal sac and duct.

dacryocystotomy: incision of the lacrimal gland or duct (also called **lacrimotomy**).

enucleation: excision of the eyeball.

evisceration: excision of the contents of the eyeball.

goniotomy (gon″ne-ot′o-me): surgical procedure in congenital glaucoma consisting of opening Schlemm's canal at the angle of the anterior chamber (**goni** here means angle).

intrastromal corneal ring (ICR): small plastic ring implanted in the cornea to correct myopia.

iridectomy: excision of part of the iris.

iridencleisis (ir″i-den-kli′sis): procedure used to reduce intraocular pressure, forming a permanent drain for the aqueous humor by strangulation of a slip of the iris in a corneal incision.

iridocorneosclerectomy (ir″i-do-kor″ne-o-skle-rek′to-me): removal of a portion of the iris, cornea, and sclera in glaucoma.

iridocyclectomy (ir″i-do-si-klek′to-me): removal of a portion of the iris and the ciliary body.

iridocystectomy (ir″i-do-sis-tek′to-me): plastic surgery on the iris, to establish an artificial pupil.

iridomesodialysis (ir″i-do-me″so-di-al′i-sis): loosening of adhesions around the inner edge of the iris (also called **iridomedialysis**).

iridosclerotomy (ir″i-do-skle-rot′o-me): incision of the sclera and of the edge of the iris in treatment of glaucoma.

iridotasis (ir″i-dot′ah-sis): stretching the iris in treatment of glaucoma.

iridotomy: formation of artificial pupil by cutting the iris (also called **iritomy**).

iritoectomy (i″ri-to-ek′to-me): removal of a portion of the iris.

keratectomy: excision of a portion of the cornea.

keratocentesis: puncture of cornea for aspiration of aqueous humor.

keratoplasty: corneal transplant or repair of the cornea.

keratotomy: incision of the cornea.

lacromotomy: incision of the lacrimal gland or duct.

laser surgery: use of an instrument that concentrates light energy into a narrow beam, so that treatment of tissue can be done so quickly that the surrounding areas are not affected; used within the eyeball to repair the retina, and also in cataract and glaucoma surgery.

orbitotomy: incision of the orbit.

peritectomy: excision of a ring of conjunctiva around the cornea, followed by cauterization of the trench made—an operation for pannus (an abnormal membrane-like vascularization of the cornea).

radial keratotomy (RK): microscopic radial incisions on the corneal surface to flatten the cornea to correct myopia.

sclerectomy: excision of part of the sclera (also called **scleroticectomy**).

scleriritomy: incision of sclera and iris in anterior staphyloma (defect in the eye inside the cornea, with protrusion of the cornea or sclera).

scleroplasty: repair of the sclera.

sclerostomy: creation of an opening through the sclera for the relief of glaucoma.

sclerotomy: incision of the sclera.

Vision Tests and Diagnostic Instruments

color perception tests: designed to reveal defects in color vision by means of standard colors presented to the individual, including:

Bodal's test—colored blocks.

Cohn's test—colored embroidery.

Holmgren's test—skeins of colored yarn.

Mauthner's test—bottles of colored liquid.

Nagel's test—printed concentric colored circles.

pseudoisochromatic test—series of printed plates composed of round dots of varied standard colors and sizes, which are arranged to be read as numbers and letters in normal color perception, which, with subsequent revisions, is the most widely used and best standardized test available (used by the ***Isbihara*** and ***A.O. Hardy-Rand-Rittler*** tests).

fluorescent eye stain: test to detect abnormalities or injuries in the cornea, and to aid in the fitting of contact lenses.

Hering's test: test of binocular vision.

magnetic resonance imaging (MRI): noninvasive method of scanning the eye by use of an electromagnetic field and high-frequency radio waves, which provides visual images on a computer screen, and magnetic tape recordings, used to detect tissue changes and eye cancers (also called ***nuclear magnetic resonance [NMR]***).

ophthalmodiaphanoscope (of-thal″mo-di-ah-fan′o-skop): instrument for viewing the interior of the eye by transmitted light.

ophthalmodynamometer (of-thal″mo-di″nah-mom′e-ter): instrument for measuring retinal arterial pressure.

ophthalmoleukoscope (of-thal″mo-lu′ko-skop): instrument that uses polarized light to test color perception.

ophthalmoscope (of-thal″mo-skop): instrument that examines the interior of the eye using a light source, a perforated mirror, and a system of lenses.

opthalmotonometer (of-thal″mo-to-nom′e-ter): instrument used to measure intraocular tension or pressure (also called ***tonometer***).

refraction: determination of type and degree of refractive deviations in the eye structures along with their correction by external lenses.

retinoscopy: detection of refractive errors by noting the movement of light shined directly on the retina (also called ***shadow test***).

scanning laser ophthalmoscope: laser device that produces a picture to diagnose retinal sections that are functioning abnormally.

Snellen eye chart: standardized visual acuity measure using block letters in successive lines of decreasing size to be read at a set distance; the most commonly used eye chart for gross screening.

sonogram: use of ultrasound to detect diseases of the eye.

visual field test: measure of the extent of retinal area within which visual stimuli can be perceived.

SENSE OF HEARING

Ear and Related Anatomic Terms

auricle: external projecting part of the ear (also called ***pinna***).

auris: term that refers to the ear.

cerumen: earwax.

cochlea (kok′le-ah): snail-shaped canal in the inner ear.

endolymph: fluid that fills the semicircular canals and the membranous labyrinth of the ear.

eustachian tube (u-sta′she-an): tube that leads from the ear to the throat (also called ***auditory tube***).

incus: anvil-shaped bone in the middle ear (also called ***anvil***).

labyrinth (lab′i-rinth): inner ear, consisting of numerous canals and membranes and the organ of hearing, the organ of Corti.

malleus: hammer-shaped bone in the middle ear (also called ***hammer***).

meatus: opening to the ear; both internal and external.

middle ear: small, air-filled tympanic cavity in the skull, between the labyrinth and tympanic membrane.

organ of Corti: spiral organ of hearing located on the basilar membrane of the cochlear membrane.

ossicles: little bones of the middle ear, including malleus, incus, and stapes.

otolith: stone in the utricle and saccule of the inner ear (***lith*** means stone).

oval window: opening between the middle ear and the inner ear.

perilymph: fluid that fills some chambers of the inner ear.

saccule: small hair-lined sac of the inner ear, which, together with the utricle and semicircular canals, is the organ for equilibrium.

semicircular canals: three membranous canals (lateral, superior, and posterior) contained within the bony semicircular structures of the labyrinth, involved with equilibrium.

stapes (sta′pez): stirrup-shaped bone in the middle ear (also called ***stirrup***).

tympanic membrane: membrane (***eardrum***) that separates the middle ear from the external ear, and transmits vibrations to ossicles.

utricle (u′tre-k′l): small hair-lined sac of the inner ear that is concerned with equilibrium.

Pathologic Conditions of the Ear
Inflammations and Infections of the Ear

eustachitis (u"sta-ki'tis): inflammation of the eustachian tube.

labyrinthitis: inflammation of the inner ear, or labyrinth.

mastoiditis: inflammation of the mastoid process behind the ear.

myringitis: inflammation of the eardrum.

otitis media, externa, and interna: inflammation of the middle ear (also called *tympanitis*), external ear, and inner ear, respectively.

panotitis: inflammation of all parts of the ear.

tympanomastoiditis: inflammation of the eardrum and mastoid.

Congenital and Developmental Disorders of the Ear

deformity of auricle: a variety of abnormal pinna formations, including pointed ear, dog-ear, and ridged ear.

macrotia: excessively large ears.

microtia: excessively small ears.

otosclerosis: hereditary disorder, with formation of spongy bone tissue around the stapes and oval window, preventing transmission of vibration to the inner ear, resulting in progressive deafness.

polyotia: presence of more than one ear on a side of the head.

Other Abnormal Conditions and Descriptive Terms of the Ear

deafness: complete or partial loss of the sense of hearing, of many different types, including:

  central deafness: disease or defect in the auditory pathways of the brain stem or cerebral hemispheres.

  conductive deafness: defective sound-conducting apparatus in the auditory meatus, eardrum, or ossicles.

  cortical deafness: caused by a lesion of the cerebral cortex.

  labyrinthine deafness: disease or defect of the labyrinth.

  sensorineural deafness: caused by lesion or dysfunction of the nerve tracts of the cochlea and nerve centers.

diplacusis (dip"lah-ku'sis): hearing of one sound as two, caused by a difference in perception between the two ears, usually related to cochlear pathology.

Meniere's syndrome: condition in which there is dizziness, nausea, tinnitus, and progressive deafness, caused by nonsuppurative disease of the labyrinth (also called *labyrinthine syndrome*).

otalgia: earache (also called *otodynia*).

otoneuralgia: neuralgia of the ear.

otopyorrhea (o"to-pi"o-re'ah): discharge of pus from the ear.

otorrhagia (ot"to-ra'je-ah): hemorrhage from the ear.

otorrhea (o"to-re'ah): discharge from the ear.

presbycusis: progressive late-life hearing loss due to inner ear and/or nerve deterioration.

tinnitus (ti-ni'tus): ringing in the ears.

tympanophonia (tim"pah-no-fo'ne-ah): condition of increased resonance in which the voice sounds unnatural to oneself, found in diseases of the middle ear or nasal fossae (also called *autophony*).

tympanosclerosis (tim"pah-no-skle-ro'sis): hardening of tympanic membrane.

vertigo: dizziness.

Oncology of the Ear

Other tumors occur in the structures of the ear, as they do in other parts of the body, but only one peculiar to the ear is given here.

acoustic neuroma: usually arising from the acoustic nerve, this tumor grows within the internal auditory meatus, encroaching upon the brain stem, and may adhere to and displace the facial nerve, and involve the trigeminal nerve.

Surgical Procedures of the Ear

fenestration (fen"es-tra'shun): formation of an opening into the labyrinth of the ear for the restoration of hearing in cases of otosclerosis.

incudectomy: removal of the incus.

labyrinthectomy (lab"i-rin-thek'to-me): excision of the labyrinth of the ear.

labyrinthotomy (lab"i-rin-thot'o-me): incision into the labyrinth.

malleotomy (mal"e-ot'o-me): dividing the malleus in cases of ankylosis of the ossicles of the middle ear.

myringectomy: excision of the tympanic membrane (also called *myringodectomy*).

myringoplasty: plastic repair of the eardrum.

myringotomy: incision of the tympanic membrane, or eardrum.

ossiculectomy (os"i-ku-lek'to-me): excision of ossicles, or small bones of the ear, incus, malleus, and stapes.

ossiculotomy: incision of the small bones of the ear.

stapedectomy (sta"pe-dek'to-me): excision of the stapes.

tympanectomy (tim"pan-ek-to-me): excision of the eardrum.

tympanolabyrinthopexy (tim″pah-no-lab″i-rin′tho-pek″se): surgical procedure to cure progressive deafness caused by otosclerosis.

tympanosympathectomy (tim″pah-no-sim″pah-thek′to-me): excising of the tympanic plexus for the relief of tinnitus.

tympanotomy: surgical puncture of the eardrum.

Hearing Tests and Diagnostic Instruments for the Ear

audiometer: instrument for measuring hearing acuity by testing the thresholds for electrically or electronically generated pure tones of varying frequency and amplitude.

audiometry: measurement of hearing by audiometer.

Bekesy audiometry (bay-kay-se): semiautomatic method in which the examinee responds by signal (button press) to indicate perception of monaural tones that cover the audiometric scale.

caloric test: test of the functioning of the inner ear by instilling hot or ice water into the ear and watching the eye movements, which normally move toward the hot and away from the cold, used for patients with ear disease, trauma, or symptoms of syncope or vertigo.

computerized tomography (CT): imaging device using x-rays at multiple angles through specific sections, analyzed by computer to provide a total picture of the part being examined (also called **computerized axial tomography** [**CAT**]).

conduction deafness tests: tests designed to determine the location of defect in the sound-conducting apparatus, including:

  bone conduction test: a vibrating tuning fork handle is placed against the skull to determine middle ear conduction loss.

  Kabaschnik's test: transfer of below-threshold vibration of a tuning fork to the nail of the examiner's finger, which closes the external auditory meatus, in which the normal ear will detect sound.

  Rinne test: compares air and bone conduction by alternate placement of a vibrating tuning fork on the mastoid process and just outside the external auditory meatus.

  Schwabach test: comparison of bone conduction efficiency of examinee with that of the examiner.

  Weber's test: bone conduction test placing vibrating tuning fork on the forehead or vertex midline and noting sound perception on right, left, or midline.

electrocochleography: test that measures the electrical current generated in the inner ear by sound stimulation.

electrodermal audiometry: the use of a mild electric shock to condition the patient to a pure tone, which then elicits an electrodermal response to measure hearing threshold.

magnetic resonance imaging (MRI): noninvasive method of scanning the tissues of the ear by means of an electromagnetic field and high frequency radio waves, which provide visual images on a computer screen, and magnetic tape recordings, to detect and locate tumors (also called **nuclear magnetic resonance [NMR]**).

SENSE OF SMELL
Nose and Related Anatomic Terms

concha (kong′kah): shell-shaped turbinate bones of the nose.

external nares: nostrils.

olfactory center: center for smell located in the brain.

olfactory epithelium: organ of odor reception located in a small area in the nasal mucosa.

septum: wall between the two nasal cavities.

vomeronasal organs: minute pits located just inside the nostrils, containing nerve cells directly connected to the olfactory bulb, and are sensitive to pheromones (sex chemicals).

Pathologic and Other Terms Relating to Sense of Smell

anosmia: absence of the sense of smell.

dysosmia (dis-oz′me-ah): defect or impairment of the sense of smell.

hyperosmia: abnormally marked sensitivity to odors (also called **hyperosphresia**).

hyposmia (hi-poz′me-ah): impairment or defect of the sense of smell.

osmesis (oz-me′sis): act of smelling.

osmesthesia (oz″mes-the′ze-ah): olfactory sensibility involving inability to perceive and distinguish odors.

osmodysphoria (oz″mo-dis-fo′re-ah): abnormal dislike of certain odors.

Laboratory Tests for Sense of Smell

Proetz test: test for acuity of smell, using different concentrations of substances with recognizable odors to the lowest concentration at which recognition occurs, which is called the **olfactory coefficient** or **minimal identifiable odor**.

SENSE OF TASTE
Taste and Related Anatomic Terms

papillae: tiny projections on the mucous membrane of the tongue that contain the taste buds.

primary tastes: the four fundamental tastes are sweet, sour, salt and bitter.

taste buds: organs of taste located mainly on the tongue.

Pathologic and Other Terms Relating to Taste

ageusia (ah-gu′ze-ah): lack or impairment of the sense of taste (also called **ageustia**; **geusia** refers to taste).

dysgeusia (dis-gu′ze-ah): abnormal or perverted sense of taste (also called **parageusia**).

hypergeusia (hi″per-gus″e-ah): excessive or abnormal acuteness of the sense of taste (also called **oxygeusia**).

hypogeusia (hi″po-gus″e-ah): impairment of the sense of taste.

TERMS REFERRING TO TOUCH AND OTHER CUTANEOUS SENSES

esthesiometer (es-the″ze-om′e-ter): instrument for measuring or mapping tactile and other cutaneous sensitivity, using both a fixed and a movable point of touch to determine how closely the points may come before they are perceived as a single stimulus, called two-point discrimination (also called **tactometer**).

free nerve endings: sensory dendritic nerve endings located close to the surface of the skin and around hair follicles.

Meissner's (tactile) corpuscle: small, oval body in the corium (layer of skin below the epidermis) with interlaced sensory fibrils and epitheloid cells believed to be receptors for light touch, along with free nerve endings.

Merkel's (tactile) disks: flattened, dome-like expansions of nerve endings in the epidermis, believed to be receptors for light touch and superficial pressure.

Pacinian corpuscle: oval sensory body located deep in the subcutaneous layer, which appears to be the receptor for heavy pressure (also called **lamellated corpuscle**).

Ruffini corpuscle: oval sensory end structure in the corium that is believed to be a receptor for warmth, which also seems to be a function of free nerve endings and capillary responses.

CHAPTER 16

The Lymphatic and Immune Systems

The Defenders of the Body

CHAPTER OVERVIEW

In this chapter we describe the lymphatic and immune systems and their component parts and mechanisms.

THE LYMPHATIC SYSTEM

The lymphatic system includes the **lymph nodes**, **spleen**, **tonsils**, and **thymus**, and has roles in the cardiovascular and immune systems. It interacts with the cardiovascular system by way of the **lymphatic vessels** which carry the fluid, called **lymph**, back to the circulation. Lymph, made up of tissue fluids, almost colorless, rich in white blood cells, similar to blood plasma in appearance and composition, is circulated through the body by the lymphatic vessels. The lymphatic system also has a crucial role in the immune system, because of its production and circulation of white blood cells.

The Lymphatic Vessels

The lymphatic vessels begin as lymphatic capillaries and form a vast network throughout the body. These capillaries join with slightly larger lymphatic vessels, which progressively repeat the process, forming larger and larger vessels. These vessels collect proteins and water, which continually filter out of the blood into the tissue fluid, and return them to the circulation. The lymphatic structure resembles that of veins, but with a beaded appearance due to sinus spaces associated with the numerous valves which prevent backflow. The lymphatic vessels collect the lymph and carry it to either the **thoracic duct** or the **right lymphatic duct**, which in turn empty into the left and right subclavian veins, respectively. In the abdominal area, the thoracic duct has a saclike expansion, the **cisterna chyli** (**cisterna** means storage tank; **chyli** refers to liquid contents), that collects and stores lymph on its way back to the venous system.

The Lymph Nodes

Along the course of the lymph vessels are numerous **lymph nodes**, enclosed in fibrous capsules (Fig. 16-1). These nodes vary in size from mere dots to larger, bean-sized and bean-shaped bodies, identified by their location. Some examples are:

submandibular—lower jaw
cervical—neck
axillary—axilla
inguinal—groin
popliteal—knee

The lymph nodes act as filters to remove bacteria and other foreign bodies or particles, including malignant cells. They may be felt, or even seen, when they are inflamed or swollen by ingested bacteria and their toxins. Another important function of the lymph nodes is the manufacture of white blood cells (lymphocytes and monocytes), making the nodes an extremely important part of the body's defense against infection.

The Spleen

The spleen is a large, flattened, oval-shaped, glandlike organ, dark red in color, located in the upper left side of the abdominal cavity, just below the diaphragm, and behind the fundus of the stomach. It is soft and pliable, and is the largest structure of the lymphoid system. Its size varies in different people and at different times in the same person. The spleen enlarges during infectious dis-

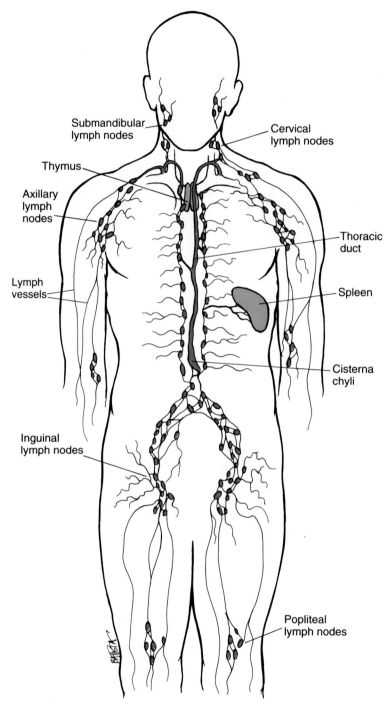

Figure 16-1.   Principal organs of the lymphatic system.

eases and decreases in size in old age. The spleen, although an extremely useful and functional organ, can be removed if necessary with no harmful effect.

The chief functions of the spleen are:

hemopoiesis—the formation of lymphocytes, monocytes, and plasma cells.

phagocytosis—the removal and destruction of microorganisms, faulty platelets, and old erythrocytes, and salvaging of globin and heme contents of the erythrocytes to be returned to the bone marrow and liver for later use.

storage area for blood in the splenic pulp.

The Tonsils

The tonsils are three pairs of small, round masses of lymphoid tissue, that filter out bacteria and other foreign-matter, and play a part in the formation of lymphocytes.

Their names and locations are:

palatine—located at the back of the throat
lingual—located at the root of the tongue
pharyngeal (also called ***adenoids***)—located at the back of the roof of the pharynx

The Thymus

The thymus is a bi-lobate, grayish-pink structure of lymph tissue, located in the mediastinum, extending into the neck, to the lower border of the thyroid gland, behind the sternum. The thymus plays an important part in the immune system as a source of lymphocyte formation (T-cells) that destroy foreign substances. Its maximum development, relative to body size, is during early childhood, and it is largest at puberty, after which it begins to atrophy, so that it has almost disappeared by extreme old age.

Review A

Complete the following:

1. The lymphatic system plays roles in the _____ and _____ systems.

2. The lymphatic system includes _____, _____, _____, and _____.

3. The lymphatic structure resembles that of _____, including _____ to prevent backflow.

4. Five areas where lymph glands are located are _____, _____, _____, _____, and _____.

5. The lymph nodes have two major functions:_____ and the manufacture of _____.

6. The largest structure of the lymphoid system is the _____.

7. One major function of this structure (in 6 above) is _____.

8. There are _____ pairs of tonsils.

9. The tonsils are the _____, _____, and _____.

10. The thymus plays an important part in the _____ system.

THE IMMUNE SYSTEM

The immune system consists of cells and chemicals that protect the body against invasion of foreign substances and maintain its general health. Weak immune-system responses can result in failure to combat infections or malignancies, whereas excessively strong responses can result in ***hypersensitivities*** or ***autoimmune disease*** reactions.

Nonspecific Immune Mechanisms

There are many mechanisms in the various systems of the body that are involved in the prevention of infection and disease. The integumentary system (Chapter 8) provides both a physical and a chemical barrier (cerumen, sebum, and sweat) thereby blocking or killing invading organisms. The cardiovascular system (Chapter 9) produces granulocytes that function in phagocytosis and detoxification of foreign proteins. The respiratory system (Chapter 10) provides chemical and mechanical barriers through the action of the mucous membranes, which trap and kill disease organisms, and coughing and sneezing mechanisms which expel them. Other mechanisms include the actions of saliva and hydrochloric acid, products of the gastrointestinal system (Chapter 11), urine from the genito-urinary tract (Chapter l2), and tears from the eyes (Chapter 15), which wash foreign substances out of the body and can limit the growth of organisms or kill them outright. The more direct functions of the lymphatic system in the destruction of invading organisms have been described above.

There are also other substances involved in protection of the body against disease. There are natural body chemicals, such as **histamines** and **prostaglandins**, which produce vasodilation and inflammation, resulting in greater blood flow. This causes a rise in the number of leukocytes, leading to increased phagocytosis. Chemicals called **pyrogens** (**pyr**—means fire) are released by invading bacteria and by the defending leukocytes. These chemicals stimulate the nervous system, affecting the body temperature and producing fever, further increasing phagocytic action.

Complement refers to a group of approximately 12 proteins normally present in the globulin of blood serum. These proteins are given the name complement because they complement (complete or perfect) antibodies that activate the proteins to produce inflammation and destroy invading cells.

Interferon is a natural cell protein protecting the body against infection, and possibly some types of cancer. Viral infection causes cells of the body to produce interferon, which attaches itself to noninfected cell surfaces. The interferon stimulates production of other antiviral proteins that directly interfere with and block further viral growth and infection.

Review B

Complete the following:

1. The immune system consists of _____ and _____ to protect the body.

2. Three systems of the body that prevent infection and disease are _____, _____, and

   _____.

3. Natural body chemicals producing vasodilation and inflammation are _____ and

   _____.

4. Chemicals producing fever are called _____.

5. _____ refers to a group of proteins present in blood serum.

Specific Immune Mechanisms

Specfic immunity is the response of the defenses of the body to specific substances that are recognized as harmful and are attacked. Substances that are capable of producing such immune-system reactions are called **antigens**. Antigens can be foreign to the body, such as bacteria, viruses, and pollen, or can be part of the body's own immune mechanisms.

There are two chief types of lymphocytes that are extremely important in the production of specific immunity, called **B-cells** and **T-cells**.

B-cells, which are formed as stem cells in the red bone marrow, migrate as immature B-cells, mainly to the lymph nodes. B-cells produce proteins called **antibodies** (**immunoglobulins**—also called **immune gamma globulins**). The immature B-cells are activated by contact with antigens. These activated B-cells quickly reproduce and develop into two types of cells, **plasma cells** and **memory cells**. The plasma cells produce an outpouring of antibodies that attack the sources of the antigens. Antibodies work by binding to antigens in the blood, preventing them from functioning. This produces inflammation, activates the globulin proteins (complements), attracts eosinophils, macrophages, monocytes, and neutrophils, resulting in phagocytosis of the invading organisms. The memory cells are stored in the lymph nodes until some of them are exposed to the specific antigen that activated their production. These then change into plasma cells, once again resulting in an outpouring of the specific antibodies that attack the source of the antigen. The remaining memory cells, with the ability to recognize the activating antigen, produce long-term immunity to that antigen (Fig. 16-2).

The initial antibody response, before memory cell development, takes some time to produce sufficient antibodies to be effective, and usually some disease develops. Little or no disease occurs after the memory cells are available to produce antibodies.

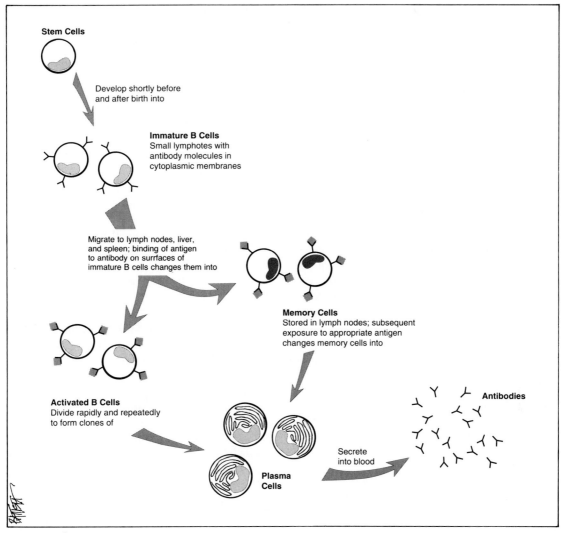

Figure 16-2. B-cell devlopment.

T-cells are also produced as stem cells in the red bone marrow, maturing in the thymus, and stored in the lymph nodes. There are three types, **T-effector**, **T-helper**, and **T-suppressor**.

T-effector cells have several functions. They produce proteins, called **lymphokines**, which stimulate inflammation and phagocytosis. They are attracted to antigens produced by viruses, tumors, or transplanted foreign tissue on the surface of cells, and dissolve those "infected" cells. Like the B-cells, T-effector cells also can become **memory cells**, responding rapidly and vigorously to the presence of previously encountered antigens on cell surfaces, also producing long-term immunity to such antigens.

T-helper cells increase the immune response of both the T-effector and the B-cells.

T-suppressor cells suppress, or limit, the immune response of the T-effector and B-cells.

The combined action of the T-helper and T-suppressor cells regulates the immune responses of the T-effector and B-cells.

A third type of lymphocyte, **null cells**, do not have the surface molecules that characterize B-cells and T-cells, and are not able to develop into memory cells. This type includes **natural killer cells** (**NK cells**) and **killer cells** (**K cells**), and like the T-effector cells, they kill the target tumor cells and viral-infected cells by lysis. Their action may be enhanced by interferon, or inhibited by prostaglandins.

Review C

Complete the following:

1. Substances that produce immune system reactions are called _____.

2. Two types of lymphocytes important in specific immunity are _____ and _____.

3. Proteins called _____ respond to antigens in the blood.

4. When activated, B-cells develop into _____ and _____cells.

5. The three types of T-cells are _____, _____, and _____.

Acquired Immunity

Long-term specific immunity develops in response to the presence of antigens that arouse the various immune system responses. Immunity may be **natural** or **artificial**; **active** or **passive**. Natural immunity develops through the body's ordinary exposure to daily living. Artificial immunity is achieved by vaccination. Active immunity develops through the body's own immune response, whereas passive immunity is achieved by antibodies transferred from an external source.

Natural, **active** immunity is illustrated by exposure to measles (without benefit of previous vaccination). The immune system fights the infection until it has been brought under control, providing long-term immunity.

Natural, **passive** immunity is illustrated by the transfer of the antibodies of a pregnant woman to the fetus, or from a mother to her breast-fed infant, which provides temporary, partial immunity.

Artificial, **active** immunity is illustrated by vaccination with weakened or dead infectious agents, or specific antigens, introduced into the body to arouse the immune system (as in vaccination for diphtheria, measles, whooping cough, etc.).

Artificial, **passive** immunity is illustrated by the introduction into the body of substances artificially produced outside of the body, such as antibiotics, gamma globulin, and interferon, providing immediate, temporary immunity.

Immunity may be short or long term, depending on the production of memory cells. Active immunity usually produces memory cells and is long-term, whereas passive immunity does not produce memory cells and is of much shorter duration.

Immune System Problems

There are two major types of immune system problems. There may be a weakness or deficiency in the effectiveness of the system, or an excessively strong reaction by the system.

Immune System Weakness or Deficiency

Problems producing deficiencies in the immune system can arise from congenital factors in which B-cells and T-cells may develop inadequately in number or effectiveness. An example of this is the condition known as **severe combined immunodeficiency disease** (see glossary). In addition, inadequacies in availability of protein, stress problems that depress antibody formation, diseases that affect the effectiveness of lymphocytes, depletion of lymphocytes and granulocytes by previous infections, and suppression of the system by drugs to prevent tissue rejection in transplants or grafts, all represent conditions in which the immune system is limited in effectiveness.

Excessively Strong Immune System Reaction

In some situations the immune system response to an antigen produces excessive inflammatory reactions and other **hypersensitivity** complications, such as those in allergic conditions like hay fever, hives, and asthma. Perhaps the greatest problem of overreaction is in **autoimmune diseases**, in which the system does not adequately distinguish between foreign antigens and those of its own cells, and the body's tissues are attacked by its own antibodies. Diseases of this sort include **rheumatoid arthritis**, where joint tissue is attacked (Ch. 17), **myasthenia gravis**, in which the action of the neurotransmitter acetylcholine is affected (Ch. 7), **thrombocytopenic purpura**, in which platelets are destroyed (Ch. 9), **multiple sclerosis**, where the myelin sheath is attacked (Ch. 14), and **systemic lupus erythematosus**, in which skin, blood vessels, kidneys and genetic material are attacked (Chapter 17).

Review D

Complete the following:

1. Immunity can be _____ or _____ and _____ or _____.

2. The transfer of antibodies by a mother to a fetus is an example of _____immunity.

3. Two types of immune system problems are _____ and _____.

4. Immunity may be short- or long-term, depending on the production of _____cells.

5. Rheumatoid arthritis is an example of a(n) _____disease.

Answers to Review Questions: The Lymphatic and Immune Systems

Review A
1. cardiovascular, immune
2. lymph nodes, spleen, tonsils, thymus
3. veins, valves
4. lower jaw, neck, axilla, groin, knee (or any other known areas)
5. remove bacteria and foreign bodies, white blood cells (lymphocytes and monocytes)
6. spleen
7. hemopoeisis, phagocytosis, storage
8. three
9. palatine, lingual, pharyngeal (or adenoids)
10. immune

Review B
1. cells, chemicals
2. (any three) integumentary, cardiovascular, respiratory, gastrointestinal, genitourinary, eyes (special senses or vision), lymphatic
3. histamines, prostaglandins
4. pyrogens
5. complement

Review C
1. antigens
2. B-cells, T-cells, null cells
3. antibodies (immunoglobulins, gamma globulins)
4. primary response
5. T-effector, T-helper, T-suppressor

Review D
1. natural, artificial; active, passive
2. natural passive immunity
3. weakness or deficiency, excessively strong reaction
4. memory
5. autoimmune

CHAPTER 16 EXERCISES

THE LYMPHATIC AND IMMUNE SYSTEMS: THE DEFENDERS OF THE BODY

Exercise 1: Complete the following:

1. The two ducts in the lymphatic system that receive the lymph and empty into the subclavian veins are called

   _____ and _____.

2. A _____ encloses lymph nodes.

3. There are _____ pairs of tonsils.

4. One function of the tonsils is _____.

5. Other than the lymphatic system, the thymus plays a part in the _____ system.

6. The largest structure of the lymphoid system is the _____.

7. The thymus is the source of _____ formation.

8. Two natural body chemicals that produce vasodilation and inflammation are _____ and

   _____.

9. A natural cell protein protecting against infection and possibly cancer is _____.

10. _____ are substances recognized as harmful and attacked by the immune system.

Exercise 2: Identify each listed part from Fig. 16-3 in numbered blanks below.

Axillary lymph nodes   Cisterna chyli
Cervical lymph nodes   Lymph vessels
Inguinal lymph nodes   Spleen
Popliteal lymph nodes   Thoracic duct
Submandibular lymph nodes   Thymus

1. _____
2. _____
3. _____
4. _____
5. _____
6. _____
7. _____
8. _____
9. _____
10. _____

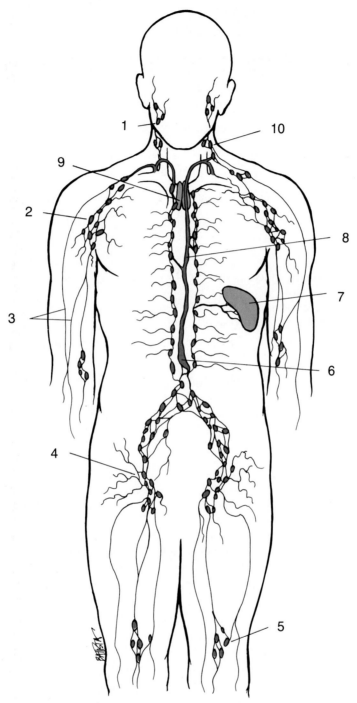

Figure 16-3.   Principal organs of the lymphatic system.

Exercise 3: Matching:

____	**1.** lymphatic vessels	**A.** filters
____	**2.** cisterna chyli	**B.** natural killer
____	**3.** spleen	**C.** firelike chemicals
____	**4.** lymph nodes	**D.** protein group
____	**5.** tonsils	**E.** beaded appearance
____	**6.** thymus	**F.** hypersensitivity
____	**7.** pyrogens	**G.** storage sac
____	**8.** complement	**H.** T-cells
____	**9.** null cells	**I.** palatine
____	**10.** allergy	**J.** glandlike

Exercise 4: Multiple choice:

1. Inflammation of lymphatic vessels is called:
   a. lymphadenitis   b. lymphangitis   c. lymphedema
2. Chemicals released by invading bacteria and defending leukocytes are:
   a. histamines   b. prostaglandins   c. pyrogens
3. B-cells produce:
   a. antibodies   b. antigens   c. complements
4. B-cells have the ability to become:
   a. memory cells   b. T-helper cells   c. stem cells
5. A type of leukocyte is:
   a. interferon   b. lymphokines   c. null cells
6. Which of the following cannot become memory cells?
   a. B-cells   b. null cells   c. T-cells
7. Which of the following kill target cells by lysis?
   a. null cells   b. B-cells   c. T-cells
8. Recovery from exposure to a disease such as measles is an example of:
   a. natural passive immunity   b. artificial active immunity   c. natural active immunity
9. Weakness of the immune system is illustrated by:
   a. auto-immune disease   b. severe combined immunodeficiency disease   c. hypersensitivities
10. Rheumatoid arthritis is a disease in which the immune system reaction is:
    a. excessively strong   b. excessively weak   c. natural passive

Exercise 5: Give the meaning of the components in the following words and then define the word as a whole. Suffixes meaning *pertaining to* or *state or condition* shown following a slash mark (/), are not to be defined separately. Before reaching for your medical dictionary, check the glossary at the end of the chapter.

1. Lymphadenitis:

lymph _____

aden _____

itis _____

_____

2. Splenectomy:

splen _____

ectomy _____

_____

3. Thymoma:

thym _____

oma _____

_____

4. Lymphocytopenia:

lympho _____

cyto _____

pen/ia _____

_____

5. Immunodeficient:

immuno _____

deficient _____

_____

Chapter 16 Crossword Puzzle

Across

1. Body chemical producing vasodilation

6. Small mass of lymphoid tissue

8. Proteins produced by T-effector cells

10. One of the functions of the spleen

11. A group of lymph nodes

14. Fever-producing chemical

15. Type of invading organism

17. Body chemicals producing vasodilation

20. One function of the spleen

20. One function of the spleen

21. Type of immunity

22. Natural cell protein

23. Type of immunity conferred by vaccination

24. Largest structure of lymphoid system

25. Type of lymphocyte that uses lysis

Down

2. A third type of lymphocyte

3. Antibody produced by B-cells

4. Blood vessel enlargement caused by natural body chemicals

5. Results in greater blood flow

7. Type of T-cell

9. Type of B-cell or T-cell that recognizes a specific antigen

12. Proteins produced by B-cells

13. Cells producing antibodies against antigen sources

16. Source of lymphocyte formation

18. Type of T-cell that increases the immune response

19. Fluid carried by lymphatic vessels

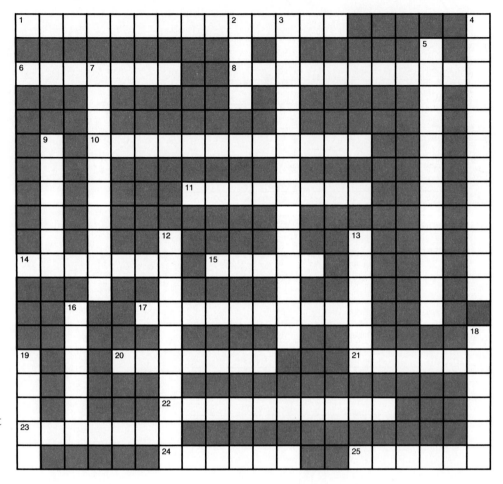

Chapter 16 Hidden Words Puzzle

```
P U L T R Y V L H M P I W M L E M Q N O R G L Z Z P U A
A U T O I M M U N E Z T X X I R Q U D Z D G J T R L L P
C P C L L X C Z O S M R O F M Z F D F P C A U E O O F X
P W L Z F B F H D H V O G P M A J Z U F A U Y C Z R O T
T E F D C N Q M C F L U P J U U Q I O I B S L Q X D C I
L W X R W J J Y K U H W C O N V G V Q B E S S C P S R Q
O W K G U M Y W S D Y A R T I F I C I A L M N I V D I K
G X Z I C Y J W L E W E J S T E B P J E K V J S V B F O
W Q L H Q U R J A V R H R E Y Q S Q Q F I B H T F E X R
P J E L M U W G L G S U B M A N D I B U L A R E X F J D
V I V P R W C F B R D Y M I D B R M S G L S S R L Q N Q
T E C W P D C K U T R K V T N C O M P L E M E N T P H W
Q C M B F P A Q R L V C Y S T P B U V L R H W A Y P E U
U C U U E I M N Q C H Y P E R S E N S I T I V E H U L R
S L Y B S F U O T S Q T L Y M P H O C Y T E I S B O B I
N X Y V D R H D K I B K C K J T G G M L X Z V Z O C O B
X U L P Y V V E V E G S Y O G A E L E T F U X P S L N K
S E J G G T M S L J R E F F E C T O R D L R Y V C W L N
V K K Y P V G Q N V L L N A N T I B O D Y Y C B B H V V
K C G N F J K J E N E P X U A I W U D S W M W X W T G E
K C D I V C K F I R V C E S T V C L T M F T Q F G H I W
H H G O E X O Y Y Y O T N L U E U I J W F E Q J E M F D
L A U G X R U L Y X G S L P R X U N D E U X Y D N A C V
N Y Q H A E F L L L D R A B A L L T A X E Q T C O R V C
C C E C N Q D O B E K N K V L N V H T H H E X T H D H B
```

Can you find the 20 words hidden in this puzzle?

HYPERSENSITIVE	IMMUNOGLOBULIN	SUBMANDIBULAR	HEMOPOIESIS
AUTOIMMUNE	COMPLEMENT	ARTIFICIAL	LYMPHOCYTE
EFFECTOR	ANTIBODY	IMMUNITY	CISTERNA
NATURAL	ANTIGEN	PASSIVE	KILLER
HELPER	ACTIVE	SERUM	NODES

CHAPTER 16 ANSWERS

Exercise 1
1. thoracic duct, right lymphatic duct
2. fibrous capsule
3. three (3)
4. plays a part in leukocyte formation, filters out bacteria and foreign matter
5. immune
6. spleen
7. lymphocyte or T-cell
8. histamines, prostaglandins
9. interferon
10. antigens

Exercise 2
1. submandibular lymph nodes
2. axillary lymph nodes
3. lymph vessels
4. inguinal lymph nodes
5. popliteal lymph nodes
6. cisterna chyli
7. spleen
8. thoracic duct
9. thymus
10. cervical lymph nodes

Exercise 3
1. E   6. H
2. G   7. C
3. J   8. D
4. A   9. B
5. I   10. F

Exercise 4
1. b   6. b
2. c   7. a
3. a   8. c
4. a   9. b
5. c   10. a

Exercise 5
1. lymphadenitis: lymph; glands; inflammation—inflammation of lymph glands
2. splenectomy: spleen; surgical removal—surgical removal of spleen
3. thymoma: thymus; tumor—tumor of the thymus
4. lymphocytopenia: lymph; cell; deficiency—deficiency of lymphocytes
5. immunodeficient: immune system; inadequate—inadequate immune system

Answers: Chapter 16 Crossword Puzzle

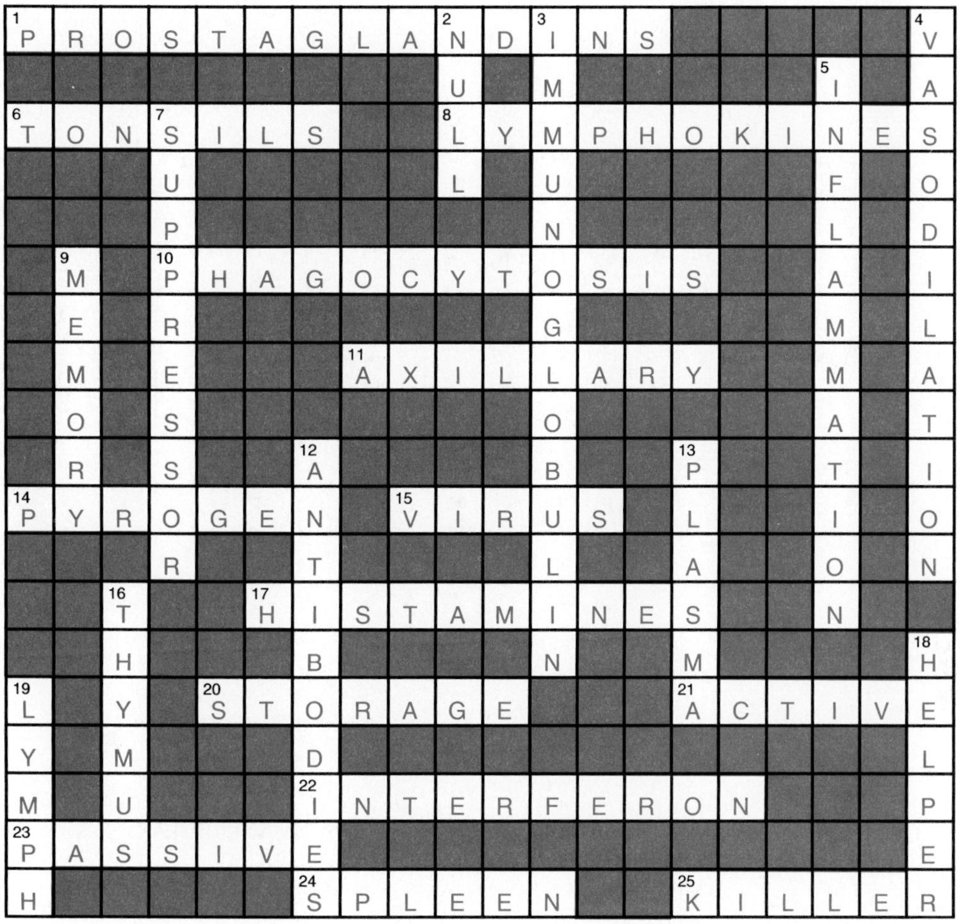

1 P	R	O	S	T	A	G	L	A	2 N	D	3 I	N	S						4 V
									U		M						5 I		A
6 T	O	N	7 S	I	L	S			8 L	Y	M	P	H	O	K	I	N	E	S
			U						L		U						F		O
			P								N						L		D
	9 M		10 P	H	A	G	O	C	Y	T	O	S	I	S			A		I
	E		R								G						M		L
	M		E				11 A	X	I	L	L	A	R	Y			M		A
	O		S								O						A		T
	R		S			12 A					B			13 P			T		I
14 P	Y	R	O	G	E	N		15 V	I	R	U	S		L			I		O
			R			T					L			A			O		N
		16 T			17 H	I	S	T	A	M	I	N	E	S			N		
		H				B					N			M					18 H
19 L		Y		20 S	T	O	R	A	G	E				21 A	C	T	I	V	E
Y		M				D													L
M		U				22 I	N	T	E	R	F	E	R	O	N				P
23 P	A	S	S	I	V	E													E
H						24 S	P	L	E	E	N			25 K	I	L	L	E	R

Answers: Chapter 16 Hidden Words Puzzle

```
. . . . . . . H . . . . . . . . . . . . . . . . . . . . . . .
A U T O I M M U N E . . . . . I . . . . . . . . . . . . . . .
. . . . . . . . . M . . . . M . . . . P . . . . . . . . . . .
. . . . . . . . O . . . M . . . . . A . . . . . . . . . . . .
. . . . . . . P . . . U . . . . . . . .S . . . . . . . . . .
. . . . . . . . O . N . . . . . . . . . S C . . . . . . . . .
. . . . . S . . A R T . I F I C I A L . . I . . . . . . . . .
. . . . . . E . . . . T E . . . . . K . . S V . . . . . . . .
. . . . . . . R . . Y . S . . . I . H T . E . . . . . . . . .
. . . . . . . S U B M A N D I B U L A R E . . . . . . . . . .
. . . . . . . . M . . . . M S . L . . R L . . . . . . . . . .
. . . . . . . . . . . C O M P L E M E N T P . . . . . . . . .
. . . . A . . . . . . U . R . A . . E . . . . . . . . . . . .
. . . . N . . H Y P E R S E N S I T I V E . . . . R . . . . .
. . . . O T . . L Y M P H O C Y T E . . . . . . . . . . . . .
. . . . D . I . . . . . G . . . . . . . . . . . . . . . . . .
. . . . E . G . . . A . L . . . . . . . . . . . . . . . . . .
. . . . S . . E F F E C T O R . . . . . . . . . . . . . . . .
. . . . . . . N A N T I B O D Y . . . . . . . . . . . . . . .
. . . . . . . . A . I . U . . . . . . . . . . . . . . . . . .
. . . . . . . . T . V . L . . . . . . . . . . . . . . . . . .
. . . . . . . . U E . I . . . . . . . . . . . . . . . . . . .
. . . . . . . . R . . N . . . . . . . . . . . . . . . . . . .
. . . . . . . . A . . . . . . . . . . . . . . . . . . . . . .
. . . . . . . . L . . . . . . . . . . . . . . . . . . . . . .
```

Words:

>	HYPERSENSITIVE	V	IMMUNOGLOBULIN	>	SUBMANDIBULAR	\ HEMOPOIESIS
>	AUTOIMMUNE	>	COMPLEMENT	>	ARTIFICIAL	> LYMPHOCYTE
>	EFFECTOR	>	ANTIBODY	V	IMMUNITY	V CISTERNA
V	NATURAL	\	ANTIGEN	\	PASSIVE	V KILLER
\	HELPER	V	ACTIVE	\	SERUM	V NODES

CHAPTER 16 GLOSSARY

Lymphatic and Immune Systems
Related Anatomic and Other Terms

active immunity: immunity developed by stimulating the body's own defenses.

adenoids: see **pharyngeal tonsils**.

antibody: a protein substance that interacts with a specific antigen to protect the body.

antigen: substance that triggers the formation of specific antibodies, which react against the antigen.

artificial immunity: immunity derived by vaccination, from a source outside the body.

B-cells: lymphocytes that form and mature in the bone marrow, producing antibodies.

celluar immunity: immunity produced by T-cell lymphocytes (also called **cell-mediated** immunity).

cisterna chyli (sis-ter′nah): saclike reservoir for collection of lymph, and origin of the thoracic duct.

complement: a group of proteins normally present in blood serum that produces inflammation and destruction of invading cells.

hemopoiesis: lymphocyte, monocyte and plasma cell formation (also called **hemapoiesis** and **hematopoiesis**).

histamine: natural body chemical that produces vasodilation and inflammation.

hilum: depression where vessels and nerves enter the spleen.

humoral immunity: immunity produced by antibodies.

hypersensitivity: excessive immune system response to antigens.

immunoglobulins: antibodies produced by B-cells (also called **immune gamma globulins**).

interferon: a natural cell protein that protects against infection by stimulating production of other antiviral proteins.

killer cell: a type of null cell lymphocyte that kills tumor and viral-infected cells by lysis.

lienic (splenic) capsule: membranous envelope enclosing the spleen.

lymph: relatively colorless tissue fluid containing leukocytes, proteins, and water.

lymphatic duct: channel conveying lymph, specifically the right and left (thoracic) lymphatic ducts.

lymphatic vessel: channel conveying lymph.

lymph follicle (fol′i-k′l): sac-like collector of lymphoid substances, chiefly beneath the mucous surfaces.

lymph nodes: gland-like masses of lymphatic tissue varying in size from dots to bean-sized bodies, identified by their locations along the course of lymphatic vessels.

lymphocytes: several types of leukocytes that either produce antibodies or carry out phagocytosis.

memory cells: lymphocytes that can recognize previously encountered antigens, and react quickly.

memory response: rapid lymphocyte response to previously encountered antigens.

monoclonal antibodies: antibodies grown (cloned) in quantity from a single cell, for vaccine use.

natural immunity: immunity produced by natural body defenses such as antibodies or killer cells.

natural killer cells: type of null cell lymphocyte that kills tumor and viral-infected cells by lysis.

null cells: lymphocytes that do not become memory cells, and destroy target cells by lysis.

passive immunity: immunity directly produced by sources external to the body.

phagocytosis: removal and destruction of foreign bodies, platelets, and erythrocytes, and salvaging of globin and heme contents.

pharyngeal tonsils: tonsils located at the back of the roof of the pharynx (also called **adenoids**.)

plasma cells: activated B-cells that produce antibodies for specific antigens.

prostaglandin: natural body chemical that produces vasodilation and inflammation.

pyrogen: chemical released by invading bacteria and defending leukocytes that stimulates the nervous system to increase body temperature.

right lymphatic duct: lymphatic duct draining the lymph from the upper right quadrant of the body.

sinusoids: sinuslike capillaries with specialized function.

spleen: largest lymphoid system structure, a flattened, oval-shaped, glandlike organ located in the upper left side of the abdominal cavity.

red splenic pulp: lymphatic tissue permeated with sinusoids filled with blood.

T-cells: lymphocytes maturing in the thymus that produce antibodies.

T-effector cells: type of T-cell that produces lymphokines, and can become memory cells.

T-helper cells: type of T-cell that increases immune responses of T-effector and B-cells.

T-suppressor cells: type of T-cell that suppresses the immune responses of T-effector and B-cells.

thoracic duct: left lymphatic duct draining lymph from all but the upper right quadrant of the body.

thymus gland: bi-lobate, grayish-pink, structure of lymph tissue in the mediastinum, that develops the T-cell lymphocytes from stem cells.

tonsils: three pairs of small, round masses of lymphoid tissue.

white splenic pulp: sheath of lymphatic tissue that surrounds the arteries of the spleen.

Pathologic Conditions

Inflammations and Infections

acquired immune deficiency syndrome (AIDS): see Chapter 17.

actinomycosis: see Chapter 17.

AIDS-related complex (ARC): see Chapter 17.

filariasis: tropical parasitic disease, transmitted by a mosquito carrying *Filaria nematode* larvae, causing granulomatous inflammation and obstruction of lymph channels, with pain, blindness, swelling of extremities, and development of elephantiasis and pachyderma (Chapter 17).

infectious mononucleosis (mon″o-nu′kle-o′sis): acute, contagious, viral infection, caused by the *Epstein-Barr* virus (may be present in latent form in most human leukocytes and activated to pathogenicity by an immune suppression response), resulting in an abnormal increase in mononuclear leukocytes in the blood (Chapter 17).

lymphadenitis (lim-fad″e-ni′tis): inflammation of the lymph nodes.

lymphangitis (lim″fan-ji′tis): inflammation of one or more lymphatic vessels.

paratyphoid fever: *Salmonella* bacterial infection similar to typhoid but not as severe, involving lymphoid mesenteric tissues and the intestines (Chapter 17).

splenitis: painful inflammatory condition of the spleen.

sporotrichosis (spo″ro-tri′ko′sis): common, chronic, fungal infection caused by an organism of *Sporotrichum*, characterized by skin ulcers and multiple subcutaneous granulomas along lymphatic channels, with rare involvement in muscles, joints, bones, and lungs.

Hereditary, Congenital, and Developmental Disorders

Gaucher's disease (go-shaz′): hereditary splenic anemia (Chapter 17).

hypertrophy of thymus: congenital enlargement of thymus.

leukocyte adhesion deficiency (LAD): a genetic defect resulting in inability of leukocytes to adhere to other cells, rendering a significant part of the immune system helpless.

severe combined immunodeficiency disease (SCID): congenital immune system deficiency disease in which the individual must be kept in a sterile environment ("bubble") to prevent illness or death from infections.

Other Lymphatic and Immune System Disorders

accessory spleen: small mass of splenic tissue, sometimes found near the spleen in a peritoneal fold.

Banti's disease: splenomegaly resulting from portal hypertension.

gammopathy: disorder in which there are abnormal levels of gamma globulin in the blood.

lymphadenectasis (lim-fad″e-nek′tah-sis): dilation of a lymph gland.

lymphadenopathy: disease of the lymph nodes.

lymphangiectasis (lim-fan″je-ek′tah-sis): swelling of lymphatic vessels.

lymphatic leukemia: leukemia combined with hyperplasia and over-activity of the lymphoid tissue (also called *lymphocytic leukemia* and *lymphoid leukemia*).

lymphedema (lim″fe-de′mah): swelling caused by blockage of the lymphatic vessels.

lymphorrhea: discharge of lymph from a cut or torn lymph vessel.

lymphostasis (lim-fos′tah-sis): obstruction to the lymph flow.

myasthenia gravis: muscular disease with suspected autoimmune involvement (Chapter 7).

multiple sclerosis: neural demyelinating disorder of suspected autoimmune origin (Chapter 14).

rheumatoid arthritis: destructive collagen disease of autoimmune origin (Chapter 17).

splenomegaly: enlargement of the spleen.

systemic lupus erythematosus (SLE): chronic disease of suspected autoimmune origin involving many organ systems individually or in a variety of combinations (Chapter 17).

thrombocytopenic purpura: systemic condition with suspected autoimmune origin (Chapter 9).

thymolysis: destruction of the thymus.

thymopathy: any disease of the thymus.

thymus hyperplasia: enlarged thymus.

Oncology*

giant follicular lymphoma* (lim-fo′mah): malignant lymphoma marked by folliclelike nodules in the lymph nodes (also called *giant follicular lymphadenopathy* and *Brill-Symmers disease*).

Hodgkin's disease*: malignant, progressive, painless condition marked by the enlargement of the spleen, lymph nodes, and lymphoid tissues (also called *granulomatous lymphoma*, *multiple lymphadenoma*, *lymphogranuloma*, and *lymphomatosis granulomatosa*).

*Indicates a malignant condition.

Kaposi's sarcoma* (kap′a-sez): malignant neoplasm affecting lymph nodes and other systems (Chapter 17).

lymphangioma (lim-fan″je-o′mah): tumor made up of newly formed lymph channels and spaces.

lymphangiosarcoma*: malignant tumor of the lymph vessels.

lymphoma*: lymphoid tissue tumors, usually malignant.

lymphomatosis* (lim″fo-mah-to′sis): development of multiple lymphomas in the body.

lymphosarcoma* (lim″fo-sar′ko′mah): general term for malignant neoplasm of lymphoid tissue.

Surgical Procedures

angiotomy: incision of a blood or lymph vessel.

lymphadenectomy (lim-fad″e-nek′to-me): excision of a lymph node.

lymphangiectomy (lim-fan″je-ek′to-me): excision of lymphatic vessels.

lymphangioplasty (lim-fan″je-o-plas″te): repair or replacement of a lymph vessel (also called *lymphoplasty*).

lymphangiotomy (lim-fan″je-ot′o-me): incision into a vessel of the lymphatic system.

lymphaticostomy (lim-fat″i-kos′to-me): making an opening into a lymphatic duct.

splenectomy: removal of the spleen.

splenopexy: fixation of a movable spleen.

splenorrhaphy: repair of the spleen.

splenotomy: incision of the spleen.

thymectomy: removal of thymus.

Laboratory Tests and Procedures

AIDS serology tests: blood tests to screen for antigens or the antibodies to the human immunodeficiency virus (HIV). Used in patient diagnosis and in screening blood for transfusion.
  Western blot test
  Enzyme-linked immunosorbent assay (ELISA)

angiotensin-converting enzyme (ACE): blood test used to assist in diagnosis of Gaucher's and Hodgkin's diseases.

complement assay: blood test to measure serum complement levels, which increase or decrease according to type of disorder (e.g., increased levels in rheumatoid arthritis, decreased levels in systemic lupus erythematosus).

Multiple-System Diseases

A Glossary of Conditions Affecting Multiple Systems

In the preceding chapters, diseases and abnormal conditions have been listed under the appropriate anatomic systems. This method of classification, however, does not take into consideration all the diseases and congenital anomalies that affect more than one system. Multiple descriptions of each disease or anomaly would be required if they appeared under individual systems. To eliminate this duplication, we have chosen to list and describe many of these diseases in this chapter.

In multiple-system diseases, a "target" organ may be involved primarily, but as the disease advances and constitutional symptoms develop, other organs become progressively affected. This is particularly true of many infections, especially immunodeficiency diseases, which begin with a symptom in one body system and progressively spread to involve other systems.

Radiologic examinations often reveal characteristic findings in organs other than the primary system under investigation. The extent of spread of the disease process is evident in many body structures far removed from the primary focus, as in acquired immune deficiency syndrome (AIDS), and lupus erythematosus (LE). It is also not unusual, in autopsies on stillborn neonates and those dying shortly after birth, to find a number of anomalies incompatible with life, including gross malformations of organs, atresia of passages, or heart defects that are not visually detected at birth.

The classification of diseases as "multiple-system" is now widespread since the advent of new and improved laboratory and radiologic procedures as well as other diagnostic tests such as computer-assisted imaging techniques. These and other advances in medical knowledge make it possible to trace the extent of involvement of multiple systems in a disease. No attempt is made here to list all the multiple-system diseases, since several medical writers have devoted separate texts to to this subject.

CHAPTER 17 GLOSSARY

MULTIPLE-SYSTEM DISEASES AND RELATED ANATOMIC TERMS

Inflammations and Infections

acquired immune deficiency syndrome (AIDS): infectious disease that produces a breakdown in the immune system and is transmitted by unprotected intercourse (anal or vaginal) with an infected person, by contact with infected blood or blood products, contaminated needles, and infected donor organs, or across the placental barrier from mother to fetus. The disease process begins with infection by a retrovirus, *Human Immunodeficiency Virus (HIV)*. This retrovirus destroys the ability of T-helper cells (a type of lymphocyte) to recognize invading pathogens, and also converts the T-cells into factories to reproduce the infecting virus, eventually leaving the body defenseless against even the most minor of infections. Eight to 12 weeks after initial infection, HIV antibodies begin to be produced, but there may be an extended incubation period that *can* last an average of 10 years, during which time the virus may remain hidden in the lymph nodes. Although most cases take several months for HIV antibodies to be detected after initial infection, some may take as long as 24 months. *AIDS-related complex (ARC)* syndrome is an early condition, in which symptoms of fatigue, weakness, fever, weight loss, diarrhea, and lymphadenopathy appear. The immune system's weakness allows many opportunistic infections to develop in one or more body systems, from sources that include protozoa, fungi, viruses, and bacteria. Life-threatening conditions common in full-blown AIDS include *Pneumocystis carinii pneumonia (PCP)*, and *Kaposi's sarcoma (KS)*. Neurologic involvement is common, including such conditions as *AIDS dementia*. Some drugs such as zidovudine (AZT), retrovir, and dideoxyinosine (DDL) are being used to inhibit progression of the disease, but there is no known cure and the current prognosis is death.

actinomycosis (ak″ti-no-mi-ko′sis): fungal infection caused by the organism *Actinomyces*, characterized mainly by abscesses or granulomas of cervicofacial lymph nodes, abdominal organs, and pulmonary tissue.

AIDS-related complex (ARC): pre-AIDS syndrome, also known as *chronic lymphadenopathy syndrome* (see **acquired immune deficiency syndrome**).

alastrim: mild form of smallpox (also called *variola minor*).

amebiasis (am″e-bi′ah-sis): protozoal infection with the microorganism *Entamoeba histolytica*, transmitted to humans by food and drink containing encysted forms of the microorganism, which affects the mucous membrane of the colon in the form of abscesses and ulcers, and may also form abscesses in the liver, thoracic cavity, lungs, and skin.

anthrax: bacterial infection of animals with the microorganism *Bacillus anthracis*, transmitted to humans by inhalation or handling of infected wool, hides, and carcasses, beginning with a lesion at the entry site of the infection, progressing to bloody, mucinous edema in many tissues and serous cavities, and may be fatal (also called *splenic fever*, *woolsorters'* or *ragsorters' disease*, and *malignant pustule*).

ascariasis (as″kah-ri′ah-sis): helminthic infection with the roundworm *Ascaris lumbricoides*, transmitted by ingestion of embryonated ova, which develop into adult worms in the intestines, but the worms may migrate to other organs.

botulism (bot′u-lizm): potent bacterial food poisoning with a high mortality rate, caused by the growth of *Clostridium botulinum* in food that has not been properly sterilized before canning or preserving. Symptoms include vomiting, abdominal pain, vision problems, central nervous system symptoms, motor disturbances, dyspepsia, coughing, dilation of the pupils, and muscle paralysis (*botulus* means sausage, and the disease derives its name from its first recognition in improperly cooked sausages).

brucellosis (broo″sel-lo′sis): bacterial infection caused by a species of *Brucella*, infecting humans through contact with infected animals or products such as meat, milk and cheese, with lesions in many organs (also known as *undulant*, *Malta*, and *Mediterranean fevers*).

candidiasis (kan″di-di′ah-sis): *Candida albicans* fungal infection, involving superficial lesions of moist areas such as the respiratory tract, vagina, and mouth (*thrush*- common in HIV infections), with rare endocardial and systemic infections (also called *moniliasis*, *candidosis*, and *oidomycosis*).

cat scratch disease: usually benign bacterial infection caused by the bite or scratch of a cat, which produces lymphadenitis, but can also become more severe and manifest as osteomyelitis, arthritis, hepatitis, pleurisy, and other conditions (also called *cat scratch fever*).

chickenpox: highly contagious childhood disease, caused *by herpes zoster virus*, with vesicular eruptions on face and trunk, and possible complications, including pneumonia, myelitis, Guillain-Barre syndrome, encephalitis, meningitis, and Reye's syndrome (also called *varicella*).

cholera (kol′er-ah): acute bacterial infection caused by *Vibrio cholerae*, contracted from contaminated water, food, hands, and utensils, beginning with an acute diarrhea and progressing to vomiting, cramps, and severe dehydration, which may result in renal failure.

chronic Epstein-Barr virus syndrome (CEBV): chronic infection caused by the *Epstein-Barr herpesvirus*, a sequel to an acute mononucleosis infection (also called ***chronic fatigue syndrome*** and ***yuppie flu***).

cryptococcosis (krip″to-kok-o′sis): a *Cryptococcus neoformans* fungal infection involving any part or organ of the body, especially brain and meninges, fatal if untreated (also called ***torulosis***).

cytomegalovirus disease (CMV): *herpes* infection with large inclusion bodies in infected cells, most often found in salivary glands, with infection ranging from asymptomatic to severe. Transmitted across the placental barrier, or, postnatally, through contact with body secretions, transfusions, renal and bone marrow transplants (post-immunosuppressive consequence), sexual relations, and kissing. It produces lesions throughout the body, particularly brain, liver, lungs, kidneys, and spleen (also called ***salivary gland virus disease***, and, in infants, ***cytomegalic inclusion disease***).

dengue (deng′e): eruptive febrile disease, caused by *Arbovirus* infection transmitted by the Aedes mosquito, with rash and systemic symptoms. Though mild, it is so painful that it has been nicknamed "breakbone fever."

dengue hemorrhagic fever shock syndrome (DHFS): severe form of dengue fever, with all its symptoms plus hemorrhage, prostration, shock and possible death. Common in tropical and subtropical regions, it is also transmitted by the Asian tiger mosquito, found in 17 of the United States.

Ebola hemorrhagic fever: named for the river in Zaire, this lethal *filovirus* (threadlike virus) infects with symptoms of headache, fever, blood clots, and hemorrhages disseminated throughout the body, ultimately leading to death.

echinococcosis (e-ki″no-kok-ko′sis): a tapeworm, *Echinococcus granulosus*, infecting humans through drinking water, food, or hands contaminated by animal feces, produces hydatid cysts in liver and lungs (also called ***hydatid disease***).

filariasis: tropical parasitic disease, transmitted by a mosquito carrying *Filaria nematode* larvae, causing granulomatous inflammation and obstruction of lymph channels, with pain, blindness, swelling of extremities, and development of elephantiasis and pachyderma.

infectious mononucleosis (mon″o-nu′kle-o′sis): acute, contagious, viral infection, caused by the *Epstein-Barr virus* (may be present in latent form in most human leukocytes and activated to pathogenicity by an immune suppression response), resulting in an abnormal increase in mononuclear leukocytes in the blood. Symptoms include fever, malaise, sore throat, lymphadenopathy, liver dysfunction, and enlarged spleen, with possible effect on the brain, meninges, and myocardium.

Kawasaki's disease: childhood disease, etiology unknown, apparently noncontagious, more common in males, usually appearing after viral infection, lasting 2 to 3 weeks, with complete recovery in almost all cases. Symptoms include fever, reddening and inflammation of eyes, nose, mouth, and throat, red rash on the trunk, swollen lymph glands and hands and feet, with desquamation of fingers and toes (complications include heart arrhythmias, heart attack, and coronary artery rupture, and may be fatal to 2% of those affected—also called ***mucocutaneous lymph node syndrome [MLNS]***).

leishmaniasis: group of diseases, caused by one of a number of species of protozoa that belong to the genus *Leishmania*, transmitted to humans by the bite of insects. Varying symptoms include splenomegaly, cutaneous lesions, ulcers, granulomas, leukopenia, lymphatic involvement, and frequent involvement of the mucosal surfaces of the nose, mouth, and upper respiratory tract, which, if untreated, may be fatal to young children.

leprosy: chronic communicable disease caused by the microorganism *Mycobacterium leprae*. Symptoms include granulomatous lesions in the skin, mucous membranes, and peripheral nervous system, which may result in progressive anesthesias, paralysis, ulceration, atrophies, gangrene, and mutilation (also called ***Hansen's disease***).

Lyme disease: tick-transmitted, *spirochete*-caused disease with symptoms of bull's-eye red rash, fever, headache, chills, nausea, vomiting, fatigue, muscle and joint pain, and swollen lymph glands, which, if not treated, progresses to a second stage that may affect joints (Lyme arthritis), the nervous system, or heart.

malaria: protozoan parasitic (*Plasmodium* genus) infection transmitted through the bite of an infected female mosquito of the genus Anopheles. Involves the liver, spleen, and bone marrow, and is characterized by recurrent attacks of chills, fever, and sweating.

mumps: contagious, viral infection affecting the salivary glands, usually the parotid, manifested by fever and inflammation, and if contracted after puberty, may affect the testes, ovaries, pancreas, and meninges (also called ***parotitis***).

paratyphoid fever: *Salmonella* bacterial infection similar to typhoid but not as severe, involving lymphoid mesenteric tissues and the intestines.

periarteritis nodosa: inflammatory disease, etiology unknown, of the coats of the small- and medium-sized arteries of the body, with multiple-organ involvement, including nodular swellings, hypertension, jaundice, hepatomegaly, motor weakness, foot and wrist drop, and skin lesions (also called **polyarteritis** and **panarteritis**).

plague: several types of bacterial infection caused by *Pasteurella pestis*, with *bubonic*, the best known type, spread by fleas of infected rodents, and characterized by buboes (enlarged lymph nodes), occurring in femoral, inguinal, axillary, and cervical areas, with infection spread by the circulation. The *pneumonic* type is spread by person-to-person contact; both types are septicemic, involving lungs and other organs.

rat-bite fever: two types, contracted from an infected rat or mouse bite: a Far Eastern type, *Spirillum minus* spirochetal infection characterized by relapsing fever, lymphadenopathy and rash, lasting 4 to 8 weeks, with relapses common (also called **sodoku**); a United States type, caused by *Streptobacillus moniliformis* bacterium, characterized by fever, headache, malaise, nausea, vomiting, and rash on soles and palms, lasting 2 weeks (also called **Haverhill fever**).

relapsing fever: spirochetal infection caused by various species of *Borrelia* and transmitted to humans by the bite of a tick or louse, characterized by petechial rashes and febrile and afebrile periods, with enlargement of the liver and spleen accompanying the fever.

rheumatic fever: delayed consequence of an upper respiratory tract infection in children, caused by *Group A hemolytic streptococci*, producing multiple focal inflammatory lesions, which may develop into migratory arthritis, carditis, chorea, erythema marginatum, and subcutaneous nodules, with the acute phase limited, but involvement of the heart may lead to permanent valvular damage.

Rocky Mountain spotted fever: tick-borne rickettsial infectious disease (*Rickettsia rickettsii*) transmitted to humans by bite, beginning with fever, myalgia, and weakness, and progressing to hemorrhagic lesions and a rash; may prove fatal without treatment (also called **mountain fever, mountain tick fever,** and **spotted fever**).

rubella: viral infection transmitted by direct contact, with symptoms of macular rash, rhinorrhea, sore throat, and conjunctivitis, and with the ability to cross the placental barrier, possibly causing infection of the fetus, which, in the first trimester, may result in a high frequency of developmental abnormalities without interrupting the pregnancy (also called **German measles**).

rubeola: highly contagious viral infection, spread by direct or indirect contact, affecting the respiratory tract and reticuloendothelial tissues, with skin eruptions in the form of red papules usually preceded by coryza, lymphadenitis, conjunctivitis, photophobia, myalgia, cough, and fever, and may be followed by complications of bacterial pneumonia, otitis media, and encephalitis (also called **measles**).

scarlet fever: bacterial infection caused by a *group A hemolytic streptococcus*, transmitted directly or indirectly, characterized by an erythematous rash, fever, enlarged cervical lymph nodes, and sore throat, and may disseminate, involving many organs (also called **scarlatina**).

schistosomiasis (skis″to-so-mi′ah-sis): helminthic infection caused by a species of fluke of the genus *Schistosoma*. Transmitted by wading or bathing in water contaminated by human waste. Characterized by pain, dysfunction, and anemia, involving the bladder, rectum, lungs, spleen, intestines and the liver and its portal venous system.

Serratia infection: a species of gram-negative bacteria, *Serratia* is responsible for nosocomial infections (acquired during hospitalization for other conditions) including respiratory and urinary tract infections, as well as bacteremia.

smallpox: acute, contagious, viral infection, transmitted by direct or indirect contact, characterized by an eruption of papules, vesicles and pustules, fever, and prostration, which may occur in hemorrhagic form in the kidneys and lungs, with possible complications of arthritis, osteomyelitis, and other conditions (also called **variola**).

sporotrichosis (spo″ro-tri′ko′sis): common, chronic, fungal infection caused by an organism of *Sporotrichum*, characterized by skin ulcers and multiple subcutaneous granulomas along lymphatic channels, with rare involvement in muscles, joints, bones, and lungs.

syphilis: contagious, sexually transmitted disease caused by the spirochete *Treponema pallidum*, which can also be transmitted transplacentally to a fetus from an infected mother (congenital syphilis). It initially produces a primary lesion (a chancre), with multiple skin eruptions, especially on the trunk in the second stage, and progressing to a tertiary (third) stage involving multiple organs of the body, especially the heart, blood vessels, and the central nervous system.

TORCH syndrome: acronym for fetal or neonatal infection by one of the following agents: *Toxoplasma gondii, Other* (90% of infections), *Rubella virus, Cytomegalovirus,* and *Herpes simplex virus*. TORCH complications may result in stillbirth, growth retardation, abortion, or premature delivery.

toxic shock syndrome (TSS): infectious condition involving a penicillin-resistant strain of *staphylococcus aureus*, characterized by fever, diffuse macular erythroderma, desquamation of palms and soles, hypotension, and involvement of three or more systems, especially gastrointestinal (vomiting or diarrhea), muscular (myalgia), mucous membranes, kidneys, liver, circulatory, and central nervous system (disorientation and alterations of consciousness). Previously, there was a higher incidence among females, linked to the use of superabsorbent tampons, which were believed to provide a growth medium for the bacteria. A change in tampon construction has dropped the female incidence markedly, and the syndrome is now mainly associated with sequellae of various surgical procedures.

toxoplasmosis: *Toxoplasma gondii* protozoal infection, carried by cats and other hosts, of two types: *lymphadenopathic*-resembling mononucleosis, with a *disseminated type* widely distributed to brain, meninges, muscles, skin, heart, lungs, and liver, with lesions in any or all, and passed from infected mother to fetus; *congenital type*, with CNS involvement, including blindness, brain defect, and death.

trench fever: *Rickettsia quintana* infection transmitted by body lice, with weakness, fever, leg pains, and a macular rash.

trypanosomiasis (tri-pan″o-so-mi′ah-sis): protozoal infection of two types: a Central and South American type (Chagas' disease) caused by *Trypanosoma cruzi*, characterized by conjunctivitis, and lesions caused by infected insect bites, and may have lymphatic, heart and brain involvement; and an African trypanosomiasis, caused by *T. gambiense* or *T. rhodesiense*, transmitted by the tsetse fly, with the central nervous system as the main target (also called *sleeping sickness*).

tsutsugamushi fever (soot″soo-gah-moosh′e): *Rickettsia tsutsugamushi* infection, transmitted from infected rodents by the bite of lice, fleas, mites or ticks, with headache, fever, chills, rash, and possible neurologic symptoms, vascular lesions, and lymphadenopathy (also called *scrub typhus*).

tularemia (too″lah-re′me-ah): bacterial infection caused by *Francisella tularensis*, which is transmitted by direct contact with infected animals, insect bite (especially tick, horsefly, or deerfly), handling contaminated animal products, or eating undercooked infected meat. It is characterized by suppurative or granulomatous lesions and septicemia, and can also involve the skin, eyes, lungs, lymph glands, and more rarely, the meninges.

typhoid fever: a bacterial infection caused by *Salmonella*, and resembling typhus, transmitted directly or indirectly, with food and water as principal vehicles. Characterized by rash, fever, cough, headache, delirium, and diarrhea, followed by splenomegaly and leukopenia and possible gastrointestinal hemorrhage or perforation.

typhus: group of rickettsial infections caused by a species of *Rickettsia*, transmitted by infected lice,

fleas, mites, and ticks, with the central nervous system as the main target, but it can involve other systems, with fatalities in 20% of untreated cases.

yaws: tropical disease caused by a spirochete, *Treponema pertenu*, produced by direct contact with a lesion (yaw) of an infected person. It is characterized by a primary lesion, followed by a secondary stage skin eruption, and tertiary lesions (gummas and ulcers) of the bones.

yellow fever: acute viral disease transmitted to humans in tropical regions by the bite of a mosquito, *Aedes aegypti*, involving the liver, gastrointestinal tract, and kidneys in a systemic spread, causing characteristic fever and jaundice.

Hereditary, Congenital, and Developmental Disorders

congenital hemihypertrophy: one-sided overgrowth of part of body.

cystic fibrosis: genetic disorder causing dysfunction of sweat glands, affecting the pancreas and respiratory system, with decreased pancreatic enzymes in feces and excessive sodium and chloride loss in sweat, characterized by excessive fat in feces, malnutrition, viscid sputum, and bronchitis (also called *mucoviscidosis* and *fibrocystic disease of the pancreas*).

Danlos' syndrome: hereditary symptom tetrad, includng excessive extensibility of joints, fragility and hyperelasticity of skin, and pseudotumors following trauma (also called *Ehlers-Danlos syndrome*).

Down's syndrome: congenital condition characterized by some degree of mental retardation, with physical features including a broad, short nose, protruding tongue, short, broad neck, prominent abdomen, short phalanges, underdeveloped genitalia, rounded face, slanted eyes, and defects that may involve the eyes, ears, heart, and extremities. Results from chromosomal aberration, especially an extra chromosome 21, which is more likely to occur in infants born to older women, or from an extra chromosome translocated to the end of a larger chromosome, and not related to maternal age (also called *mongolism* and *trisomy 21*).

Fanconi's syndrome: rare, recessive, familial disease characterized by congenital hypoplasia of bone marrow with various congenital defects of the musculoskeletal and genitourinary systems; also a form of rickets beginning in early life, marked by hypophosphatemia, acidosis, and renal glycosuria.

fetal alcohol syndrome (FAS): developmental anomalies of the fetus, with growth deficiencies, limb and cranio-facial defects, and mental retardation, caused by chronic alcoholism of the mother.

fragile X syndrome: the second most common diagnosable cause of mental retardation after Down's syndrome, with macro-orchidism, craniofacial abnormalities, and neurologic problems, primarily affecting males, but carried by the mother.

gargoylism: inherited type of dwarfism involving bone and other tissue, caused by a disturbance in carbohydrate metabolism, which appears to be the result of an absence of one or more of a group of enzymes that break down mucopolysaccharides. Noticeable physical characteristics appear early in life, including large head, coarse facial features, broad saddle nose, wide nostrils, thick lips and tongue, and an open-mouth expression, followed by dwarfism, skeletal deformities, mental retardation, hepatosplenomegaly, corneal opacities, deafness, and cardiovascular defects (also called ***Hurler's syndrome*** and ***mucopolysaccharidosis***).

Gaucher's disease (go-shaz′): hereditary splenic anemia, with Gaucher's cells found in the brain, pituitary gland, hypothalamus, kidneys, lungs, adrenals, thymus, and intestinal lymphatics, and lesions from tumorlike accumulations of these cells in the bones.

hepatolenticular degeneration (hep″ah-to-len-tik′u-lar): familial disorder of copper metabolism, with cirrhosis of liver, splenomegaly, and degenerative brain changes.

Klinefelter's syndrome (klin-fel′terz): gonadal abnormality caused by chromosomal aberrations of 47 chromosomes with an XXY sex chromosome, producing testicular dysgenesis and azoospermia, with possible gynecomastia and mental deficiency.

Laurence-Moon-Biedl syndrome: autosomal recessive syndrome composed of a number of anomalies, consisting of obesity, hypogenitalism, retinitis pigmentosa, mental deficiency, skull defects, and sometimes, webbed fingers and toes.

Lindau-von Hippel disease: hereditary condition involving angioma of the cerebellum, usually associated with hemangioma of the retina, polycystic pancreas and kidneys (also called ***cerebroretinal angiomatosis*** and ***von Hippel-Lindau disease***).

Marfan's syndrome: hereditary condition involving some skeletal, vascular and/or ophthalmic defects, such as long, thin extremities and fingers, loose joints, aortal aneurysm, and lens ectopia.

neurofibromatosis type 1 (NF-1): genetic disorder, with 50% probability of transmission by a gene-carrying parent. Half of all cases are not inherited, but arise from a spontaneous genetic mutation. The condition is characterized by cafe-au-lait spots, neurofibromas in many systems of the body, skeletal dysplasias, and optic gliomas, with no known cure or effective treatment (also known as ***von Recklinghausen's disease***).

neurofibromatosis type 2 (NF-2): less common form of neurofibromatosis, characterized by bilateral acoustic neuromas, presenile cataracts, gliomas, and meningiomas, often leading to deafness (also called ***central neurofibromatosis*** and ***bilateral acoustic neurofibromatosis***).

Niemann-Pick disease: hereditary disturbance of infantile phosphatide metabolism, marked by anemia and a leukocytosis with an increase in lymphocytes, neural involvement, and an enlarged liver and spleen (also called ***lipid histiocytosis*** and ***Neimann's disease***).

phenylketonuria (PKU) (fen″il-ke″to-nu′re-ah): autosomal recessive congenital disorder of phenylalanine metabolism with phenylpyruvic acid present in the urine. It is characterized by central nervous system symptoms with resultant mental deficiency; treatable, when detected early, to minimize deterioration.

porphyria (por-fi′re-ah): group of rare inherited disorders characterized by excessive production of porphyrins in the hematopoietic tissues of the bone marrow and liver, producing pigmentation of the face, facial deformation, hairiness in some cases, sensitivity to light (particularly sunlight), vomiting, and intestinal disturbances. Patients must avoid sunlight and are treated by injections of heme, a blood product. The condition has been linked, in theory, to the development of the werewolf and vampire myths (deformed features, drinking of blood, hairiness, going out only at night), including the finding that garlic (which supposedly repels these creatures) contains a substance that exacerbates the condition.

Prader-Willi syndrome: congenital metabolic condition caused by lack of normal secretion of gonadotropic pituitary hormone, producing hypotonia, short stature, obesity, hyperphagia, sexual infantilism, and mental retardation.

progeria, juvenile: rare disorder, etiology not well established, in which growth ceases and premature aging signs appear. Includes symptoms such as graying of the hair, wrinkling of skin, generalized fibrosis and tissue atrophy, atherosclerosis, and connective tissue tumors, with death occurring early in life (also known as ***Hutchinson-Gilford syndrome***).

proteus syndrome: condition affecting multiple systems, especially characterized by lumps and tumors producing varying degrees of disfigurement (also known as ***Elephant man's disease***—previously confused with neurofibromatosis).

Turner's syndrome: female gonadal abnormality, caused by chromosomal aberration of a total of 45 chromosomes with only one X chromosome, producing an XO female karyotype. Characterized by features of hypogonadism after puberty, such as amenorrhea, lack of breast development, delayed epiphyses closure, possible dwarfism, mental deficiency, cardiovascular anomalies, and deafness.

Werner's syndrome: hereditary syndrome of adults producing premature senility, premature gray hair, spindly appearance of extremities, glossy skin, loss of subcutaneous fat tissue, hyperkeratosis with skin ulceration, cataracts, arteriosclerosis, diabetes, and underdevelopment of the sexual organs.

Williams syndrome: rare congenital disorder, characterized by slow growth, mental retardation, pixie-like features, aortic stenosis, and abnormalities of other organs (also called ***pixie disease***).

Other Multiple-System Disorders

amyloidosis: accumulation of waxy starchlike glycoprotein in body tissues, causing dysfunction; due to heredity, a primary disturbance of endogenous protein metabolism, or following another disease.

beriberi (ber″e-ber′e): vitamin B$_1$ (thiamine) deficiency disease, occurring chiefly in the Far East, resulting from a diet of polished rice, with symptoms including edema, cardiac pathology, and neuritis.

Caisson disease: condition producing nitrogen bubbles in body tissues, affecting aviators, deep-sea divers, and others who work at great depths; due to rapid pressure changes, causing disorientation, pain, and syncope (also called ***bends*** or ***decompression sickness***).

calcinosis: condition of unknown etiology, with deposition of calcium salts in skin, muscles, tendons, nerves, and bones.

cheilosis (ki-lo′sis): disease of riboflavin deficiency, characterized by fissures and scaling of the lips.

collagen diseases: group of conditions in which collagen tissue is involved, occurring in rheumatic fever, systemic lupus erythematosus, scleroderma, and dermatomyositis, and other connective tissue diseases.

Cushing's syndrome: pituitary basophilism, with excessive secretion of adrenocortical hormone, characterized by obesity, moon-face, oligomenorrhea in women, and lowered testosterone levels in men, with additional involvement of osteoporosis, hypertension, kyphosis, polycythemia, and muscular weakness in both sexes (also called ***hypercortisolism***).

Dercum's disease: condition occurring mainly in females, accompanied by painful fatty swellings and nerve lesions, which may cause death from lung complications (also called ***adiposis dolorosa***).

erythroblastosis fetalis (e-rith″ro-blas-to′sis): excessive destruction of red blood cells, with overdevelopment of the erythropoietic tissues, or organs. It becomes evident late in fetal life, or soon after birth, as a result of transplacental passage of an anti-Rh antibody produced in an Rh-negative mother as a reaction to the Rh-positive red cells of the fetus, or by a transfusion of Rh-positive blood, with a possibility of also having an ABO incompatibility (also called ***hemolytic disease of the newborn***).

gout: condition in which there are urate deposits in the cartilages of the joints and an excess of uric acid in the blood, manifested by acute arthritic attacks, with some forms of gout involving severe constitutional disturbances, including renal impairment.

hemochromatosis: disorder of iron metabolism that may arise from exogenous, idiopathic, or hereditary causes, characterized by bronze pigmentation of the skin, diabetes mellitus, and hepatomegaly, with deposition of iron in parenchymal cells throughout much of the body, with liver cells particularly affected, and cirrhosis usually present (also called ***bronze diabetes***).

ochronosis: inherited or exogenous metabolic condition involving lack of homogentisic acid-oxidase activity in the kidney and liver, preceded by alkaptonuria, with a peculiar discoloration of the tissues of the body, due to the deposit of alkapton bodies in the sweat glands, sclera, cornea, conjunctiva, eyelids, and ears, as well as in the cardiovascular and genitourinary systems.

plumbism (plum′bizm): form of poisoning caused by the absorption of lead or one of the salts of lead. Symptoms include loss of appetite, colic, insomnia, headache, and dizziness, and more severe conditions extending to albuminuria, hypertension, anemia, and neuropathy with paralysis. It is commonly found in children who eat lead paint chips in poorly maintained lead-painted quarters, with resulting encephalopathy and secondary mental retardation (***plumbum*** means lead).

polycythemia vera: disease, etiology unknown, involving increase in red blood cell mass and total blood volume, producing splenomegaly, flushed face, and ecchymosis of the skin, with symptoms including headache, vertigo, and epistaxis (also called ***Osler's disease***).

Reye's syndrome: acute, noncontagious, childhood condition of unknown etiology (failure of the immune system is suspected, along with toxins that might unbalance metabolism and lead to liver damage). It is characterized by encephalopathy and fatty hepatomegaly, with brain swelling and central nervous system damage, generally following viral infections, especially influenza A and B strains, and chickenpox, and usually beginning with fever, vomiting, fatigue, apathy, and progressing, if untreated, to coma and death in 75% of cases (with some studies linking aspirin medication for viral conditions to toxicity that produces liver and brain damage).

sarcoidosis: chronic disorder, etiology unknown, characterized by multisystem granulomatous formations in mucous membranes, lacrimal and salivary glands, liver, spleen, lungs, skin, and lymph nodes.

scleroderma: disease involving hardening and shrinking of connective tissues, manifested by dermal fibrosis and fixation of the skin to underlying organs or structures, characterized by weakness, joint pains, edema of hands, and Raynaud's phenomenon. This syndrome is characterized by paroxysmal ischemia of the digits, progressing to systemic organ changes affecting skin, heart, esophagus, kidneys, lungs, etc., and can appear in a diffuse form with progressive fibrosis of internal organs, as well as of the skin of the trunk, face, and extremities (also called *systemic sclerosis*).

sudden infant death syndrome (SIDS): condition, etiology unknown, of a seemingly healthy infant who, when placed in a crib for rest or sleep, is later found dead. General agreement is that no single mechanism is responsible, but that SIDS babies may have defects of adaptation, with current views focusing on abnormal sleep patterns related to disturbed autonomic activity, on vagus nerve and cardiorespiratory reactions, and immunologic, metabolic, and endocrine factors (monitoring systems have been developed that set off alarms when the breathing pattern is interrupted for an excessive period—also called *crib death*).

systemic lupus erythematosus (SLE): chronic disease of suspected autoimmune origin involving many organ systems individually or in a variety of combinations, including a generalized connective tissue disease for which diagnosis is made by the LE test and antinuclear antibody test (ANA). Most patients have arthralgia, less than half have the classic butterfly rash, some have renal disease, some

have pleural effusion, and, commonly, anorexia, nausea, vomiting, abdominal pain, and lymphadenopathy are present. Exposure to sunlight or ultraviolet radiation exacerbates the disease.

Oncology*

adenocarcinoma*: malignant epithelial neoplasm appearing throughout the different systems of the body, such as salivary glands, bronchi, large intestine, connective tissue, kidneys, etc.

carcinomatosis*: widespread dissemination of cancer throughout the body (also called *carcinosis*).

Kaposi's sarcoma* (kap′a-sez): malignant neoplasm occurring in the skin, and metastasizing to the lymph nodes and viscera, beginning with purplish papules on the feet that slowly spread, occurring most often in men, and associated with malignant lymphoma, diabetes, and other disorders (also called *multiple idiopathic hemorrhagic sarcoma*; see also under *acquired immune deficiency syndrome*).

Laboratory Tests and Procedures

antinuclear antibody test (ANA): blood test to measure levels of ANA. Increased levels are positive for systemic lupus erythematosus, rheumatoid arthritis, chronic hepatitis, periarteritis nodosa, dermatomyositis, scleroderma, infectious mononucleosis, Raynaud's disease, and other diseases.

lupus erythematosus test (LE cell prep): blood test to diagnosis and monitor treatment for systemic lupus erythematosus.

sweat electrolytes test: detects elevations of sodium and chloride levels in sweat, for diagnosis of cystic fibrosis.

trypsin activity test: test on fecal matter to detect trypsin, for diagnosis of fibrocystic disease of sweat glands and other organs.

*Indicates a malignant condition.

Section V

Adding to the Structure

This is the last of the five sections of LEARNING MEDICAL TERMINOLOGY. This section completes the building process by including additional enrichment material.

This section contains the appendices, with the first appendix listing commonly used abbreviations and symbols. The second and third appendices include combining forms that relate to numbers, and the metric system and English equivalents for linear measures, weights, volumes, and temperatures. The fourth appendix lists the various board-regulated medical specialties in the United States. The last two appendices contain samples of various types of hospital records and reports, as well as medical insurance forms, with general instructions for their completion and use.

375

A

Abbreviations and Symbols

A

A accommodation; acetum; angstrom unit; anode; anterior

a accommodation; ampere; anterior; area

aā of each

A₂ aortic second sound

ABGs arterial blood gases

ABO three basic blood groups

AC alternating current; air conduction; axiocervical; adrenal cortex

a.c. before meals *(ante cibum)*

acc. accommodation

ACE adrenocortical extract

ACh acetylcholine

ACH adrenocortical hormone

ACTH adrenocorticotropic hormone

AD right ear *(auris dextra)*

ad lib. as much as desired *(ad libitum)*

add add to

ADH antidiuretic hormone

ADHD attention-deficit hyperactivity disorder

ADS antidiuretic substance

A/G; A-G ratio albumin-globulin ratio

Ag silver

ah hypermetropic astigmatism

AHF antihemophilic factor

AI aortic insufficiency

AIDS acquired immune deficiency syndrome

aj ankle jerk

Al aluminum

alb albumin

ALH combined sex hormone of anterior lobe of hypophysis

ALL acute lymphocytic leukemia

ALS amyotrophic lateral sclerosis

ALT alanine aminotransferase (formerly SGPT)

alt. dieb. every other day *(alternis diebus)*

alt. hor. alternate hours *(alternis horis)*

alt. noct. alternate nights *(alternis noctes)*

Am mixed astigmatism

A.M.A.; a.m.a. against medical advice

AML acute myelocytic leukemia

amp ampule

ana so much of each

AO anodal opening; atrioventricular valve openings

AOP anodal opening picture

AOS anodal opening sound

A-P; AP; A/P anterior-posterior

A.P. anterior pituitary gland

A & P auscultation and percussion

APA antipernicious anemia factor

AQ achievement quotient

Aq water *(aqua)*

ARC AIDS related complex; anomalous retinal correspondence

ARDS acute respiratory distress syndrome

arg silver

AS left ear *(auris sinistra)*

As arsenic

ASD atrial septal defect

ASH asymmetric septal hypertrophy

AsH hypermetropic astigmatism

ASHD arteriosclerotic heart disease

AsM myopic astigmatism

ASS anterior superior spine

AST aspartate aminotransferase (formerly SGOT)

Ast; As. astigmatism

ATS anxiety tension state; antitetanic serum

AU Angstrom unit

Au gold

A-V; AV; A/V arteriovenous; atrioventricular

Av average; avoirdupois

AVR aortic valve replacement

ax axis; axillary

B

B boron; bacillus

Ba barium

BAC buccoaxiocervical

Bact bacterium

BBB blood-brain barrier; bundle branch block

BBT basal body temperature

BE barium enema

Be beryllium

BFP biologically false positivity (in syphilis test)

Bi bismuth

bib. drink

bid; b.i.d. twice a day *(bis in die)*

BM bowel movement

BMR basal metabolic rate

BMT bone marrow transplant

BP blood pressure; buccopulpal

bp boiling point

BPH benign prostatic hypertrophy

BRP bathroom privileges
BSA body surface area
BSP bromsulphalein
BUN blood urea nitrogen
BWS battered woman syndrome

C

C carbon; centigrade; Celsius
c̄ with
C$_{alb}$ albumin clearance
C$_{cr}$ creatinine clearance
C$_{in}$ inulin clearance
CA chronologic age; cervicoaxial
C$_a$ calcium; cancer
CABG coronary artery bypass graft
CaCO$_3$ calcium carbonate
CAD coronary artery disease
Cal large calorie
cal small calorie
Cap. let him take *(capiat)*
CBC; cbc complete blood count
CC chief complaint
cc cubic centimeter
CCl$_4$ carbon tetrachloride
CCU coronary care unit
cf compare; bring together
CFT complement-fixation test
cg; cgm centigram
CH crown-heel (length of fetus)
CHCl$_3$ chloroform
CH$_3$COOH acetic acid
CHD coronary heart disease
ChE cholinesterase
CHF congestive heart failure
C$_5$H$_4$N$_4$O$_3$ uric acid
C$_2$H$_5$OH ethyl alcohol
CH$_2$O formaldehyde
CH$_3$OH methyl alcohol
Cl chlorine
CLD chronic liver disease
CLL chronic lymphocytic leukemia
cm centimeter
CMR cerebral metabolic rate
c.m.s. to be taken tomorrow morning *(cras mane sumendus)*
CMV cytomegalovirus
c.n. tomorrow night *(cras nocte)*
CNS central nervous system
c.n.s. to be taken tomorrow night *(cras nocte sumendus)*
CO carbon monoxide
CO$_2$ carbon dioxide
Co cobalt
COPD chronic obstructive pulmonary disease
CPC clinicopathologic conference
CPD cephalopelvic disproportion

CPR cardiopulmonary resuscitation
CR crown-rump (length of fetus)
C-section cesarean section
CSF cerebrospinal fluid
CSM cerebrospinal meningitis
CT; CAT computerized (axial) tomography scan
Cu copper
CuSO$_4$ copper sulfate
CVA cerebrovascular accident; costovertebral angle
CVD cardiovascular disease
cyl cylinder

D

D dose; vitamin D; right *(dexter)*
DAH disordered action of the heart
D/C discontinue
D & C dilation (dilatation) and curettage
DC direct current
DCA deoxycorticosterone acetate
deg degeneration; degree
det. let it be given *(detur)*
dg decigram
dieb. tert. every third day *(diebus tertiis)*
diff differential blood count
dil dilute; dissolve
dim one half
DCE discoid lupus erythematosus
DNA deoxyribonucleic acid
DOA dead on arrival
DOB date of birth
DPT diphtheria, pertussis, tetanus (vaccine)
DRG diagnosis-related group
dr dram; ℥
DSM Diagnostic and Statistical Manual of Mental Disorders
DTR deep tendon reflex
DTs delerium tremens
Dx diagnosis

E

E eye
EAHF eczema, asthma, and hayfever
EBV Epstein-Barr virus
ECG; EKG electrocardiogram; electrocardograph
ECT electroconvulsive therapy
ED erythema dose; effective dose
ED$_{50}$ median effective dose
EDC estimated date of confinement
EEG electroencephalogram; electroencephalograph
EENT eye, ear, nose, and throat
Em emmetropia
EMB eosin-methylene blue
EMC encephalomyocarditis
EMF erythrocyte maturation factor
EMG electromyogram

EMS Emergency Medical Service
ENT ear, nose, and throat
EOM extraocular movement
EPR electrophrenic respiration
ER emergency room (hospital); external resistance
ERG electroretinogram
ERPF effective renal plasma flow
ERT estrogen replacement therapy
ESR erythrocyte sedimentation rate
EST electroshock therapy
Et ethyl
ext extract

F

F Fahrenheit; field of vision; formula
FA fatty acid
FANA fluorescent antinuclear antibody (test)
F & R force and rhythm (pulse)
FBS fasting blood sugar
FD fatal dose; focal distance
Fe iron
FeCl$_3$ ferric chloride
FH family history
Fl; fld fluid
fl dr; fl. dr. fluid dram
fl oz; fl. oz. fluid ounce
FR flocculation reaction
FSH follicle-stimulating hormone
ft foot
FUO fever of undetermined origin

G

GA gingivoaxial
galv galvanic
GB gallbladder
GBS gallbladder series
GC gonococcus; gonorrheal
GFR glomerular filtration rate
GH growth hormone
GI gastrointestinal
GL greatest length (small flexed embryo)
GLA gingivolinguoaxial
Gm; gm gram
GP general practitioner; general paresis
gr grain(s)
grad by degrees (*gradatim*)
Grav I, II, III, etc. pregnancy one, two, three, etc. (*gravida*)
GSW gunshot wound
gt drop (*gutta*)
GTT glucose tolerance test
gtt drops (*guttae*)
GU genitourinary
Gyn; gyn gynecology

H

H hydrogen
Hb; Hgb hemoglobin
H$_3$BO$_3$ boric acid
HBV hepatitis B-virus vaccine
HCG human chorionic gonadotropin
HCl hydrochloric acid
HCN hydrocyanic acid
H$_2$CO$_3$ carbonic acid
HCT; Hct hematocrit
HD hearing distance
h.d. at bedtime (*hora decubitus*)
HDL high-density lipoprotein
HDLW distance at which a watch is heard by the left ear
HDRW distance at which a watch is heard by the right ear
He helium
HEENT head, ear, eye, nose, and throat
Hg mercury
HIV human immunodeficiency virus
HNO$_3$ nitric acid
H$_2$O water
H$_2$O$_2$ hydrogen peroxide
HOP high oxygen pressure
h.s. at bedtime (*hora somni*)
H$_2$SO$_4$ sulfuric acid
Ht; ht total hyperopia; height
Hy hyperopia

I

I iodine
^{131}I radioactive isotope of iodine (atomic weight 131)
^{132}I radioactive isotope of iodine (atomic weight 132)
IBD inflammatory bowel disease
ICS; IS intercostal space
ICSH interstitial cell-stimulating hormone
ICT inflammation of connective tissue
ICU intensive care unit
Id. the same (*idem*)
IH infectious hepatitis
IM intramuscular; infectious mononucleosis
IOP intraocular pressure
IQ intelligence quotient
IU immunizing unit
IUD intrauterine device
IV intravenous
IVP intravenous pyelogram
IVT intravenous transfusion
IVU intravenous urogram; intravenous urography

K

K potassium
k constant
Ka cathode; kathode

KBr potassium bromide
kc kilocycle
KCl potassium chloride
kev kilo electron volts
Kg kilogram
KI potassium iodide
kj knee jerk
km kilometer
KOH potassium hydroxide
KUB kidney, ureter, and bladder
kv kilovolt
kw kilowatt

L

L left; liter; length; lumbar; lethal; pound
L & A light and acccmmodation
lb pound *(libra)*
LB large bowel (x-ray film)
LBBB left bundle branch block
LCM left costal margin
LD lethal dose; perception of light difference
LDL low-density lipoprotein
LE lupus erythematosus
l.e.s. local excitatory state
LFD least fatal dose of a toxin
LFTs liver function tests
LH luteinizing hormone
Li lithium
LIF left iliac fossa
lig ligament
Liq liquor
LLL left lower lobe (of lung)
LLQ left lower quadrant
LMP last menstrual period
LP lumbar puncture
LPF leukocytosis-promoting factor
LTH luteotrophic hormone
LUL left upper lobe (of lung)
LUQ left upper quadrant
LV left ventricle
L & W living and well

M

M myopia; meter; muscle; thousand
m meter
MA mental age
mag large *(magnus)*
MBD minimal brain dysfunction
uc microcurie
uu micromicron
mcg; ug microgram
MCH mean corpuscular hemoglobin
MCHC mean corpuscular hemoglobin concentration
mc; mCi millicurie
MCV mean corpuscular volume

Me methyl
MED minimal erythema dose; minimal effective dose
mEq millequivalent
mEq/L milliequivalent per liter
ME ratio myeloid-erythroid ratio
Mg magnesium
mg milligram
MHD minimal hemolytic dose
mmHg millimeters of mercury
MI myocardial infarction
MID minimum infective dose
ML midline
ml milliliter
MLD median lethal dose; minimum lethal dose
MM mucous membrane
mm millimeter; muscles
mu millimicron
Mn manganese
mN millinormal
MRI magnetic resonance imaging
MS multiple sclerosis; mitral stenosis; morphine sulphate
MSL midsternal line
MT medical technologist; tympanic membrane *(membrane tympani)*
mu mouse unit
MVP mitral valve prolapse
My myopia

N

N nitrogen
n normal
Na sodium
NaBr sodium bromide
NaCl sodium chloride
Na$_2$C$_2$O$_4$ sodium oxalate
Na$_2$CO$_3$ sodium carbonate
NAD no appreciable disease
NaF sodium fluoride
NaHCO$_3$ sodium bicarbonate
Na$_2$HPO$_4$ sodium phosphate
NaI sodium iodide
NaNO$_3$ sodium nitrate
Na$_2$O$_2$ sodium peroxide
NaOH sodium hydroxide
Na$_2$SO$_4$ sodium sulfate
NCA neurocirculatory asthenia
Ne neon
NH$_3$ ammonia
Ni nickel
NPN nonprotein nitrogen
NPO; n.p.o. nothing by mouth *(non per os)*
NRC normal retinal correspondence
NTP normal temperature and pressure
NYD not yet diagnosed

O

O oxygen; oculus; pint
O₂ oxygen; both eyes
O₃ ozone
OB obstetrics
OBS organic brain syndrome
OD right eye *(oculus dexter)*; optical density; overdose
o.d. once a day *(omni die)*
Ol oil *(oleum)*
o.m. every morning *(omni mane)*
o.n. every night *(omni nocte)*
OPD outpatient department
OR operating room
OS left eye *(oculus sinister)*
os opening; mouth; bone
OT occupational therapy
OTD organ tolerance dose
OU each eye *(oculus uterque)*
oz ounce; ℥

P

P phosphorus; pulse; pupil
P₂ pulmonic second sound
P-A; P/A; PA posterior-anterior
P & A percussion and auscultation
PAB; PABA para-aminobenzoic acid
Pap test Papanicolaou smear
Para I, II, III, etc. live births: unipara, bipara, tripara, etc.
PAS; PASA para-aminosalicylic acid
Pb lead
PBI protein-bound iodine
p.c. after meals *(post cibum)*
PCP *Pneumocystis carinii pneumonia*
PCV packed cell volume
PD pupillary distance; prism diopter
PDA patent ductus arteriosus
PDR *Physician's Desk Reference*
PE physical education; physical examination
PEG pneumoencephalography
PET positron emission tomography
PFF protein-free filtrate
PGA pteroylglutamic acid (folic acid)
PH past history
pH hydrogen ion concentration (alkalinity and acidity measure)
pharm; phar. pharmacy
PI previous illness
PID pelvic inflammatory disease
PK psychokinesis
PKU phenylketonuria
PL light perception
PM post-mortem; evening
PMB polymorphonuclear basophil leukocytes
PME polymorphonuclear eosinophil leukocytes

PMI point of maximal impulse
PMN polymorphonuclear neutrophil leukocytes
PN percussion note
PNH paroxysmal nocturnal hemoglobinuria
PO; p.o. orally *(per os)*
p/o postoperative
PPD purified protein derivative (test for tuberculosis)
Pr presbyopia; prism
PRN; p.r.n. as required *(pro re nata)*
pro time prothrombin time
PSA prostate specific antigen
PSP phenosulfonphthalein
PT physical therapy
Pt platinum; patient
pt pint
PTA plasma thromboplastin antecedent
PTC plasma thromboplastin component
Pu plutonium
PUO pyrexia of unknown origin
PVC premature ventricular contraction
PZI protamine zinc insulin

Q

Q electric quantity
q. every; each
q.d. every day *(quaque die)*
q.h. every hour *(quaque hora)*
q.h.s. each bedtime *(quaque hora somni)*
qid; q.i.d. four times daily *(quater in die)*
q.l. as much as desired *(quantum libet)*
q.n. every night *(quaque nocte)*
qns quantity not sufficient
q.o.d. every other day *(quaque otro die)*
q.p. as much as desired *(quantum placeat)*
q.s. sufficient quantity
qt quart
Quat four *(quattuor)*
q.v. as much as you please *(quantum vis)*

R

R respiration; right; *Rickettsia;* roentgen
Rx take
Ra radium
rad unit of measurement of the absorbed dose of ionizing radiation
RAI radioactive iodine
RAIU radioactive iodine uptake
RBC; rbc red blood cell; red blood count
RCD relative cardiac dullness
RCM right costal margin
RE right eye; reticuloendothelial tissue; reticuloendothelial cell
Re rhenium
rect rectified
reg umb umbilical region
REM rapid eye movement

rep. let it be repeated *(repetatur)*
RES reticuloendothelial system
RF rheumatoid factor
Rh symbol of rhesus factor; symbol for rhodium
RhA rheumatoid arthritis
RHD relative hepatic dullness
RIA radioimmunoassay
RLL right lower lobe (of lung)
RLQ right lower quadrant
RM respiratory movement
RML right middle lobe (of lung)
Rn radon
RNA ribonucleic acid
R/O rule out
ROM range of motion
RPF renal plasma flow
RPM; rpm revolutions per minute
RPS renal pressor substance
RQ respiratory quotient
RT radiation therapy
RUL right upper lobe (of lung)
RUQ right upper quadrant

S

S sulfur
S. sacral
s̄ without *(sine)*
S-A; S/A; SA sinoatrial
SB small bowel (x-ray film)
SC closure of semilunar valves
Se selenium
SD skin dose
Sed rate; SR sedimentation rate
seq. luce. the following day *(sequenti luce)*
SGOT serum glutamic oxaloacetic transaminase (see *AST*)
SGPT serum glutamic pyruvic transaminase (see *ALT*)
SH serum hepatitis
Si silicon
SLE systemic lupus erythematosus
Sn tin
SOB shortness of breath
sol solution
sp spirit
SPECT single-photon emission computed tomography
sp. gr. specific gravity
Sr strontium
s̈s one half *(semis)*
Staph staphylococcus
Stat; stat immediately *(statim)*
STD sexually transmitted disease
STH somatotrophic hormone
Strep streptococcus
STS serologic test for syphilis
sym symmetrical

T

T temperature; thoracic
t temporal
T$_3$ triiodothyronine
T$_4$ thyroxine
TA; TAT toxin-antitoxin
T & A tonsillectomy and adenoidectomy
tab tablet
TAM toxoid-antitoxoid mixture
TB tuberculin; tuberculosis; tubercle bacillus
TE tetanus
TEM triethylene melamine
TENS transcutaneous electrical nerve stimulation
Th thorium
TIA transient ischemic attack
TIBC total iron-binding capacity
T.V. tidal volume
tid; t.i.d. three times daily *(ter in die)*
Tl thallium
TLC tender, loving care
Tm maximal tubular excretory capacity (kidneys)
TP tuberculin precipitation
TPI *treponema pallidum* immobilization (test for syphilis)
TPR temperature, pulse, and respiration
tr tincture
TRU turbidity reducing unit
TS test solution
TSH thyroid-stimulating hormone
TUR; TURP transurethral resection of prostate
Tx treatment

U

U uranium; unit
UA urinalysis
UBI ultraviolet blood irradiation
UIBC unsaturated iron-binding capacity
Umb; umb umbilicus
ung ointment *(unguentum)*
URI upper respiratory infection
US ultrasonic
USP *U.S. Pharmacopeia*
ut. dict. as directed *(ut dictum)*
UTI urinary tract infection
UV ultraviolet

V

V vanadium; vision; visual acuity
v volt
VA visual acuity
VC vital capacity
VD venereal disease
VDA visual discriminatory acuity
VDG venereal disease-gonorrhea
VDM vasodepressor material

VDRL Venereal Disease Research Laboratories (test for syphilis)
VDS venereal disease-syphilis
VEM vasoexciter material
VF field of vision
VHD valvular heart disease
VIA virus inactivating agent
VLDL very-low-density lipoprotein
VMA vanillylmandelic acid
VR vocal resonance
VS vital signs;volumetric solution
Vs venisection
VsB bleeding in arm *(venaesectio brachii)*
VSD ventricular septal defect
VW vessel wall

W

w watt
WBC; wbc white blood cell; white blood count
WD well-developed
WL wavelength
WN well-nourished
WR Wassermann reaction
Wt; wt weight

X

x-ray roentgen ray

Z

z symbol for atomic number
Zn zinc

Symbols

> Greater than
< Less than
♀ Female
♂ Male

B

Latin and Greek Combining Forms for English Numbers

Number	Latin term	Greek term
one	uni-	mon-, mono-
two	duo-	dy-, dyo-
three	tri-	tri-
four	quadri-, quadr-	tetr-, tetra-
five	quinqu-	pent-, penta-
six	sex-	hex-, hexa-
seven	sept-, septi-	hept-, hepta-
eight	octo-	oct-, octa-, octo-
nine	novem-, nonus-	ennea-
ten	deca-, decem-	dek-, deka-
one half	semi-	hemi-
one and one half	sesqui-	
one hundred	centi-	hect-, hecto-, hecato-
one thousand	milli-	kilo-
one-hundredth part	centi-	
one-thousandth part	milli-	
first	primi-	prot-, proto-
second	secundi-	deut-, deuto-, deutero
third	tert-	trit-, trito-
fourth	quart-	
fifth	quint-	
ninth	non-, nona-	
twice, duplication	di-, dis-	dys-

C

The Metric System and Equivalents

The basis of measurement in science is a standard one, the metric system, in which the chief units are the meter, the gram, and the liter, which are always multiplied and divided by 10.

Although the English system is still used in the United States, the metric system is the preferred system in medicine because of its logic and accuracy.

UNITS OF LENGTH

Metric linear decimal scale and English (U.S.) equivalents

10 millimeters	= 1 centimeter	= 0.3937 inches
10 centimeters	= 1 decimeter	= 3.937 inches
10 decimeters	= 1 meter	= 39.37 inches (3.2808 feet)
10 meters	= 1 dekameter	= 10.936 yards
10 dekameters	= 1 hectometer	= 19.884 rods
10 hectometers	= 1 kilometer	= 0.62137 mile
10 kilometers	= 1 myriameter	= 6.2137 miles

1 inch	= 2.54 centimeters or 25.4 millimeters
1 foot	= 3.048 decimeters or 304.8 millimeters
1 yard	= 0.9144 meter or 914.40 millimeters
1 rod	= 0.5029 dekameter
1 mile	= 1.6093 kilometers

UNITS OF VOLUME

Metric liquid measure capacity and English (U.S.) equivalents

1 milliliter (cc)		= 16.23 minims or 0.2705 fluidram or 0.0338 fluidounce
1 liter		= 33.8148 fluidounces or 2.1134 pints or 1.0567 quarts or 0.2642 gallon
1 fluidram		= 3.697 milliliters
1 fluidounce		= 29.573 milliliters
1 pint	= 16 ounces	= 473.166 milliliters or 0.473 liter
1 quart	= 2 pints	= 946.332 milliliters or 0.946 liter
1 gallon	= 4 quarts	= 3.785 liters

UNITS OF WEIGHT

Metric weights and English (U.S.) equivalents

1 milligram	= 0.001 gram	= 0.015 grain
1 centigram	= 0.01 gram	= 0.154 grain
1 decigram	= 0.10 gram	= 1.543 grains
1 gram	= (1 gram)	= 0.035 ounce
1 dekagram	= 10 grams	= 0.353 ounce
1 hectogram	= 100 grams	= 3.527 ounces
1 kilogram	= 1000 grams	= 2.205 pounds
1 grain	= 0.0648 gram	
1 ounce	= 28.349 grams	
1 pound	= 0.453 kilogram	

TEMPERATURE EQUIVALENTS

Conversion rules

To convert Fahrenheit to Centigrade (Celsius), subtract 32 from the Fahrenheit temperature and multiply that figure by 5/9.

To convert Centigrade (Celsius) to Fahrenheit, multiply the Centigrade temperature by 9/5 and add 32 to the total.

D

Medical Specialties

The American Board of Medical Specialties (ABMS) is concerned with establishing and maintaining standards of medical specialty practice. There are 23 individual boards that certify physicians choosing to practice in 24 specialty areas (Neurology and Psychiatry are separate specialties under one board).

AMERICAN BOARDS OF MEDICAL SPECIALTIES

American Board of Allergy and Immunology (A Conjoint Board of the American Board of Internal Medicine and the American Board of Pediatrics)
American Board of Anesthesiology
American Board of Colon and Rectal Surgery
American Board of Dermatology
American Board of Emergency Medicine
American Board of Family Practice
American Board of Internal Medicine
American Board of Neurological Surgery
American Board of Nuclear Medicine (A Conjoint Board of the American Boards of Internal Medicine, Pathology, and Radiology, and sponsored by the Society of Nuclear Medicine)
American Board of Obstetrics and Gynecology
American Board of Ophthalmology
American Board of Orthopaedic Surgery
American Board of Otolaryngology
American Board of Pathology
American Board of Pediatrics
American Board of Physical Medicine and Rehabilitation
American Board of Plastic Surgery
American Board of Preventive Medicine
American Board of Psychiatry and Neurology
American Board of Radiology
American Board of Surgery
American Board of Thoracic Surgery
American Board of Urology

MEDICAL SPECIALTIES

Allergy and Immunology (AI) are those specialties concerned with the identification and treatment of allergies and the study of immunity to disease. The physicians are called *allergists* and *immunologists*.

Anesthesiology (AN) is the branch of medicine devoted to the administration of a drug or gas to induce partial or complete loss of sensation with or without loss of consciousness. The physician is called an *anesthesiologist*.

Colon and Rectal Surgery (CR) is the surgical specialty dealing with surgery of the colon (large intestine) and the rectum and anus. The physician is a *proctologist*.

Dermatology (D) is the branch of medicine devoted to the study of the skin and its diseases. The medical specialist is called a *dermatologist*.

Emergency Medicine (EM) is the branch of medicine devoted to diagnosing, treating, and stabilizing trauma or crisis conditions.

Family Practice (FP) is the branch of medicine dealing with the care of all members of the family regardless of age or sex. The practitioner is often compared with one in general practice.

Internal Medicine (IM) is the branch of medicine dealing with diseases not usually treated surgically. The practicing physician is an *internist*.
Subspecialties of *Internal Medicine* are:

Cardiology is the study of diseases of the heart. The physician is a *cardiologist*.

Endocrinology is the study of the endocrine glands and their internal secretions. The physician is an *endocrinologist*.

Geriatrics or Gerontology is the study and treatment of diseases of the aged. The physician is a *geriatrician* or *gerontologist*.

Neurological Surgery (NS) is the surgical specialty concerned with surgical procedures on the nervous system. The physician is a *neurosurgeon*.

Nuclear Medicine (NM) is the branch of medicine concerned with the development and use of radioactive equipment and substances in diagnosis and treatment.

Obstetrics and Gynecology (OG) is the branch of medicine concerned with the care of women.

Obstetrics is devoted to the care of women during pregnancy, labor, delivery, and puerperium (the physician is an *obstetrician*).

Gynecology is devoted to the treatment of diseases of women, especially those of the genital, urinary, or rectal areas (the physician is a *gynecologist*).

Ophthalmology (OP) is the branch of medicine devoted to the treatment of disorders of the eye. The physician is an *ophthalmologist*.

Orthopaedic Surgery (OS) is the surgical specialty concerned with prevention and correction of deformities by use of surgical procedures. The physician is an *orthopedist*.

Otolaryngology (OT) is the medical specialty dealing with the study and treatment of diseases of the ear (otology), nose (rhinology), and throat (laryngology). The physician is an *otolaryngologist*.

Pathology (PA) is the branch of medicine that studies the causes and effects of disease and the resulting changes in structure and function. The physician is a *pathologist*.

Pediatrics (PD) is the branch of medicine concerned with care and treatment of children. The physician is a *pediatrician*. A subspecialty of pediatrics is:

Neonatology the branch of medicine that deals with the diseases and abnormalities of the newborn infant. The physician is a *neonatologist*.

Physical Medicine and Rehabilitation (PMR) is the branch of medicine devoted to the study and treatment of disease by mechanical and physical means.

Plastic Surgery (PL) is the surgical specialty concerned with restoration and repair of physical damage and defects.

Preventive Medicine (PRM) is the branch of medicine dealing with the prevention of both physical and mental illness.

Psychiatry (P) and Neurology (N) is the branch of medicine concerned with the structure and functioning of the nervous system and its diseases. Subspecialties include:

Psychiatry is devoted to diagnosis, treatment, and prevention of mental illness. The physician is a *psychiatrist*.

Neurology is devoted to the study of the nervous system and its diseases. The physician is a *neurologist*.

Radiology (R) is the branch of medicine concerned with the use of roentgen rays (x-rays) for diagnostic and therapeutic purposes. The physician is a *radiologist*.

Surgery (S) is the branch of medicine that treats deformities, defects, injury, and disease by use of surgical procedures. The physician is a *surgeon*.

Thoracic Surgery (TS) is the surgical specialty concerned with surgical procedures of the thorax (chest).

Urology (U) is the branch of medicine dealing with the study of the urinary tract in both sexes, and the male genital tract. The physician is a *urologist*.

E

Hospital Records and Reports

There are many different medical reports that are part of a patients hospital record, such as the diagnostic evaluation and pathologic and x-ray findings.

A notation of surgical instruments, techniques, and medications used is a part of hospital records, and the medical secretary must consult reference sources and medical dictionaries to spell these names correctly. Names of drugs, in particular, change from year to year, but each medical records department will have a copy of the *Physicians' Desk Reference (PDR)*, as well as a list of approved drugs published by the American Medical Association. The names of surgical instruments and techniques may also be found in various references available in the medical records department. Correct identification and spelling should present no problem when sources for reference are available.

Not all reports follow the same format. Each facility has specific forms for particular reports. The sampling in this appendix is to familiarize the reader with a variety of records and reports.

ADMISSION NOTE
Neurologic Hospital Report

This 5-year-old black male child was admitted to the emergency room shortly after being involved in a two-car accident. Apparently, the patient was thrown about 20 feet from the car into a ditch. He was unconscious when removed from the ditch by ambulance drivers shortly after the accident. He was then taken to a nearby hospital, where he was examined. It is reported that the patient appeared to be having intermittent convulsive activity and that his pupils were midposition and reactive, with the left pupil possibly larger than the right. He was transferred to the Neurologic Hospital for further evaluation.

On admission to the emergency room of the Neurologic Hospital, he is said to have been having seizure activity, or at least some activity of rigid contraction of muscles, more or less in extension but with no true *clonic* seizure activity, and vomiting.

When seen by a neurosurgeon a short while later, the patient was not having any seizure activity but was actu-

ally making some semi-purposive movements with his extremities. He moved his extremities reflexly in response to pain, the movement being generally somewhat extensor in type but not true *decerebrate rigidity. Babinski's signs* were easily elicited. The patient was *comatose* but not groaning. He had rapid breathing with a definite tendency toward periodicity, suggesting *Cheyne-Stokes respiration.*

The patient's pupils were midposition and promptly reactive to light. They were sometimes equal in size, and sometimes the left was slightly larger than the right. *Optic fundi* and *otoscopic* examinations were negative. There was a 4 cm *semilunar* laceration in the right *parietal* region.

The left side of the thorax was dull to percussion, but the breath sounds were equal on the two sides. Abdomen was lax. There was no evidence of *intracranial* bleeding. There was a *contusion* of the right elbow and a contusion of the posterior thorax bilaterally that appeared a short while later. From the beginning, a dark discoloration was noted in the midthorax posteriorly. There was no *crepitus* on palpation over the thorax.

There was a healed incision from a cutdown on the *left greater saphenous vein* in the past, and there was a *pilonidal* dimple.

Impression:

1. Cerebral contusion
2. Scalp laceration
3. Skull fracture (by x-ray examination)

CASE HISTORY

Admission Note:

This 65-year-old white female was admitted because of persistent *epigastric* and lower *substernal* pain off and on for the last 1 month. It is especially bad in the night, waking her up with an indigestion type of discomfort in the lower sternal area. After she gets up and walks around, she feels better. She has had a *myocardial infarction* in the past. She had a posterior myocardial infarction and since that time has been relatively symptom-free except for occasional *angina*. She had been taking nitroglycerine with some relief for angina. However, the pain was relieved usually by sitting up or changing positions. Because it was felt this could be cardiac or gastrointestinal or *hiatus hernia*, she was admitted to the hospital for a complete work-up. She has had no nausea, vomiting, diarrhea, black bowel movements, etc.

Past History:
Essentially negative except for myocardial infarct.

Review of Systems:
HEENT: Negative; no complaints.
Pulmonary: Negative; no cough, sputum, *hemoptysis*.
Cardiovascular: *Angina pectoris* with some nitroglycerine for relief.
GI: See admission note.
GU: Negative; no frequency, burning, *dysuria*.
Neuromuscular and arthritic: Has had some generalized arthritic discomfort off and on. However, has had no specific gallop or *rheumatoid arthritis*, mostly *osteoarthritis* symptoms.

Social History:
Does not drink or smoke.

Family History:
Essentially negative.

Physical Examination:
General: Well-developed, well-nourished. BP 128/ 80, pulse 84.
HEENT: Eyes, ears, nose, mouth, and pharynx are negative. Fundi reveals some arteriosclerotic changes.
Neck: Negative.
Lungs: Clear to percussion and auscultation.
Heart: Normal sinus rhythm, no murmers. Tones good.
Abdomen: Liver and spleen are not palpable. Some slight tenderness in the epigastrium. Lower abdominal examination is negative.
Extremities: Reveal good peripheral pulses. Reflexes are equal and active throughout.

Impression:
Rule out gastrointestinal disease.
Rule out *hiatus hernia*.
Rule out *duodenal ulcer*.
Arteriosclerotic heart disease with myocardial infarction in the past.

DISCHARGE SUMMARY

Final Diagnosis: *Idiopathic* convulsive disorder.

Chief Complaint: This is a second College Hospital admission for this 40-year-old black male who enters with the chief complaint of blacking out.

History of Present Illness: The patient was in excellent health until the day of admission when, without any warning or *aura*, he developed *tonic* and *clonic* muscle activity with complete loss of consciousness and his eyes rolled back (this was observed by his wife). This lasted less than 5 minutes. There was no tongue biting or *incontinence* of urine or stool. He returned to consciousness but with severe headaches and was confused and disoriented for about 45 minutes. He was first taken to Metropolitan Hospital, then College Hospital Emergency Room where a variety of tests were done including EKGs, times 2, which apparently were nonrevealing. He was sent to Dr. A's office. While waiting to see Dr. A, he suddenly felt sick to his stomach and had loss of consciousness and had a similar but less violent episode, again followed by confusion. He was then returned to the College Hospital Emergency Room for admission. For the past few days prior to admission the patient had been eating very little and working very hard. He had no prior history of preceding hunger, sickness, weakness, or *diaphoresis*. There was no history of any seizures or head trauma, febrile or serious childhood illness. The only medicine he takes is a nerve pill 4 times a day and a sleeping pill. The patient drank heavily until 10 years ago, one-half case of beer per day, but has not had any ethanol since. The patient was in an auto accident 5 days prior to admission but without any head trauma. Denies any history of diabetes.

Past History: The patient had a *varicose* vein stripping 1 year ago. Denies any allergies. Medications are as above. No blood transfusions.

Review of Systems: The patient has had a *pruritic erythematous* localized rash over the right arm for several weeks.

Family History: Father is 77 years old, has high blood pressure and congestive heart failure. Mother is 74 years old, has low blood pressure. Brother is 36 years old, alive and well. There is no family history of seizure disorders. The patient works for the Smith and Co., Manufacturers. He smoked 2 packs of cigarettes per day for 10 years; quit 19 years prior to admission.

Physical Examination: The patient is a well-nourished, well-developed male complaining of headache and diffuse myalgia. BP is 150/65; pulse is 96 and regular; respiration 12; he is *afebrile.*

HEENT: Reveals that there are no *bruits.* Pupils are equal and reactive. Fundi reveal sharp discs. Ears are normal.

Neck: Supple, carotids 2+ and equal, no jugular venous distension. Thyroid is not enlarged.

Skin: Reveals times 2 times 2 crowded *erythematous papules* on the right arm anteriorly; no nodes palpable.

Chest: Clear to *percussion* and *auscultation.*

Heart: Reveals PMI 8 cm left of midsternal line in fourth intercostal space. S_1 and S_2 are normal. Physiologic split of S_2. There is a loud apical S_4.

Abdomen: Soft and nontender without any *organomegaly* or masses. Bowel sounds are normal. Pulses are 2+.

Extremities: Reveal no *cyanosis,* clubbing, or edema. Pulses are full.

Rectal: Is normal.

Neurologic: Reveals patient is alert, oriented, intelligent, good recent and remote memory but slight confusion (for example, he could not remember his age). Speech was slightly slurred. Cranial nerves were intact. Motor coordination was intact as was sensory exam. DTRs were 3+ uniformly. Toes were downgoing. Gait was normal.

Laboratory Tests and Results: Admitting CBC was normal as was profile. EKG was also within normal limits.

Hospital Course: The patient had a brain scan and echo; both were within normal limits. LP was attempted but was unsuccessful. However, after the LP the patient developed severe *orthostatic,* throbbing-type headache which finally remitted prior to discharge. Cervical spine films were also normal. EEG reveals a large amount of low voltage symmetric alpha rhythm. There were also a few bursts of medium voltage beta delta waves on frontal and temporal areas. EEGs were consistent with a seizure disorder. The patient was started on Dilantin 100 mg, p.o., t.i.d., without any further seizure activity in the hospital.

Discharge Program: The patient was discharged to be followed by his doctor with medicine including Dilantin 100 mg p.o., t.i.d, and Benadryl 50 mg p.o., q.i.d for rash.

PHYSICAL EXAMINATION

General: An elderly, somewhat overweight, white male who is not acutely ill.

HEENT and Neck: Ears are negative; pupils react well; fundi show about a 1+ *sclerosis* of *retinal vessels;* no *papilledema* is noted. *Pharynx* is negative. *Thyroid* seems to be normal, but there are several tumor-like masses in the *supraclavicular* region on both sides. These masses are fairly movable, nonpainful, and do not seem to be tied down to surrounding tissue.

Chest: Respiration equal on both sides; lungs fairly clear, with only an occasional *rale* in the base.

Heart: By *percussion,* heart would seem to be enlarged slightly to the left; rate is 92/min and regular. The blood pressure is 130/70. There is a Grade IV *systolic murmur* at the *aortic* area, transmitted upward to the vessels of the neck and also transmitted downward toward the *apex. Apical* murmer does not follow the transmission around to the *axilla,* as seen with *mitral* lesions. I believe the aortic lesion is the main one here. The pulse is rather slow rising, consistent with *aortic stenosis.*

Abdomen: Right lower quadrant scar, inverted Y appearance from a *strangulated hernia* and *appendectomy.* Inguinal regions contain some slightly enlarged lymph glands on both sides. Abdomen shows a normal-sized liver. To the right of the scar, there seems to be an *incisional hernia* that protrudes slightly through the weakened abdominal wall. Spleen is definitely enlarged and comes down about two fingers on inspiration.

Genitalia: Testicles normal.

Rectal: Enlargement of the prostate gland (1+).

Impression: Congestive heart failure due to *arteriosclerotic* heart disease with *aortic stenosis,* calcific in type. Lymphatic pathology, type unknown.

SURGICAL PROCEDURES
Number 1

Surgical Procedure: *D & C,* total abdominal *hysterectomy,* bilateral *salpingo-oophorectomy,* and *lysis* of adhesions.

Procedure: The patient was placed in the *lithotomy* position on the operating table, and the *perineum* and *vagina* were prepared with Ioprep. Pelvic examination revealed the presence of a *marital introitus,* with normal external *genitalia.* There was good anterior and posterior support of the vaginal wall. The vagina was clean and well *epithelized,* as was the *cervix,* which was normal in appearance. *Bimanual* examination revealed an irregularly enlarged *uterus* the size of an 8-week *gestation*. The *adnexal* areas could not be identified as such. The operative site was draped with sterile towels and sheets, and the interior lip of the cervix was grasped with a sharp-tooth *tenaculum*. The *endometrial* cavity was sounded to a depth of 4½ inches, after which the *endocervical canal* was dilated with a No. 20 Hank dilator. *Endometrial curettage* was performed, revealing *submucous leiomyomata*. The dilation and curettage (D & C) was then dispensed with.

The anterior abdominal wall was prepared with Io-prep; the operative site was draped with sterile towels and sheets; and a Pfannenstiel incision was then made. The anterior *aponeurotic* flap was elected off the *rectus,* and the *peritoneal* cavity was entered in a longitudinal fashion. Examination of the pelvis revealed an irregularly enlarged uterus covered with *submural* and *subserous leiomyomata*. There were also a number of adhesions between the bowel and the anterior abdominal wall from a previous appendectomy site. *Lysis* of adhesions was carried out to free up the bowel, after which the *infundibulopelvic* ligaments were incised, the anterior leaves to the round ligaments, the posterior leaves to the *uterosacral* ligaments. The round ligaments were then ligated with No. 1 chromic catgut suture. An elliptic incision was carried out between the two round ligaments in such a way as to elevate the bladder flap away from the lower *uterine* segment of the uterus. The uterine vessels were visualized, bilaterally clamped with Dr. Long clamps, cut, and ligated with No. 1 chromic catgut suture. The lower portion of the broad ligaments was bilaterally clamped with Dr. Long clamps, cut and ligated with No. 1 chromic catgut suture. The *cardinal ligaments* were identified, bilaterally clamped with Dr. Long clamps, cut, and ligated with No. 1 chromic catgut suture. At this point it was noted that the *vagina* had been entered, and the *cervix* was then circumcised from the posterior vaginal vault. Aldridge sutures were placed at the angles, using No. 1 chromic catgut suture, after which the vagina was closed in a purse-string fashion with a running No. 1 chromic catgut suture.

Examination of the operative pedicles revealed good *hemostasis* to be present, although it was estimated that the total blood loss during the operative procedure was around 750 ml. A unit of blood was started at this point, and the *peritoneum* was closed, extraperitonealizing the entire operative site with chromic catgut suture. The *rectosigmoid* was then placed in the pelvis, and the peritoneum was picked up and closed in a running fashion. The *aponeuroses* of the *external-internal oblique* muscles were reapproximated, using interrupted No. 00 cotton suture. The subcutaneous and subcuticular tissues were reapproximated, using running No. 1 Dermalon suture.

Telfa and drygauze dressings were placed over the incision, after which the patient was returned to the recovery room in excellent condition.

Number 2

Preoperative Diagnosis: Anterior mediastinal mass; rule out malignancy.

Postoperative Diagnosis: Anterior mediastinal mass; malignant; probably carcinoma; rule out *lymphoma.*

Operation: *Mediastinoscopy* with biopsy of anterior mediastinal mass and frozen section.

Anesthesia: General.

Incision: Low cervical transverse incision.

Findings: Several enlarged lymph nodes in the anterior mediastinum just to the left of the trachea with a large, hard, necrotic appearing mass, just to the right and just over the trachea.

Procedure: After an adequate level of anesthesia was reached, the patient was prepared and draped in the usual sterile fashion. The above-mentioned incision was then made and carried down through the subcutaneous tissue, down through the *platysma. Hemostasis* was made and verified using curved Kellys and *electrocautery.* This brought into view the strap muscles, which were divided in a vertical direction using blunt and sharp dissection. Hemostasis was again made and verified using curved Kellys. The *isthmus of the thyroid* was visualized and an inferior thyroid vessel was clamped, cut and ligated, and tied with a No. 000 suture ligature of catgut. We then viewed the trachea and, using blunt dissection, the mediastinum was opened, just anterior to the trachea, with the above-mentioned findings. A large 1 × 1½ × ½ cm of soft lymph node was removed just from the right of the trachea and sent out for frozen section. Frozen section revealed a malignancy, probably carcinoma, but with no chance of it being a lymphoma. While waiting for the results of the lymph node dissection, two more biopsies were taken from a hard, necrotic mass, just to the right of the trachea. Hemostasis was verified at this point and the strap muscles were approximated using interrupted sutures of No. 000 Tab-Dek. The platysma was then approximated using interrupted sutures of No. 4/0 Tab-Dek and the skin was approximated using interrupted suture of No. 4/0 Tab-Dek. The dressing was placed on the wound, and the patient left the operating room in satisfactory condition.

Packs: None.

Drains: None.

Fluids: 1000 cc of D5 and lactated Ringer's.

Estimated Blood Loss: 50 cc.

Number 3

Preoperative Diagnosis: Hodgkin's disease.

Postoperative Diagnosis: Same.

Operation: Exploratory laparotomy for staging of Hodgkin's disease with *splenectomy,* liver biopsy, and *periaortic node biopsy*

Anesthesia: General

Incision: Midline

Findings: Enlarged spleen and a slightly mottled liver and a large periaortic lymph node.

Procedure: The patient was prepped and draped in the usual manner following successful general anesthesia. A midline incision was made down through the skin and subcutaneous tissue into the anterior fascia. The fascia was incised sharply and the abdomen was entered with hemostasis achieved by fine ligatures. Exploration of the abdomen revealed the above findings. At this time attention was turned toward the splenectomy. This was achieved by first dissecting on the gastrohepatic ligament for the splenic artery, which was difficult to find. Subsequently, the stomach was retracted superiorly and the lesser sac was entered. Dissection on top of the pancreas at this time revealed the splenic artery, and it was ligated in continuity with a No. 00 Poly-Dek ligature. Following this the spleen was dissected from its position by both blunt and sharp dissection brought into the midline abdominal wound. The pedicle of the spleen was then divided between large hemo clips without difficulty and the spleen was removed. A pack was placed in the left upper quadrant in the splenic bed and attention was turned toward a liver biopsy. Two sutures of No. 0 chromic were then placed in a figure-of-eight horizontal fashion such that a v was created at the edge of the liver and the liver between these two sutures was excised sharply. Another hemostatic suture was taken in the liver to ensure there would be no bleeding. Attention was then turned to the dissection of the periaortic region and lymph node biopsy. By the use of sharp and blunt dissection a portion of a large node in this

region of the celiac plexus was excised. Small bleeders were suture ligated and a pack was placed here. Prior to closure all the packs were removed. There was no evidence of bleeding and the abdominal wall was then closed with interrupted figure-of-eight Tom Jones No. 0 Tycron suture and the skin approximated with No. 4/0 silks.

Packs: None.

Drains: None

Tubes: NG tube in place.

The patient tolerated the procedure well and received 600 cc of lactated Ringer's. Estimated blood loss was 600 cc. Sponge count was correct, times two.

REPORTS OF ELECTROCARDIOGRAMS WITH CASE HISTORIES

During a cardiac cycle, the electrical changes in the heart will cause five distinct movements of the galvanometer string in the normal electrocardiogram. Three are directed upward, and two are directed downward. These five movements are designated as P, Q, R, S, and T. P, R, and T are directed upward, and Q and S are directed downward. The P wave is produced by spread of excitation wave over the *auricle.* The Q, R, S, and T movements, or deflections, are produced by the *ventricles;* the Q, R, S waves during the spread, and the T wave during the retreat, of the excitation wave. The P-R interval is the beginning of P to the beginning of QRS. The S-T interval is the interval elapsing between the end of the S wave and beginning of T.

Number 1

History: This 35-year-old white male was admitted to the hospital with symptoms of 6 weeks duration, consisting of *malaise,* fever, and aching of various joints. Prior to admission he became *dyspneic* and had to sit up to breathe. A *systolic* murmer was noted on the day of admission. Physical examination revealed a temperature of 102° F; pulse rate of 130; respirations, 24; blood pressure 90/60 mm Hg. Lungs were clear to *auscultation* and *percussion.* The heart was not enlarged, but there was a harsh *systolic* murmur in the *mitral* area. No *diastolic* murmur or thrill was noted. Abdomen and extremities were negative. Repeated blood cultures were positive for a *Streptococcus* of the *viridans* group, and the patient was given penicillin. *Tachycardia* persisted, and he developed congestive heart failure and died after an illness of approximately 4½ months.

Electrocardiogram: The QRS was 0.11 sec, and the right axis deviation was marked. Two days later the electrocardiogram showed a sinus rhythm with a rate of 84 per min. The P waves were low and the P-R interval was 0.24 sec. The QRS occupied 0.15 sec. The initial R wave in leads I and II was followed by a deep, wide S wave. In lead III the R wave was wide and was followed by an inverted T wave. The T waves were upright in leads I and II. The V leads were not taken. The initial axis of the QRS was calculated to be plus 76 degrees, and the final axis was calculated to be minus 178 degrees. The mean QRTS axis was calculated to be plus 172 degrees. The tracing was classified as a Type II right *intraventricular conduction block.*

Following autopsy the final anatomic diagnosis was considered to be rheumatic heart disease with *mitral* and *aortic valvulitis;* and *subacute bacterial endocarditis (Streptococcus),* with cardiac enlargement and Type II right *intraventricular conduction block* and congestive heart failure resulting from *myocardial* degeneration.

Number 2

History: This 36-year-old white female was admitted to the hospital because of *tachycardia* and a slightly elevated blood pressure on routine examination, which led to an electrocardiogram revealing a left intraventricular conduction block. She gave a history of exertional *dyspnea* and *palpitation* and at times a tight feeling in the interior chest. An occasional skipped beat was noted, especially at night. There had been no *orthopnea, angina* or *hemoptysis.* Past history revealed the usual childhood diseases, with no scarlet fever or known rheumatic fever. She did have a history of one episode of *gonorrhea* and had been treated for *arthritis.* She also gave a history of *asthmatic* attacks following colds. Further, she had had *lymphocytic choriomeningitis,* with no complications or *sequelae* noted.

Physical examination revealed blood pressure of 140/90 mm Hg on the left and 146/96 mm Hg on the right. Weight was 135 pounds, and height was 63 inches. Temperature was 99° F; pulse rate, 100; and respirations, 18. Fundoscopic examination was normal. Lungs were normal to auscultation and percussion. The heart was not enlarged to inspection, palpation, or percussion. Heart sounds were of good quality, with no murmurs. *Blood urea nitrogen* level was 11.4 mg/100 ml; *cholesterol* level was 167 mg/100 ml; *fasting blood* sugar level was 98 mg/100 ml; *hemoglobin* level was 97%; and total *leukocyte count was 8,900, with 68% neutrophils,* 24% *lymphocytes,* 6% *monocytes,* 1% *eosinophils,* and *basophils.*

Electrocardiogram: This revealed a sinus rhythm with a rate of 84 per min. The P waves were normal. The P-R interval was 0.14 sec, and the QRS occupied 0.13 sec, with a wide notched R_1, and R_2. The R_3 was wide, and S_3 constituted the final portion of the QRS. The T waves were upright in the limb leads. The chest leads revealed a delay in the intrinsicoid deflection of 0.08 sec in V_6. The initial axis of the QRS was calculated to be plus 50 degrees, and the final axis was calculated to be 0 degree. The mean axis of the QRS was calculated at plus 41 degrees. The tracing was classified as Type III left intraventricular conduction block.

Interpretation: At the time of discharge, her diagnosis was considered by exclusion to be *arteriosclerotic* heart disease; *coronary artery sclerosis;* and a Type III left intraventricular conduction block.

REPORTS OF ELECTROENCEPHALOGRAMS WITH CASE HISTORIES

Changes in electrical potential of the brain can be recorded by applying electrodes to the scalp and obtaining tracings of brain wave activity, which is called an electroencephalogram. The patterns of these brain wave tracings can be related to neurologic conditions, alterations of consciousness, and mental states, and are used for diagnosing seizure and brain stem disorders, and brain lesions or tumors.

Number 1

History: This 32-year-old black female had a skull fracture 3 years ago with unconsciousness for about 3 days. She began to have blackouts late this year, which have persisted and are now increasing in frequency, with up to three per week (they formerly occurred every 3 months). Severe headache for 5 to 10 minutes occurred during the first attack. The impression was a *chronic brain syndrome* associated with *trauma.*

Encephalogram: *Monopolar* leads from right and left *frontal, parietal, occipital, temporal,* and *anterior temporal* areas, bilaterally. *Bipolar* leads were also run. It was necessary to give sedation for sleep record.

Record: The waking frequency is a well-defined 9 per sec. Sleep shows random slowing. There are no *paroxysmal dysrhythmias* or *asymmetries.* Overventilation produced no buildup.

Interpretation: Normal EEG.

Number 2

History: This 38-year-old white male stated he had had two *grand mal seizures* recently, occurring five months apart. He stated he had incurred a head injury at the age of 6 when he was hit on the head by a baseball.

Encephalogram: Monopolar and bipolar leads were placed on frontal, parietal, occipital, temporal, and anterior temporal areas.

Record: The basic waking alpha is 10 per sec. Light sleep frequencies show rather low-voltage (flat) random slowing with variable frequencies and occasional (1 to 3 per sec) waves (14 per sec spindles are average). There are no asymmetries. On two isolated occasions, larval "slow" spikes appeared in the right temporal and anterior temporal leads. Overventilation produced marked buildup and 2 to 4 per sec slow waves.

Interpretation: Borderline normal record. Two questionable isolated spikes seen in the right temporal and right anterior temporal areas.

RADIOLOGIC REPORTS
Number 1

Salpingogram: Examination of the female pelvis after the transvaginal injection of contrast material shows that the uterine outline shows an *"arcuate"* uterine configuration. Some dilation and filling of the *endocervical* portion of the uterus are consistent with a local *endocervicitis.* Both fallopian tubes fill but the fimbriated end of the right tube is closed and forms a *hydrosalpinx.* A large dilated hydrosalpinx is also observed on the left, but after the injection of a second volume of dye a small amount of free peritoneal spillage is demonstrated.

Impression:

1. *Arcuate* uterus.
2. *Endocervicitis.*
3. The presence of a small *hydrosalpinx* is seen on the right, which is completely blocked.
4. A large hydrosalpinx is present on the left, but a small quantity of dye spills into the peritoneal cavity.

Number 2

Barium Enema, Large Bowel: There has been a history of surgical intervention in the large bowel. On the filled film there are *diverticula* present in the *distal descending* and *sigmoid* regions, as well as in the *ascending colon.* There is overlapping of bowel in the *transverse colon,* and whether this represents redundancy or a side-to-side *anastomosis* could not be determined either fluroscopically or radiographically. On the evacuation film there is noted contrast medium extending outside the bowel wall in the region of the *sigmoid diverticula,* and the possibility that these represent abscesses resulting from diverticulitis must be considered. The *terminal ileum* is visualized. No filling defects are seen.

Number 3

Gallbladder: The gallbladder is faintly visualized. No obvious stone is identified. The *cystic* and *common ducts* are seen and are within normal limits. There is good contraction following the fatty stimulus. Opaque medium is seen in the region of the *cecum* and *ascending colon.* The findings suggest a poorly functioning gallbladder.

Number 4

Retrograde Aortogram: The retrograde aortogram gives good visualization of the aorta and its arterial branches. There is noted persistent narrowing in the first portion of the left *renal* artery, with some *poststenotic* dilation. The right renal artery shows no gross abnormality.

PATHOLOGY REPORTS
Number 1

Gross: The specimen consists of approximately 10 ml of yellowish-white, very mucoid material (sputum), which is submitted for *cytologic* examination.

Microscopic: The *Papanicolaou smear* of sputum reveals sheets and strands of *mucus,* as well as a few *exfoliated stratified squamous epithelial cells* and some *bronchial epithelial cells.* No cells resembling carcinoma are seen within this sputum.

Diagnosis: Papanicolaou smear of sputum negative for maglignancy.

Number 2

Gross: This specimen consists of three irregular pieces of liver tissue measuring 1 to 2 cm in length and 1 cm in width. They have a yellowish-tan color and are rubbery in consistency. The *hepatic* lobules are fairly distinct.

There is also a *vermiform appendix* measuring 12 cm in length and 0.8 cm in diameter. The *serosal* surface is smooth and glistening. The vessels appear markedly dilated and congested. On cut section, the appendiceal wall is 2 mm in thickness. The lumen is filled with a greenish-brown *fecal* material. The mucosa is moderately congested. No ulcerations are seen. The attached *mesoappendix* is 1 cm in width.

Microscopic: Section of the liver reveal a normal *lobular* pattern. The liver cells are pale because of a moderate increase in *glycogen* content. The *portal* spaces have a light increase in *lymphocytes;* the *biliary ducts* and *portal veins* have normal features.

Sections of the appendix reveal an intact normal *mucosa.* The *lumen* is *patent* and filled with fecal material. In the *submucosa* there is a moderate increase in the fibrous tissue. The *lymphatic* tissue shows several *germinal* centers. The *muscularis* and *serosal* layers are unremarkable.

Diagnosis: Liver with mild *cholangitis; fibrosis* of appendix.

Number 3

Specimen: Rectal biopsy.

Preoperative Diagnosis: *Ulcerative colitis.*

Postoperative Diagnosis: Parasitic infestation.

Specimens
Gross description: The specimen is submitted as "rectal biopsy". It consists of two fragments of gray-tan tissue, which measures 4 × 3 × 1 mm each. The entire specimen is submitted in a single cassette.

Microscopic: Sections show *rectal mucosa* and small portion of underlying *submucosa* and *muscularis mucosa.* A focal area of chronic inflammation is seen in the submucosa. This inflammation is composed of *plasma cells, lymphocytes,* and *eosinophils.* In this area, mucosal gland architecture has been interrupted and many of the glands show regenerative epithelium. No crypt abscesses are seen. There is no evidence of granulomatous disease. These changes are compatible with but not diagnostic of *ulcerative colitis.*

Diagnosis: Chronic inflammation of rectum.

AUTOPSY REPORTS
Number 1
Male 68 years.

Clinical Diagnosis: Abdominal aneurysm.

Primary:
1. *Arteriosclerosis* of thoracic and abdominal aorta, coronary arteries (advanced), and renal and mesenteric arteries (moderate)
2. Old occlusion of circumflex branch of left coronary artery
3. Replacement of lower abdominal aorta by aorta-iliac bypass graft, bilaterally patent
4. Old *dissecting aneurysm* of ascending aorta with large (1 × 1.8 cm.) orifice
5. Dilation of aortic annulus, moderate (90 mm). (History of murmur of aortic insufficiency, significance unclear in light of dissecting aneurysm)
6. Small *fenistration* of aortic valve and patent guarded *foramen ovale*
7. Dilation and hypertrophy of left ventricle of heart (750 gm)
8. *Subendocardial myocardial infarct, anteroseptal* and *posterolateral,* old, with questionable valve (clinical history of rheumatic heart and recent small *apical infarct*)
9. Pulmonary congestion and edema
10. *Arteriolar nephrosclerosis,* moderate
11. Splenomegaly (350 gm)
12. Chronic passive congestion of liver and spleen

Accessory
1. *Diverticulosis* of sigmoid colon and rectum
2. Pulmonary *emphysema*, diffuse, moderate
3. *Cholelithiasis*
4. Calcification in pulmonary hilar lymph nodes
5. *Osteoporosis,* moderately advanced
6. Small *adenocarcinoma* of the prostate in left posterior lobe
7. Nodular *hyperplasia* of prostate with dilation and trabeculation of the bladder, advanced.

Number 2
Female 74 years.

Clinical Diagnosis: Congestive heart failure.

Primary:

1. Rheumatic *valvulitis* (mitral disease) (T-32, F-9136)
2. *Cardiomegaly,* moderate (450 gm) (T-32, M-7200)
3. Pulmonary *thromboemboli,* multiple, with infarcts of lower lobes of both lungs (T-28, M-5470, T-28, M-3710)
4. *Hydrothorax* (1800 cc right side, 300 cc left side)
5. Fibrous pleural adhesions, upper lobes, bilateral
6. Acute passive congestion of the liver and spleen, severe

Bacteriology   Culture: Blood   (heart):   no growth.

Summary: This 74-year-old female was admitted 2 weeks ago in terminal stage of congestive heart failure secondary to rheumatic valvular disease involving the mitral valve with moderate cardiomegaly (450 gm). The lung changes show multiple thrombeoemboli with segmental infarcts as well as fibrosis of lung parenchyma (popliteal veins do not show any thrombi). The changes in the *viscera* are secondary to passive congestion.

F

Medical Insurance

The importance of processing medical insurance claims has increased tremendously during the past few years because a large percentage of the population now is covered by either a service or an indemnity-type insurance with commercial firms, the Medicare program of the Social Security Administration, or a state-sponsored Medicaid program.

Due to the proliferation of computerized records, it is becoming more necessary for personnel in hospitals and offices to be computer-literate.

GENERAL RULES

When a patient is admitted to an outpatient clinic, an emergency room, or a hospital or consults a physician, it is necessary to establish immediately whether the patient has medical insurance. If he or she does, the name and address of the insured must be recorded exactly as they appear on the insurance identification card. In addition, the patient's age, policy number, insurer, and, if applicable, the group number and name of the employer, union, or association through which the person is insured also must be recorded.

AUTHORIZATION FOR RELEASE OF INFORMATION

An "authorization for release of information" appears on many insurance company forms, and only if it is signed by the patient will the physician or hospital representative discuss the patient's case with the insurance claims adjuster.

AUTHORIZATION FOR ASSIGNMENT OR PAYMENT

In policies written by commercial companies, where there are provisions for certain services by physicians and hospitals, the patient should sign the authorization to pay the hospital or physician directly. Be sure the form is dated. This authorization appears on many insurance forms, but if there is none on the form, have the patient sign and date one that you have for this purpose.

MULTIPLE INSURANCE POLICIES

It is important to learn the names of all companies by which the patient is insured. Many insurance policies allow only a small amount toward hospital room charges and services, whereas others allow larger benefits. Some insurance policies carry a pro rata clause or rider, which distributes the charges among different companies, with each paying a fair share of the expenses involved, in instances of multiple coverage. The patient may also be eligible for collection from a number of policies for any one illness. Claim forms for each of these policies will have to be filled out. It is important to note which insurance is primary and which is secondary.

WORKMEN'S COMPENSATION OR OTHER EMPLOYER LIABILITY LAWS

It is always necessary to ascertain whether the patient's illness or injury is incident to employment, because it may be covered under Workmen's Compensation laws or other employer liability laws. The forms for claims under Workmen's Compensation or other employer liability laws are processed in much the same manner as all other medical claims.

SPECIAL POINTS FOR PROCESSING MEDICAL CLAIMS

After the type of coverage is determined and the necessary authorizations obtained, there usually is no further need to be concerned with the insurance until the time comes for processing the claim. Before typing any claim form, thoroughly read the instructions and all questions and be sure you understand them. Never leave any blank spaces.

Keep two points in mind when insurance forms are filled out: the welfare of the patient and the fees you expect to collect from the insurance company. Reimbursements from insurance companies are benefits for the patient as well as sources of income for the physician.

All questions that arise over a claim should be referred to the proper insurance company for settlement because their agents know the conditions and stipulations of the policy. If additional information is needed to clarify a point, your office will be contacted.

When filing a hospital claim, include records of all diagnostic procedures, room fees, drug charges, surgical and medical procedures, uses of respirators, kidney dialysis machines or any other therapy (Fig. F-1).

In a medical office, patient records should contain all information necessary to file claims.

A primary consideration in filling out insurance claims is the need to use standardized, approved medical coding or terminology for all diagnoses and procedures. (Coding is in the *International Classification of Diseases* code books or, in the case of Medicare claims, in the current *Common Procedural Coding System).*

Accuracy is essential in completing any insurance form, including spelling names and copying numbers correctly. Some policies contain a clause stating that if a claim is not filed within a prescribed time period, benefits are disallowed, making timeliness of utmost importance. Copies of all completed claims filed must be kept for the record and to settle any disputes that may arise.

SPECIFIC MEDICAL CLAIM FORMS

This section contains a sample universal form HCFA-1500 (Health Insurance Claim Form) used in filing claims for commercial insurance, Medicare, Medicaid, and CHAMPUS (the Civilian Health and Medical Program of the Uniformed Services) (Fig. F-2, *A* and *B*). BlueCross and Blue Shield forms vary, and questions about processing these forms should be referred to the regional Blue-Cross or Blue Shield office (Fig. F-3, *A* and *B*).

MEDICARE

Medicare is the government health insurance program for persons 65 years of age or older, as well as certain disabled persons under age 65 covering approved hospital and medical costs.

The hospital insurance (part A) helps pay for hospital patient care, post-hospital care in a skilled nursing facility, and post-hospital home health care. The hospital and the extended-care facility must be approved by and be a participating member of Medicare.

The medical insurance (part B) helps pay for physician services, outpatient hospital services, and various approved medical services and supplies not covered by part A Medicare insurance.

Medicare specifies charges for diagnostically related groups (DRGs) and pays 80% of approved charges, with the balance paid by the patient or other insurance.

Forms are subject to revision from time to time, but copies of the latest forms and information can be sent directly to your office. Preprinted forms with physician name and provider number are available for a fee. Increasingly, Medicare encourages claims to be filed electronically by computer using Medicare-developed software.

All Medicare insurees have health insurance cards, with their name and identification number.

CHAMPUS

The Civilian Health and Medical Program of the Uniformed Services (CHAMPUS) is a federally sponsored, comprehensive health benefits program for dependents of uniformed services personnel, retired uniformed services personnel, and their dependents. It provides civilian health care with much of the cost paid by the government (see Fig. F-2, *A* and *B*).

HOSPITAL INSURANCE FORM	HIF (69)
GROUP OR INDIVIDUAL	

Spaced for Typewriter – Marks for Tabulator Appear on this Line

PATIENT'S NAME AND ADDRESS	DATE OF BIRTH
INSURED'S NAME IF PATIENT IS A DEPENDENT	INSURED'S SOC. SEC. NUMBER
NAME OF INSURANCE COMPANY	POLICY NUMBER

IF GROUP INSURANCE, NAME OF POLICYHOLDER (i.e. Employer, Union or Association through whom insured)

I HEREBY AUTHORIZE PAYMENT directly to the below named hospital of the hospital insurance benefits otherwise payable to me but not to exceed the balance due of the hospital's regular charges for this period of hospitalization. I understand I am financially responsible to the hospital for charges not covered by this authorization.

SIGNED (INSURED PERSON)

DATE

I HEREBY AUTHORIZE RELEASE OF INFORMATION, requested on this form, by the below named hospital.

SIGNED (PATIENT, OR PARENT IF MINOR)

DATE

DATE ADMITTED	TIME ADMITTED	AM PM	DATE DISCHARGED	TIME DISCHARGED	AM PM

COMPLAINT

DATE OF FIRST SYMPTOMS

DIAGNOSIS FROM RECORDS (IF INJURY GIVE DATE, PLACE OF ACCIDENT)

IS CONDITION DUE TO INJURY OR SICKNESS ARISING OUT OF PATIENT'S EMPLOYMENT?   Yes ☐   No ☐

OPERATIONS OR OBSTETRICAL PROCEDURES PERFORMED (NATURE AND DATE)

OTHER HOSPITAL COVERAGE: YES ☐ NO ☐ (IF "YES" NAME OF CARRIER)	IF PATIENT HAD OTHER THAN SEMI-PRIVATE ROOM, INDICATE MOST COMMON SEMI-PRIVATE DAILY RATE $................

HOSPITAL CHARGES: (COMPLETE THIS SECTION OR ATTACH COPY OF BILL WITH A DETAILED BREAKDOWN OF CHARGES)

ROOM AND BOARD			
	Ward	_____Days at $_____ Total	$_____
	Semi-Private	_____Days at $_____ Total	_____
	Private	_____Days at $_____ Total	_____
	Intensive Care Unit	_____Days at $_____ Total	_____
	Extended Care Facility	_____Days at $_____ Total	_____

OTHER CHARGES		
	Operating or Delivery Room	_____
	Anesthesia	_____
	X-Ray	_____
	Laboratory	_____
	EKG BMR	_____
	Physical Therapy	_____
	Medical and Surgical Supplies	_____
	Pharmacy (Except Take-Home Drugs)	_____
	Inhalation Therapy	_____
	Intravenous Solutions	_____
	TOTAL	$_____

TOTAL CHARGES $ _____
PAYMENT CREDITS–PATIENT $ _____
PAYMENT CREDITS–OTHER CARRIER (S) $ _____
BALANCE DUE $ _____

THIS FORM APPROVED BY THE HEALTH INSURANCE COUNCIL AND ACCEPTED FOR USE BY HOSPITALS BY THE AMERICAN HOSPITAL ASSOCIATION.

HOSPITAL

ADDRESS

TAKEN FROM RECORDS	SIGNED BY
ON: 19	

MEMORANDUM REGARDING DISPOSITION OF THIS FORM ON REVERSE SIDE

Figure F-1.   Individual Hospital Insurance Form.

Figure F-2A,   **Health Insurance Claim Form (Universal).**

```
                                                        HEALTH INSURANCE CLAIM FORM

                      REFERS TO GOVERNMENT PROGRAMS ONLY
```

MEDICARE AND CHAMPUS PAYMENTS: A patient's signature requests that payment be made and authorizes release of medical information necessary to pay the claim. If item 9 is completed, the patient's signature authorizes releasing of the information to the insurer or agency shown. In Medicare assigned or CHAMPUS participation cases, the physician agrees to accept the charge determination of the Medicare carrier or CHAMPUS fiscal intermediary as the full charge, and the patient is responsible only for the deduct- ible, coinsurance, and noncovered services. Coinsurance and the deductible are based upon the charge determination of the Medicare carrier or CHAMPUS fiscal intermediary if this is less than the charge submitted. CHAMPUS is not a health insurance program and renders payment for health benefits provided through membership and affiliation with the Uniformed Services. Information on the patient's sponsor should be provided in those items captioned "Insured;" i.e., items 3, 6, 7, 8, 9 and 11.

```
          SIGNATURE OF PHYSICIAN OR SUPPLIER (MEDICARE AND CHAMPUS)
```

I certify that the services shown on this form were medically indicated and necessary for the health of the patient and were personally rendered by me or were rendered incident to my professional service by my employee under immediate personal supervision, except as otherwise expressly permitted by Medicare or CHAMPUS regulations.

For services to be considered as 'Incident' to a physician's professional services, 1) they must be rendered under the physician's immediate personal supervision by his/her employee, 2) they must be an integral, although incidental part of a covered physician's service, 3) they must be of kinds commonly furnished in physician's offices, and 4) the services of nonphysicians must be included on the physician's bills.

For CHAMPUS claims, I further certify that neither I nor any employee who rendered the services are employees or members of the Uniformed Services (refer to 5 USC 5536).

No Part B Medicare benefits may be paid unless this form is received as required by existing law and regulations (20 CFR 422 510).

NOTICE: Any one who misrepresents or falsifies essential information to receive payment from Federal funds requested by this form may upon conviction be subject to fine and imprisonment under applicable Federal laws.

```
    NOTICE TO PATIENT ABOUT THE COLLECTION AND USE OF MEDICARE AND CHAMPUS INFORMATION
```

We are authorized by HCFA and CHAMPUS to ask you for information needed in the administration of the Medicare and CHAMPUS programs. Authority to collect information is in section 205 (a), 1872 and 1875 of the Social Security Act as amended and 44 USC 3101, 41 CFR 101 et seq and 10 USC 1079 and 1086.

The information we obtain to complete Medicare and CHAMPUS claims is used to identify you and to determine your eligibility. It is also used to decide if the services and supplies you received are covered by Medicare or CHAMPUS and to insure that proper payment is made.

The information may also be given to other providers of services, carriers, intermediaries, medical review boards and other organizations of Federal agencies as necessary to administer the Medicare and CHAMPUS programs. For example, it may be necessary to disclose information about the benefits you have used to a hospital or doctor.

With the one exception discussed below, there are no penalties under Social Security or CHAMPUS law for refusing to supply information. However, failure to furnish information regarding the medical services rendered or the amount charged would prevent payment of Medicare or CHAMPUS claims. Failure to furnish any other information, such as name or claim number, would delay payment of the claim.

It is mandatory that you tell us if you are being treated for a work related injury so we can determine whether workers' compensation will pay for treatment. Section 1877 (a) (3) of the Social Security Act provides criminal penalties for withholding this information.

```
                MEDICAID PAYMENTS (PROVIDER CERTIFICATION)
```

I hereby agree to keep such records as are necessary to disclose fully the extent of services provided to individuals under the State's Title XIX plan and Medical Assistance Program and to furnish information regarding any payments claimed for providing such services as the State Agency, its designee, or Health and Human Services may request. I further agree to accept, as payment in full, subject to audit, the amount paid by the Medicaid (Medical Assistance) program for those claims submitted for payment under that program, with the exception of authorized deductibles, coinsurance, copayment and spenddown.

SIGNATURE OF PHYSICIAN (OR SUPPLIER): I certify that (1) the services listed on the reverse side were medically indicated and necessary to the health of this patient and were personally rendered by me or under my personal direction; (2) the charges for such services are just, unpaid, actually due according to law and program policy and not in excess of regular fees; (3) the information provided on the reverse side of this claim is true, accurate and complete. I agree to comply with the provisions of the Civil Rights Act of 1964 and Section 504 of the Rehabilitation Act of 1973.

I understand that payment and satisfaction of this claim will be from Federal and/or State funds, and that any false claims, statements, or documents, or concealment of a material fact, may be prosecuted under applicable Federal or State laws.

Figure F-2B, Health Insurance Claim Form (Universal) (cont'd).

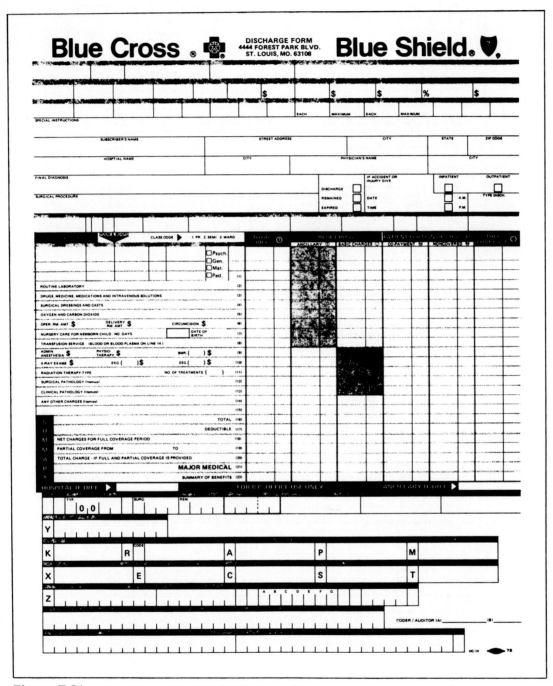

Figure F-3A,   Blue Cross-Blue Shield Discharge Form.

Saint Louis
BLUE SHIELD PLAN
MISSOURI MEDICAL SERVICE
P.O. BOX 14656 • ST. LOUIS, MISSOURI 63172

A Non-Profit Medical Surgical Service Program

PHYSICIAN'S SERVICE REPORT

RECIPROCITY

IF WORKMEN'S COMPENSATION DO NOT SEND REPORT TO BLUE SHIELD.
IF YOUR PATIENT IS NOT A MEMBER OF ST. LOUIS BLUE SHIELD, AND YOUR PATIENT'S IDENTIFICATION CARD DOES NOT
INDICATE ⟺ (RECIPROCITY) PLEASE SEND THIS REPORT DIRECTLY TO THE BLUE SHIELD PLAN TO WHICH THE PATIENT BELONGS.

NUMBER

| PATIENT'S LAST NAME | FIRST NAME | M. INITIAL | BIRTH DATE (Month Day Year) | SEX 1=MALE 2=FEMALE | GROUP NO | CERTIFICATE OR IDENT. NO |

| YOUR PATIENT ACCOUNT NO. | RELATIONSHIP 1=SUBSCRIBER 2=SPOUSE 3=CHILD 4=OTHER (SPECIFY) | IF IN HOSPITAL SHOW HOSPITAL NAME | ADMISSION DATE | DISCHARGE DATE | ADMITTING DR 1=YES 2=NO |

SUBSCRIBER'S LAST NAME   FIRST NAME   M. INITIAL   PHYSICIAN'S NAME AND ADDRESS

STREET ADDRESS

CITY   STATE   ZIP CODE

1=YES 2=NO   DOES PATIENT HAVE MEDICARE PART B?   COVERAGE CODE

WAS THIS A TRAUMATIC ACCIDENTAL INJURY?   1=YES 2=NO   DATE OF ACCIDENT MO. DAY YR   DESCRIPTION OF ACCIDENT   PATIENT SOCIAL SEC. NO.

DOES THIS PATIENT HAVE OTHER GROUP MEDICAL—SURGICAL COVERAGE?
1=YES 2=NO 3=UNKNOWN

PATIENT'S SIGNATURE (IF AVAILABLE)   1=YES 2=NO   OCCUPATIONAL ILLNESS OR INJURY?

ICDA CODE OR DIAGNOSIS OR NATURE OF ILLNESS OR INJURY REQUIRING SERVICES OR SUPPLIES (PATIENT'S CHIEF COMPLAINT OR SET OF SYMPTOMS)   1=YES 2=NO   COMPLICATION OF PREGNANCY?

DID ANOTHER PHYSICIAN RENDER SERVICES DURING THIS ADMISSION?   DID YOU USE OUTSIDE LABORATORY?   CHARGES TO YOU

1=YES 2=NO   GIVE NAME, ADDRESS AND SPECIALTY   1=YES 2=NO   GIVE NAME, ADDRESS AND CHARGES

DATES OF SERVICE						SERVICE		PROCEDURE CODE	NO VISITS	DESCRIBE SURGICAL OR MEDICAL PROCEDURES AND OTHER SERVICES OR SUPPLIES FURNISHED FOR EACH DATE GIVEN.	TOTAL CHARGES	FOR OFFICE USE ONLY			
FROM			TO			PL OF	TYPE OF					A.P.	C.C.	D.C	A.R.
MO.	DAY	YR.	MO.	DAY	YR.										

I, A DULY LICENSED PHYSICIAN, PERSONALLY PERFORMED OR SUPERVISED THE ABOVE SERVICES.

DATE SIGNED

TOTAL CHARGES	
AMOUNT PAID	
BALANCE DUE	

SPECIMEN

PHYSICIAN'S SIGNATURE

PLACE OF SERVICE
1. IN-PATIENT HOSPITAL
2. OUT-PATIENT HOSPITAL
3. OFFICE
4. HOME
8. EXTENDED CARE FACILITY
9. AMBULANCE
0. OTHER
A. INDEPENDENT LAB

TYPE OF SERVICE
A. MEDICAL EMERGENCY
B. CONCURRENT MEDICAL CARE
C. PSYCHIATRIC CARE
D. PHYSICAL THERAPY
E. RADIATION THERAPY
G. PROSTHETIC DEVICES
H. OTHER SERVICES OR SUPPLIES

J. HOME CARE SERVICE
M. VISION CARE
Q. CHEMOTHERAPY
T. RADIOIMMUNOASSAY
V. HEARING CARE

2. SURGICAL
3. OBSTETRICAL
4. ANESTHESIA
5. DIAGNOSTIC X-RAY
6. MEDICAL CARE

7. DENTAL
8. PATHOLOGY OR LAB
9. CONSULTATION
0. SURGICAL ASSISTANT

Figure F-3B, Blue Cross-Blue Shield Discharge Form (cont'd).

Bibliography

Ackerman D: A natural history of the senses, New York, 1990, Random House.

American Psychiatric Association: Diagnostic and statistical manual of mental disorders, ed 4, Washington, DC, 1994, American Psychiatric Association.

Asimov I: Isaac Asimov's book of facts, New York, 1979, Grosset & Dunlap.

Anderson KN, Anderson LE, and Glanze WD: Mosby's medical, nursing and allied health dictionary, ed 4, St Louis, 1994, Mosby.

Austrin MG: Sony medical transcription program, 1974, Sony Corp of America.

Berne RM and Levy MN: Cardiovascular physiology, ed 6, St Louis, 1992, Mosby.

Carson RC, Butcher JN, and Coleman JC: Abnormal psychology and modern life, ed 8, Glenview, Ill, 1987, Scott, Foresman & Co.

Department of Health and Human Services, Health Care Financing Administration: Guide to health insurance for people with medicare, Baltimore, Md.

Department of Health and Human Services, Social Security Administration: Your medicare handbook, Baltimore, Md.

Dorland's illustrated medical dictionary, ed 27, Philadelphia, 1988, WB Saunders Co.

Finegold M: Diagnostic microbiology, ed 7, St Louis, 1986, The CV Mosby Co.

Fordney MT: Insurance handbook for the medical office, Philadelphia, 1988, WB Saunders Co.

Ganong WF: Review of medical physiology, Los Altos, Calif, 1989, Lange Medical Publications.

Gilroy J and Holliday PL: Basic neurology, New York, 1982, Macmillan Publishing Co.

Gleitman H: Psychology, ed 2, 1986, WW Norton.

Gould JA III, editor: Orthopaedic and sports physical therapy, ed 2, St Louis, 1990, Mosby.

Groer ME and Shekleton ME: Basic pathophysiology: a conceptual approach, ed 3, St Louis, 1989, The CV Mosby Co.

Guyton AC: Textbook of medical physiology, ed 7, Philadelphia, 1986, WB Saunders Co.

Irwin S and Tecklin JS, editors: Cardiopulmonary physical therapy, ed 2, St Louis, 1990, Mosby.

Jaffe MS and Melson KA: Laboratory and diagnostic cards: clinical implications and teaching, St Louis, 1988, The CV Mosby Co.

Kuby J: Immunology, Salt Lake City, 1992, WH Freeman & Co.

McAleer N: The body almanac, 1985.

Miller FF and Keane CB: Encyclopedia and dictionary of medicine, nursing, and allied health, ed 4, Philadelphia, 1987, WB Saunders Co.

Nurnberg M and Rosenblum M: All about words: an adult approach to vocabulary building, Englewood Cliffs, NJ, 1966, Prentice-Hall.

Pagana KD and Pagana TJ: Mosby's diagnostic and laboratory test reference, St Louis, 1992, Mosby-Yearbook, Inc.

Perry AG and Potter PA: Clinical nursing skills and techniques, ed 2, St Louis, 1990, The CV Mosby Co.

Schroeder SA and others, editors: Current medical diagnosis and treatment, Norwalk, Conn, 1990, Appleton & Lange.

Seeley RR, Stephens TD, and Tate P: Anatomy and physiology, ed 2, St Louis, 1992, Mosby.

Selye H: The stress of life, New York, 1956, McGraw-Hill Book Co.

Stedman's medical dictionary, ed 24, Baltimore, 1982, The Williams & Wilkins Co.

Taber's cyclopedic medical dictionary, ed 15, Philadelphia, 1985, FA Davis Co.

Thibodeau GA and Patton KT: The human body in health and disease, St Louis, 1992, Mosby-Yearbook, Inc.

Thibodeau GA and Patton KT: Structure and function of the body, ed 9, St Louis, 1992, Mosby-Yearbook, Inc.

Thompson JM and others: Mosby's manual of clinical nursing, ed 2, St Louis, 1989, The CV Mosby Co.

Tilkian SM, Conover MB, and Tilkian AG: Clinical implications of laboratory tests, ed 4, St Louis, 1987, The CV Mosby Co.

Umphred DA, editor: Neurological rehabilitation, ed 2, St Louis, 1990, Mosby.

Varmus HE and Weinberg RA: Genes and the biology of cancer, Holmes, Pa, 1992, Scientific American Library.

Wilson EO: The diversity of life, Cambridge, Mass, 1992, Harvard University Press

Periodicals
The American Scientist
Discover
The Journal of the American Medical Association
The New England Journal of Medicine
Nursing
RN
Science
Scientific American

Index

A

A blood type, 147
A-, 11
Ab-, 11
AB blood type, 147
Abbreviations and symbols, 377-383
Abdomen and thorax, terms related to, 57
Abdominal aorta, descending, 150
Abdominal aortography, 173
Abdominal cavity, 200-201
Abdominal muscles, 106-107, 119
  lateral, 56, 57
Abdominal viscera, transposition of, 216
Abdominocentesis, 218
Abducens nerve, 290, 303
Abduction, 75, 118
Abductor muscles, 118
ABO blood grouping, 147
Abortion, 255
  spontaneous, 254
Abruptio placentae, 253
Abscess, Brodie's, 94
-ac, 15
Acanthokeratodermia, 134
Accessory spleen, 364
Accommodation, 321, 322, 338
Accordion graft, 137
Acetabulum (acetabula), 72, 91
Achalasia, 216
Achilles tendon, 108, 118
Achilles tendon reflex, 292
Achlorhydria, 216
Acholia, 216
Achondroplasia, 94
Achromatopia, 340
Achromatopsia, 340
Achylia, 216
Acidophil, 276
Acne, 134
Acne rosacea, 135
Acoustic nerve, 290, 303
Acoustic neurofibromatosis, bilateral, 371
Acoustic neuroma, 344
Acquired immune deficiency syndrome, 366-367
Acquired immunity, 352
Acrocephaly, 94
Acromegaly, 94, 278
Acromial process, 91
Acromioclavicular joint, 93
Acromion, 68, 91
Acrophobia, 314
Actinic dermatitis, 134
Actinic keratosis, 136
Actinomycosis, 367
Activated partial thromboplastin time, 173
Active immunity, 352, 362
Ad-, 11
Adam's apple, 176

Addis count, 249
Addison's disease, 278
Adduction, 75, 118
Adductor brevis muscle, 108, 118
Adductor longus muscle, 108, 118
Adductor magnus muscle, 108, 118
Adductor muscles, 108, 118
Aden/o-, 26
Adenocarcinoma, 373
  adrenal gland, 279
Adenocystic carcinoma, 193
Adenohypophysis, 276
Adenoids, 349
Adenoma
  basophilic, 279
  bronchial, 193
  chromophobic, 279
  eosinophilic, of pituitary gland, 279
  feminizing, of adrenal gland, 279
  Hurthle cell, of thyroid gland, 279
  virilizing, of adrenal gland, 279
Adenomyosarcoma, 248
Adenomyosis of uterus, 253
Adenosis, sclerosing, 254
Adhesions of iris, 340
Adip/o-, 40
Adipose tissue, 52, 63, 124
Adiposis dolorosa, 372
Adiposogenital dystrophy, 278
Adjectival roots and combining forms, 36-39
Admission note, 388-389
Adrenal cortex, 266, 277
  hormones of, 264
Adrenal cortical carcinoma, 279
Adrenal glands, 266-267, 276
  feminizing adenocarcinoma of, 279
  feminizing adenoma of, 279
  hormones of, 264
  virilizing adenocarcinoma of, 279
  virilizing adenoma of, 279
Adrenal hyperplasia, congenital, 278
Adrenal medulla, 266, 277
  hormones of, 264
Adrenalectomy, 279
Adrenaline, 264, 267, 276
Adrenalitis, 278
Adren/o-, 26
Adrenalopathy, 276
Adrenocortical hyperfunction, 278
Adrenocortical hypofunction, 278
Adrenocorticotrophin, 276
Adrenocorticotropic hormone, 263, 265
Adrenocorticotropin, 263, 265
Adrenogenital syndrome, 278
Adrenoleukodystrophy, 306
Adrenopathy, 276
Aerophagia, 216
Affective disorders, 313, 314

Afferent neurons, 281, 303
Age-related macular degeneration, 340
Ageusia, 345
Ageustia, 345
Agglutination inhibition test, 256
Agglutinin, trichina, 122
Aglossia, 216
Agoraphobia, 314
Agranulocytes, 146
Agranulocytosis, 170
Agraphia, 315
AIDS, 366-367
AIDS-related complex, 367
AIDS serology tests, 365
Air cells, ethmoidal, 190
Aknephascopia, 340
-al, 15
Ala (alae), 326
Ala nasi, 189
Alar cartilage, 93
Alastrim, 367
Albers-Schonberg disease, 95
Albinism, 136, 340
Albuminuria, 247
Albus, 40
Alcoholic hallucinosis, acute, 313
Alcoholic psychoses, 313
Aldosterone, 264, 266, 276
Aldosterone assay, 280
Aldosteronism, 278
Aleukemic leukemia, 170
Alexia, 315
-algia, 15
Algophobia, 314
Alimentary tract, 195, 196, 213; see also
      Gastrointestinal system
Alkaline phosphatase, total, 222
Alkalosis, altitude, 170
Allergic dermatitis, 134
Allergic rhinitis, 191
Allergy, 386
  skin, 134-135
Allograft, 96
Alopecia, 136
Alpha-fetoprotein, 256
Altered pupillary reflexes, 340
Altitude alkalosis, 170
Alveolar cell carcinoma, 193
Alveolar ducts, 177, 189
Alveolar nerve, 303
Alveolar sacs, 177
Alveolectomy, 219
Alveolus (alveoli), 177, 189, 213
Alzheimer's disease, 308
Ambi-, 11
Ambly-, 340
Amblyopia, 340
Amebiasis, 367

405

Amelia, 94
Ameloblastoma, 218
Amenorrhea, 253
Amentia, 315
American boards of medical specialties, 386
Ametro, 340
Ametropia, 340
Aminotransferases, 222
Ammonia, serum, 312
Amnesia, 315
  retrograde, 310
Amniocentesis, 256
Amniography, 256
Amnion, 234, 251
Amniotic fluid, 234
Amniotomy, 255
Amphetamines, 318
Amphi-, 11
Amphiarthroses, 73, 93
Ampho-, 11
Ampulla, 213
Amyelencephalia, 306
Amyelia, 306
Amygdala, 287
Amylase, 222, 223
Amyl/o-, 40
Amyloid beta-protein precursor test, 311
Amyloidosis, 371
Amyoplasia congenita, 94
Amyotonia, congenital, 121
Amyotrophia, 121
Amyotrophic lateral sclerosis, 309
Amyotrophy, 121
An-, 11
Ana-, 11, 50
Anabolism, 50
Anal canal, 201, 213
Analgesia, 315
Anastomosis (anastomoses), 91, 172, 220-221
  within periosteum, 66
Anatomic planes, 55
Anatomic positions, 55, 56
Anatomy, 49
  external, roots and combining forms related to,
    23-24
  internal, roots and combining forms related to,
    26-28
Ancylostomiasis, 215
Androgen, 229, 264, 266
Androsterone, 276
Anemias, 169-170
Anencephalia, 94, 306
Anencephaly, 306
Anepia, 315
Anergic, 315
Anesthesia, 315
Anesthesiology, 386
Aneurysm, 170
Aneurysmectomy, 172
Aneurysmoplasty, 172
Aneurysmorrhaphy, 172
Aneurysmotomy, 172
Angialgia, 170
Angiectasis, 171
Angiectomy, 172
Angina, 170
Angina pectoris, 170
Angi/o-, 26
Angiocardiogram, 173
Angiocardiography, radionuclide, 174
Angiodynia, 170
Angiogram, 173
Angiography
  celiac, 222
  cerebral, 311-312
  renal, 250

Angiomatosis, cerebroretinal, 371
Angiomatosis retinae, 341
Angiomegaly, 170
Angionecrosis, 170
Angioneurectomy, 172
Angioneurotic edema, 134
Angioneurotomy, 172
Angioparalysis, 170
Angioplasty, 172
  coronary, percutaneous ltransluminal, 173
  excimer laser, 173
Angiorrhaphy, 172
Angiosclerosis, 171
Angiostenosis, 171
Angiostomy, 172
Angiotensin-converting enzyme, 365
Angiotomy, 172, 364
Anhidrosis, 134
Aniridia, 340
Aniseikonia, 340
Anisopia, 340
Ankle bones, 66
Ankyl/o-, 36
Ankyloglossia, 216
Ankylosis, 97
  artificial, 96
Annular pancreas, 216
Anomia, 315
Anophthalmia, 340
Anophthalmos, 340
Anoplasty, 219
Anorchism, 253
Anorexia, 216, 273
Anorexia nervosa, 313
-anosmia, 345
Anosognosia, 315
Antagonists, 101, 118
Ante-, 11
Antebrachial vein, 168
Anterior, 54
Anterior commissure, 286, 301
Anthracosis, 192
Anthrax, 367
Anti-, 11
Antianxiety drugs, 318
Antibody(ies), 350, 362
  humoral, 362
  monoclonal, 363
Antideoxyribonuclease B, 249
Antidepressant drugs, 318
Antidiuretic hormone, 263, 264, 265, 276-277
Antigen, 147, 362
  Australian, 222
  carcinoembryonic, 222
  prostate specific, 256
  Rh, 147
Antimanic drugs, 318
Antinuclear antibody test, 373
Antipsychotic drugs, 318
Antisepsis, 3
Antisocial personality disorder, 313, 314
Antrum, 213
Anuresis, 247
Anuria, 247
Anus, 201, 213
Anusitis, 215
Anxiety disorders, 313, 314
Anxiety states, 313
A.O. Hardy-Rand-Rittler test, 342
Aorta, 142, 149, 166
  ascending, 149
  coarctation of, 170
  descending, 150
  dextroposition of, 170
  transposition of, 170
Aortic arch, 149, 166

Aortic insufficiency, 171
Aortic valve, 164
Aortitis, 168
Aortography, abdominal, 173
Aortotomy, 172
Ap-, 11
Apathy, 315
Apex nasi, 189
Apex pulmonis, 189
Aphakia, 340
Aphasia, 309
Aphonia, 191, 315
Aphthous stomatitis, 134, 215
Apicostomy, 220
Aplastic anemia, 169
Apnea, 191
Apo-, 11
Apocrine sweat gland, 125, 133
Apolipoprotein test, 173
Aponeurosis, 99, 118
Appendage, atrial, 164
Appendectomy, 219
Appendicitis, 215
Appendicular skeleton, 66-68, 72-73
Appendix, 213
  vermiform, 201
Apraxia, 315
Aqua, 39
Aquaphobia, 314
Aqueduct of Sylvius, 285, 302
Aqueous chamber, 338
Aqueous humor, 320, 321, 338
Arachnitis, 305
Arachno, 283
Arachnodactylia, 95
Arachnodactyly, 94
Arachnoid, 283, 301
Arachnoiditis, 305
Arcus senilis, 340
Areola, 133, 233, 250
Areolar tissue, 52, 63, 124
Argininosuccinic lyase, 222
Arms, muscles of, 104
Arnold-Chiari syndrome, 306
Arrector pili muscle, 124, 133
Arrest, cardiac, 171
Arrhenoblastoma, 254
Arrhythmia, 171
Arterial plethysmography, 173
Arteriectomy, 172
Arteri/o-, 26
Arteriography, renal, 250
Arteriolar nephrosclerosis, 247
Arterioles, 143, 166
Arteriol/o-, 26
Arteriolonecrosis, 171
Arteriolosclerosis, 171
Arteriomalacia, 171
Arterionecrosis, 171
Arterioplasty, 172
Arteriorrhaphy, 172
Arteriosclerosis, 171-172
Arteriospasm, 171
Arteriostenosis, 171
Arteriotomy, 173
Arteritis, 168
Artery (arteries), 143, 149-151, 166-167; see also
    specific artery
Arthr-, 73
Arthralgia, 97
Arthrectomy, 96
Arthritis, 94
  rheumatoid, 352, 364
Arthr/o-, 26
Arthrocele, 97
Arthrocentesis, 96

Arthrodesis, 96
Arthrodynia, 97
Arthrography, 97
Arthrolithiasis, 97
Arthrology, 73, 93
Arthroneuralgia, 97
Arthroonychodysplasia, 95
Arthropathy, 97
Arthroplasty, 96
Arthrosclerosis, 97
Arthroscopy, 97
Arthrosis, 97
Arthrotomy, 96
Articular cartilage, 73, 93
Articular disks, 73
Articulation, 93
Artificial ankylosis, 96
Artificial cardiac pacemaker, 173
Artificial immunity, 352, 362
Artificial skin graft, 137
Arytenoid cartilage, 176, 189
Arytenoidectomy, 193
Arytenoiditis, 190
Arytenoidopexy, 193
Asbestosis, 192
Ascariasis, 215, 367
Ascending aorta, 149
Ascending colon, 201
Ascending pharyngeal artery, 166
Ascending tracts, 301
Aschoff's node, 164
Ascites, 216
Aspartate aminotransferase, 173
Aspergilloma, 190
Aspermia, 253
Asphyxia, 192
Aspiration, 193
    bone marrow, 97, 173
    puncture for, 218
Assignment, authorization for, 397
Asthenia, 315
Asthma, 192
Astigmatism, 340
Astragalus bone, 73, 91
Astraphobia, 314
Astro-, 282, 303
Astroblastoma, 310
Astrocytes, 282, 303
Astrocytoma, 310
Ataxia, 309
    cerebral, 309
    Friedreich's, 307
Ataxia telangiectasia, 306
Ataxic cerebral palsy, 309
-ate, 15
Atel-, 306
Atelectasis, 192
Atelencephalia, 306
Atelomyelia, 306
Atelorachidia, 306
Atherectomy, coronary, directional, 173
Atherosclerosis, 171
Athetoid cerebral palsy, 309
Athetos, 309
Athetosis, 309
Atlanto-, 91
Atlantoaxial joint, 93
Atlas, 71, 91
Atonic pseudoparalysis, 121
Atresia, 216
    of vagina, 253
Atria, 151
Atrial appendage, 164
Atrial myxoma, 172
Atri/o-, 26
Atriotomy, 173

Atrioventricular bundle, 142, 164
Atrioventricular node, 142, 164
Atrioventricular valves, 164
Atrium (atria), 141, 151, 164
Atrophy, muscular; see Muscular atrophy
Attention deficit disorder, 316
Attention deficit hyperactivity disorder, 313
Audi-, 324
Audi/o-, 33
Audiometer, 344
Audiometry, 344, 345
Auditory meatus, external, 324
Auditory nerve, 290, 303
Auditory ossicles, 324
Auditory tube, 343
Aura, 309
Auricle, 324, 343
Auricular, 57
Auricular muscle group, 103
Auricular nerve, posterior, 303
Auricular posterior artery, 166
Auricular vein, 167
Auriculares muscle group, 118
Auriculotemporal nerve, 304
Auris, 324, 343
Auscultation, 194
Australian antigen, 222
Aut-, 11
Autism, 315
Auto-, 11, 315
Autodermic skin graft, 137
Autoeroticism, 315
Autoimmune disease, 349, 352
Automatism, 315
Autonomic nervous system, 142, 292, 301
Autophony, 344
Autopsy reports, 395-396
AV node, 142, 164
Aversion therapy, 318
Avoidant personality disorder, 313
Axial skeleton, 66-71
Axial tomography, computerized; see Computerized
        axial tomography
Axillary, 56, 57
Axillary artery, 150, 166
Axillary lymph nodes, 347
Axillary vein, 151, 167
Axis, 71, 91
Axon, 63, 281, 303
Azotemia, 247
Azygos vein, 167
Azygous, 102

B

B blood type, 147
Babinski reflex, 292
Back
    median region of, 56, 57
    muscles of, 104
Bacteremia, 169
Bacterial skin infections, 135
Bacterial vaginitis, 252
Bagassosis, 192
Balance, sense of, 327
Balanitis, 247
Balan/o-, 26
Balanus, 229
Ball-and-socket joints, 74, 93
Ballistocardiogram, 173
Banti's disease, 364
Barium enema, 222
Bartholinitis, 252
Bartholin's glands, 232, 250-251
Basal cell carcinoma, 136
Basal layer of skin, 124, 134

Basalis vein, 167
Basedow's disease, 278
Basia, 309
Basilar artery, 166
Basilar membrane, 325
Basilic vein, 151, 167, 168
Basiotripsy, 255
Basophilic adenoma, 279
Basophils, 146, 165, 277
B-cells, 350, 362
    development of, 351
Beau's lines, 136
Beck Depression Inventory, 314
Bedsore, 134
Behavior modification, 318
Behavior therapy, 318
Bekesy audiometry, 344
Bell's palsy, 309
Bender Visual Motor Gestalt Test, 315
Bends, 372
Benton Test of Visual Retention-Revised, 315
Benzodiazepines, 318
Beriberi, 371-372
Berylliosis, 192
Bestiality, 315
Bi-, 11, 102
Biceps, 118
Biceps brachii muscle, 104
Biceps femoris muscle, 108, 119
Biceps reflex, 292
Bicuspid, 213
Bicuspid valve, 141, 164
Bifid clitoris, 253
Bilateral acoustic neurofibromatosis, 371
Bile, 213
Bile duct(s), 202
    common, 202, 214
Biliary, 213
Biliary system, 202
Bilirubin, 222
Bio-, 33
Biology, 49
Biopsy, 122, 137, 222
    bone marrow, 97
    chorionic villus, 256
    excisional, 137
    punch, 137
Bipolar disorder, 313
Bladder, 246
    urinary, 227
Bleb, 134
Blennorrhagia, 247
Blennorrhea, 247
Blepharectomy, 341
Blepharitis, 339
Blephar/o-, 23, 320
Blepharon, 338
Blepharoplasty, 341
Blepharorrhaphy, 341
Blepharospasm, 340
Blepharosphincterectomy, 341
Blepharotomy, 341
Blindness, 340-341
Blister, 134
Block, heart, 171
Blood, 52, 144-147
    ABO grouping of, 147
    circulation of, 148
    clotting mechanism of, 147
    Rh factor in, 147
    terms related to, 165
Blood cells, 144-147
Blood count, 174
Blood culture, 173
Blood poisoning, 169
Blood pool imaging, 174

Blood pressure, 147
Blood sampling, percutaneous umbilical, 256
Blood tests related to gastrointestinal system, 222
Blood types, 147
Blood vessels
    major, 149-151
    terms related to, 165
    types of, 143
Blue Cross-Blue Shield discharge form, 401-402
Bodal's test, 342
Body fluids, roots and combining forms related to,
    39
Body regions, 56-57
Bolus, 49
Bone(s), 52
    cancellated, 65
    cancellous, 65
    classification of, 66-69
    composition of, 65
    cranial, 70
    cuboid, 91
    facial, 70
    flat, 66
    of foot, 73
    growth of, 66
    of hands, 72
    innominate, 72
    irregular, 66
    long, 66
    of lower extremities, 72-73
    marble, 95
    sesamoid, 92
    short, 66
    skull, principal, 70
    structural descriptive terms of, 69
    structure of, 65-66
    of upper extremities, 72
    wrist, 72
Bone conduction tests, 345
Bone marrow, 65
Bone marrow aspiration, 97, 173
Bone marrow biopsy, 97
Bone marrow transplantation, 173
Bone scan, 97
Bone tissue, compact, 65
Bone x-ray, 97
Bony tissue, 63
Borderline personality disorder, 313
Botulism, 367
Botulus, 367
Bourneville's disease, 308
Bowman's capsule, 224, 226, 246
Brachial artery, 150, 166
Brachial plexus, 291
Brachialis muscle, 104, 118
Brachi/o-, 23
Brachiocephalic artery, 149, 166
Brachiocephalic vein, 151, 167
Brachioradialis muscle, 118
Brachy-, 36
Brachytherapy, volumetric interstitial, 311
Brady-, 36
Bradycardia, 171
Bradykinesia, 315
Bradylalia, 309
Bradyphrenia, 315
Bradypragia, 315
Bradypsychia, 315
Brain, 284-287, 301
Brain elecrical activity map, 311
Brain scan, 311
Brainstem, 284-285
Breasts, 232-233
    fibrocystic disease of, 252
    lactating, 231
Brenner tumor, 254

Brev/i-, 36
Bridge of nose, 189, 326
Brief Psychiatric Rating Scale, 314
Brill-Summers disease, 364
Broca's speech area, 286
Brodie's abscess, 94
Bromsulphalein, 222
Bronch/i-, 26
Bronchial adenoma, 193
Bronchial tree, 177, 189
Bronchial vein, 167
Bronchiectasis, 190
Bronchiolar carcinoma, 193
Bronchioles, 177, 189
Bronchioli, 189
Bronchiolitis, 190
Bronchiol/o-, 26
Bronchitis, 190
Bronch/o-, 26
Bronchocephalitis, 191
Bronchogenic carcinoma, 193
Bronchogram, 194
Broncholithiasis, 192
Bronchoplasty, 193
Bronchoplegia, 192
Bronchopneumonia, 190-191
Bronchorrhagia, 192
Bronchorrhaphy, 193
Bronchorrhea, 192
Bronchoscopy, 194
Bronchosinusitis, 191
Bronchospasm, 192
Bronchostenosis, 192
Bronchostomy, 193
Bronchotomy, 193
Bronchus (bronchi), 177, 189
Bronze diabetes, 372
Brown-Sequard syndrome, 309
Brucellosis, 367
Brunner's glands, 214
Buccal, 57
Buccal smear, 137
Buccal surface of tooth, 213
Buccinator muscle, 103, 118
Buccinator nerve, 304
Bucc/o-, 23
Bulb of eye, 320
Bulbar paralysis, progressive, 310
Bulbourethral glands, 229, 250
Bulimia, 216, 313
Bulla, 134
Bundle
    atrioventricular, 164
    of His, 142, 164
Bursa(e), 74, 93
Bursectomy, 96
Bursitis, 74, 94
Bursotomy, 96
Butyrophenomes, 318
Bypass graft, coronary artery, 173
Byssinosis, 192

C

Cachexia, 216, 278, 279
Caffey's disease, 95
Caisson disease, 372
Calcaneal tendon, 118
Calcaneo-astragaloid joint, 93
Calcaneocuboid joint, 93
Calcaneofibular joint, 93
Calcaneonavicular joint, 93
Calcaneoscaphoid joint, 93
Calcaneotibial joint, 93
Calcaneum, 91
Calcaneus, 68, 73, 91

Calcified cartilage, 93
Calcinosis, 372
Calcinosis cutis, 136
Calcitonin, 264, 266, 277
Calculus (calculi), 216
    renal, 247
    urinary, 248
Calix, 246
Callosities, 136
Caloric test, 344
Calvaria, 91
Calyx (calyces), 224, 246
Canal, 69
    of Schlemm, 322, 338
Cancellated bone, 65
Cancellous bone, 65
Candidiasis, 367
    genital, 252
Candidosis, 252, 367
Canine tooth, 196
Canker sores, 134, 215
Canth/, 341
Canthectomy, 341
Cantholysis, 341
Canthoplasty, 341
Canthotomy, 341
Canthus (canthi), 322, 338
Capillary(ies), 143, 165, 328
Capillary fragility test, 173
Capitate bone, 72, 91
Capit/o-, 23
Capsulectomy, 341
Capsulorrhaphy, 96
Capsulotomy, 96, 341
Carbon dioxide, 189
Carbuncle, 135
Carcinoembryonic antigen, 222
Carcinoma
    adenocystic, 193
    adrenal cortical, 279
    alveolar cell, 193
    basal cell, 136
    bronchiolar, 193
    bronchogenic, 193
    cervical, 254
    epidermoid, 137, 193
    epithelial, 136
    hair-matrix, 136
    Hurthle cell, of thyroid gland, 279
    hypernephroid, 248
    intraepidermal, 136
    lenticular, 136-137
    neomammary, 254
    oat cell, 193
    renal cell, 248
    signet ring cell, 218
    small cell, 193
    squamous cell, 137, 193
    transitional cell, 248
    tuberous, 137
    verrucous, 137
Carcinoma acutaneum, 136
Carcinomatosis, 373
Carcinosis, 373
Cardiac arrest, 171
Cardiac catheterization, 173
Cardiac cycle, 142-143
Cardiac edema, 171
Cardiac hypertrophy, 171
Cardiac murmur, 171
Cardiac muscle, 100, 118, 141; see also heart
Cardiac muscle tissue, 52, 53, 63
Cardiac pacemaker, artificial, 173
Cardiac prosthesis, 173
Cardiac sphincter muscle, 199
Cardiac vein, 167

Cardialgia, 171
Cardiectasis, 171
Cardi/o-, 26
Cardiocentesis, 173
Cardiodynia, 171
Cardiohepatomegaly, 171
Cardiology, 386
Cardiomalacia, 171
Cardiomegaly, 171
Cardiomyoliposis, 171
Cardionecrosis, 171
Cardioptosis, 171
Cardiotomy, 173
Cardiovascular system, 54, 141-174
    hereditary, congenital, and developmental
        disorders of, 170
    inflammations and infections of, 168-169
    laboratory tests and procedures on, 173-174
    oncology related to, 172
    pathologic conditions of, 168-169
    surgical procedures on, 172-173
Carditis, 169
Caries, 94, 216
Carotenemia, 171
Carotid arteries, 149, 150, 166
Carotid body tumor, 172
Carpal bones, 66, 67, 69, 72
Carpectomy, 96
Carp/o, 23
Carpometacarpal joint, 93
Carpus, 91
Cartilage, 52, 93; *see also* specific cartilage
    laryngeal, 175-176
    terms related to, 93
Cartilaginous joints, 73
Case history, 388-389
Cat scratch disease, 367
Cat scratch fever, 367
CAT; *see* Computerized axial tomography
Cata-, 11, 50
Catabolism, 50
Catalepsy, 315
Cataphasia, 315
Cataract, 341
    congenital, 340
Cataract implant, 341
Catatonia, 315
Catatonic schizophrenia, 314
Catecholamine test, 280
Catheterization, cardiac, 173
Catheterized urine specimen, 249
Cathexis, 315
Cauda, 54, 291
Cauda equina, 291, 304
Caudal, 54
Caus-, 33
Caut-, 33
Cavernous urethra, 227
Cavity; *see* specific cavity
Cecal junction, 201
Cecectomy, 219
Cecocolostomy, 220
Cecoileostomy, 220
Cecopexy, 220
Cecorrhaphy, 218
Cecostomy, 220
Cecum, 201, 213
Cel-, 36
-cele, 15, 169
Celiac, 213
Celiac angiography, 222
Celiac trunk, 166
Celiocentesis, 218
Celioenterotomy, 219
Celiogastrotomy, 219
Celiorrhaphy, 218

Celiotomy, 219
Cell-mediated immunity, 362
Cell(s), 49, 50-51
    air, ethmoidal, 190
    blood, 144-147
    composition of, 50-51
    diagram of, 50
    hair, of ear, 325
    interstitial, 229
    killer (K), 351, 363
    Leydig, 229, 250
    memory, 350, 351, 363
    natural killer (NK), 351, 363
    null, 351, 363
    osseous, 92
    plasma, 350, 363
    Sertoli's, 250
    stem, 144
    structures of, 50
Cell body, 281
Cellular immunity, 362
Cellulitis, 135, 252
Cementoma, 218
Cementum, 196
-centesis, 15, 218
Central deafness, 344
Central incisors, 196
Central nervous system, 283-286, 301
Central neurofibromatosis, 371
Centrosome, 63
Cephalalgia, 309
Cephalic vein, 151, 167
Cephalin-cholesterol flocculation, 222
Cephal/o-, 23
Cephalocele, 307
Cephalodynia, 309
Cephalon, 302
Cerebellar artery, 166
Cerebellar hemispheres, 285
Cerebellar vein, 167
Cerebell/o-, 26
Cerebellomedullary malformation syndrome, 306
Cerebellum, 285, 302
Cerebral angiography, 311-312
Cerebral aqueduct, 285, 302
Cerebral artery, 166
Cerebral ataxia, 309
Cerebral cortex, 286, 302
Cerebral fissures, 286
Cerebral hemispheres, 286
Cerebral hemorrhage, 308
Cerebral palsy, 309
    Lesch-Nyhan, 307
Cerebral sphingolipidosis, 307
Cerebral vein, 167
Cerebralgia, 309
Cerebr/i-, 26
Cerebr/o-, 26
Cerebromeningitis, 305
Cerebroretinal angiomatosis, 371
Cerebrospinal fluid, 287, 302
Cerebrospinal fluid scan, 312
Cerebrospinal fluid tests, 312
Cerebrospinal syphilis, 305
Cerebrospinal system, 301
Cerebrovascular accident, 308
Cerebrum, 286, 302
Cerumen, 40, 125, 343
Ceruminous glands, 125
Cervical artery, transverse, 167
Cervical lymph nodes, 347
Cervical plexus, 291
Cervical vein, 167
Cervical vertebrae, 68, 71
Cervicectomy, 255
Cervicitis, 252

Cervic/o-, 23
Cervix, 232, 251
    carcinoma of, 254
    hypoplasia of, 253
Cesarean section, 255
Chagas' disease, 370
CHAMPUS, 403
Charcot-Marie-Tooth disease, 307
Charcot's disease, 309
Cheeks, 195-196
Cheilitis, 215
Cheil/o, 23
Cheiloplasty, 219
Cheilorrhaphy, 218
Cheilosis, 372
Cheilotomy, 219
Cheir/o-, 23
Chest x-ray, 194
Chiasm, 302
Chiasma, optic, 286, 302, 322, 339
Chickenpox, 367
Chiggers, 135
Chilblain, 134
Chil/o-, 23
Chir/o-, 23
Chlamydia, 252
Chlor/o-, 40
Chloros, 40
Choana, 189
Choanae osseae, 189
Chol-, 202
Cholangiocholecystocholedochectomy, 219
Cholangioenterostomy, 220
Cholangiogastrostomy, 220
Cholangiography, 222
Cholangiohepatoma, 218
Cholangiojejunostomy, 220
Cholangiolitis, 215
Cholangioma, 218
Cholangiostomy, 220
Cholangiotomy, 219
Cholangitis, 215
Chole-, 39, 202
Cholecyst, 213
Cholecyst-, 202
Cholecystectomy, 219
Cholecystenterostomy, 220
Cholecystitis, 215
Cholecystocolostomy, 220
Cholecystoduodenostomy, 220
Cholecystogastrostomy, 220
Cholecystography, 222
Cholecystoileostomy, 220
Cholecystojejunostomy, 220
Cholecystolithotripsy, 221
Cholecystomy, 219
Cholecystopexy, 220
Cholecystorrhaphy, 218
Cholecystotomy, 219
Choledochectomy, 219
Choledoch/o-, 26
Choledochocholedochostomy, 220
Choledochoduodenostomy, 220
Choledochoenterostomy, 220
Choledochogastrostomy, 220
Choledochoileostomy, 220
Choledochojejunostomy, 220
Choledocholithotomy, 219
Choledocholithotripsy, 221
Choledochoplasty, 219
Choledochorrhaphy, 218
Choledochostomy, 220
Choledochotomy, 219
Choledochus, 213
Cholelithiasis, 216
Cholelithotomy, 219

Cholelithotripsy, 221
Cholelithotrity, 221
Cholera, 367
Cholesterol, 144
    total, 222
Cholesterol test, 173
Cholesteroleresis, 216
Cholesterolosis, 216
Cholesterosis, 216
Chol/o-, 39
Chondralgia, 97
Chondrectomy, 96
Chondr/i-, 26
Chondr/io-, 26
Chondritis, 94
Chondr/o-, 26
Chondro-osteodystrophy, 95
Chondroblastoma, 96
Chondrodynia, 97
Chondrofibroma, 96
Chondroid, 97
Chondroma, 96
Chondromalacia, 96
Chondromatosis, 96
Chondromyoma, 96
Chondromyxoid fibroma, 96
Chondromyxoma, 96
Chondromyxosarcoma, 96
Chondronecrosis, 97
Chondroporosis, 97
Chondrosarcoma, 96
Chondrotomy, 96
Chordae tendineae, 164
Chorditis, 191
Chord/o-, 26
Chordotomy, 311
Chorea, 307, 309
Choriocarcinoma, 254
Chorioepithelioma, 254
Choriomeningitis, 305
Chorion, 234, 251
Chorionic gonadotropin, 277
    human, 234
Chorionic villus biopsy, 256
Chorionic villus sampling, 256
Chorioretinitis, 339
Choroid, 320, 321, 338
Choroid vein, 167
Choroiditis, 339
Chromaffinoma, 311
Chrom/o-, 40
Chromophobe, 277
Chromophobic adenoma, 279
Chromosomes, 50-51, 63
Chronic fatigue syndrome, 367
Chronic obstructive pulmonary disease, 192
Chyle, 39, 213
Chyli, 347
Chylous ascites, 216
Chyme, 199, 213
Cicatrix (cicatrices), 134
Ciliary body, 320, 321, 339
Cili/o-, 23
Cilium (cilia), 125, 133, 189, 320, 338
Cingulate gyrus, 287
Circular fibers of stomach wall, 199
Circulation of blood, 148
Circulatory disturbances, 308
Circum-, 11
Circumcision, 255
Circumduction, 75
Circumflex vein, 167
Cirrhos, 40
Cirrhosis, 216
Cisterna, 303, 347
Cisterna chyli, 347, 362

Citrate agar hemoglobin electrophoresis, 173-174
Clas-, 33
Claustrophobia, 314
Clavicle, 67, 69, 71, 72, 91
Clavicotomy, 96
Clavicular, 56, 57
-cle, 15
Clear layer of skin, 124, 134
Cleft palate, 216
Cleid/o-, 26
Cleidocranial dysostosis, 95
-cleisis, 255
Client-centered therapy, 318
Climacteric, 233, 251
Clitoridectomy, 255
Clitoris, 232, 251
    bifid, 253
    dorsal veins of, 167
Closed fracture, 95
Clotting, blood, mechanism for, 147
Clubfoot, 95
Clubhand, 95
Co-, 11
Coagulation, disseminated intravascular, 169
Coagulation tests, 174
Coal worker's pneumoconiosis, 192
Coarctation of aorta, 170
Coats of stomach, 199
Coccidioidomycosis, 191
Coccidioidomycosis antibodies, 312
Coccyalgia, 97
Coccygectomy, 96
Coccygeus muscle, 118
Coccygodynia, 97
Coccyodynia, 97
Coccyx, 68, 71, 91
Cochlea, 325, 343
Cochlear canal, 325
Cochlear nerve, 290, 303
Codman's tumor, 96
Coel-, 36, 169
Cognitive therapy, 319
Cohn's test, 342
Cold, sense of, 327, 328
Colectomy, 219
Colic, 216
    renal, 248
Colic artery, 166
Colic vein, 151, 167
Colitis, 215, 216
Collagen, 40
Collagen diseases, 372
Collateral, 282, 303
Collaterals, 64
Collecting tubules, 226, 227, 246
Colles' fracture, 95
Colloid, 265, 277
Colocecostomy, 220
Colocentesis, 218
Colocolostomy, 220
Colon, 200, 201, 213
    spastic, 215
Colon and rectal surgery, 386
Colonoscopy, 222
Colopexy, 220
Coloproctostomy, 220
Color perception tests, 342
Colorectostomy, 220
Colorrhaphy, 218
Colors, roots and combining forms related to, 40
Colosigmoidostomy, 220
Colostomy, 220
Colotomy, 219
Colpectomy, 255
Colp/o-, 26, 169
Colpocleisis, 255

Colpohysterectomy, 255
Colpohysteropexy, 255
Colpohysterotomy, 255
Colpomyomectomy, 255
Colpoperineoplasty, 255
Colpoperineorrhaphy, 255
Colpopexy, 255
Colpoplasty, 255
Colpopoiesis, 255
Colporrhaphy, 255
Colpotomy, 255
Columnar epithelial tissue, 51, 52
Columnar epithelium, 64
Com-, 11
Coma, 309
Combined fatty acids test, 223
Combining forms, roots and, 23-28, 33-41
Comitans vein, 167
Comminuted fracture, 95
Commissural tracts, 286
Commissure, 302
    anterior, 286, 301
    posterior, 286, 302-303
Common bile duct, 202, 214
Common carotid artery, 149, 150
Common iliac artery, 151
Common iliac vein, 151, 167
Compact bone tissue, 65
Complement, 350, 362
Complement assay, 365
Complement C3, 222
Complete blood count, 174
Compound fracture, 95
Compulsive personality disorder, 313
Computed tomography, single photon emission,
    312
Computerized axial tomography, 97, 122, 137, 174,
    194
Computerized tomography, 97, 122, 137, 174, 194,
    222, 249, 256, 280, 312, 344
Con-, 11
Concentration test, 249
Concha(e), 189
    nasal, 70, 326, 345
Conchae nasalis, 93, 189
Conduction, heat loss through, 123
Conduction deafness, 344
Conduction deafness tests, 344-345
Conduction system of heart, 142, 143
Condyle(s), 69, 72, 91
Condylectomy, 96
Condyloid joints, 74
Condyloma acuminatum, 252
Cones and rods, 320, 322, 339
Confabulation, 315
Congenital adrenal hyperplasia, 278
Congenital amyotonia, 121
Congenital cardiovascular disorders, 170
Congenital cataract, 340
Congenital disorders, terms related to, 94-95
Congenital goiter, 278
Congenital hemihypertrophy, 370
Congenital hypertrophic pyloric stenosis, 216
Congenital megacolon, 216
Congenital multiple-system diseases, 370-371
Congenital muscle disorders, 121
Congenital skin disorders, 136
Congestive heart failure, 171
Conjunctiva, 320, 321, 339
Conjunctivitis, 339
Conjunctivoplasty, 341
Conn's syndrome, 278
Connective tissue, 51-52, 64
Connector neurons, 281
Connectors, 303
Constipation, 216

Constrictor pharyngis muscles, 118
Contact dermatitis, 134
Contagious conjunctivitis, acute, 339
Contingency management, 318
Contra-, 11
Contracture
　Dupuytren's, 121
　Volkmann's, 121
Conus arteriosus, 164
Convection, heat loss through, 123
Convergence, 322
Convergent strabismus, 341
Conversion disorder, 313
Convolution(s), 302
　of cerebrum, 286
Cooley's anemia, 170
Coombs' test, 174
Copper, 223
Copro-, 315
Coprolalia, 315
Coproporphyrin, 223
Cor, 165
Cor pulmonale, 171
Cordectomy, 193
Cordopexy, 193
Cords, vocal, 190
Cor/e-, 23, 340
Corectomedialysis, 342
Corectopia, 340
Coreoplasty, 342
Coretomedialysis, 342
Corium, 133
Cornea, 320, 321, 339
Corneal opacity, 341
Corneal ring, 342
Corneal ulcer, 341
Corniculate cartilage, 176
Cornu, 286, 302
Cornua, 286, 302
Cor/o-, 23
Coronal plane, 55
Coronal suture, 69, 70, 91
Coronary angioplasty, percutaneous transluminal,
　　173
Coronary arteries, 149, 165, 166
Coronary artery bypass graft, 173
Coronary artery procedure, Vineberg, 173
Coronary atherectomy, directional, 173
Coronary vein, 151, 165
Corpora cavernosa penis, 250
Corpus (corpora), 251
Corpus callosum, 286, 302
Corpus cavernosum clitoridis, 251
Corpus hemorrhagicum, 253
Corpus luteum, 231, 233, 251
Corpus luteum hormone, 277
Corpus spongiosum penis, 250
Corpuscles
　lamellated, 346
　malpighian, 246
　Meissner's, 327, 345-346
　Pacinian, 327-328, 346
　renal, 224, 226, 246
　Ruffinian, 328, 346
Cortex
　adrenal, 266, 277
　　hormones of, 264
　cerebral, 286, 302
　renal, 224, 246
Corti, organ of, 325, 343
Cortical blindness, 340
Cortical deafness, 344
Cortical hyperostosis, infantile, 95
Corticoids, 266
Corticospinal tracts, 291
Corticosterone, 264, 266, 277

Cortisol, 264, 266, 277
Cortisol tests, 280
Costal cartilage, 67, 71, 93
Costalgia, 192
Costectomy, 96
Cost/o-, 26
Costosternal joint, 93
Costovertebral junction, 93
Cowper's glands, 229, 250
Coxa valga, 95
Coxa vara, 95
Coxal, 56, 57, 93
Coxalgia, 97
Coxarthritis, 94
Coxitis, 94
Coxodynia, 97
Coxotomy, 96
C-peptide test, 222
Cranial, 54
Cranial bones, 70
Cranial nerves, 289-291, 303-304
Craniectomy, 311
Craniocele, 307
Cranioclasis, 96
Craniofacial dysostosis, 95
Craniomeningocele, 307
Craniopharyngioma of pituitary gland, 279
Cranioplasty, 96, 311
Craniorachischisis, 95, 307
Craniostosis, 95
Craniotomy, 96, 311
Craniotrypesis, 96
Cranisacral system, 292
Cranium, 67, 69
Creatine phosphokinase, 122
Creatinine clearance, endogenous, 250
Creatinine test, 249
Crenioclasis, 255
Crepitus, 216
Crest, 69
Cretinism, 278
Crib death, 373
Cricoid cartilage, 176, 189
Cricoidectomy, 193
Cricothyrotomy, 193
Cricotomy, 193
Crista, 69
Crohn's disease, 215
Croup, 192
Crouzon's disease, 95
Crown of tooth, 196
Cry/o-, 36
Crypt/o-, 36
Cryptococcosis, 367
Cryptorchidism, 253
Cryptorchism, 253
Crystalline lens, 320, 339
CT; see Computerized tomography
Cubital, 93
Cubital vein, 168
Cubitus, 91
Cuboid bone, 73, 91
Cuboidal epithelial tissue, 51
Cuboidal epithelium, 64
Cuboidonavicular joint, 93
-cule, 15
Culture
　blood, 173
　stool, 223
　throat, 194
　tissue, 137
Cuneiform bones, 73, 91
Cuneiform cartilage, 176
Cuneocuboid joint, 93
Cuneonavicular joint, 93
Cuneoscaphoid joint, 93

Curettage, dilatation and, 255
Curvatures of stomach, 199
Cushing's syndrome, 278, 372
Cusp, 165
Cuspid, 214
Cutaneous papilloma, 136
Cutaneous vein, 167
Cutis graft, 137
Cutis hyperelastica, 136
Cyan/o-, 40
Cyanosis, 134, 171
Cyclodialysis, 342
Cyclodiathermy, 342
Cyclopia, 340
Cyclothymia, 315
Cyclothymic disorder, 313
Cyema, 251
Cyesis, 251
Cylindruria, 247
Cynophobia, 314
Cyst(s)
　dentigerous, 218
　nabothian, 253-254
　nasopharyngeal, 192
　parovarian, 254
　sebaceous, 137
Cystadenoma, 254
Cystauchenotomy, 248
Cystectomy, 248
Cystendesis, 248
Cyst/i-, 26
Cystic artery, 166
Cystic duct, 202
Cystic fibrosis, 370
Cystic mastitis, chronic, 252
Cystic vein, 151, 167
Cysticercosis, 215
Cystidolaparotomy, 248
Cystidotrachelotomy, 248
Cystitis, 247
Cyst/o-, 26
Cystocele, 247
Cystocolostomy, 220
Cystogram, 250
Cystolithectomy, 248
Cystolithotomy, 248
Cystopexy, 248
Cystoplasty, 248
Cystoproctostomy, 248
Cystorectostomy, 248
Cystorrhaphy, 248
Cystoscope, 250
Cystostomy, 248
Cystotomy, 248
Cystotrachelotomy, 248
Cyt-, 49
-cyte, 15
Cyt/o-, 26
Cytomegalic inclusion disease, 368
Cytomegalovirus disease, 367-368
Cytoplasm, 50, 64

D

Dacry/o-, 39
Dacryadenitis, 339
Dacryoadenectomy, 342
Dacryoadenitis, 339
Dacryocystectomy, 342
Dacryocystitis, 339
Dacryocystorhinostomy, 342
Dacryocystosyringotomy, 342
Dacryocystotomy, 342
Dactyl/o-, 23
Danlos' syndrome, 370
Darier's disease, 136

Darkfield examination, 256
De-, 11
Deafness, 344
Death, crib, 373
Decerebration, 309
Decidua, 251
Decidual endometritis, 252
Decompression sickness, 372
Decubitus ulcer, 134
Deep veins, 151
Deferential artery, 166
Deficiency anemia, 170
Deficiency and metabolic diseases, terms related to, 96
Degenerative chorea, 307
Degenerative dementias, primary, 308
Degenerative muscle disorders, 121
Deja entendu, 315-316
Deja vu, 316
Delayed skin graft, 137
Delirium, 309
Delirium tremens, 313
Deltoid muscle, 104, 118
Delusion, 316
Dementias, 308, 309
Dendrites, 281, 303, 327
Dengue, 368
Dengue hemorrhagic fever shock syndrome, 368
Dense fibrous connective tissue, 52
Dense fibrous tissue, 64
Dental caries, 216
Dent/i-, 23
Dentigerous cyst, 218
Dentin, 198, 214
Dent/o-, 23, 195
Deoxyribonucleic acid, 50, 64
Dependent personality disorder, 313
Depressive disorder, major, 313
Depressive personality disorder, 313
DER, 97
Dercum's disease, 372
Dereism, 316
Derm/a-, 23, 133
Dermabrasion, 137
Dermatitis, 134, 135
Dermatitis herpetiformis, 134
Dermatitis medicamentosa, 135
Dermatitis multiformis, 134
Dermatitis venenata, 134
Dermat/o-, 23
Dermatocellulitis, 135
Dermatoconiosis, 135
Dermatofibroma, 136
Dermatographia, 135
Dermatoheteroplasty, 137
Dermatology, 123, 386
Dermatomyositis, 120
Dermatophytosis, 135
Dermatosis, 135
Dermis, 124, 133
Derm/o-, 23
Dermomycosis, 135
Descending aorta, 150
Descending colon, 201
Descending tracts, 302
Descriptive and diagnostic terms, 97
Desensitization, systematic, 318
Desert fever, 191
Desmoid tumor, 121
Deuteranomaly, 340
Deuteranopia, 340
Developmental disorders, terms related to, 94-95
Deviated septum of nose, 192
Dextrocardia, 170
Dextroposition of aorta, 170
Di-, 11

Dia-, 11, 302
Diabetes, bronze, 372
Diabetes insipidus, 278
Diabetes mellitus, 278
Diabetic retinopathy, 341
Diacetic acid, 223
Diagnostic and descriptive terms, 97
Diaphragm, 106, 118, 119, 178, 190
    pituitary, 261
Diaphysis (diaphyses), 65, 66, 91
Diarrhea, 216
Diarthroses, 73, 93
Diastasis, 307
Diastematomyelia, 307
Diastole, 142, 165
Diastolic blood pressure, 147
Diastomyelia, 307
Dichromatopsia, 340
Dick test, 137
Diencephalon, 285-286, 302
Differential blood count, 174
Diffuse interstitial pulmonary fibrosis, 192
Diffusion-weighted magnetic resonance imaging, 312
Digestive process, 200
Digestive tract, 195, 196, 213; see also
            Gastrointestinal system
    subdiaphragmatic organs of, 200
Digital vein, 167
Dilatation and curettage, 255
Diodrast clearance, 250
Diphtheria, 191
Diplacusis, 344
Diplegia, 309
Dipl/o-, 36, 341
Diplopia, 341
Dipsomania, 316
Directional coronary atherectomy, 173
Directions, 54, 55
Dis-, 11
Discharge form, Blue Cross-Blue Shield, 401-402
Discharge summary, 389-390
Discogram, 97
Discoid lupus erythematosus, 135
Disease; see specific disease
Disks
    articular, 73
    intervertebral, 71
Disorganized schizophrenia, 314
Disorientation, 316
Displacement(s)
    suture of, 218-219
    of uterus, 253
Disseminated intravascular coagulation, 169
Disseminated sclerosis, 309
Dissociative disorder, 313
Distal, 54
Distal convoluted tubules, 226, 227, 246
Distomiasis, 215
Diurnus, 317
Diverticulitis, 215
Diverticulosis, 217
Diverticulum, Meckel's, 216
DNA, 50, 64
Dolich/o-, 36
Dolichostenomelia, 95
Donor, universal, 147
Donto-, 195
Dorsal position, 56
Dorsalis pedis artery, 166
Dors/i-, 23
Dors/o-, 23
Double fracture, 95
Down's syndrome, 313, 370
Drainage, puncture for, 218
Dropsy, 217

Drug dependency, 316
Dual energy radiography, 97
Duchenne's muscular dystrophy, 121
Duchenne's paralysis, 310
-duct-, 33
Ducts, 133; see also specific duct
Ductule, 133
Ductus, 133
Ductus arteriosus, 165, 190
    patent, 170
Ductus deferens, 229, 250
Duhring's disease, 134
Dukes' classification of colorectal tumors, 218
Duodenal glands, 214
Duodenectomy, 219
Duodenitis, 215
Duoden/o-, 26
Duodenoenterostomy, 220
Duodenoileostomy, 220
Duodenojejunostomy, 220
Duodenorrhaphy, 218
Duodenostomy, 221
Duodenotomy, 219
Duodenum, 199, 200, 201, 214
Dupuytren's contracture, 121
Dura mater, 261, 283, 302
Duraplasty, 311
Dwarfism, 278
-dynia, 15
Dys-, 11
Dysarthria, 316
Dysbasia, 309
Dyschondroplasia, 95
Dysentery, 215
Dysgerminoma, 254
Dysgeusia, 345
Dysgraphia, 316
Dyskeratosis, 134
Dyskinesia, 309
Dyslexia, 316
Dyslogia, 318
Dysmenorrhea, 253
Dysosmia, 345
Dysostosis, 95
Dyspareunia, 253
Dyspepsia, 217
Dysphasia, 309
Dysphonia, 192, 316
Dysphoria, 316
Dysplasia
    ectodermal, 136
    fibrous, 95
Dyspnea, 192
Dyspraxia, 309
Dysthymia, 316
Dysthymic disorder, 313
Dystrophy
    adiposogenital, 278
    muscular; see Muscular dystrophy
    Zimmerlin's, 121
Dysuria, 247

E

E-, 11
Ear, 324, 343-344
Eardrum, 343
Eastern equine encephalitis, 305
Eating disorder, 313
Ebola hemorrhagic fever, 368
Ec-, 11
Eccentrochondroplalsia, 95
Ecchymosis (ecchymoses), 134
Eccrine sweat gland, 125, 133
Echinococcosis, 368
Echocardiography, 174

Echoencephalogram, 312
Echolalia, 316
Echopathy, 316
Echo-planar imaging, 312
Eclipse blindness, 340
Ect-, 12
-ectas-, 33
Ecthyma, 135
Ecto-, 12
Ectoderm, 251
Ectodermal dysplasia, 136
-ectomy, 15, 218
Ectopia
    of lens, 340
    renal, 247
    of testis, 253
Ectopic, 251
Ectopic pregnancy, 251
Ectropion uveae, 340
Eczema, 135
-edem-, 33
Edema
    angioneurotic, 134
    cardiac, 171
    pulmonary, 192
Efferent neurons, 281, 303
Egocentric, 316
Ehlers-Danlos syndrome, 136, 370
Eisenmenger's complex, 170
Ejaculatory ducts, 229, 250
Elastic cartilage, 93
Elbow, tennis, 74
Electrocardiograms, reports of, with case histories,
        392-393
Electrocardiograph, 174
Electrocochleography, 345
Electroconvulsive therapy, 318
Electrodermal audiometry, 345
Electroencephalograms, reports of, with case
        histories, 393-394
Electroencephalograph, 312
Electromyography, 122
Electrophoresis, citrate agar hemoglobin, 173-174
Elephant man's disease, 371
Ele/o-, 40
Em-, 12
Embolectomy, 173
Embolism, 171
Embryo, 234, 251
Embryology, 49
Embryoma of kidney, 248
Embryonic stage of pregnancy, 234
Embryotomy, 255
Embryotoxon, 340
Emergency medicine, 386
Emesis, 217
-emesis, 15
-emia, 15
Emmetropia, 339
Emmetros, 339
Empathy, 316
Emphraxis, 172
Emphysema, 192
Employer liability laws, 397
Empyema, 192
En-, 12
Enamel of tooth, 198, 214
Encephalitis, 305
Encephal/o-, 26
Encephalocele, 307
Encephalomalacia, 308
Encephalomeningitis, 305
Encephalomyelitis, 305
Encephalomyelocele, 307
Enchondromatosis, 95
End-, 12

Endarteritis, 169
Endarteritis deformans, 169
Endarteritis obliterans, 169
Endo-, 12, 51
Endocarditis, 169
Endocardium, 141, 165
Endocervix, 251
Endocrine gland(s), 201, 261
    hormones of, 264
    location of, 262
Endocrine system, 54, 261-280
    hereditary, congenital, and developmental
        disorders of, 278
    inflammations and infections of, 278
    laboratory tests and procedures of, 280
    oncology of, 279
    surgical procedures of, 279-280
Endocrinology, 386
Endoderm, 251
Endogenous creatinine clearance, 250
Endolymph, 325, 343
Endometritis, 252
Endometrium, 232, 251
    hyperplasia of, 253
Endoplasmic reticulum, 50
Endorphins, 302
Endoscope examinations, 222
Endoscopy, 97, 194
Endothelium, 51, 64
Enema, barium, 222
Enophthalmos, 341
-ent, 15
Ent-, 12
Enteritis, 215
Enter/o-, 26, 201
Enteroanastomosis, 221
Enterobiasis, 215
Enterocholecystostomy, 220
Enterocholecystotomy, 219
Enterocolitis, 215
    necrotizing, neonatal, 216
Enterocolostomy, 221
Enterocystocele, 217
Enteroenterostomy, 221
Enterogastritis, 215
Enterohepatitis, 215
Enterolith, 217
Enteropexy, 220
Enteroptosis, 217
Enterorrhaphy, 218
Enterostomy, 221
Enterotomy, 219
Ento-, 12
Entoderm, 251
Entomophobia, 314
Enucleation, 342
Enzyme(s), 64
    angiotensin-converting, 365
    in gastric juice, 199
Enzyme-linked immunosorbent assay, 365
Eosinophilic adenoma of pituitary gland, 279
Eosinophils, 146, 165
Ep-, 12
Ependyma, 302
Ependymitis, 305
Ependymoblastoma, 310
Ependymoma, 310
Epi-, 12, 51
Epicardium, 141, 165
Epicondyle, 91
Epidermal necrolysis, toxic, 135
Epidermis, 124, 133
Epidermoid carcinoma, 137, 193
Epidermolysis bullosa, 136
Epidermomycosis, 135
Epididymectomy, 255

Epididymis (epididymides), 229, 250
Epididymitis, 252
Epididymotomy, 255
Epididymovasotomy, 255
Epidural hematoma, 308
Epigastric, 56, 57
Epigastric artery, 166
Epigastric vein, 167
Epigastrium, 214
Epiglottidectomy, 193
Epiglottiditis, 191
Epiglottis, 190
Epiglottis cartilage, 176
Epiglottitis, 191
Epilepsy, 307
Epinephrine, 264, 267, 276
Epiphyses, 66
Epiphysial cartilage, 93
Epiphysis, 91
Epiphysis cerebri, 267
Epiphysitis, 94
Episcleritis, 339
Episi/o-, 26
Episioplasty, 255
Episiorrhaphy, 255
Episiotomy, 255
Epispadias, 247
Epistaxis, 169, 192
Epithalamus, 285, 302
Epithelial carcinoma, 136
Epithelial tissue, 51, 52
Epithelioma, 136
Epithelium, 64
    olfactory, 326, 345
Epstein-Barr virus, 368
Epstein-Barr virus syndrome, chronic, 367
Epulis, 218
Equilibrium, sense of, 325
Equina, 291
-er, 15
Erb-Duchenne paralysis, 309
Erb-Landouzy disease, 121
Erb's disease, 121
Erb's paralysis, 121, 305, 309
Erect, 56
Erector spinae muscle, 118
-erg-, 101
-ergic, 315
Erotic, 316
Erotomania, 316
Erotophobia, 314
Eructation, 217
Erysipelas, 135
Erythema, 134
Erythema infectiosum, 135
Erythema pernio, 134
Erythemia, 171
Erythr/o-, 40
Erythroblastosis fetalis, 372
Erythrocyte sedimentation rate, 174
Erythrocytes, 144, 146, 165
Erythrocytopenia, 171
Erythrocytosis, 169, 171
Erythropenia, 171
Erythropoiesis, 165
-esis, 15
Eso-, 36
Esophageal artery, 166
Esophageal vein, 167
Esophagectomy, 219
Esophagitis, 215
Esophagoduodenostomy, 221
Esophagoenterostomy, 221
Esophagogastrostomy, 221
Esophagojejunostomy, 221
Esophagoplasty, 219

Esophagoscopy, 222
Esophagostomy, 221
Esophagotomy, 219
Esophagus, 175, 199, 214
-esthes-, 33
Esthesiometer, 345
Estrogen, 230, 264, 267
Estrogen receptor test, 280
Estrogenic hormones, 277
Estrus, 251
Ethmoid bone, 70, 92
Ethmoid sinuses, 70, 190
Ethmoidal air cells, 190
Ethmoidectomy, 193
Eu-, 12
Eulenburg's disease, 121
Euphoria, 316
Eury-, 36
Eustachian tube, 175, 324, 343
Eustachitis, 343
Euthymia, 316
Euthyroid, 277
Evaporation, heat loss through, 123
Eversion, 75
Evisceration, 342
Ex-, 11
Exanthem, 134
Exanthema, 134
Excimer laser angioplasty, 173
Excisional biopsy, 137
Exfoliation, 134
Exfoliative dermatitis, 135
Exhalation; see Expiration
Exhibitionism, 316
Exo-, 12
Exocrine glands, 133, 201
Exophthalmos, 278
Exostosis, 95
Exotropia, 341
Expiration, 175, 178, 190
Expiratory pressure, maximum, 194
Expiratory reserve volume, 179, 190
Expiratory volume, timed forced, 194
Extension, 75
Extensor muscles, 119
    of arms and hands, 104
Exteriorize, 221
External, 54
External anatomy, roots and combining forms
        related to, 23-24
External auditory meatus, 324
External carotid artery, 149, 150
External ear, 324
External iliac artery, 151
External iliac veins, 151
External jugular vein, 151
External nares, 326, 345
External oblique muscles, 106
External os, 232, 251
External sphincter muscle, 201
Externus, 102
Extra-, 12
Extrapyramidal tracts, 291
Extremities
    lower, bones of, 72-73
    upper, bones of, 72
Extrinsic muscles of eye, 320, 339
Extro-, 12
Eye, 320-322
    hereditary, congenital, and developmental
        disorders of, 340
    inflammations and infections of, 339
    oncology of, 341
    pathologic conditions relating to, 339-341
    structures of, 320-322
    surgical and other procedures of, 341-342

Eye chart, Snellen, 343
Eye stain, fluorescent, 342
Eyeball, 320
Eyelids, 320

F

Facet, 69
Facial bones, 70
Facial muscles, 103, 104
Facial nerve, 290, 304
Facial vein, 168
Faci/o-, 23
Factitious disorders, 313
    by proxy, 313
Fallopian tubes, 230, 231-232, 251
Fallot, tetralogy of, 170
Fallot's tetrad, 170
False ribs, 71
False vocal cords, 176
Familial spinal muscular atrophy, 121
Family practice, 386
Fanconi's syndrome, 370
Farmer's lung, 192
Fascia, 99, 119
Fascia lata femoris, 119
Fasciculus (fasciculi), 119
Fasciectomy, 121
Fasciitis, 120
Fasciodesis, 121
Fascioplasty, 121
Fasciorrhaphy, 121
Fasciotomy, 121
Fascitis, 120
Fatigue syndrome, chronic, 367
Fatty acids test, combined, 223
Fauces, 195, 214
Fecalith, 217
Feces, incontinence of, 217
Felon, 135
Female pelvic floor, muscles of, 107
Female reproductive organs, 230-233
Female reproductive system, inflammations and
        infections of, 252
Feminizing adenocarcinoma of adrenal gland, 279
Feminizing adenoma of adrenal gland, 279
Femoral artery, 151, 166
Femoral nerve, 304
Femoral veins, 151, 168
Femur, 66, 67, 68, 69, 72, 92
Fenestration, 344
Ferrum, 40
Fertilization, 232
Fetal alcohol syndrome, 370
Fetal stage of pregnancy, 234
Fetus, 234, 251
Fibers
    of cytoplasm, 50
    muscle, 100
    Purkinje, 142
Fibrillation, 171
Fibrin, 147
Fibrinogen, 147
Fibr/o-, 26
Fibroadenoma, 254
Fibrocystic disease
    of breast, 252
    of pancreas, 370
Fibroma, chondromyxoid, 96
Fibromuscular, 119
Fibrosarcoma, odontogenic, 218
Fibrosis
    cystic, 370
    pulmonary, 192
Fibrous connective tissue, dense, 52
Fibrous dysplasia, 95

Fibrous joints, 73
Fibrous thyroiditis, 278
Fibrous tissue, dense, 64
Fibula, 67, 68, 69, 73, 92
Fifth disease, 135
Filariasis, 363, 368
Filiform papillae, 196
Fimbria(e), 232, 251
Fimbriated, 230
Fingers, bones of, 72
Fiss-, 33
Fissure, 134, 302
    cerebral, 286
Fistula, 217
Fixator muscles, 119
Flagellantism, 316
Flat bones, 66
-flect-, 33
-flex-, 33
Flexion, 75
Flexor muscles, 119
    of arms and hands, 104
Floaters, 341
Floating ribs, 71
Flooding, 318
Fluid(s)
    body, roots and combining forms related to, 39
    synovial, 98
Fluorescent eye stain, 342
Focal epilepsy, 307
Focal sclerosis, 309
Folie a deux, 316
Follicle(s), 125, 133, 230
    graafian, 233, 251
    hair, 125
    lymph, 363
Follicle-stimulating hormone, 263, 264, 277
Follicular lymphoma, giant, 364
Fong's disease, 95
Fontanel(s), 69, 92
Fontanelle, 92
Food poisoning, 215
Foot
    bones of, 73
    Morton's, 94
    muscles of, 108
Foramen, 69
Foramen magnum, 70, 92, 302
Foramen ovale cordis, 165
Foramina, 66
Forearm, bones of, 72
Foreign body in gastrointestinal system, 222-223
Foreskin, 229, 250
-form, 15
Fossa, 69
Fourth ventricle, 302
Fovea, 69, 339
Fovea centralis, 322
Fowler's position, 56
Fractures, terms related to, 95-96
Fragile X syndrome, 313, 370
Fragilitas ossium, 95
Free nerve endings, 327, 3435
Free sensory nerve endings, 327
Frenulum, lingual, 196
Friedreich's ataxia, 307
Frohlich's syndrome, 278
Frontal bone, 69, 70, 92
Frontal lobe of cerebral cortex, 286
Frontal plane, 55
Frontal sinuses, 70, 190
Frontalis muscle, 103
Frostbite, 135
Fugue, 316
Functional magnetic resonance imaging, 174
Functional residual capacity, 194

Fundus of stomach, 199
Fungal skin infections, 135
Fungiform papillae, 196
Furuncle, 135
Furunculosis, 135
Fused kidney, 247

G

Galact/o-, 39
Galactophorous ducts, 251
Galea aponeurotica, 103, 119
Gallbladder, 202, 214
Gamma globulins, immune, 350, 363
Gammopathy, 364
Gangliectomy, 311
Gangliocytoma, 310
Ganglion (ganglia), 282, 302
Ganglionectomy, 311
Ganglioneuroma, 310
Ganglionitis, 305
Gargoylism, 95, 370
Gastralgia, 217
Gastrectomy, 219
Gastric artery, 166
Gastric glands; see Stomach, glands of
Gastric juice, 199
Gastric vein, 151, 168
Gastritis, 215
Gastr/o-, 26, 199
Gastroanastomosis, 221
Gastrocnemius muscle, 108, 119
Gastrocolostomy, 221
Gastroduodenal artery, 166
Gastroduodenitis, 215
Gastroduodenostomy, 221
Gastroenteritis, 215
Gastroenterocolitis, 215
Gastroenterocolostomy, 221
Gastroenterostomy, 221
Gastroepiploic artery, 166
Gastroepiploic vein, 151, 168
Gastroesophageal reflux disorder, 217
Gastrogastrostomy, 221
Gastrohepatitis, 215
Gastroileitis, 215
Gastroileostomy, 221
Gastrointestinal series, 222
Gastrointestinal system, 54, 195-223
　foreign body in, 222-223
　hereditary, congenital, and developmental
　　disorders of, 216
　inflammations, infections, and toxic conditions
　　of, 215-216
　oncology of, 218
　structures and functions of, 195-202
　subdiaphragmatic digestive tract organs of, 200
Gastrojejunostomy, 221
Gastrolith, 217
Gastropexy, 220
Gastroplasty, 219
Gastroptosis, 217
Gastropylorectomy, 219
Gastrorrhaphy, 218
Gastroscopy, 222
Gastrostomy, 221
Gastrotomy, 219
Gaucher's disease, 364, 370
Gay, 316
Gemellus (gemelli) muscle, 119
Gemellus inferior muscle, 108
Gemellus superior muscle, 108
General adaptation system, 318
Generalized anxiety disorder, 313
-genesis, 15
Genital candidiasis, 252

Genital herpes, 252
Genital wart, 252
Genitofemoral nerve, 304
Genitourinary system, 54, 224-257
　hereditary, congenital, and developmental
　　disorders of, 247
　inflammations and infections of, 247
　oncology related to, 248, 254
　radiographic studies of, 256-257
　surgical and other procedures on, 248-249
Gen/o-, 33
Genu recurvatum, 95
Genu valgum, 95
Genu varum, 95
Genupectoral position, 56
Geriatrics, 386
German measles, 369
Gerontology, 386
Geusia, 345
Giant follicular lymphoma, 364
Giant urticaria, 134
Giantism, 95, 278
Giardiasis, 215
Gigantism, 95
Gilbert's disease, 216
Gingiva(e), 195, 196, 214
Gingivitis, 215
Gingiv/o-, 23
Gladiolus, 92
Gland; see specific gland
Glans penis, 229, 250
Glaucoma, 341
-glia, 53
Gliding joints, 74
Gli/o-, 26
Glioblastoma multiforme, 310
Glioma, 310
　of nose, 193
　of pineal gland, 279
Glioma multiforme, 310
Glioneuroma, 310
Globin, 144
Globoid cell leukodystrophy, 307
Globulin, thyroxine-binding, 280
Glomerular capsule, 224, 226
Glomerulonephritis, 247
Glomerulus (glomeruli), 227, 246
Glossectomy, 219
Glossitis, 215
Gloss/o-, 23
Glossolalia, 316
Glossopalatine arch, 214
Glossopharyngeal nerve, 290, 304
Glossoplasty, 219
Glossorrhaphy, 218
Glottis, 175, 176, 190
Glucagon, 201, 264, 267
Glucocorticoids, 264, 266, 277
Glucose, qualitative, 223
Glucose test, 250
Glucose tolerance test, 174
　oral, 223
Glucosuria, 247
Gluteal artery, 166
Gluteal muscle group, 108, 119
Gluteal nerve, 304
Gluteal vein, 168
Gluteus maximus muscle, 108, 119
Gluteus medius muscle, 108, 119
Gluteus minimus muscle, 108, 119
Glyc/o-, 36, 40
Glycogenosis, 216
Glycohemia, 3
Glycosuria, 247
Glycuresis, 247
Gnath/o-, 23

Gnosia, 315
Goetsch's skin reaction, 280
Goiter, 278
Golgi apparatus, 50, 64
Gonadotropic hormones, 263, 264, 277
Gonadotropin, chorionic, 277
　human, 234
Gonads, 228, 267
　hormones of, 264
Goni-, 342
Goniotomy, 342
Gonorrhea, 252
Gout, 372
Graafian follicles, 233, 251
Gracilis, 102
Gracilis muscle, 102, 108, 119
Graft
　bypass, coronary artery, 173
　skin, 137
-gram, 15
Grand mal epilepsy, 307
Granular layer of skin, 124, 134
Granulocytes, 144, 146, 165
Granulocytopenia, 171
Granulocytopoiesis, 165
Granulocytosis, 171
Granulomatous lymphoma, 364
Granulopenia, 171
Granulosa cell tumor, 254
-graph, 15
-graphy, 15
Graves' disease, 278
Gravid, 251
Gravida I, 251
Gravida, 251
Great saphenous vein, 151, 168
Great vessels, transposition of, 170
Greater curvature of stomach, 199
Greater multangular bone, 72
Greater omentum, 200
Greater trochanter, 67, 72
Greater vestibular glands, 232, 251
Greek combining forms for English numbers, 384
Greenstick fracture, 95
Growth of bone, 66
Growth hormone, 261, 263, 277
Guaiac test, 223
Guanase, 222
Guillain-Barre syndrome, 305
Gums, 196
Gyn-, 317
Gynecomastia, 253
Gynephobia, 314
Gyrus (gyri), 286, 287, 302

H

Hair, 125
Hair bulb, 133
Hair cells of ear, 325
Hair follicle, 125, 133
Hair shaft, 125, 134
Hair-matrix carcinoma, 136
Halitosis, 217
Hal/o-, 40
Hallucination, 316
Hallucinosis, alcoholic, acute, 313
Hallux valgus, 95
Hallux varus, 95
Halstead-Reitan neuropsychological battery, 315
Hamate bone, 72, 92
Hamstring muscle group, 108, 119
Hand
　bones of, 72
　muscles of, 104
Hansen's disease, 368

Hapl/o-, 36
Haplology, 316
Hard palate, 195
Harelip, 216
Hashimoto's diseae, 278
Haverhill fever, 369
Haversian canals, 92
HDL, 144
Head
    of bone, 69
    terms related to, 57
Health insurance claim form, universal, 399-400
Hearing, sense of, 324-325, 327
Hearing tests and diagnostic instruments for ear,
        344-345
Heart, 141
    action of, nerve function in, 142
    chambers of, 141, 142
    conduction system of, 142, 143
    homograft replacement of, 173
    nodes of, 164, 165
    structure of, 141-142
    valves of, 141-142, 164, 165
Heart block, 171
Heart failure, congestive, 171
Hebephrenic schizophreia, 314
Hedonia, 316
Hem/a-, 39
Hemangiectasis, 171
Hemangioma, 172
Hemapoiesis, 362
Hemarthrosis, 97, 169
Hematemesis, 169
Hematencephalon, 169
Hemat/o-, 39
Hematocele, 169, 253
Hematocoelia, 169
Hematocolpos, 169, 253
Hematocrit, 174
Hematocytopenia, 171
Hematocytosis, 171
Hematoma, 169, 308
Hematometra, 169, 253
Hematomphalocele, 169
Hematomyelia, 169
Hematopenia, 171
Hematopericardium, 169
Hematopoiesis, 145, 165, 362
Hematopoietic tissue, 52
Hematorrhachis, 169
Hematorrhea, 169
Hematosalpinx, 169, 253
Hematospermatocele, 169
Hematotympanum, 169
Hematuria, 169, 247
Heme, 40, 144, 165
Hemeralopia, 340
Hemi-, 12
Hemicraniectomy, 311
Hemicraniotomy, 311
Hemidecortication, 311
Hemihypertrophy, congenital, 370
Hemimelia, 95
Hemiplegia, 309
Hemisphere, 302
Hemispherectomy, 311
Hemithyroidectomy, 279
Hem/o-, 39
Hemochromatosis, 217, 372
Hemocytoblasts, 144
Hemodialysis, 248
Hemoglobin, 144, 146, 165
Hemoglobin electrophoresis, citrate agar, 173-
        174
Hemoglobin test, 250
Hemoglobinemia, 171

Hemogram, 174
Hemolith, 171
Hemolysis, 174
Hemolytic anemia, 170
Hemolytic disease of newborn, 372
Hemoperitoneum, 217
Hemophilia, 170
Hemophthalmia, 169
Hemophthalmos, 169
Hemophthalmus, 169
Hemopneumothorax, 192
Hemopoiesis, 165, 349, 362
Hemoptysis, 169, 192
Hemorrhages, 169, 308
Hemorrhagic colitis, 215
Hemorrhagic pachymeningitis, 308
Hemorrhagic sarcoma, multiple idiopathic, 373
Hemorrhagic telangiectasia, hereditary, 170
Hemorrhoidal artery, 166
Hemorrhoidal vein, 168
Hemorrhoidectomy, 173, 219
Hemosalpinx, 169
Hemothorax, 169, 192
Henle, loop of, 227, 246
Heparin, 165
Hepat-, 201
Hepatectomy, 219
Hepatic artery, 166
Hepatic ducts, 202
Hepatic portal circulation, 148
Hepatic portal vein, 151, 168
Hepatic vein, 151, 168
Hepat/ico-, 26
Hepaticocholangioenterostomy, 221
Hepaticoduodenostomy, 221
Hepaticoenterostomy, 221
Hepaticogastrostomy, 221
Hepaticojejunostomy, 221
Hepatitis, 215
Hepat/o-, 26
Hepatocarcinoma, 218
Hepatocholangiostomy, 221
Hepatoduodenostomy, 221
Hepatolenticular degeneration, 371
Hepatoma, 218
Hepatomalacia, 217
Hepatomegaly, 217
Hepatopexy, 220
Hepatorrhaphy, 218
Hepatosplenomegaly, 217
Hepatotomy, 219
Hereditary disorders, terms related to, 94-95
Hereditary hemorrhagic telangiectasia, 170
Hering's test, 342
Hermaphroditism, 253
Hernia, 217
Hernioplasty, 219
Herniorrhaphy, 218
Herpes, 135
Herpes febrilis, 135
Herpes genitalis, 135, 252
Herpes simplex, 215
Herpes zoster, 305
Herpes zoster virus, 367
Heter/o-, 36
Heterodermic skin graft, 137
Heterolalia, 316
Heterophasia, 316
Heterotopia, 307
Hiatal hernia, 217
Hiccough, 192
Hiccup, 192
Hickory-stick fracture, 95
Hidradenoma, 136
Hidr/o-, 39
High-density lipoprotein, 144, 174

Hilus
    of kidney, 224, 246
    of lung, 190
    of spleen, 362
Hindbrain, 284
Hinge joints, 74, 93
Hip joint, 93
Hippocampal gyrus, 287
Hippocampus, 287, 302
Hirschsprung's disease, 216
Hirsutism, 134, 279
His, bundle of, 142, 164
Histamines, 350, 362
Histiocytosis, lipid, 371
Hist/o-, 26
Histology, 49
Histoplasmosis, 191
Histrionic personality disorder, 313
Hives, 135
Hodgkin's disease, 364
Hoffmann-Werdnig's syndrome, 121
Holmgren's test, 342
Hom/eo-, 36
Homeostasis, 292
Hom/o-, 36
Homograft replacement of heart, 173
Homosexuality, 316
Hordeolum, 339
Hormone(s), 40, 261, 263, 264, 265, 277; *see also*
        specific hormone
Horner's syndrome, 309
Horns of spinal cord, 287
Horseshoe kidney, 247
Hospital insurance form, individual, 398
Hospital records and reports, 388-396
Housemaid's knee, 74
Human chorionic gonadotropin, 234
Human immunodeficiency virus, 366-367
Human papilloma virus, 252
Humeroradial junction, 93
Humeroscapular junction, 93
Humeroulnar junction, 93
Humerus, 66, 67, 68, 69, 72, 92
Humoral antibody, 362
Huntington's chorea, 307
Hurler's syndrome, 95, 313, 370
Hurthle cell adenoma of thyroid gland, 279
Hurthle cell carcinoma of thyroid gland, 279
Hutchinson's teeth, 216
Hutchinson-Gilford syndrome, 371
Hyalin, 40
Hyaline cartilage, 93
Hyaline membrane disease, 192
Hyal/o-, 40
Hydatid disease, 368
Hydatidiform mole, 253
Hydrarthrosis, 97
Hydrencephalocele, 307
Hydrencephalomeningocele, 307
Hydr/o-, 36, 39
Hydrocele, 253
Hydrocephalocele, 307
Hydrocephalus, 307
Hydrochloric acid in gastric juice, 199
17-Hydrocorticosteroid test, 280
Hydrocortisone, 264, 266, 277
Hydromeningocele, 307
Hydromyelia, 307
Hydromyelocele, 307
Hydromyelomeningocele, 307
Hydronephrosis, 247
Hydrophobia, 306
Hydropneumothorax, 192
Hydrops, 217
Hydrorrhea gravidarum, 253
Hydrothorax, 192

5-Hydroxyindoleacetic acid, 223
Hydroxyproline, 97
Hymen, 232, 251
Hymenectomy, 255
Hymenotomy, 255
Hyoid bone, 69, 70, 92
Hyp-, 12
Hypalgesia, 316
Hyper-, 12
Hyperbilirubinemia, 216
Hypercalciuria, 247
Hypercementosis, 217
Hyperchlorhydria, 217
Hypercholesterolemia, 217
Hypercholia, 217
Hypercortisolism, 278, 372
Hypergeusia, 345
Hyperglycemia, 217
Hyperhidrosis, 134
Hyperinsulinism, 217
Hyperkeratosis, 134
Hyperkinesis, 316
Hyperkinetic disorder, 316
Hypermetropia, 341
Hypernephroid carcinoma, 248
Hyperopia, 341
Hyperorexia, 216
Hyperosmia, 345
Hyperosphresia, 345
Hyperostosis, cortical, infantile, 95
Hyperparathyroidism, 279
Hyperpathia, 309
Hyperphrenia, 316
Hyperplasia
  adrenal, congenital, 278
  endometrial, 253
  thymus, 364
Hyperpnea, 192
Hyperpragia, 316
Hypersensitivity, 349, 352, 362
Hypersplenism, 217
Hypertension, 147, 171
Hypertensive retinopathy, 341
Hyperthyroidism, 279
Hypertrophic pyloric stenosis, congenital, 216
Hypertrophy
  cardiac, 171
  prostatic, 253, 254
  of thymus, 364
Hypertropia, 341
Hyperventilation, 192
Hypervitaminosis, 217
Hypnosis, 316
Hypo-, 12
Hypoalgesia, 316
Hypochlorhydria, 217
Hypocholesteremia, 217
Hypochondria, 316
Hypochondriac, 56, 57
Hypochromic microcytic anemia, 170
Hypochylia, 217
Hypoesthesia, 316
Hypogastric, 56, 57
Hypogastric nerve, 304
Hypogastric vein, 168
Hypogastrium, 214
hypogeusia, 345
Hypoglossal nerve, 291, 304
Hypoglycemia, 217
Hypogonadism, 278
Hypokinesia, 316
Hypomania, 316
Hypoparathyroidism, 278
Hypopharynx, 190
Hypophrasia, 316
Hypophyseal cachexia, 279

Hypophysectomy, 279
Hypophysis, 261, 276; see also Pituitary gland
Hypophysis cerebri, 277
Hypoplasia of cervix, 253
Hypopyon, 341
Hyposmia, 345
Hypospadias, 247
Hypotension, 147, 171
Hypothalamus, 261, 265, 285-286, 287, 302
  hormones of, 264
Hypothyroidism, 279
  infantile, 278
Hypotropia, 341
Hypovitaminosis, 217
Hysterectomy, 255
Hyster/o-, 26, 232
Hysterogram, 256
Hysterolaparotomy, 255
Hysterolith, 253
Hysteromyotomy, 255
Hysteropexy, 255
Hysterorrhaphy, 255
Hysterorrhexis, 253
Hysterosalpingography, 256
Hysterosalpingostomy, 255
Hysterostoscopy, 256

I

-ia, 15
-iasis, 15
-iatr/o-, 34
-ible, 15
-ic, 15
Ichthyosis congenita, 136
Id, 316
Idiopathic muscular atrophy, 121
Idiopathic polyneuritis, acute, 305
-ile, 15
Ileal artery, 166
Ileal vein, 168
Ileectomy, 219
Ileitis, 215
Ile/o-, 26
Ileocecal valve, 201, 214
Ileocecostomy, 220
Ileocolic artery, 166
Ileocolic valve, 214
Ileocolic vein, 151, 168
Ileocolitis, 215
Ileocolostomy, 221
Ileoileostomy, 221
Ileoproctostomy, 221
Ileorrhaphy, 219
Ileosigmoidostomy, 221
Ileostomy, 221
Ileotomy, 219
Ileum, 200, 201, 214
Ileus, 217
Iliac, 56, 57
Iliac arteries, 151, 166
Iliac crest, 201
Iliac veins, 151, 167, 168
Iliacus muscle, 119
Ili/o-, 26
Iliocostalis cervicis muscle, 119
Iliocostalis dorsi muscle, 119
Iliocostalis lumborum muscle, 119
Iliocostalis muscle, 119
Iliohypogastric nerve, 304
Ilioinguinal nerve, 304-305
Iliolumbar artery, 166
Iliolumbar vein, 168
Iliopsoas muscle, 108, 119
Ilium, 67, 68, 72, 92
Im-, 12

Imaging
  blood pool, 174
  magnetic resonance; see Magnetic resonance imaging
Immune deficiency syndrome, acquired, 366-367
Immune gamma globulins, 350, 363
Immune mechanisms
  nonspecific, 349-350
  specific, 350-351
Immune system, 54, 349-365
  hereditary, congenital, and developmental disorders of, 365
  inflammations and infections of, 363
  laboratory tests and procedures of, 365
  oncology of, 364
  problems with, 352
  surgical procedures on, 364
  weakness of deficiency of, 352
Immune system reaction, excessively strong, 352
Immunity, 352, 362
Immunodeficiency disease, severe combined, 352, 364
Immunodeficiency virus, human, 366-367
Immunoglobulins, 350, 362
Immunology, 386
Immunosorbent assay, enzyme-linked, 365
Impacted fracture, 96
Impetigo, 135
Impetigo contagiosa, 135
Implant, cataract, 341
Impotence, 253
Impulses, nerve, 281
In-, 12
Incest, 316
Incisors, 196
Incomplete fracture, 96
Incontinence, 247
  of feces, 217
Incudectomy, 344
Incus, 92, 324, 343
Individual hospital insurance form, 398
Industrial dermatitis, 135
Inertia, 316
Infantile autism, 315
Infantile cortical hyperostosis, 95
Infantile hypothyroidism, 278
Infants, progressive spinal muscular atrophy of, 121
Infarct, 171
Infarction
  myocardial, 172
  renal, 248
Infections, 94
Infectious mononucleosis, 363, 368
Infectious polyneuritis, 305
Inferior, 54
Inferior mesenteric vein, 151
Inferior vena cava, 168
Inflammations, 94
Influenza, 191
Information, release of, authorization for, 397
Infra-, 12
Infraclavicular, 56, 57
Infrahyoid muscles, 119
Infraorbital, 57
Infraorbital nerve, 304
Infrascapular, 56, 57
Infraspinatus muscle, 119
Infundibulum (infundibula), 232, 261, 277
  of heart, 164
Inguinal, 56, 57
Inguinal canals, 229
Inguinal lymph nodes, 347
Inhalation; see Inspiration
Injuries, suture of, 218-219
Inner canthus, 322
Inner ear, 324, 325

Innervative muscle disorders, 121
Innominate artery, 149, 166
Innominate bone, 67, 72, 92
Innominate vein, 151, 167
Inorganic matter, 64
Insertion of muscle, 99
Insomnia, 316
Inspiration, 175, 178, 190
    muscle of, 190
Inspiratory capacity, 194
Inspiratory muscles, 119
Inspiratory pressure, maximum, 194
Inspiratory reserve volume, 179, 190
Insula, 286
Insular sclerosis, 309
Insulin, 201, 264, 267
Insulin clearance, 122
Insulin coma therapy, 318
Insulin shock, 217
Insulin test, 222
Insurance, medical, 397-403
Insurance form, individual hospital, 398
Insurance policies, multiple, 397
Integumentary system, 54, 123-137
Inter-, 12
Interatrial septum, 141
Intercarpal joint, 93
Intercostal artery, 166
Intercostal muscles, 106, 119
Intercostal vein, 168
Intercostobrachial nerve, 305
Interferon, 350, 363
Interlobular vein, 168
Intermediate basilic vein, 168
Intermediate cuneiform bone, 73
Intermediate nerve, 304
Internal, 54
Internal anatomy, roots and combining forms
        related to, 26-28
Internal carotid artery, 149, 150
Internal iliac artery, 151
Internal iliac vein, 151
Internal jugular vein, 151
Internal mechanisms of body, 139-257
Internal medicine, 386
Internal oblique muscles, 106
Internal os, 232, 251
Internal spermatic artery, 166
Internal sphincter muscle, 201
Internal thoracic artery, 166
Internal thoracic vein, 168
Interneurons, 281
Interossei muscles, 119
Interosseus nerve, 305
Interphalangeal joint, 93
Interscapular, 56, 57
Interspinales muscle group, 119
Interstitial cells, 229
Interstitial pulmonary fibrosis, diffuse, 192
Intertarsal joint, 93
Interventricular, 165
Interventricular septum, 141
Intervertebral disks, 71
Intervertebral vein, 168
Intestinal artery, 166
Intestinal glands, 214
Intestine
    large, 200, 201
    small, 199, 201
Intimal layer of artery, 143
Intoxication, pathologic, 313
Intra-, 12
Intracranial hemorrhage, 308
Intradermal tests, 137
Intraepidermal carcinoma, 136
Intraepidermal epithelioma, 136

Intraocular pressure, 322, 339
Intrastromal corneal ring, 342
Intravascular coagulation, disseminated, 169
Intravenous pyelogram, 250
Intrinsic factor in gastric juice, 199
Intro-, 12
Introverted, 316
Intubation, 193
Intussusception, 217
Inulin clearance, 227
Inversion, 75, 316
Invertebrate, 64
Involuntary muscle, 100, 119
Involuntary muscle tissue, 64
Iodine, 277
    protein-bound, 266, 280
Iridectomy, 342
Iridectropium, 340
Iridencleisis, 342
Irid/o-, 24
Iridocorneosclerectomy, 342
Iridocyclectomy, 342
Iridocyclitis, 339
Iridocyclochoroiditis, 339
Iridocystectomy, 342
Iridodialysis, 342
Iridokeratitis, 339
Iridomedialysis, 342
Iridomesodialysis, 342
Iridosclerotomy, 342
Iridotasis, 342
Iridotomy, 342
Iris, 320, 322, 339
    adhesions of, 340
Iritis, 339
Iritoectomy, 342
Iritomy, 342
Irregular bones, 66
Irritable bowel syndrome, 215
Ischemia, 171
Ischemic attack, transient, 172
Ischemic muscular atrophy, 121
Ischemic optic neuropathy, anterior, 340
Ischium, 67, 68, 72, 92
Ishihara test, 342
Islands (islets)
    of Langerhans, 201, 214, 267, 277
        hormones of, 264
    of Reil, 286
-ism, 15, 49-50
Is/o-, 36
-ist, 15
Isthmectomy, 279
Isthmus, 265, 286
-ites, 15
-itis, 15
-ity, 15
-ize, 15

J

Jacksonian seizure, 309
Jadassohn-Lewandowsky syndrome, 136
Jansky-Bielschowsky disease, 307
Jaundice, 217
Jejunal vein, 168
Jejunectomy, 219
Jejunitis, 215
Jejun/o-, 26
Jejunocolostomy, 221
Jejunoileitis, 215
Jejunoileostomy, 221
Jejunojejunostomy, 221
Jejunorrhaphy, 219
Jejunostomy, 221
Jejunotomy, 219

Jejunum, 200, 201, 214
Joint capsule, 73
Joint cavity, 73
Joints, 72, 73-74; see also specific joint
    terms related to, 93-94
Jugular veins, 151, 168
Juvenile progeria, 371

K

K cells, 351, 363
Kabaschnik's test, 345
Kanner's syndrome, 315
Kaposi's sarcoma, 364, 367, 373
Karyotyping, 256
Kawasaki's disease, 368
Keloid, 134
Kerat-, 124
Keratectomy, 342
Keratin, 134
Keratinized, 124
Keratitis, 339
Kerat/o-, 26
Keratocentesis, 342
Keratoconjunctivitis, 339
Keratoiridocyclitis, 339
Keratoiritis, 339
Keratoplasty, 342
Keratosis
    actinic, 136
    seborrheic, 137
Keratosis follicularis, 136
Keratotomy, 342
    radial, 342
Ketosteroids tests, 280 17-
Kidney, 224-227, 246, 247, 248; see also renal
        entries
    composition and structure of, 224, 225
    functional unit of, 224-227
    functions of, 227
Killer cells, 351, 363
Kin/e-, 34
Kinesis, 315
Kin/o-, 34
Kinky hair disease, 307
Klepto, 316
Kleptomania, 316
Klinefelter's syndrome, 371
Klippel-Feil syndrome, 95
Knee, housemaid's, 74
Knee jerk reflex, 292
Knee joint, 93
Knee-chest position, 56
Knepha, 340
Knuckle joints, 74
Koilonychia, 136
Korsakoff's psychosis, 313
Krabbe's diseae, 307
Kraurosis vulvae, 253
Kufs' disease, 307
Kynophobia, 314
Kyphosis, 97

L

Labia, 195, 214
Labia majora, 232, 251
Labia minora, 232
Labi/o-, 24
Laboratory tests, terms related to, 97-98
Labyrinth, 325, 343
Labyrinthectomy, 344
Labyrinthine deafness, 344
Labyrinthine syndrome, 344
Labyrinthine vein, 168
Labyrinthitis, 343
Labyrinthotomy, 344

Lac-, 39
Lacrima, 39
Lacrimal bones, 70, 92
Lacrimal glands, 320, 322, 339
Lacrimal nerve, 304
Lacrimotomy, 342
Lacromotomy, 342
Lactating breast, 231
Lactation, 253
Lactic dehydrogenase isoenzymes, 222
Lactiferous ducts, 251
Lactogenic hormone, 263, 265, 277
Lacuna (lacunae), 92
-lalia, 309
Lambdoid suture, 70, 92
Lamella (lamellae), 92
Lamellated corpuscle, 346
Lamina, 92
Laminectomy, 96
Laminotomy, 96
Landry's paralysis, 305
Landry-Guillain-Barre-Strohl syndrome, 305
Langerhans, island (islets) of, 201, 214, 267, 277
    hormones of, 264
Lapar/o-, 24
Laparorrhaphy, 218
Laparotomy, 219
Lapis, 40
Large intestine, 200, 201
Laryngalgia, 192
Laryngeal artery, 166
Laryngeal nerve, 304
Laryngeal papillomatosis, 193
Laryngeal vein, 168
Laryngectomy, 193
Laryngitis, 191
Laryng/o-, 27
Laryngofissure, 193
Laryngopharyngectomy, 193
Laryngopharyngitis, 191
Laryngopharynx, 190
Laryngophthisis, 191
Laryngoplasty, 193
Laryngoplegia, 192
Laryngoptosis, 192
Laryngorrhagia, 192
Laryngoscope, 193
Laryngoscopy, 194
Laryngospasm, 192
Laryngostasis, 192
Laryngostenosis, 192
Laryngostomy, 193
Laryngotomy, 193
Laryngotracheitis, 191
Laryngotracheobronchitis, 191
Laryngotracheotomy, 193
Laryngovestibulitis, 191
Larynx, 175-176, 190
Laser surgery, 342
Lateral, 54
Lateral abdominal, 56, 57
Lateral condyles, 72
Lateral cuneiform bone, 73
Lateral incisors, 196
Lateral malleolus, 73
Lateral recumbent position, 56
Lateral sclerosis, amyotrophic, 309
Lateral thoracic vein, 168
Lateral ventricle, 286, 302
Later/o-, 24
Latin combining forms for English numbers, 384
Latissimus, 102
Latissimus dorsi muscle, 104, 119
Laurence-Moon-Biedl syndrome, 371
LDL, 144
LE cell prep, 373

Leg, muscles of, 107-108
Legionellosis, 191
Legionnaires' disease, 191
Lei/o-, 36
Leiomyoma, 121
Leiomyoma cutis, 136
Leiomyosarcoma, 121
Leischmaniasis, 368
Length, units of, 385
Lens, 322, 339
    crystalline, 320, 339
    ectopia of, 340
Lenticular carcinoma, 136-137
Lenticular opacity, 341
Lentiform bone, 72, 92
Leprosy, 368
Lept/o-, 36
Leptomeningitis, 305
Leptomeninx (leptomeninges), 284, 302
Lesbian, 316
Lesch-Nyhan cerebral palsy, 307
Lesions, suture of, 218-219
Lesser curvature of stomach, 199
Lesser multangular bone, 72
Lesser omentum, 200
Lesser trochanter, 67, 72
Lethargy, 317
Leuc/o-, 40
Leucotomy, 311
Leukemias, 170, 364
Leukemia cutis, 170
Leuk/o-, 40
Leukocytes, 144, 146, 165
    polymorphonuclear, 165
Leukocyte adhesion deficiency, 364
Leukocytopenia, 171
Leukocytopoiesis, 165
Leukocytosis, 169
Leukodystrophy, globoid cell, 307
Leukoerythroblastosis, 170
Leukopenia, 171
Leukoplakia, 217
Leukopoiesis, 165
Leukorrhea, 253
Leukotomy, 311
Levator ani muscle, 107, 119
Levator coccygeus muscle, 107
Levator palpebrae muscle, 339
Levator scapulae muscle, 119
Lev/o-, 36
-lexia, 315
Leydig's cells, 229, 250
Libido, 317
Lieberkuhn's glands, 214
Lienal vein, 168
Lienic capsule, 363
Lien/o-, 27
Ligaments, 73, 99, 119
    suspensory, 320, 321, 339
Ligneous thyroiditis, 278
Limbic system, 287, 302
-limia, 313
Lindau-von Hippel disease, 371
Line, 69
Lingua, 214
Lingual artery, 166
Lingual frenulum, 196
Lingual nerve, 196, 304
Lingual tonsils, 349
Lingual vein, 168, 196
Lingu/o-, 24
Linguopapillitis, 215
Lipid, 40
    in blood, 144
Lipid histiocytosis, 371
Lip/o-, 40

Lipochondrodystrophy, 95
Lipoprotein tests, 174
Lipoproteins, 144
Lips, 195
-lith, 325, 343
Lithium carbonae, 318
Lith/o-, 40
Lithopedion, 253
Lithotripsy, 248
Liver, 201-202, 214
Liver function tests, 222
Living matter, characteristics of, 49-50
Lobectomy, 279, 311
Lobotomy, 311
    prefrontal, 318
Lockjaw, 306
Logographia, 317
-logy, 16
Long bone x-ray, 97
Long bones, 66
Long thoracic nerve, 305
Longissimus, 102
Longissimus capitas muscle, 119
Longissimus cervicis muscle, 119
Longissimus muscles, 119
Longissimus thoracic muscle, 119
Longitudinal fibers of stomach wall, 199
Longus, 102
Loop of Henle, 227, 246
Lorain-Levi syndrome, 278
Lordosis, 97
Loreta's method, 222
Lou Gehrig's disease, 309
Louis-Bar syndrome, 306
Low-density lipoprotein, 144, 174
Lower extremities, bones of, 72-73
Lower respiratory tract, organs of, 177-178
Lumbago, 97
Lumbar, 56, 57
Lumbar artery, 166
Lumbar puncture, 97
Lumbar vein, 168
Lumbar vertebrae, 68, 71
Lumbosacral joint, 93
Lumbosacral plexus, 291
Lumbricale muscle group, 119
Lumpectomy, 255
Lunate bone, 72, 92
Lunula, 134
Lung(s), 177-178
    farmer's, 192
    lobes of, 178
Lung capacity, total, 194
Lung scan, 194
Lunula, 134
Lupus erythematosus
    discoid, 135
    systemic, 352, 364, 373
Lupus erythematosus test, 373
Lutein, 40
Luteinizing hormone, 263, 264, 277
Luteinizing hormone assay, 280
Luteum, 251
Lyme disease, 368
Lymph, 363
Lymph follicle, 363
Lymph nodes, 347, 363
Lymphadenectasis, 364
Lymphadenectomy, 364
Lymphadenitis, 363
Lymphadenopathy, 364
    follicular, giant, 364
Lymphadenopathy syndrome, chronic, 367
Lymphangiectasis, 364
Lymphangiectomy, 364
Lymphangioma, 364
Lymphangioplasty, 364

Lymphangiosarcoma, 364
Lymphangiotomy, 364
Lymphangitis, 363
Lymphatic duct, 347, 363
Lymphatic leukemia, 364
Lymphatic system, 54, 347-365
   hereditary, congenital, and developmental
      disorders of, 364-365
   inflammations and infections of, 363
   laboratory tests and procedures of, 365
   oncology of, 364
   organs of, 348
   surgical procedures on, 364
Lymphatic vessels, 347, 363
Lymphaticostomy, 364
Lymphedema, 364
Lymph/o-, 27, 39
Lymphoblasts, 144
Lymphocytes, 144, 146, 165, 363
Lymphocythemia, 171
Lymphocytic leukemia, 364
Lymphocytopenia, 171
Lymphocytosis, 171
Lymphogranuloma, 364
Lymphogranuloma inguinale, 252
Lymphogranuloma venereum, 252
Lymphoid leukemia, 364
Lymphokines, 351
Lymphoma, 364
Lymphomatosis, 364
Lymphomatosis granulomatosa, 364
Lymphomatous thyroiditis, chronic, 278
Lymphopathia venereum, 252
Lymphoplasty, 364
Lymphopoiesis, 165
Lymphorrhea, 364
Lymphosarcoma, 364
Lymphostasis, 364
Ly/o-, 34
Lys/o-, 34
Lysosomes, 50, 64

M

Macr/o-, 36
Macrobrachia, 95
Macrocephalia, 307
Macrocephaly, 95, 307
Macrocheilia, 216
Macrocyte, 165
Macrocytic anemia, 170
Macroglossia, 216
Macrognathia, 95
Macropodia, 95
Macrostomia, 216
Macrotia, 343
Macula, 134, 339
Macula lutea, 322, 339
Macular degeneration, age-related, 340
Maculopathy, 341
Magnetic resonance, nuclear; *see* Magnetic
     resonance imaging
Magnetic resonance imaging, 98, 122, 174, 194, 222,
     250, 256-257, 280, 312, 342, 345
   diffusion-weighted, 312
   functional, 174
   perfusion, 312
Magnetoencephalography, 312
Major depressive disorder, 313
Mal-, 37
Malac/o-, 37
Malar bones, 70, 92, 93
Malaria, 368
Male pelvic floor, muscles of, 107
Male reproductive organs, 228-229

Male reproductive system, inflammations and
     infections of, 252
Malignant pustule, 367
Malingering, 317
Malleolar artery, 166
Malleolus, 73, 92
Malleotomy, 344
Malleus, 92, 324, 343
Malocclusion, 217
Malpighian corpuscle, 246
Malta fever, 367
Mamae, 251
Mamilliplasty, 255
Mamm/a-, 24
Mammalgia, 253
Mammary, 56, 57
Mammary artery, 166
Mammary glands, 232, 251
Mammary vein, 168
Mammectomy, 255
Mammilitis, 252
Mamm/o-, 24
Mammography, 257
Mammotomy, 255
Mandible, 67, 69, 70, 92
Mandibular nerve, 290, 304
Mania, 313
Manic-depressive, 313
Mantoux test, 137
Manubrium (manubria), 92
Marasmus, 217
Marble bones, 95
Marfan's syndrome, 94-95, 371
Marie's sclerosis, 307
Marie-Strumpell disease, 94
Marrow, bone, 65
   aspiration of, 97
   biopsy of, 97
Masochism, 317
Masseter muscles, 103, 119
Mastadenitis, 252
Mastalgia, 253
Mastectomy, 255
   radical, 256
Mastication, muscles of, 103
Mastitis, 262
   cystic, chronic, 252
Mast/o-, 24
Mastodynia, 253
Mastoid process, 92
Mastoid sinuses, 70
Mastoiditis, 343
Mastopexy, 255
Mastoplasty, 255
Mastoptosis, 253
Mastorrhagia, 253
Mastotomy, 255
Matter
   inorganic, 64
   living, characteristics of, 49-50
   organic, 64
Mauthner's test, 342
Maxilla, 67
Maxillary artery, 166
Maxillary bones, 70
Maxillary nerve, 290, 304
Maxillary sinuses, 70, 190
Maximum expiratory pressure, 194
Maximum inspiratory pressure, 194
Measles, 369
Meatus, 69, 324, 343
   auditory, external, 324
   urinary, 227
Meckel's diverticulum, 216
Medial, 54
Medial arteriosclerosis, 172

Medial condyles, 72
Medial cuneiform bone, 73
Medial layer of artery, 143
Medial malleolus, 73
Median antebrachial vein, 168
Median cubital vein, 168
Median nerve, 305
Median plane, 55
Median region of back, 56, 57
Mediastinal vein, 168
Mediastinitis, 191
Mediastinum, 178, 190
Medical claims, processing, 397, 403
Medical insurance, 397-403
Medical specialties, 386-387
Medical terminology
   basic foundation of, 1-46
   introduction to, 3-9
   learning, specific suggestions for, 4
   plurals of, 4
   pronunciation of, 4
   spelling, 4
Medical vocabulary, building, 10-22
Medicare, 403
Mediterranean fever, 367
Medius, 102
Medulla
   adrenal, 266, 277
     hormones of, 264
   renal, 224, 246
Medulla oblongata, 284, 302
Medullary artery, 167
Medullary carcinoma, 254
Medullary cavity, 65
Medullary pyramids, 224
Medullated nerves, 303
Medulloblastoma, 310
Medulloepithelioma, 310
Meg/a-, 37
Megacephaly, 307
Megacolon, congenital, 216
Megakaryoblasts, 144
Megakaryocytes, 147, 165
Meg/alo-, 37
Megalocornea, 340
Megalocyte, 165
Megalogastria, 216
Megaloglossia, 216
Megalophthalmos, 340
Meg/aly-, 37
Meissner's corpuscles, 327, 345-346
Melanin, 124, 134
Melan/o-, 40
Melanocyte-stimulating hormone, 263, 265
Melanocytic nevus, 137
Melanoma, 137
Melatonin, 264, 267
Melena, 169
Mel/i-, 40
Mel/o-, 24
Membrane
   basilar, 325
   mucous, 190
   nuclear, 50
   nucleated, 303
   plasma, 50
   synovial, 73
   tectorial, 325
   tympanic, 324, 343
Membranous urethra, 227
Memory cells, 350, 351, 363
Memory response, 363
Men-, 233
Menarche, 233
Meniere's syndrome, 344
Meningematoma, 310

Meningeorrhaphy, 311
Meninghematoma, 310
Meningioma, 310
Meningitis, 305
Mening/o-, 27
Meningocele, 307
Meningoencephalitis, 305
Meningoencephalocele, 307
Meningoencephalomyelitis, 305
Meningofibroblastoma, 310
Meningomyelitis, 305
Meningomyelocele, 307
Meningomyeloradiculitis, 305
Meningoradiculitis, 305
Meninx (meninges), 283, 302
Menkes' syndrome, 307
Menometrorrhagia, 253
Menopause, 233, 251
Menorrhagia, 169, 253
Menoschesis, 25
Menostasis, 253
Mensis (menses), 233, 251
Menstrual cycle, 233
Menstruation, 232, 251
    stages of, 233, 234
Mental region, 57
Mental retardation, 313
Merkel's disks, 327
Mes-, 12
Mesencephalon, 285
Mesenteric artery, 166
Mesenteric vein, 151, 168
Mesentery, 200, 214
Meso-, 12, 51
Mesoderm, 251
Mesopexy, 220
Mesothelium, 51, 64
Meta-, 12, 49
Metabolic and deficiency diseases, terms related to,
    96
Metabolism, 49-50, 64
Metacarpals, 67, 69, 72, 92
Metacarpophalangeal joint, 93
Metaphysis, 92
Metatarsalgia, 94
Metatarsals, 67, 69, 73, 92
Metatarsectomy, 96
Metatarsophalangeal joint, 93
Methoxy-hydroxymandelic acid, 122 3-
Methylphenidates, 318
Metr/a-, 27
Metratrophia, 253
Metric system and equivalents, 385
Metritis, 252
Metr/o-, 27, 232
Metroperitonitis, 252
Metrophlebitis, 252
Metrorrhagia, 169, 253
Metrorrhexis, 253
Metrosalpingitis, 252
Metrostenosis, 253
Micr-, 12
Micro-, 12
Microbiophobia, 314
Microcephalia, 307
Microcephalus, 307
Microcephaly, 307
Microcornea, 340
Microcytic anemia, hypochromic, 170
Microgastria, 216
Microglia, 282, 303
Microgyrus, 308
Micromyelia, 308
Microphakia, 340
Microphthalmos, 340
Microstomia, 216

Microtia, 343
Midbrain, 284, 285, 302
Middle ear, 324, 343
Midline, 55
Midsagittal, plane, 55
Millon Clinical Multiaxial Inventory, 314
Mineralocorticoids, 264, 266, 277
Minimal identifiable odor, 345
Minnesota Multiphasia Personality Inventory, 314
Mi/o-, 37
Misogyny, 317
Misopedia, 317
Mitochondria, 50, 64
Mitosis, 51, 64
Mitral valve, 141, 164
Mitral valve prolapse, 171
Moebius syndrome, 308
Mogi-, 317
Mogilalia, 317
Molars, 196
    sectioned, 198
Mole, hydatidiform, 253
Molecule, 64
Molilalia, 317
Monckeberg's arteriosclerosis, 171-172
Mongolism, 370
Monilia, 252
Moniliasis, 367
Monoamine oxidase inhibitors, 318
Monoblasts, 144
Monoclonal antibodies, 363
Monocytes, 144, 146, 165
Monocytic leukemia, 170
Monocytopenia, 172
Monocytopoiesis, 165
Monocytosis, 172
Mononucleosis, infectious, 363, 368
Monoplegia, 309
Mons pubis, 232, 251
Morph/o-, 34
Morquio's syndrome, 95
Morton's disease, 94
Morton's foot, 94
Morton's neuralgia, 94
Morton's toe, 94
Motor nerves, 100
Motor neurons, 281
Mountain fever, 369
Mountain tick fever, 369
Mouth, 195-198
Movement, types of, 75
MRI; see Magnetic resonance imaging
Mucin in gastric juice, 199
Mucocele, 217
Mucocutaneous lymph node syndrome, 368
Mucopolysaccharidosis, 370
Mucosa, nasal, 175
Mucous colitis, 215
Mucous lining coat of stomach wall, 199
Mucous membrane, 190
Mucoviscidosis, 370
Mucus, 39
Mucus test, 223
Mult-, 12
Multangular bone, 72
Multi-, 12
Multifidus spinae muscle, 119
Multi-infarct dementia, 309
Multiplane imager, 312
Multiple idiopathic hemorrhagic sarcoma, 373
Multiple insurance policies, 397
Multiple lymphoma, 364
Multiple sclerosis, 309, 352, 364
Multiple system diseases, 366-373
Mumps, 368
Munchausen by proxy disorder, 313

Munchausen syndrome, 313
Murmur, cardiac, 171
Muscle fibers, 100
Muscle groups, 103-108
Muscle tissue, 52
    cardiac, 52, 53, 63
    involuntary, 64
    types of, 53
    voluntary, 64
Muscles, 99; see also specific muscle
    abdominal, 106-107, 119
    of arms and hands, 104
    attachment of, 101
    of back, 104
    cardiac, 100
    classification of, 100
    composition of, 100
    degenerative and innervative disorders of, 121
    descriptive and diagnostic terms, 122
    facial, 103, 104
    of foot, 108
    hereditary, congenital, and developmental
        disorders of, 121
    inflammations and infections of, 120
    of inspiration, 190
    laboratory tests on, 122
    of mastication, 103
    movement of, 101
    naming, 101-102
    of neck and shoulder, 103-104
    oncology of, 121
    of pelvic floor, 107
    of scalp, 103
    skeletal, 100
    superficial, of body, 105, 106
    surgical procedures involving, 121-122
    of thigh and leg, 107-108
    of thorax, 106
    visceral, 100
Muscular atrophy, 121
Muscular coat of stomach wall, 199
Muscular dystrophy, 121
Muscular structures, 99-100
Muscular system, 54, 99-122
Musculocutaneous nerve, 305
Musophobia, 314
My/o-, 27
Myalgia, 122
Myasthenia gravis, 121, 352, 364
Myatonia congenita, 121
Myectomy, 121
Myel-, 305
Myelin sheath, 282, 303
Myelinated nerves, 303
Myelitis, 305
Myel/o-, 27
Myeloblastic leukemia, 170
Myeloblasts, 144
Myelocele, 308
Myelocystocele, 308
Myelocystomeningocele, 308
Myelodysplasia, 308
Myelography, 312
Myelomeningocele, 308
Myeloneuritis, 306
Myelophthisic anemia, 170
Myeloplegia, 309
Myeloradiculitis, 306
Myeloradiculodysplasia, 308
Myeloschisis, 308
Myelosyphilis, 306
Myoblastoma, 121
Myoblastomyoma, 121
Myocardial infarction, 172
Myocarditis, 169
Myocardium, 141, 165

Myocellulitis, 120
Myochorditis, 120
Myoclonus, 122
Myodiastasis, 122
Myodynia, 122
Myodystonia, 122
Myodystrophia, 121
Myoedema, 122
Myofascitis, 120
Myofibroma, 121
Myofibrosis, 121
Myogelosis, 122
Myoglobin, 122
Myokinesimeter, 122
Myokinesis, 122
Myology, 99, 122
Myolysis, 122
Myoma, 121
Myomalacia, 122
Myomelanosis, 122
Myometritis, 252
Myometrium, 232, 251
Myonecrosis, 122
Myoparalysis, 121
Myopathy, 122
Myopia, 341
Myoplasty, 121
Myorrhaphy, 121
Myosarcoma, 121
Myosclerosis, 122
Myositis, 120
Myositis ossificans, 120
Myospasm, 122
Myosuture, 121
Myotasis, 122
Myotenositis, 120
Myotenotomy, 121-122
Myotomy, 122
Myotonia, 121
Myotonia acquista, 121
Myotonia congenita, 121
Myotonia hereditaria, 121
Myringectomy, 344
Myringitis, 343
Myring/o-, 27
Myringodectomy, 344
Myringoplasty, 344
Myringotomy, 344
Mysophobia, 314
Myxedema, 279
Myx/o-, 39
Myxoma, atrial, 172

N

Nabothian cyst, 253-254
Nagel's test, 342
Nail-patella syndrome, 95
Nails, 126
    spoon, 136
Narcissism, 317
Narcissistic personality disorder, 313
Narco-, 309
Narcolepsy, 309
Naris (nares), 190, 326, 345
Nasal bones, 67, 70
Nasal cartilage, 93
Nasal concha(e), 70, 326
Nasal mucosa, 175
Nasal septum, 190, 326, 345
    deviated, 192
Nasal turbinates, 70, 326
Nasal vein, 168
Naso, 175
Nas/o-, 24, 326
Nasopharyngeal cyst, 192

Nasopharyngitis, 191
Nasopharynx, 175, 190
Nasosinusitis, 191
Natrium, 40
Natural immunity, 352, 363
Natural killer cells, 351, 363
Nausea, 217
Navel, 252
Navicular bone, 72, 73, 92
Neck and shoulder, muscles of, 103-104
Necr/o-, 37
Necrobiosis lipoidica, 136
Necrobiosis lipoidica diabeticorum, 136
Necrolysis, epidermal, toxic, 135
Necromania, 317
Necrophilia, 317
Necrophobia, 314
Necrosadism, 317
Necrotizing enterocolitis, neonatal, 216
Negativism, 317
Negativistic personality disorder, 313
Neimann's disease, 371 see also Niemann-Pick
Neo-, 12
Neomammary carcinoma, 254
Neonatal necrotizing enterocolitis, 216
Neonate, 251
Neonatology, 387
Nephrectomy, 248
Nephritis, 247
Nephr/o-, 27, 224
Nephroangiosclerosis, 247
Nephroblastoma, 248
Nephrocapsectomy, 248
Nephrocystanastomosis, 248
Nephrolith, 247
Nephrolithiasis, 247
Nephrolithotomy, 248
Nephromalacia, 247
Nephromegaly, 247
Nephron, 224, 225, 246
Nephropexy, 248
Nephroptosis, 247
Nephropyelitis, 247
Nephropyelolithotomy, 248
Nephrorrhagia, 247
Nephrorrhaphy, 248
Nephrosclerosis, arteriolar, 247
Nephrosis, 247
Nephrosplenopexy, 248
Nephrostomy, 248
Nephrotomy, 248
Nephrotresis, 248
Nephrotuberculosis, 247
Nephroureterectomy, 249
Nephroureterocystectomy, 249
Nerve endings, free, 345
    sensory, 327
Nerve fibers, 282
Nerve function in heart action, 142
Nerve impulses, 281
Nerve pathways, 291
Nerve trunk, 303
Nerves, 282; see also specific nerve
    controlling respiration, 179
    motor, 100
    structure and function of, 281-282
Nervous system, 54, 281-319
    autonomic, 142, 292, 301
    central, 283-286, 301
    characteristics of, 281-282
    hereditary, congenital, and developmental
        disorders of, 306-308
    inflammations and infections of, 305-306
    laboratory tests and procedures on, 311-312
    parasympathetic, 288, 292, 301
    pathologic conditions of, 305-310

Nervous system—cont'd
    peripheral, 289-292, 301
    surgical procedures of, 311
    sympathetic, 288, 292, 301
Nervous tissue, 53, 64
Neuralgia, 309
    Morton's, 94
Neurectomy, 311
Neurilemma, 282, 303
Neurilemoma, 310
Neurinoma, 310
Neuritis, 306
    optic, 339
Neur/o-, 27, 53
Neuroamebiasis, 306
Neuroanastomosis, 311
Neuroblastoma, 310
Neurochorioretinitis, 306
Neurocytoma, 310
Neurodynia, 309
Neuroepithelioma, 310
Neurofibroma, 310
Neurofibromatosis, 308, 371
Neurofibromatosis type 1, 371
Neurofibromatosis type 2, 371
Neuroglia, 53, 282, 303
Neurogliocytoma, 311
Neuroglioma, 311
Neurohypophysis, 276, 277
Neurolemma, 303
Neurolemmoma, 310
Neurologic and psychiatric conditions, tests for,
    314-315
Neurologic hospital report, 388
Neurological surgery, 386
Neurology, 387
Neurolysis, 311
Neuroma, acoustic, 344
Neuromyelitis, 306
Neuromyositis, 306
Neurons, 53, 281, 303
Neuropathy, optic, anterior ischemic, 340
Neuroplasty, 311
Neuropsychological tests, 315
Neuroradiography, stereotaxic, 312
Neurorrhaphy, 311
Neurosis, 317
Neurosurgery Center comprehensive examination
    of aphasia, 315
Neurotomy, 311
Neurotransmitter, 282, 303
Neurotransmitter reuptake inhibitors, 318
Neurotripsy, 311
Neutrocytopenia, 172
Neutropenia, 172
Neutrophil, 165
Neutrophila, 146
Nevus, 137
Newborn, hemolytic disease of, 372
Niemann-Pick disease, 371 see also Neimann's
Nipha, 341
Niphablepsia, 340-341
Nipple, Paget's disease of, 254
Nitrogen, total, 223
NK cells, 351, 363
NMR; see Magnetic resonance imaging
Noctiphobia, 314
Nocturnus, 317
Node(s)
    atrioventricular, 142
    of heart, 164, 165
    lymph, 347, 363
    Ranvier's, 303
    sinoatrial, 142
Nodule, 134
-nomia, 315

Nonspecific immune mechanisms, 349-350
Nonstriated muscle, 100
Noradrenaline, 264, 267, 277
Norepinephrine, 264, 267, 277
Nose, 175, 326
    glioma of, 193
    polyposis of, 193
Noso, 315
Nosophilia, 317
Nostrils, 326
Nuchal, 56, 57
Nuclear magnetic resonance; see Magnetic
        resonance imaging
Nuclear medicine, 386
Nuclear membrane, 50
Nucleated membrane, 303
Nuclei, 64
    nerve, 282
Nucleolus (nucleoli), 51, 64
Nucleus, 64, 302
    of cells, 50
Null cells, 351, 363
Nutrient artery, 166-167
Nyctalopia, 341
Nyctophobia, 314
Nymphomania, 317
Nys-, 341
Nystagmus, 341

O
-o, 23
O blood type, 147
Oat cell carcinoma, 193
Oblique external abdominal muscle, 119
Oblique fibers of stomach wall, 199
Oblique internal abdominal muscle, 119
Oblique muscles, 106
Obsessive-compulsive disorder, 313
Obstetrics and gynecology, 387
Obstipation, 217
Obturator artery, 167
Obturator externus muscle, 108, 119
Obturator internus muscle, 108, 119
Obturator nerve, 305
Obturator vein, 168
Occipital, 57
Occipital artery, 167
Occipital bone, 68, 70, 92
Occipital fontanel, 69
Occipital lobe of cerebral cortex, 286
Occipital vein, 168
Occipitalis muscle, 103
Occipit/o-, 24
Occipitofrontal muscle, 119
Occipitofrontal muscle group, 103
Occlusion, 172
Occupational dermatitis, 135
Ochronosis, 372
Ocul-, 103
Ocular muscles, 320
Ocul/o-, 24, 320
Oculomotor nerve, 290, 304
Odont/o-, 24
Odontogenic fibrosarcoma, 218
Odontoma, 218
-oid, 15
Oidomycosis, 367
-ola, 15
-ole, 15
Olecranon processes, 72, 92
    of ulna, 68
Ole/o-, 40
Olfact, 326
Olfactory bulb, 326
Olfactory center, 345
    in brain, 326

Olfactory coefficient, 345
Olfactory epithelium, 326, 345
Olfactory nerve, 289, 304
Olfactory receptors, 175
Olig/o-, 37
Oligodendroblastoma, 311
Oligodendroglia, 282, 303
Oligodendroglioma, 311
Oligodontia, 216
Oligohydramnios, 254
Oligomenorrhea, 254
Oligopepsia, 217
Oligophrenia, 317
Oligospermia, 254
Oligotrophy, 217
Oliguria, 247
Ollier's disease, 95
-oma, 16
Omentectomy, 219
Omentopexy, 220
Omentorrhaphy, 219
Omentum, 200, 214
Om/o-, 24
Omohyoid muscle, 119
Omphalectomy, 219
Omphal/o-, 24
Omphalus, 251, 252
Oncology, terms related to, 96
Onych/o-, 24
Onychomycosis, 135
Onychoosteodysplasia, 95
Onychophagy, 317
Oophorectomy, 255
Oophoritis, 252
Oophor/o-, 27
Oophorocystectomy, 255
Oophorohysterectomy, 255
Oophoropexy, 255
Oophoroplasty, 255
Oophorosalpingectomy, 255
Oophorosalpingitis, 252
Oophorostomy, 255
Oophorotomy, 255
-op/ia, 34
Opacity
    corneal, 341
    lenticular, 341
Open heart surgery, 173
Ophidiophobia, 314
Ophthalmia, 339
Ophthalmic artery, 167
Ophthalmic nerve, 290, 304
Ophthalmic vein, 168
Ophthalmitis, 339
Ophthalm/o-, 24, 320
Ophthalmodiaphanoscope, 343
Ophthalmodynamometer, 343
Ophthalmoleukoscope, 343
Ophthalmology, 387
Ophthalmoplegia, 341
Ophthalmoscope, 343
Ophthalmotonometer, 343
Opisth/o-, 37, 309
Opisthognathism, 95
Opisthotonos, 309
Oppenheim's disease, 121
Optic, 320, 339
Optic chiasma, 286, 302, 322, 339
Optic disk, 322
Optic nerve, 289-290, 304, 320, 322
Optic neuritis, 339
Optic neuropathy, anterior ischemic, 340
Opt/ico-, 34
Opt/o-, 34
-or, 15
Oral cavity, 195-198

Oral glucose tolerance test, 223
Orb, 339
Orbicularis, 102
Orbicularis oculi muscle, 103, 119
Orbicularis oris muscle, 103, 119
Orbit, 67, 339
Orbital, 57
Orbitalis muscle, 119
Orbitotomy, 342
Orbits, 70
Orchi/do-, 27
Orchidorrhaphy, 255
Orchiectomy, 255
Orchi/o-, 27
Orchiopexy, 255
Orchioplasty, 255
Orchis-, 250
Orchitis, 252
Organ, 49
    of Corti, 325, 343
Organelles, 50
Organic disorder, 314
Organic matter, 64
Organs, 54
    of lower respiratory tract, 177-178
    of lymphatic system, 348
    reproductive
        female, 230-233
        male, 228-229
    of upper respiratory tract, 175-176
    vomeronasal, 345
Origin of muscle, 99
Ornithine carbamoyl transferase, 222
Or/o-, 24
Oropharynx, 175, 190, 195, 214
Orth/o-, 37
Orthopaedic surgery, 387
Orthopnea, 192
Os, 232, 251
Os pubis, 92
Os triquetrum, 92
Osche/o-, 27
-osis, 15
Osler's disease, 372
Osmesis, 345
Osmesthesia, 345
Osmodysphoria, 345
Oss-, 65
Ossein, 92
Oss/eo-, 27
Osseous cell, 92
Osseous tissue, 65; see also Bone
Osseous tuberculosis, 94
Oss/i-, 27
Ossicles, 69, 92, 324, 343
    auditory, 324
Ossiculectomy, 344
Ossiculotomy, 344
Ost-, 65
Ostalgia, 97
Ost/e-, 27
Ostealgia, 97
Ostearthrotomy, 96
Ostectomy, 96
Osteitis, 94
Ost/eo-, 27
Osteoarthritis, 3, 94
Osteoblastoma, 96
Osteoblasts, 65, 66, 92
Osteochondritis, 94
Osteochondroma, 96
Osteoclasia, 97
Osteoclasis, 96
Osteoclasts, 66, 92
Osteocyte, 92
Osteodiastasis, 97

Osteodynia, 97
Osteodystrophy, 97
  renal, 96
Osteogenesis, 92
Osteogenesis imperfecta, 95
Osteogenetic, 97
Osteoid, 97
Osteology, 65
Osteolysis, 97
Osteoma, 96
Osteomalacia, 96, 97
Osteomyelitis, 94
Osteonecrosis, 97
Osteoneuralgia, 97
Osteopathy, 97
Osteopetrosis, 95
Osteoplasty, 96
Osteopoikilosis, 95
Osteoporosis, 96
Osteorrhagia, 97
Osteorrhaphy, 96
Osteosarcoma, 96
Osteosclerosis, 97
Osteospongioma, 96
Osteotomy, 96
Ostomies, 220-221
Otalgia, 344
Otitis externa, 343
Otitis interna, 343
Otitis media, 343
Ot/o-, 24, 324
Otodynia, 344
Otolaryngology, 387
Otoliths, 325, 344
-otomy, 218
Otoneuralgia, 344
Otopyorrhea, 344
Otorrhagia, 344
Otorrhea, 344
Otosclerosis, 343
-ous, 15
Oval window, 325, 343
Ovarian artery, 167
Ovarian vein, 168
Ovariectomy, 255
Ovariocentesis, 255
Ovariostomy, 255
Ovariotomy, 255
Ovary(ies), 230-231, 251
  hormones of, 264
Oviducts, 251
Ovotestis, 253
Ovulation, 233
Ovum (ova), 230, 251
Oxy-, 37
Oxycephaly, 94
Oxygen, 190
Oxygeusia, 263, 345
Oxytocin, 263, 264, 265
Oxyuriasis, 215

P

Pacemaker, 142, 165
  artificial cardiac, 173
Pachy-, 37
Pachyleptomeningitis, 306
Pachymeningitis, 306
  hemorrhagic, 308
Pachymeninx (pachymeninges), 302
Pachyonychia congenita, 136
Pacinian corpuscles, 327-328, 346
Paget's disese of nipple, 254
Pain, sense of, 327, 328
Palate, 92, 195, 214
  cleft, 216

Palatine arches, 195, 214
Palatine bones, 70
Palatine nerve, 304
Palatine tonsils, 349
Palatine vein, 168
Palat/o-, 27
Palatoglossus muscle, 119
Palatopharyngeus muscle, 119
Palatoplasty, 219
Pale/o-, 37
Pali-, 317
Palilalia, 317
Pallor, 134
Palpebra(e), 320, 338, 339
Palpitation, 172
Palsy, 309
  cerebral, 309
    Lesch-Nyhan, 307
Pan-, 12
Panarteritis, 169, 368
Pancreas, 201, 213, 214, 267
  annular, 216
  fibrocystic disease of, 370
  hormones of, 264
Pancreatectomy, 219
Pancreatic juice, 201
Pancreatic polypeptide, 264, 267
Pancreatic vein, 151, 168
Pancreaticoduodenal artery, 167
Pancreaticoduodenal vein, 168
Pancreaticoduodenostomy, 221
Pancreaticogastrostomy, 221
Pancreaticojejunostomy, 221
Pancreatitis, 215
Pancreatomy, 219
Pancreatotomy, 219
Panhysterectomy, 255
Panic disorder, 313
Pannus, 341
Panophthalmitis, 339
Panoplegia, 309
Panotitis, 343
Pansinusitis, 191
Pap smear, 256
Papanicolaou smear, 256
Papilla(e), 196
  hair, 125
  renal, 224, 246
  of tongue, 326, 345
Papill/o-, 24
Papilloma, cutaneous, 136
Papilloma virus, human, 252
Papillomatosis, laryngeal, 193
Papule, 134
Para, 251, 266
Para-, 12
Para I, 251
Paracentesis, 218
Paraganglioma, 311
Parageusia, 345
Paragraphia, 317
Parakeratosis, 135
Paralalia, 317
Paralgesia, 317
Paralogia, 317
Paralysis, 309
  bulbar, progressive, 310
  Duchenne's, 310
  Erb-Duchenne, 309
  Erb's, 121, 305, 309
  Landry's, 305
  spastic, 121
Paralysis agitans, 310
Paramyotonia congenita, 121
Paranoia, 313
Paranoid personality disorder, 313

Paranoid schizophrenia, 314
Paraparesis, 310
Paraphasia, 310
Paraphilia, 313, 315, 316, 317
Paraphrasia, 310
Paraplegia, 310
Parasites test, 223
Parasitic skin infections, 135
Parasympathetic division of autonomic nervous
    system, 142
Parasympathetic nervous system, 288, 292, 301
Parathyroid glands, 266, 277
  hormones of, 264
Parathyroid hormone, 264, 266, 277
Parathyroid tetany, 279
Parathyroidectomy, 279
Paratyphoid fever, 363, 368
Paraurethral glands, 251
Paresis, 310
Parietal artery, 150, 151
Parietal bones, 68, 69, 70, 92
Parietal layer of heart, 141
Parietal lobe of cerebral cortex, 286
Parietal peritoneum, 200
Parietal pleura, 178, 190
Parkinson's disease, 310
Parkinsonism, 310
Paronychia, 135
Parotid salivary gland, 214
Parotid vein, 168
Parotidectomy, 219
Parotitis, 215, 368
Parovarian cyst, 254
Paroxysmal tachycardia, 172
Parrot fever, 191
Parturition, 251
Passive immunity, 352, 363
Passive-aggressive personality disorder, 313
Patch test, 137
Patella, 67, 69, 72-73, 92
Patent ductus arteriosus, 170
Pathologic conditions, terms related to, 94-96
Pathologic intoxication, 313
Pathology, 49, 387
Pathology reports, 394-395
Pavor, 317
Pavor diurnus, 317
Pavor nocturnus, 317
Payment, authorization for, 397
Pectineus muscle, 119
Pectoralis major muscle, 104, 119
Pectoralis minor muscle, 119
-pedia, 317
Pediatrics, 387
Pediculosis, 135
Pellagra, 217
Pelvic floor, muscles of, 107
Pelvic girdle, 69, 72, 92
Pelvic inflammatory disease, 252
Pelvis, 66
  renal, 224, 247
Pemphigus, 136
-penia, 16
Penis, 227, 229, 250
  dorsal veins of, 167
Peptic glands, 214
Peptic ulcer disease, 215
Per-, 13
Percussion, 194
Percutaneous transhepatic cholangiography, 222
Percutaneous transluminal coronary angioplasty,
    173
Percutaneous umbilical blood sampling, 256
Perfusion magnetic resonance imaging, 312
Peri-, 13
Periarteritis, 169

Periarteritis nodosa, 368
Pericardiac vein, 168
Pericardial space, 141
Pericardicentesis, 173
Pericardiectomy, 173
Pericardiocentesis, 173
Pericardiotomy, 173
Pericarditis, 169
Pericardium, 141, 165
Perihepatitis, 215
Perilymph, 343
Perilymph fluid, 325
Perimeningitis, 306
Perimetrium, 232
Perineal prostatectomy, 255
Perinephritis, 247
Perineum, 107
Periodontal diseae, 215
Periodontium, 196, 198
Periosteomyelitis, 94
Periosteum, 65-66, 92
Periostitis, 94
Peripheral nervous system, 289-292, 301
Perisplenitis, 169
Peristalsis, 195, 199, 214
Peritectomy, 342
Peritoneocentesis, 218
Peritoneum, 200, 214
Peritonitis, 215
Pernicious anemia, 170
Peroneal artery, 167
Peroneal nerve, 305
Peroneal vein, 168
Peroneus brevis muscle, 108, 119
Peroneus longus muscle, 108, 119
Peroneus tertius muscle, 108, 119
Peroophoritis, 252
Personality, sociopathic, 314
Personality disorders, 313
Pertussis, 191
Petechia(e), 134
Petechial hemorrhages, 169
Petit mal epilepsy, 307
Petrous, 40
-pexis, 16
-pexy, 16, 218
-phagia, 16
Phag/o-, 34, 50
Phagocytosis, 50, 64, 165, 349, 363
Phagomania, 313
-phagy, 16
Phalanx (phalanges), 67, 69, 72, 73, 92
Phall/o-, 24
Phan/ero-, 34
Phantom limb phenomenon, 317
Pharmacologic methods of treatment, 318
Pharyngeal artery, 166
Pharyngeal tonsils, 349, 363
Pharyngeal vein, 168
Pharyngectomy, 219
Pharyngitis, 191
Pharyng/o-, 27
Pharyngolaryngitis, 191
Pharyngopalatine arch, 214
Pharyngoplasty, 220
Pharyngorhinitis, 191
Pharyngotomy, 219
Pharynx, 175, 190, 199, 214
-phas-, 34
Phenomenon, Raynaud's, 172
Phenothiazines, 318
Phenylketonuria, 371
Pheochromocytoma, 279
Phil-, 34
Phimosis, 254
Phlebangioma, 172

Phlebectasia, 172
Phlebectasis, 172
Phlebemphraxis, 172
Phlebitis, 169
Phleb/o-, 27
Phlebolithiasis, 172
Phlebophlebostomy, 173
Phleboplasty, 173
Phleborrhaphy, 173
Phlebosclerosis, 172
Phlebostenosis, 172
Phobia, 314
-phobia, 16
Phobic disorders, 313
Phosphaturia, 247
Phrenectomy, 311
Phrenemphraxis, 311
Phren/i-, 27
Phrenia, 315
Phrenic artery, 167
Phrenic nerve, 190, 305
  respiration, 179
Phrenic vein, 168
Phrenicectomy, 193, 311
Phreniclasia, 311
Phren/ico-, 27
Phreniconeurectomy, 311
Phrenicotomy, 193, 311
Phrenicotripsy, 311
Phren/o-, 27
Physical examination, 390
Physical medicine and rehabilitation, 387
Physiology, 49
Phytobezoar, 217
Pia mater, 283, 302
Pia-arachnoid, 284, 302
Pica, 317
Pick's diseae, 310
Pil/o-, 24
Pineal body, 267, 271
Pineal gland, 267
  glioma of, 279
  hormones of, 264
Pinealectomy, 279
Pinealoma, 279
Pinkeye, 339
Pinna, 324, 343
Piriformis muscle, 108, 119
Pisiform bone, 72, 92
Pituicyte, 277
Pituitary cachexia, 279
Pituitary diaphragm, 261
Pituitary gland, 261-265, 277
  craniopharyngioma of, 279
  eosinophilic adenoma of, 279
Pituitary stalk, 261
Pivot joints, 74, 93
Pixie disease, 371
Placenta, 234, 251
  velamentous, 254
Placenta accreta, 254
Placenta bipartita, 254
Placenta circumvallata, 254
Placenta previa, 254
Placenta tripartita, 254
Plague, 368
Planes, anatomic, 55
Planing, skin, 137
Plasma, 39, 144, 165
Plasma cells, 350, 363
Plasma membrane, 50
Plasma volume, 222
Plasmacytoma, 172
Plasmocyte, 165
Plastic surgery, 387
-plasty, 16, 218

Platelets, 144, 147, 165
Platy-, 37
Platysma muscle, 103, 119
-plegia, 34
Ple/o-, 37
Plethysmography
  arterial, 173
  venous, 174
Pleura, 190
  parietal, 178, 190
  visceral, 177, 190
Pleuracentesis, 193
Pleuracotomy, 193
Pleural cavity, 178, 190
Pleuralgia, 192
Pleurectomy, 193
Pleurisy, 191
Pleur/o-, 27
Pleurocentesis, 193
Pleurodynia, 192
Pleuroparietopexy, 193
Pleuropericarditis, 191
Pleuropneumonia, 191
Plexus, 168, 291, 303
Plumbism, 372
Plumbum, 372
Plurals, 4
-pnea, 16
Pneum/a-, 27
Pneum/ato-, 27
Pneum/o-, 27
Pneumocentesis, 193
Pneumoconiosis, 192
Pneumocystis carinii pneumonia, 191, 367
Pneumoencephalography, 312
Pneumohemothorax, 192
Pneumohydrothorax, 192
Pneumolithiasis, 192
Pneumomalacia, 192
Pneumomediastinum, 192
Pneumomelanosis, 192
Pneumonectomy, 193
Pneumonia, 191
  Pneumocystis carinii, 191, 367
Pneumonitis, 191
Pneum/ono-, 27
Pneumonocirrhosis, 192
Pneumonopexy, 193
Pneumonorrhaphy, 193
Pneumonotomy, 193
Pneumopleuritis, 191
Pneumopyothorax, 192
Pneumorrhagia, 192
Pneumothorax, 192
Pod/o-, 24
-poiesis, 34
Poikil/o-, 37
Poisoning
  blood, 169
  food, 215
Polio, 306
Poli/o-, 40
Polioencephalitis, 306
Polioencephalomeningomyelitis, 306
Poliomyelencephalitis, 306
Poliomyelitis, 306
Poliomyeloencephalitis, 306
Poly-, 13
Polyarteritis, 169, 368
Polycoria, 340
Polycystic kidney disease, 247
Polycythemia, 172
Polycythemia vera, 172, 372
Polydipsia, 217, 219
Polyemia, 172
Polymastia, 253

Polymorphonuclear leukocyte, 165
Polymyalgia rheumatica, 120
Polyneuritis, 305, 306
Polyneuropathy, 305
Polyneuroradiculitis, 306
Polyorchism, 253
Polyotia, 344
Polyp, 193, 218
Polyphagia, 217
Polyposis, 218
    of nose, 326
Polyradiculitis, 305, 306
Polyserositis, 169
Polythelia, 253
Polyuria, 247, 279
Pons, 284-285, 302
Popliteal artery, 151, 167
Popliteal lymph nodes, 347
Popliteal muscle, 119
Popliteal vein, 151, 168
Porencephalia, 308
Porencephaly, 308
Poriomania, 317
Pornographomania, 317
Porphyria, 371
Portal vein, 168
Positions, anatomic, 55, 56
Positron emission computerized tomography, 174
Positron emission tomography, 174
Positron emission transaxial tomography, 312
Post-, 13
Posterior, 54
Posterior commissure, 286, 302-303
Posterior pituitary gland, 262, 263, 265
Posterior trunk, terms related to, 56, 57
Postmenstrual stage, 233
Postpartum hemorrhage, 169
Post-traumatic stress disorder, 313, 314
Potential space, 178, 190
Pott's disease, 94
PPD test, 137
Prader-Willi syndrome, 371
Pragmatagnosia, 310
Pre-, 13
Prefixes, 10-14
Prefrontal area, 286
Prefrontal lobotomy, 318
Pregnancy, 233-234
    ectopic, 251
Pregnancy tests, 256
Premenstrual stage, 233
Premenstrual syndrome, 254, 317
Premolars, 196
Premotor area, 286
Prepuce, 229, 250
Presbycusis, 344
Presbyopia, 341
Presenile dementia, 308
Presentation, 251
Pressure
    blood, 147
    pulse, 147
    sense of, 327
Preventive medicine, 387
Priapism, 252
Primary degenerative dementias, 308
Primary tastes, 345
Prime movers, 101
Primigravida, 251
Primipara, 251
Pro-, 13
Process, 69
    acromial, 91
    mastoid, 92
    olecranon, 72, 92
    of ulna, 68

Process—cont'd
    styloid, 93
    xiphoid, 67, 92
Proctalgia, 217
Proctectomy, 219
Proctitis, 215
Proct/o-, 27
Proctocele, 217
Proctococcypexy, 220
Proctopexy, 220
Proctoplasty, 220
Proctoptosis, 217
Proctorrhaphy, 219
Proctoscopy, 222
Proctosigmoidectomy, 219
Proctosigmoidoscopy, 222
Proctostomy, 221
Proctotomy, 219
Proctotoreusis, 221
Proerythroblasts, 144
Proetz test, 345
Progeria, juvenile, 371
Progesterone, 230, 264, 267, 277
Prognathism, 95
Progressive bulbar paralysis, 310
Progressive spinal muscular atrophy of infants, 121
Prolactin, 263, 265, 277
Prolapse
    mitral valve, 171
    of uterus, 254
Pronation, 75
Pronator quadratus muscle, 119
Pronator teres muscle, 104, 119
Prone position, 56
Propanediols, 318
Prostaglandins, 350, 363
Prostate gland, 229, 250
    transurethral resection of, 256
Prostate specific antigen, 256
Prostatectomy, 255, 256
Prostatic acid phosphatase, 256
Prostatic carcinoma, 254
Prostatic hypertrophy, 253, 254
Prostatic urethra, 227
Prostatitis, 252
Prostatomy, 256
Prostatotomy, 256
Prostatovesiculectomy, 256
Prosthesis, cardiac, 173
Protanomalopsia, 340
Protanomaly, 340
Protanopia, 340
Protein, 222
Protein-bound iodine, 266, 280
Proteus syndrome, 371
Prothrombin, 147, 165
Prothrombin time, 174
Proximal, 54
Proximal convoluted tubule, 226, 227
Prozac, 318
Pruritus ani, 217
Pruritus vulvae, 254
Pseud-, 13
Pseudo-, 13
Pseudocyesis, 317
Pseudographia, 317
Pseudohermaphroditism, 253
Pseudohypertrophic muscular atrophy, 121
Pseudohypertrophic muscular dystrophy, 121
Pseudoisochromatic test, 342
Pseudologia, 317
Pseudomania, 317
Pseudoparalysis, atonic, 121
Pseudorickets, 96
Pseudostratified epithelial tissue, 51, 52
Psittacosis, 191

Psoas major muscle, 119
Psoas minor muscle, 119
Psoriasis, 136
Psychalia, 317
Psyche, 317
Psychiatric conditions, 312-314
    tests for, 314-315
    treatment methods for, 318-319
Psychiatry, 387
Psychoanalytic therapy, 319
Psychogenic, 317
Psycholepsy, 317
Psychomotor epilepsy, 307
Psychopathic personality, 314
Psychosis (psychoses), 313, 317
Psychosomatic, 314
Psychotherapies, 318
Psychotic disorder, 314
Pterygoid muscles, 103
Ptosis, 341
-ptosis, 16
Ptyalectasis, 221
Ptyalin amylase, 214
Ptyal/o-, 39
Ptysis, 169
Pubic, 56, 57
Pubiotomy, 97
Pubis, 67, 72, 92
Pudendal artery, 167
Pudendal nerve, 305
Pudendal vein, 168
Pudendum, 251
Puerperal eclampsia, 254
Pulm/o-, 27
Pulmonary artery, 142, 167
    transposition of, 170
Pulmonary circulation, 148
Pulmonary disease, chronic obstructive, 192
Pulmonary edema, 192
Pulmonary fibrosis, 192
Pulmonary function tests, 194
Pulmonary stenosis, 170
Pulmonary valve, 165
Pulmonary vein, 151, 168
Pulmonary volumes, 194
Pulp, splenic, 363
Pulp cavity of tooth, 198
Pulpitis, 215
Pulse, 147
Pulse pressure, 147
Punch biopsy, 137
Puncture, lumbar, 97
Pupil, 320, 322, 339
Pupillary reflex, 292
    altered, 340
Purkinje fibers, 142
Purpura, 134
    thrombocytopenic, 172, 352, 364
Purpura fulminans, 172
Pus, 39, 223
Pustule, 134
    malignant, 367
Pyel/o-, 27
Pyelitis, 247
Pyelocystanastomosis, 249
Pyelocystitis, 247
Pyelocystostomosis, 249
Pyelogram, 250
Pyelolithotomy, 249
Pyelonephrosis, 247
Pyelophlebitis, 169
Pyeloplasty, 249
Pyelostomy, 249
Pyelotomy, 249
Pyeloureterolysis, 249
Pyeloureteroplasty, 249

Pyknodysostosis, 95
Pyloric sphincter muscle, 199
Pyloric stenosis, congenital hypertrophic, 216
Pyloric vein, 151
Pylorodiosis, 221-222
Pyloroplasty, 220
Pylorospasm, 217
Pylorostomy, 221
Pylorotomy, 219
Pylorus, 214
    of stomach, 199
Py/o-, 39
Pyocolpos, 252
Pyometra, 252
Pyonephritis, 247
Pyonephrosis, 247
Pyosalpinx, 252
Pyothorax, 192
Pyr-, 350
Pyramidal muscle, 119
Pyramidal tracts, 291
Pyramidale bone, 72, 92
Pyrogens, 350, 363
Pyromania, 317
Pyuria, 248

Q

Q fever, 191
Quadratus, 102
Quadratus femoris muscle, 108, 120
Quadratus lumborum muscle, 120
Quadri-, 102
Quadriceps femoris muscle group, 108
Quadriceps femoris muscle, 120
Qualitative glucose, 223

R

Rabies, 306
Rachicentesis, 311
Rachi/o-, 27
Rachiocentesis, 311
Rachiotomy, 96
Rachitomy, 96
Radial artery, 150, 167
Radial keratotomy, 342
Radial nerve, 305
Radiation, heat loss through, 123
Radical mastectomy, 256
Radicotomy, 311
Radiculectomy, 311
Radiculitis, 306
Radiculo-, 305
Radiculoganglionitis, 305
Radiculomeningomyelitis, 306
Radiculoneuritis, 305
Radioactive iodine uptake, 280
Radiocarpal joint, 93
Radiographic studies of genitourinary system, 256-257
Radiography, dual energy, 97
Radioimmunoassay, 256
Radiologic reports, 394
Radiologic studies, 222-223
Radiology, 387
Radiomyelitis, 306
Radionuclide angiocardiography, 174
Radioreceptor assay, 256
Radioulnar joint, 94
Radius, 67, 68, 69, 72, 92
Ragsorters' disease, 367
Rales, 192
Ranvier's node, 303
Rat-bite fever, 368-369
Rationalization, 317
Raynaud's disease, 172

Raynaud's phenomenon, 172
Re-, 13
Receptors, 303
Recipient, universal, 147
Records, hospital, 388-396
Rectal columns, 201
Rect/o-, 27
Rectocele, 217
Rectosigmoid, 214
Rectostomy, 221
Rectum, 201
Rectus, 102
Rectus abdominis muscle, 106, 120
Rectus capitis muscle, 120
Rectus femoris muscle, 108, 120
Recumbent position, lateral, 56
Red bone marrow, 65
Red splenic pulp, 363
Reflex action, 292, 303
Reflex arc, 292
    in spinal cord, 291
Reflexes, 292
    pupillary, altered, 340
Reflux, 199
Refracting media, 320, 339
Refraction, 322, 343
Regional enteritis, 215
Regions, body, 56-57
Reil, island of, 286
Relapsing fever, 369
Release of information, authorization for, 397
Renal; see also Kidney
Renal angiography and arterioigraphy, 250
Renal artery, 167
Renal calculi, 247
Renal cell carcinoma, 248
Renal colic, 248
Renal corpuscle, 224, 226, 246
Renal cortex, 224, 246
Renal ectopia, 247
Renal infarction, 248
Renal medulla, 224, 246
Renal osteodystrophy, 96
Renal papillae, 224, 246
Renal pelvis, 224, 247
Renal pyramid; see Renal medulla
Renal rickets, 96
Renal scan, 250
Renal sinus, 224, 247
Renal tubule, 224, 226, 246, 247
Renal vein, 168
Ren/i-, 27
Ren/o-, 27
-reno-, 224
Replacement of heart, homograft, 173
Reports, hospital, 388-396
Reproductive organs
    female, 230-233
    male, 228-229
Reproductive system
    inflammations and infections of, 252
    laboratory tests and procedures of, 256
Resection, transurethral, of prostate, 256
Residual capacity, functional, 194
Residual schizophrenia, 314
Residual volume, 179, 190, 194
Resonance, magnetic, nuclear; see Magnetic
    resonance imaging
Respiration, 71, 190
    process of, 178-179
Respiratory cycle, 178-179
Respiratory system, 54, 175-194
    inflammations and infections of, 190-191
    laboratory and examination procedures on, 194
    oncology of, 193
    pathologic conditions of, 190-193

Respiratory system—cont'd
    structures and functions of, 175-178
    surgical procedures on, 193-194
Respiratory tract
    lower, organs of, 177-178
    upper, organs of, 175-176
Respiratory volumes, 179, 190
Rest in respiratory cycle, 178
Retardation, mental, 313
Retention, 248
Reticular activating system, 284
Reticulocyte, 165
Reticulocyte count, 174
Reticulocytopenia, 172
Reticulopenia, 172
Reticulum, endoplasmic, 50
Retina, 320, 322, 339
Retinal detachment, 341
Retinitis, 339
Retinitis pigmentosa, 340
Retinoblastoma, 341
Retinochoroiditis, 339
Retinopathy
    diabetic, 341
    hypertensive, 341
Retinoscopy, 343
Retro-, 13
Retrograde amnesia, 310
Retrograde pyelogram, 251
Retropharynx, 190
Retropubic prostatectomy, 256
Reye's syndrome, 306, 372
Rh factor, 147
Rh negative blood, 147
Rh positive blood, 147
Rhabdomyoblastoma, 121
Rhabdomyochondroma, 121
Rhabdomyoma, 121
Rhabdomyomyxoma, 121
Rhabdomyosarcoma, 121
Rhachis, 169
Rheumatic fever, 369
Rheumatoid arthritis, 352, 364
Rheumatoid factor, 98
Rhinilith, 192
Rhinitis, 3, 191
Rhin/o-, 24, 175, 326
Rhinodynia, 192
Rhinolaryngitis, 191
Rhinopharyngitis, 191
Rhinoplasty, 193
Rhinosalpingitis, 191
Rhizomeningomyelitis, 306
Rhizotomy, 311
Rhod/o-, 40
Rhomboideus, 102
Rhomboideus major muscle, 120
Rhomboideus minor muscle, 120
Rhonchus, 193
Ribonucleic acid, 50, 64
Ribosomes, 50, 64
Ribs, 69, 71, 178
Rickets, 96, 217
Riedel's struma, 278
Rigid cerebral palsy, 309
Ringworm, 135
Rinne test, 345
Risorius muscle, 103, 120
RNA, 50, 64
Rocky Mountain spotted fever, 369
Rods and cones, 320, 322, 339
Root, tooth, 196
Roots and combining forms, 23-28, 33-41
Rorschach test, 315
Rosacea, 135
Rotary joints, 74

Rotation, 75
Rough endoplasmic reticulum, 50
Round window, 325
-rrhage, 16
-rrhagia, 16
-rrhaphy, 16, 218
-rrhea, 16
-rrhexis, 16
Rubacell test, 174
Rubella, 369
Rubeola, 369
Ruber, 40
Rubor, 40
Rudimentary uterus, 253
Ruffinian corpuscles, 328, 346
Rugae, 214, 227
Rupture, 217
    suture of, 218-219

S

SA node, 142
Sacchar/i-, 40
Sacchar/o-, 40
Saccule, 325, 343
Sacral, 56, 57
Sacral artery, 167
Sacral vein, 168
Sacr/o-, 27
Sacrococcygeal joint, 94
Sacroiliac joint, 94
Sacrospinalis muscle, 118
Sacrum, 67, 68, 71, 92
Sadism, 317
Sadomasochism, 317
Sagittal plane, 55
Sagittal suture, 70, 92
Sal, 40
Saliva, 198, 214
Salivary gland virus disease, 368
Salivary glands, 214
Salmonellosis, 215-216
Salpingectomy, 256
Salpingitis, 252
Salping/o-, 27
Salpingocele, 254
Salpingo-oophorocele, 254
Salpingo-oophorectomy, 255
Salpingoovariectomy, 255
Salpingopexy, 256
Salpingorrhaphy, 256
Salpingostomatomy, 256
Salpingostomy, 256
Salpingotomy, 256
San Joaquin Valley fever, 191
Sangui-, 39
Sanguin/o-, 39
Saphenous nerve, 305
Saphenous veins, 151, 168
Sarc/o-, 27
Sarcoidosis, 372
Sarcolemma, 100, 120
Sarcoma
    Kaposi's, 364, 367, 373
    multiple idiopathic hemorrhagic, 373
Sarcoplasm, 100, 120
Sartorius muscle, 108, 120
Scabies, 135
Scalded skin syndrome, 135
Scale, 134
Scalenus, 102
Scalenus muscle, 120
Scalp, muscles of, 103
Scan
    bone, 97
    lung, 194
    renal, 250

Scanning laser ophthalmoscope, 343
Scaphocephaly, 95
Scaphoid bone, 72, 73, 92
Scapula (scapulae), 66, 68, 69, 72, 92
Scapular, 56, 57
Scapular nerve, dorsal, 304
Scapular vein, 151
Scapuloclavicular joint, 94
Scapulohumeral junction, 93
Scapulopexy, 97
Scarlatina, 369
Scarlet fever, 369
Schick test, 137
Schist/o-, 34
Schistosomiasis, 369
Schiz/o-, 34
Schizoaffective disorder, 314
Schizoid personality disorder, 313
Schizophrenia, 314
Schizophrenic disorder, 314
Schizotypal personality disorder, 313
Schlemm, canal of, 322, 338
Schwabach test, 345
Schwann, sheath of, 282, 303
Schwann cells, 282
Schwannoma, 310
Sciatic nerve, 305
Sclera, 320-321, 339
Sclerectomy, 342
Scleriritomy, 342
Scleritis, 339
Scler/o-, 37
Sclerochoroiditis, 339
Scleroconjunctivitis, 339
Scleroderma, 372
Sclerokeratitis, 339
Scleroplasty, 342
Sclerosing adenosis, 254
Sclerosis, 307, 308, 309
    multiple, 352, 364
    systemic, 372
Sclerostomy, 342
Scleroticectomy, 342
Sclerotomy, 342
Scoli/o-, 37
Scoliosis, 97
-scope, 16
Scopophilia, 318
-scopy, 16
Scratch test, 137
Scrotoplasty, 256
Scrotum, 228-229, 250
Scrub typhus, 370
Scurvy, 96, 217
Seasonal affective disorder, 279
Sebaceous cyst, 137
Sebaceous glands, 124, 125, 134
Seborrheic dermatitis, 135
Seborrheic keratosis, 137
Seborrheic wart, 137
Sebum, 40, 125, 134
Secondary bronchi, 177
Secretin, 201, 214
Sedimentation rate, erythrocyte, 174
Segmental fracture, 95
Seizure, jacksonian, 309
Self-defeating personality disorder, 313
Sella turcica, 261
Semen, 229, 250
Semi-, 13
Semicircular canals, 325, 343
Semi-Fowler's position, 56
Semilunar bone, 72, 92
Semilunar cartilage, 93
Semilunar valve, 142, 165
Semimembranosus muscle, 108, 119, 120

Seminal fluid tests, 257
Seminal vesicles, 229, 250
Seminal vesiculitis, 252
Seminiferous tubules, 229, 250
Seminoma, 254
Seminuria, 254
Semispinalis muscle, 120
Semitendinosus muscle, 108, 119, 120
Senile dementia, 309
Senilis, 340
Senility, 310
Senses, special, 54, 320-346
Sensorineural deafness, 344
Sensory nerve endings, free, 327
Sensory neurons, 281, 303
Septal cartilage, 93
Septectomy, 194
Septicemia, 169
Septum
    interatrial, 141
    interventricular, 141
    of limbic system, 287
    nasal, 190, 326, 345
        deviated, 192
Serous coat of stomach wall, 199
Serratia infection, 369
Serratus, 102
Serratus anterior muscle, 120
Serratus muscle group, 120
Serratus posterior inferior muscle, 120
Serratus posterior superior muscle, 120
Sertoli's cells, 250
Serum, 39
Serum ammonia, 312
Serum enzyme tests, 174
Sesamoid bone, 92
Severe combined immunodeficiency disease, 352, 364
Sex hormones, 264, 266
Sexually transmitted diseses, 252-253
Shadow test, 343
Shaft, hair, 125, 134
Shaken infant syndrome, 310
Sheath of Schwann, 303
Sheehan's syndrome, 279
Shigellosis, 216
Shin splints, 120
Shingles, 305
Shock, insulin, 217
Short bones, 66
Shoulder and neck, muscles of, 103-104
Shoulder girdle, 92
Sialadenitis, 216
Sial/o-, 39
Sialoadenectomy, 219
Sialoadenotomy, 219
Sialodochoplasty, 220
Sialography, 223
Sialolithotomy, 219
Sickle cell anemia, 170
Siderosis, 192
Siemerling-Creutzfeldt disease, 306
Sigmoid, 214
Sigmoid artery, 167
Sigmoid colon, 201
Sigmoid vein, 151, 168
Sigmoidectomy, 219
Sigmoidopexy, 220
Sigmoidoproctostomy, 221
Sigmoidorectostomy, 221
Sigmoidoscopy, 222
Sigmoidosigmoidostomy, 221
Sigmoidostomy, 221
Sigmoidotomy, 219
Signet ring cell carcinoma, 218
Silicosis, 192

Silver-fork fracture, 96
Simmonds' disease, 279
Simple epithelial tissue, 51, 52
Sim's position, 56
Single photon emission computed tomography, 312
Sinistr/o-, 37
Sinoatrial node, 142, 165
Sinus(es), 69
   ethmoid, 70, 190
   frontal, 70, 190
   mastoid, 70
   maxillary, 70, 190
   renal, 224, 247
   sphenoid, 70, 190
   venous, 151
Sinusitis, 191
Sinusoid, 165, 363
Sinusoidal capillary, 165
Sinusotomy, 194
-sis, 15
Sitomania, 313
Skeletal muscle, 100
Skeletal muscle tissue, 52, 53
Skeletal system, 54, 65-98
Skeleton, 65-66
   anterior view of, 67
   appendicular, 66-68, 72-73
   axial, 66-71
   posterior view of, 68
Skene's gland, 251
Skin, 123
   and accessory structures, 123-137
   bacterial, fungal, viral, and parasitic infections of,
      135-136
   composition of, 124, 125
   grafts of, 137
   hereditary, congenital, and developmental
      disorders of, 136
   inflammations and allergies of, 134-135
   laboratory tests involving, 137
   oncology involving, 136-137
   pathologic conditions of, 134-136
   structure of, 124
   surgical procedures on, 137
Skin graft, 137
Skin tag, 136
Skull, 69
   coronal section through, 283
   principal bones and sutures of, 70
Skull x-ray, 98
Sleeping sickness, 370
Small cell carcinoma, 193
Small intestine, 199, 201
Small saphenous vein, 151, 168
Smallpox, 369
Smear
   buccal, 137
   Papanicolaou, 256
Smell, sense of, 326, 327
Smooth endoplasmic reticulum, 50
Smooth muscle, 100
Snellen eye chart, 343
Snow blindness, 341
Sociopathic personality, 314
Sodoku, 368
Sodomy, 317
Soft palate, 195
Solar blindness, 340
Soleus muscle, 108, 120
Soma, 291
Somatization disorder, 314
Somat/o-, 24
Somatoform disorders, 313
Somatotrophin, 277
Somatotropin, 261, 263, 277
Somnambulism, 317

Sonogram, 343
Sophomania, 317
Sores, canker, 134
Sorting tests, 315
Space, pericardial, 141
Spasm/o-, 34
Spastic cerebral palsy, 309
Spastic colon, 215
Spastic paralysis, 121
Spatial vectorcardiogram, 174
Special senses, 54, 320-346
Specific immune mechanisms, 350-351
Specimen, urine, catheterized, 249
Speech area, Broca's, 286
Spel-, 308
Spelencephaly, 308
Spelling, 4
Spermatic artery, 166
Spermatic cords, 229, 250
Spermatic vein, 168
Spermatid, 250
Spermatoblast, 250
Spermatocele, 254
Spermatozoon (spermatozoa), 229, 250
Spermaturia, 254
Sphenoid bone, 70, 92
Sphenoid sinuses, 70, 190
Sphincter, 214
Sphincter ani muscle, 107
Sphincter muscles, 120, 199
   rectal, 201
Sphincteroplasty, 220
Sphincterotomy, 219
Sphingolipidosis, cerebral, 307
Spielmeyer-Vogt disease, 307
Spina bifida, 308
Spina bifida occulta, 308
Spinal accessory nerve, 290, 304
Spinal cord, 287, 288, 303
   reflex arc in, 291
Spinal muscular atrophy
   familial, 121
   of infants, progressive, 121
Spinal nerves, 287, 288, 290, 291, 304-305
Spinal vein, 168
Spinal x-ray, 98
Spine, 69
Splanchn/ee-, 27
Splanchn/o-, 27
Splanchnoptosis, 218
Spleen, 347-349, 363
   accessory, 364
Splenectomy, 364
Splenic artery, 167
Splenic capsule, 363
Splenic fever, 367
Splenic pulp, 363
Splenic vein, 151, 168
Splenitis, 363
Splenius capitis muscle, 120
Splenius cervicis muscle, 120
Splenius muscle group, 120
Splen/o-, 27
Splenomegaly, 364
Splenopexy, 364
Splenoportography, 223
Splenorrhaphy, 364
Splenotomy, 364
Splintered fracture, 96
Spondylarthritis, 94
Spondylitis, tuberculous, 94
Spondyl/o-, 27
Spondylodesis, 97
Spondylosyndesis, 97
Spongioblastoma, 311
Spongiocytoma, 311

Spongiosis, 134
Spontaneous abortion, 254
Spoon nails, 136
Sporotrichosis, 363, 369
Spotted fever, 369
Sprue, 218
Squamous cell carcinoma, 137, 193
Squamous epithelial tissue, 51, 52
Squamous epithelium, 64
Squamous suture, 92
Srongyloidiasis, 216
Stain, eye, fluorescent, 342
Stannosis, 192
Stapedectomy, 344
Stapes, 92, 324, 343
Stargardt's disease, 341
-stasis, 34
Stein-Leventhal syndrome, 254
Stellwag's sign, 341
Stem cell leukemia, 170
Stem cells, 144
Sten/o-, 37
Stenosis, 216, 218
   pulmonary, 170
Stere/o-, 37
Stereotaxic neuroradiography, 312
Sterility, 254
Sternal, 56, 57
Sternal cartilage, 93
Stern/o-, 27
Sternoclavicular joint, 72, 94
Sternocleidal joint, 94
Sternocleidomastoid muscle, 103, 120
Sternocostal joint, 94
Sternohyoid muscle, 119
Sternothyroid muscle, 119
Sternotomy, 97
Sternum, 66, 67, 69, 71, 92
Steth/o-, 24
Stigma, 340
Stimulant drugs, 318
Stokes-Adams syndrome, 172
Stom-, 24
Stomach, 199, 214
Stomatic/o-, 24
Stomatitis, 215, 216
   aphthous, 134
Stomat/o-, 24
Stomatoplasty, 220
-stomy, 16, 218
Stool culture, 223
Stool tests, 223
Strabismus, 341
Stratified epithelial tissue, 51, 52
Stratified epithelium, 64
Stratum corneum, 124, 134
Stratum germinativum, 124, 134
Stratum granulosum, 124, 134
Stratum lucidum, 124, 134
Stress, 318
Stress test, thallium, 174
Striated, 64
Striated muscle, 100
Stroke, 308, 321
Struma, 278
   Riedel's, 278
Struma lymphomatosa, 278
Styloid process, 93
Sub-, 13
Subarachnoid, 303
Subarachnoid cisterns, 303
Subarachnoid hemorrhage, 308
Subarachnoid space, 284
Subclavian artery, 150, 167
Subclavian vein, 151, 168
Subclavius muscle, 120

Subcostal artery, 167
Subcostal muscles, 120
Subcutaneous, 134
Subdural hematoma, 308
Subdural hemorrhage, 308
Subdural space, 284, 303
Subinguinal, 56, 57
Sublingual salivary glands, 196, 214
Submandibular lymph nodes, 347
Submandibular salivary glands, 214
Submaxillary, 57
Submaxillary salivary glands, 196, 214
Submental, 57
Submucous coat of stomach wall, 199
Subscapular artery, 167
Subscapularis muscle, 120
Substance abuse disorders, 314
Substantia spongiosa ossium, 93
Subthalamus, 303
Sudden infant death syndrome, 372-373
Sudor, 39
Sudoriferous glands, 125, 134
Suffixes, 14-17
Sulcus (sulci), 69, 286, 303
Super-, 13
Supercilium (supercilia), 125, 134, 320, 339
Superficial muscles of body, 105, 106
Superficial veins, 151
Superior, 54
Superior mesenteric vein, 151
Superior nasal concha, 326
Superior vena cava, 168
Superior vena cava syndrome, 172
Supernumerary, 134, 253
Supernumerary kidney, 247
Supination, 75
Supinator muscle, 120
Supine position, 56
Supra-, 13
Supraclavicular, 56, 57
Supraorbital, 57
Supraorbital vein, 168
Suprarenal glands, 276, 277
Suprarenal vein, 168
Suprascapular, 56, 57
Supraspinatus muscle, 120
Surgery, 387
    laser, 342
Surgical procedure notes, 390-392
Surgical procedures, terms related to, 96-97
Suspensory ligament, 320, 321, 339
Suture, 69
    coronal, 69, 70, 91
    lambdoid, 70, 92
    sagittal, 70, 92
    skull, principal, 70
    squamous, 92
Swallowing, 199
Sweat electrolytes test, 373
Sweat glands, 125
    apocrine, 125, 133
Sylvius, aqueduct of, 285, 302
Sym-, 13
Symbols, abbreviations and, 377-383
Sympathectomy, 311
Sympathetectomy, 311
Sympathetic division of autonomic nervous system,
    142
Sympathetic nervous system, 288, 292, 301
Sympathicectomy, 311
Sympathicoblastoma, 311
Sympathicotripsy, 311
Sympathoblastoma, 311
Sympathogonioma, 311
Symphysis pubis, 72, 93, 232
Syn-, 13, 101

Synapse, 282, 303, 310
Synarthroses, 73, 94
Synchondrotomy, 97
Syndactylia, 95
Syndesmopexy, 97
Syndrome; see specific syndrome
Synechia, 341
Synergists, 101, 120
Synorchidism, 253
Synorchism, 253
Synosteotomy, 97
Synovectomy, 97
Synovial, 94
Synovial fluid, 98
Synovial joints, 73
Synovial membrane, 73
Synovioma, 96
Synovitis, 94
Syphilis, 252, 369
    cerebrospinal, 305
Syringobulbia, 308
Syringocele, 308
Syringocystadenoma, 136, 137
Syringoencephalomyelia, 308
Syringomyelia, 308
Syringomyelocele, 308
Systematic desensitization, 318
Systemic circulation, 148
Systemic lupus erythematosus, 352, 364, 373
Systemic sclerosis, 372
Systems 49, 54; see also specific system
Systole, 142, 165
Systolic blood pressure, 147

T

T-cells, 350, 351, 363
T-effector cells, 351, 363
T-helper cells, 351, 363
T-suppressor cells, 351, 363
Tabes dorsalis, 310
Tachy-, 37
Tachycardia, 172
Tactometer, 345
Talipes, 95
Tal/o-, 24
Talocalcaneal joint, 94
Talofibular joint, 94
Talonavicular joint, 94
Taloscaphoid joint, 94
Talus bone, 68, 73, 91, 93
Tarsals, 66, 67, 69, 73, 93
Tars/o-, 24
Tarsometatarsal joint, 94
Tarsorrhaphy, 341
Tarsotomy, 341
Taste(s)
    primary, 345
    sense of, 326, 327
Taste buds, 197, 326, 345
Tawara's node, 164
Tay-Sachs disease, 307, 308
Tear apparaatus, 320
Tears, 322
Tectorial membrane, 325
Telangiectasia, hereditary hemorrhagic, 170
Tel/e-, 37
Tel/o-, 37
Temperature equivalents, 385
Temporal artery, 167
Temporal bones, 70, 93
Temporal lobe of cerebral cortex, 286
Temporal vein, 168
Temporomandibular joint, 94
Temporoparietal muscle group, 103
Tenalgia, 122

Tend/o-, 27
Tendon, 99
    Achilles, 108, 118
    calcaneal, 118
Tendovaginitis, 120
Tenesmus, 218
Tennis elbow, 74
Ten/o-, 27
Tenodesis, 122
Tenodynia, 122
Tenomyotomy, 122
Tenonitis, 120
Tenontitis, 120
Tenont/o-, 27
Tenontomyotomy, 122
Tenoplasty, 122
Tenorrhaphy, 122
Tenositis, 120
Tenostosis, 120
Tenosuture, 122
Tenosynovectomy, 122
Tenosynovitis, 94, 120
Tenotomy, 122
Tenovaginitis, 120
Tensor fasciae latae muscle, 108, 120
Teratoma, 254
Teres, 102
Teres major muscle, 104, 120
Teres minor muscle, 120
Terminal twig, 282, 303
Terminology, medical; see Medical terminology
Test; see specific test
Testicles, 228, 250
Testicular artery, 166
Testis (testes), 228-229, 250
    ectopia of, 253
    hormones of, 264
Testosterone, 229, 264, 267, 277
Tetanus, 306
Tetany, 122, 279
Tetralogy of Fallot, 170
Thalamus, 285, 303
Thalassemia, 170
Thallium stress test, 174
Thanatophobia, 314
Thecoma, 254
Theleplasty, 255
Thel/o-, 24
Thematic Apperception Test, 315
Theo-, 318
Theomania, 318
Therm/o-, 37
Thigh, muscles of, 107-108
Thioxanthenes, 318
Third ventricle, 303
Thomsen's disease, 121
Thoracentesis, 193
Thoracic aorta, descending, 150
Thoracic artery, 166, 167
Thoracic cavity, 178
Thoracic duct, 363
Thoracic nerve
    long, 305
    respiration and, 179
Thoracic surgery, 387
Thoracic vein, 151, 168
Thoracic vertebrae, 68, 71
Thorac/o-, 24
Thoracocentesis, 193
Thoracoepigastric vein, 168
Thoracolumbar system, 301
Thoracoplasty, 194
Thoracostomy, 193
Thoracotomy, 193
Thorax, 178
    muscles of, 106

Thorax—cont'd
  terms related to, 57
Throat culture, 194
Thrombectomy, 173
Thrombin, 147, 165
Thromboangiitis, 169
Thrombocytes, 144, 147, 165
Thrombocytopenic purpura, 172, 352, 364
Thrombolysis, 174
Thrombophlebitis, 169
Thromboplastin, 165
Thromboplastin time, activated partial, 173
Thrombosis, 172
Thrombus, 172
Thymectomy, 364
Thymia, 316
Thym/o-, 27
Thymolysis, 364
Thymopathy, 364
Thymosin, 264, 267
Thymus gland, 267, 349, 363
  hormones of, 264
  hyperplasia of, 364
  hypertrophy of, 364
Thyr/o-, 27
Thyrocervical trunk, 167
Thyrohyoid muscle, 119
Thyroid artery, 167
Thyroid cartilage, 176
Thyroid crisis, 279
Thyroid gland, 265-266, 277
  hormones of, 264
  Hurthle cell adenoma of, 279
Thyroid hormone, 264, 265
Thyroid hormone tests, 280
Thyroid scan, 280
Thyroid stimulation test, 280
Thyroid storm, 279
Thyroid ultrasonography, 280
Thyroid vein, 168
Thyroidectomy, 280
Thyroiditis, 278
Thyroidotomy, 280
Thyroid-stimulating hormone, 263, 264, 277
Thyrolytic, 279
Thyropathy, 279
Thyroprivia, 279
Thyrotoxic crisis, 279
Thyrotrophin, 277
Thyrotropic hormone, 263, 264
Thyrotropin, 277
Thyroxin, 277
Thyroxine, 264, 265, 277
Thyroxine-binding globulin, 280
TIA, 172
Tibia, 67, 68, 69, 72, 73, 93
Tibial artery, 151, 167
Tibial nerve, 305
Tibial vein, 168
Tibialis anterior muscle, 108, 120
Tibialis posterior muscle, 108, 120
Tibiofibular joint, 94
Tibiotarsal joint, 94
Tic, 122
-tic, 15
Tidal volume, 179, 190, 194
Timed force expiratory volume, 194
Tinea, 135
Tinea capitis, 135
Tinea cruris, 135
Tinea pedis, 135
Tinnitus, 344
-tion, 15
Tissue, 49, 51-54, 63-65
  adipose, 124
  areolar, 63, 124

Tissue culture, 137
-to, 40
Toe, Morton's, 94
-tome, 16
Tomography
  computerized; see Computerized tomography
  positron emission, 174
  positron emission transaxial, 312
-tomy, 16
Tone, muscle, 100, 120
Tongue, 196, 197, 214, 326
Tonometer, 343
Tonsils, 349, 363
Tooth (teeth), 196-198
  buccal surface of, 213
  Hutchinson's, 216
Top/o-, 34
TORCH syndrome, 369
Torpor, 310
Torticollis, 120
Torulosis, 367
Total alkaline phosphatase, 222
Total cholesterol, 222
Total lung capacity, 194
Total nitrogen, 223
Total urine volume, 250
Touch, sense of, 327-328
Tourette's disease, 310
Tourette's syndrome, 310
Toxic epidermal necrolysis, 135
Toxic shock syndrome, 369
-toxon, 340
Toxoplasmosis, 369
Trachea, 177, 190
Tracheal rings, 190
Tracheal vein, 168
Tracheitis, 191
Trachelectomy, 255
Trachel/o-, 24
Tracheloplasty, 256
Trachelorrhaphy, 256
Trachelotomy, 256
Trache/o-, 27
Tracheobronchitis, 191
Tracheoplasty, 194
Tracheorrhagia, 193
Tracheorrhaphy, 194
Tracheostenosis, 193
Tracheostomy, 194
Tracheotomy, 194
Trachoma, 339
Tractotomy, 311
Trance and possession disorder, 314
Trans-, 13
Trans-esophageal echocardiography, 174
Transferrin, 222
Transhepatic cholangiography, percutaneous, 222
Transient ischemic attack, 172, 308
Transitional cell carcinoma, 248
Transitional epithelial tissue, 51
Transitional epithelium, 64
Transplantation, bone marrow, 173
Transposition
  of abdominal viscera, 216
  of aorta and pulmonary artery, 170
  of great vessels, 170
Transrectal ultrasonography, 257
Transsexual, 318
Transurethral resection of prostate, 256
Transverse cervical artery, 167
Transverse colon, 200, 201
Transverse fracture, 96
Transverse plane, 55
Transversus, 102
Transversus abdominis muscle, 106, 120
Transvestism, 318

Trapezium bone, 72, 93
Trapezius muscle, 104, 120
Trapezoid bone, 72, 93
Tremor, 309
Trench fever, 369
Trench mouth, 216
Trendelenburg position, 56
Tri-, 102
Triceps brachii muscle, 104, 120
Trichina agglutinin, 122
Trichiniasis, 120
Trichinosis, 120
Trich/o-, 24
Trichomoniasis, 253
Trichophagia, 318
Trichotillomania, 318
Trichuriasis, 216
Tricuspid valve, 141-142, 164
Tricyclic antidepressants, 318
Trigeminal nerve, 290, 304
Triglycerides, 144, 174
Triiodothyronine, 264, 265, 277, 280
Triquetrum bone, 72, 93
Trisomy 21, 370
Tritanomaly, 340
Tritanopia, 340
Tritanopsia, 340
Trochanter, 69, 93
  greater, 67, 72
  lesser, 67, 72
Trochlear nerve, 290, 304
Troph/o-, 34
Tropias, 341
-tropic, 261
-tropin, 261
True ribs, 71
True vocal cords, 176
Trumpeter muscle, 103, 118
Trunk
  anterior, terms related to, 56
  celiac, 166
  posterior, terms related to, 56, 57
  thyrocervical, 167
Trypanosomiasis, 370
Trypsin activity, 223
Trypsin activity test, 373
Tsutsugamushi fever, 370
Tubercle, 69
Tuberculosis, 191
  osseous, 94
Tuberculous spondylitis, 94
Tuberosity, 69
Tuberous carcinoma, 137
Tuberous sclerosis, 308
Tubes
  eustachian, 175
  fallopian (uterine), 230, 231-232, 251
Tubule(s)
  collecting, 246
  renal, 224, 226, 246, 247
  seminiferous, 229, 250
  uriniferous, 247
Tularemia, 370
Tumor; see specific tumor
Tunica, 165
Tunica adventitia, 143, 165
Tunica externa, 143
Tunica externa vasorum, 165
Tunica intima, 143
Tunica intima vasorum, 165
Tunica media, 143
Tunica media vasorum, 165
Turbinate, 93
  nasal, 70, 326
Turner's syndrome, 371
Twilight blindness, 340

Tympanectomy, 344
Tympanic canal, 325
Tympanic cavity, 324
Tympanic membrane, 324, 343
Tympanic nerve, 304
Tympanitis, 343
Tympanolabyrinthopexy, 344
Tympanomastoiditis, 343
Tympanophonia, 344
Tympanosclerosis, 344
Tympanosympathectomy, 344
Tympanotomy, 344
Typhoid fever, 370
Typhus, 370
Tyrosinemia, 216

U

Ulcer, 218
  corneal, 341
  decubitus, 134
Ulcerative colitis, 215, 216
-ule, 15
Ulna, 67, 68, 69, 72, 93
Ulnar artery, 150, 167
Ulnar nerve, 305
Ulnar vein, 168
Ultra-, 13
Ultrasonography, 257
  thyroid, 280
  transrectal, 257
-ulum, 15
-ulus, 15
Umbilical, 56, 57
Umbilical blood sampling, percutaneous, 256
Umbilical cord, 251
Umbilicus, 252
Unciform bone, 92, 93
Uncus, 287
Undifferentiated schizophrenia, 314
Undulant fever, 367
Universal donor, 147
Universal health insurance claim form, 399-400
Universal recipient, 147
Upper extremities, bones of, 72
Upper respiratory tract, organs of, 175-176
Uraturia, 248
Ur/e-, 39
Ur/ea-, 39
Uremia, 248
Ur/eo-, 39
Uresis, 247
Ureter, 224, 247
Ureteralgia, 248
Ureterectasis, 248
Ureterectomy, 249
Ureteritis, 247
Ureter/o-, 27
Ureterocolostomy, 249
Ureterocystanastomosis, 249
Ureterocystoneostomy, 249
Ureterocystostomy, 249
Ureteroenteroanastomosis, 249
Ureteroenterostomy, 249
Ureterolith, 248
Ureterolithiasis, 248
Ureterolithotomy, 249
Ureterolysis, 248, 249
Ureteroneocystostomy, 249
Ureteroneopyelostomy, 249
Ureteronephrectomy, 249
Ureteropelvineostomy, 249
Ureteroplasty, 249
Ureteroproctostomy, 249
Ureteropyelitis, 247
Ureteropyeloneostomy, 249

Ureteropyelonephritis, 247
Ureteropyelonephrostomy, 249
Ureteropyeloplasty, 249
Ureteropyelostomy, 249
Ureteropyosis, 247
Ureterorectoneostomy, 249
Ureterorectostomy, 249
Ureterorrhagia, 248
Ureterorrhaphy, 249
Ureterosigmoidostomy, 249
Ureterostenosis, 248
Ureterostomy, 249
Ureterotomy, 249
Ureterotrigonoenterostomy, 249
Ureterotrigonosigmoidostomy, 249
Ureteroureterostomy, 249
Ureterovesicostomy, 249
Ureters, 227
Urethra, 227, 247
Urethralgia, 248
Urethrectomy, 249
Urethremorrhagia, 248
Urethremphraxis, 248
Urethritis, 247
Urethr/o-, 27
Urethrocystitis, 247
Urethrocystopexy, 249
Urethrodynia, 248
Urethroplasty, 249
Urethrorrhagia, 248
Urethrorrhaphy, 249
Urethrorrhea, 248
Urethrostaxis, 248
Urethrostomy, 249
Urethrotomy, 249
Ur/in-, 39
Urinary bladder, 227
Urinary calculus, 248
Urinary meatus, 227
Urinary system, 224-228
  laboratory tests and procedures for, 249-250
Urine
  normal, characteristics of, 227-228
  total volume, 250
Urine specimen, catheterized, 249
Urine tests, 223
Uriniferous tubule, 247
Ur/ino-, 39
Ur/o-, 39
Urobilinogen, 223
Urology, 387
Urticaria, 134, 135
Uterine artery, 167
Uterine tubes, 230, 231-232, 251
Uterine vein, 168
Uterus, 232, 251, 253, 254
Utricle, 325, 343
Uvea, 339
Uveitis, 339
Uvula, 195, 214

V

Vagina, 232
  atresia of, 253
Vaginal orifice, 232
Vaginismus, 254
Vaginitis, 252
Vagotomy, 311
Vagus, 190
Vagus nerve, 190, 290, 304
  respiration and, 179
Vallate papillae, 196
Valley fever, 191
Valve(s)
  heart, 141-142, 164, 165

Valve(s)—cont'd
  ileocecal, 201, 214
  ileocolic, 214
  pulmonary, 165
Valvotomy, 173
Valvuloplasty, 173
Valvulotomy, 173
Vanillylmandelic acid, 280
Varicella, 367
Varicella-zoster, 305
Varico, 172
Varicocele, 254
Varicose, 172
Variola, 369
Variola minor, 367
Vas, 165
Vas deferens, 229, 250
Vascular abnormalities, 172
Vasectomy, 256
Vas/o-, 28
Vasoconstriction, 172
Vasodilation, 172
Vasopressin, 263, 265, 277
Vasospasm, 172
Vasotomy, 256
Vastus, 102
Vastus intermedius muscle, 108, 120
Vastus lateralis muscle, 108, 120
Vastus medialis muscle, 108, 120
Vectorcardiogram, spatial, 174
Veins, 143, 150, 151, 167-168
Velamentous placenta, 254
Vena cava (venae cavae), 143, 151, 168
Venae cerebri, 167
Venae cordis, 167
Venae vasorum, 168
Ven/e-, 28
Venereal Disease Research Laboratory test, 174, 257
Venereal wart, 252
Ven/i-, 28
Venipuncture, 173
Ven/o-, 28
Venography, 174
Venosclerosis, 172
Venous plethysmography, 174
Venous sinuses, 151
Ventr/i-, 24
Ventricle
  lateral, 286, 302
  fourth, 302
  third, 302
Ventriculocisternostomy, 311
Ventriculostomy, 311
Ventriculotomy, 173
Ventr/o-, 24
Venules, 143, 168
Verbal roots and combining forms, 33-35
Vermiform appendix, 201
Vermis, 285, 303
Verruca, 136
Verrucous carcinoma, 137
Vertebrae, 66, 71, 93
Vertebral artery, 150, 167
Vertebral column, 67, 69, 71
Vertebral vein, 168
Vertebrate, 64
Vertigo, 344
Vesical vein, 168
Vesicle, 134
  seminal, 229, 250
Vesic/o-, 28
Vesiculectomy, 256
Vesiculitis, seminal, 252
Vesiculotomy, 256
Vestibular canal, 325
Vestibular glands, 232, 251

Vestibular nerve, 290, 303
Vestibule, 190, 232, 325
Villi, 201, 214-215
Vincent's stomatitis, 216
Vineberg coronary artery procedure, 173
Viral skin infections, 135-136
Virilism, 279
Virilizing adenocarcinoma of adrenal gland, 279
Virilizing adenoma of adrenal gland, 279
Virus
    Epstein-Barr, 368
    herpes zoster, 367
    human immunodeficiency, 366-367
    human papilloma, 252
Viscera, abdominal, transposition of, 216
Visceral artery, 150, 151
Visceral layer of heart, 141
Visceral muscle, 100
Visceral muscle tissue, 52, 53
Visceral peritoneum, 200
Visceral pleura, 177, 190
Viscer/o-, 28
Visceroptosis, 218
Vision
    mechanism of, 322
    sense of, 320-323, 327
Vision tests and diagnostic instruments, 342-343
Visual field test, 343
Visual fields and pathways, 323
Vital capacity, 179, 190, 194
Vitamin B tests, 312
Vitelliform, 339
Vitiligo, 136
Vitreous body, 320, 322
Vitreous humor, 339
Vocabulary, medical, building, 10-22
Vocal cords, 176, 190
Voicebox, 190
Volar vein, 168
Volkmann's contracture, 121
Volume(s)
    pulmonary, 194

Volume(s)—cont'd
    respiratory, 179, 190
    units of, 385
Volumetric interstitial brachytherapy, 311
Voluntary muscle, 100, 120
Voluntary muscle tissue, 64
Volvulus, 218
Vomer, 70, 93
Vomeronasala organs, 345
Vomiting, 218
Von Graefe's sign, 341
von Hippel-Lindau disease, 371
Von Recklinghausen's disease, 371
Voyeurism, 318
Vulva, 232
Vulvectomy, 256
Vulvitis, 252

W

Wall-eye, 341
Warmth, sense of, 327, 328
Wart, 136
    genital, 252
    seborrheic, 137
    venereal, 252
Weber's test, 345
Wechsler Adult Intelligence Scale-Revised, 315
Weight, units of, 385
Werdnig-Hoffman syndrome, 121
Werner's syndrome, 371
Wernicke's disease, 310
Western blot test, 365
Wheal, 135
White splenic pulp, 363
Williams syndrome, 371
Wilms' tumor, 248
Windpipe, 190
Woolsorters' disease, 367
Workmen's compensation, 397
Wounds, suture of, 218-219

Wrist, 72
    bones of, 66, 72
Wryneck, 120

X

Xanth/o-, 40
Xanthoma, 136
Xenophobia, 314
Xer/o-, 37
Xeroderma pigmentosum, 136
Xerophthalmia, 341
Xerophthalmus, 341
Xiphoid process, 67, 92
X-ray
    bone, 97
    chest, 194
    long bone, 97
    skull, 98
    spinal, 98
X-ray scans, 223

Y

-y, 15
Yaws, 370
Yellow bone marrow, 65
Yellow fever, 370
Yellow nail syndrome, 136
Yuppie flu, 367

Z

Zimmerlin's dystrophy, 121
Zona fasciculata, 266
Zona glomerulosa, 266
Zona reticularis, 266
Zoophobia, 314
Zoosadism, 318
Zygomatic bone, 70, 92, 93
Zygomatic nerve, 304
Zygote, 252